# FIRST AID FOR THE®

# FAMILY MEDICINE BOARDS

**TAO LE, MD, MHS**

Assistant Clinical Professor
Chief, Section of Allergy and Clinical Immunology
Department of Medicine
University of Louisville

**CHRISTINE DEHLENDORF, MD**

Fellow in Family Medicine
Department of Family and Community Medicine
University of California, San Francisco

**MICHAEL MENDOZA, MD, MPH**

Clinical Assistant Professor
Department of Family Medicine
Pritzker School of Medicine
The University of Chicago

**CYNTHIA Y. OHATA, MD**

Clinical Instructor
Department of Family Medicine
University of Washington

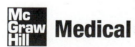 **Medical**

New York / Chicago / San Francisco / Lisbon / London / Madrid / Mexico City
Milan / New Delhi / San Juan / Seoul / Singapore / Sydney / Toronto

**First Aid for the® Family Medicine Boards**

1 2 3 4 5 6 7 8 9 0   QPD/QPD   0 9 8 7

ISBN 978-0-07-147771-0
MHID 0-07-147771-3

### NOTICE

Medicine is an ever-changing science. As new research and clinical experience broaden our knowledge, changes in treatment and drug therapy are required. The authors and the publisher of this work have checked with sources believed to be reliable in their efforts to provide information that is complete and generally in accord with the standards accepted at the time of publication. However, in view of the possibility of human error or changes in medical sciences, neither the authors nor the publisher nor any other party who has been involved in the preparation or publication of this work warrants that the information contained herein is in every respect accurate or complete, and they disclaim all responsibility for any errors or omissions or for the results obtained from use of the information contained in this work. Readers are encouraged to confirm the information contained herein with other sources. For example and in particular, readers are advised to check the product information sheet included in the package of each drug they plan to administer to be certain that the information contained in this work is accurate and that changes have not been made in the recommended dose or in the contraindications for administration. This recommendation is of particular importance in connection with new or infrequently used drugs.

This book was set in Electra LH by Rainbow Graphics.
The editors were Catherine A. Johnson and Penny Linskey.
The production supervisors were Phil Galea and Tom Kowalczyk.
Project management was provided by Rainbow Graphics.
Quebecor Dubuque was printer and binder.

This book is printed on acid-free paper.

**Library of Congress Cataloging-in-Publication Data**

First aid for the family medicine boards / Tao T. Le ... [et al.].
    p. ; cm.
  Includes index.
  ISBN-13: 978-0-07-147771-0 (pbk. : alk. paper)
  ISBN-10: 0-07-147771-3 (pbk. : alk. paper)
  1. Family medicine—Examinations, questions, etc. 2. Physicians—Certification—United States. 3. American Board of Family Medicine. I. Le, Tao.
  [DNLM: 1. Family Practice—United States—Outlines. 2. Specialty Boards—United States—Outlines. WB 18.2 F5264 2008]
  RC58.F54 2008
  616.0076--dc22
                                         2007027564

To our families, friends, and loved ones, who endured and assisted in the task of assembling this guide.

and

To the contributors to this and future editions, who took time to share their knowledge, insight, and humor for the benefit of residents.

# CONTENTS

# CONTRIBUTORS

**Tina M. Brueschke, MD, MHSA**

PrairieView Family Medicine
Elburn, Illinois

**Christina S. Chen, MD**

Resident in Family Medicine
Department of Family Medicine
University of Washington

**Graham Dresden, MD**

Resident in Family Medicine
Department of Family Medicine
University of Washington

**Michael P. Grace, MD**

Resident in Family Medicine
Department of Family Medicine
University of Washington

**Corrilynn O. Hileman, MD**

Fellow in Infectious Disease
Department of Internal Medicine
Case Western Reserve University

**Craig M. Hileman, MD**

Clinical Associate
Department of Family Medicine
Case Western Reserve University

**Matthew B. Jaffy, MD**

Clinical Instructor
Department of Family Medicine
University of Washington

**Brian Kim, MD**

Resident in Family Medicine
Department of Family Medicine
University of Washington

**Sarah S. Lowenthal, MD**

Chief Resident in Family Medicine
Department of Family and Community Medicine
University of California, San Francisco

**Miranda D. Lu, MD**

Resident in Family Medicine
Department of Family Medicine
University of Washington

**Eve Paretsky, MD**

Resident in Family Medicine
Department of Family Medicine
University of Washington

**Amanda Lee Price, MD**

Resident in Family Medicine
Department of Family Medicine
University of Washington

**Reina Rodriguez, MD**

Chief Resident in Family Medicine
Department of Family and Community Medicine
University of California, San Francisco

**Cynthia L. Salinas, MD**

North Willow Grove Family Medicine
Assistant Physician, Department of Family Medicine
Abington Memorial Hospital

**Sarah-Anne Schumann, MD**

Clinical Associate
Department of Family Medicine
Pritzker School of Medicine
The University of Chicago

**Umang Sharma, MD**

Resident in Family Medicine
Department of Family Medicine
University of Washington

**Shira Shavit, MD**

Associate Director
Correctional Medicine Consultation Network
Assistant Clinical Professor
Department of Family and Community Medicine
University of California, San Francisco

**Tara A. Shaw, MD**

Family Medicine/Sports Medicine
The Permanente Medical Group, Inc.
Vallejo, California

**Jessica Stanton, MD**

Sutter Medical Center of Santa Rosa
Santa Rosa, California

**Stephen S. Stukovsky, MD**

Resident
Department of Family Medicine
University of Washington

**Debra Stulberg, MD**

Instructor
Department of Family Medicine
Pritzker School of Medicine
The University of Chicago

**Andrea Michele Taylor, MD**

Resident in Family Medicine
Department of Family Medicine
University of Washington

**Grace Chen Yu, MD**

Clinical Faculty
San Jose–O'Connor Hospital Family Medicine Residency
Adjunct Clinical Instructor, Stanford University School of Medicine

# ASSOCIATE CONTRIBUTORS

**Diana Antoniucci, MD**
Assistant Professor
Department of Medicine
University of California, San Francisco

**Karen Earle, MD**
Medical Director, Center of Diabetes Services
Department of Internal Medicine
California Pacific Medical Center

# FACULTY REVIEWERS

**A. Eric Anderson, MD**

Clinical Assistant Professor of Medicine
Department of Medicine, Division of Nephrology
    and Hypertension
University of Washington

**Shieva Khayam-Bashi, MD**

Associate Clinical Professor
Department of Family & Community Medicine
University of California, San Francisco School of Medicine

**J. Mark Beard, MD**

Assistant Professor
Department of Family Medicine
University of Washington

**Roy Henderson, MD**

Sports Medicine Fellowship Director
MacNeal Family Medicine Residency Program
Berwyn, Illinois

**John Hickner MD, MSc**

Professor
Department of Family Medicine
Pritzker School of Medicine
The University of Chicago

**Jane H. Huntington, MD**

Associate Professor
Department of Family Medicine
University of Washington

**David P. Losh, MD**

Professor
Department of Family Medicine
University of Washington

**Timothy McGonagle, MD**

Neurologic Care Associates, PC
Teaching Faculty, MacNeal Memorial Hospital
    Residency Programs

**Thomas A. Neal, MD**

Assistant Clinical Professor
Department of Family and Community Medicine
University of California, San Francisco

**William E. Neighbor Jr., MD**

Associate Professor
Department of Family Medicine
University of Washington

**Andrew D. Schechtman, MD, FAAFP**

Faculty
San Jose–O'Connor Hospital Family Medicine Residency
Adjunct Clinical Instructor
Stanford University School of Medicine

**William Shore, MD**

Professor
Department of Family and Community Medicine
University of California, San Francisco

**Justin Strote, MD**

Fellow
Division of Cardiology
University of Washington

**Lisa Vargish, MD**

Instructor and Clerkship Director
Department of Family Medicine
Pritzker School of Medicine
The University of Chicago

**Norma Jo Waxman, MD**

Associate Clinical Professor
Department of Family and Community Medicine
University of California, San Francisco

**Lisa Winston, MD**

Assistant Clinical Professor
Department of Medicine, Division of Infectious Diseases
University of California, San Francisco

# PREFACE

With *First Aid for the Family Medicine Boards,* we hope to provide residents and clinicians with the most useful and up-to-date preparation guide for the American Board of Family Medicine (ABFM) certification and recertification exams. This new addition to the *First Aid* series represents an outstanding effort by a talented group of authors and includes the following:

- A practical exam preparation guide with resident-tested test-taking and study strategies
- Concise summaries of thousands of board-testable topics
- Hundreds of high-yield tables, diagrams, and illustrations
- Key facts in the margins highlighting "must know" information for the boards
- Mnemonics throughout, making learning memorable and fun
- Timely updates and corrections through the First Aid Team's blog at **www.firstaidteam.com.**

We invite you to share your thoughts and ideas to help us improve *First Aid for the Family Medicine Boards.* See How to Contribute, p. xv.

| | |
|---|---|
| *Louisville* | Tao Le |
| *San Francisco* | Christine Dehlendorf |
| *Chicago* | Michael Mendoza |
| *Seattle* | Cynthia Y. Ohata |

# ACKNOWLEDGMENTS

This has been a collaborative project from the start. We gratefully acknowledge the thoughtful comments, corrections, and advice of the residents, international medical graduates, and faculty who have supported the authors in the development of *First Aid for the Family Medicine Boards.*

For support and encouragement throughout the process, we are grateful to Thao Pham, Selina Franklin, and Louise Peterson. Thanks to Albert Yu, MD and Richard Wilson, MD for their feedback. Thanks to our publisher, McGraw-Hill, for the valuable assistance of their staff. For enthusiasm, support, and commitment to this challenging project, thanks to our editor, Catherine Johnson. For outstanding editorial work, we thank Andrea Fellows. A special thanks to Rainbow Graphics for remarkable production work.

| | |
|---|---|
| *Louisville* | Tao Le |
| *San Francisco* | Christine Dehlendorf |
| *Chicago* | Michael Mendoza |
| *Seattle* | Cynthia Y. Ohata |

# HOW TO CONTRIBUTE

To continue to produce a high-yield review source for the ABIM exam, you are invited to submit any suggestions or corrections. We also offer **paid internships** in medical education and publishing ranging from three months to one year (see next page for details). Please send us your suggestions for

- Study and test-taking strategies for the ABFM
- New facts, mnemonics, diagrams, and illustrations
- Low-yield topics to remove

For each entry incorporated into the next edition, you will receive a $20 gift certificate, as well as personal acknowledgment in the next edition. Diagrams, tables, partial entries, updates, corrections, and study hints are also appreciated, and significant contributions will be compensated at the discretion of the authors. Also let us know about material in this edition that you feel is low yield and should be deleted.

The preferred way to submit entries, suggestions, or corrections is via the First Aid Team's blog at **www.firstaidteam.com.** Please include name, address, institutional affiliation, phone number, and e-mail address (if different from the address of origin). Please submit at:

**www.firstaidteam.com**

Otherwise, please send entries, neatly written or typed or on disk (Microsoft Word), to:

**First Aid for the Family Medicine Boards**
**914 North Dixie Avenue, Suite 100**
**Elizabethtown, KY 42701**
**Attention: Contributions**

## NOTE TO CONTRIBUTORS

All entries become property of the authors and are subject to editing and reviewing. Please verify all data and spellings carefully. In the event that similar or duplicate entries are received, only the first entry received will be used. Include a reference to a standard textbook to facilitate verification of the fact. Please follow the style, punctuation, and format of this edition if possible.

## INTERNSHIP OPPORTUNITIES

The author team is pleased to offer part-time and full-time paid internships in medical education and publishing to motivated physicians. Internships may range from three months (e.g., a summer) up to a full year. Participants will have an opportunity to author, edit, and earn academic credit on a wide variety of projects, including the popular *First Aid* series. Writing/editing experience, familiarity with Microsoft Word, and Internet access are desired. For more information, submit a résumé or a short description of your experience along with a cover letter to **www.firstaidteam.com.**

# CHAPTER 1

# Guide to the ABFM Examination

*The majority of patients will be aware of your certification status.*

## INTRODUCTION

For residents, the American Board of Family Medicine (ABFM) certification exam represents the culmination of 3 years of hard work, and for those taking the recertification exam, 7-10 years after that. However, the process of certification and recertification does not merely represent yet another in a series of expensive tests. To your patients and their families, it means that you have attained the level of clinical knowledge and competency required to provide good clinical care.

In this chapter, we talk more about the ABFM exam and provide you with proven approaches to conquering the exam. For a detailed description of the exam, visit **www.theabfm.org.** The ABFM also provides information about specific study strategies that have worked for candidates who failed the exam initially and went on to pass successfully. These are detailed at https://www.theabfm.org/cert/fail-safe.pdf.

## ABFM—THE BASICS

*Register before March to avoid late fees.*

### How Do I Register to Take the Exam?

You can register for the ABFM exam online at www.theabfm.org. Available dates for the test are generally in July and August. Individuals who complete residency training after June 30 or who do not pass the exam in the summer may be eligible to take the test during the winter.

Those who are certifying for the first time must have a user name and password supplied by their residency program. The registration deadline in 2006 was February 28, with increasing late fees for each subsequent month. The latest date to register is generally in June. The registration fee in 2006 was $1,050.

Check the ABFM Web site for the latest information on registration deadlines, fees, and policies. Note that the deadlines and schedules for the Certificates of Added Qualifications vary.

### What If I Need to Cancel the Exam or Change Test Centers?

The ABFM currently provides partial refunds if a cancellation is received before certain deadlines (in 2006 this was the end of June). You can also change your test center and test dates before a specific deadline. Check the ABFM Web site for the latest on refund and cancellation policies as well on current procedures.

### How Is the ABFM Test Structured?

The **ABFM** certification/recertification exam is currently a one-day computer-based test administered at approximately 200 test centers around the country. For questions about the computer-based format, see the Frequently Asked Questions and practice exam on the ABFM Web site. The test is distributed by subject matter as described on the ABFM Web site at https://www.theabfm.org/cert/CertRecertExaminationOutline.pdf. The exam itself is divided into a morning and an afternoon session. The morning session is three and one-half hours long and consists of 120 multiple-choice questions and two 45-minute modules selected by the candidate at the time of application. The modules are described in detail on the Web site; briefly, they are Ambulatory Family Medicine, Child and Adolescent Care, Geriatrics, Women's Health, Maternity Care, Emergent/Urgent Care, Hospital Medicine, and Sports Medicine. The afternoon session is three hours and fifteen minutes long and consists of 160 multiple-choice questions. Twenty of these questions are being tested and are not included in the scoring—but you will not know which questions these are! Overall, you will have approximately one minute to answer each question.

### What Types of Questions Are Asked?

All questions are **single-best-answer** types only. You will be presented with a scenario and a question followed by five options. Most questions on the exam are vignette based. A substantial amount of extraneous information may be given, or a clinical scenario may be followed by a question that could be answered without actually requiring that you read the case. As with other board exams, there is no penalty for guessing. Questions can pertain to the diagnosis, treatment, or prevention of disease.

*Most questions on the ABFM exam are case based.*

### How Are the Scores Reported?

Both the scoring and the reporting of test results have varied but may take up to three months. Your score report will give you a "pass/fail" decision, the overall number of questions answered correctly with a corresponding percentile, and the number of questions answered correctly with a corresponding percentile for more than 40 different subject areas. Results from all candidates who took the test are presented alongside your results for each subject area. In 2005, the pass rate for the certification exam was 93%; for the recertification exam, the pass rate was 94%.

### THE RECERTIFICATION EXAM

The recertification exam is one part of the Maintenance of Certification for Family Physicians (MC-FP). The exam must be completed every seven years or, as of January 2007, every ten years. Additional components of the MC-FP include self-assessment modules and continuing medical education.

### TEST PREPARATION ADVICE

The good news about the ABFM exam is that it tends to focus on the diagnosis and management of disease and conditions that you have likely seen as a resident—and that you should expect to see as a family physician. Assuming that you have performed well as a resident, *First Aid* and a good source of practice questions may be all you need to pass. However, you might also consider using *First Aid* as a **guide** and using multiple resources, including a standard textbook, journal review articles, and a concise electronic text such as *UpToDate*, as part of your studies. Original research articles are low yield, and very new research (i.e., research conducted less than 1–2 years before the exam) will not be tested. In addition, a number of high-quality board review courses are offered around the country. Such courses are costly but can help those who need some focus and discipline.

*The ABFM tends to focus on the horses, not the zebras.*

*Use a combination of First Aid, textbooks, journal reviews, and practice questions.*

Ideally, you should start your preparation early in your **last year of residency,** especially if you are starting a demanding job or fellowship right after residency. Cramming during the period between the end of residency and the exam is **not advisable.**

As you study, concentrate on the **nuances of management,** especially for difficult or complicated cases. For **common diseases,** learn both common and **uncommon presentations;** for **uncommon diseases,** focus on the **classic presentations** and manifestations. Draw on the experiences of your residency training to anchor some of your learning. When you take the exam, you will realize that you've seen most of the clinical scenarios in the course of your three years of clinic and hospital medicine.

Depending on the modules you choose in the morning session, you may want to focus on specific chapters and sections in the *First Aid for the Family Medicine Boards:*

- **Ambulatory Family Medicine:** Community Medicine, Cardiology (hypertension, dyslipidemia, CHF), Endocrinology (diabetes), Gastroenterology, Pulmonary Medicine, Dermatology, and Reproductive Health (gynecology).
- **Child and Adolescent Care:** Pediatric and Adolescent Medicine, Reproductive Health (gynecology), and Hematology and Oncology (anemia, leukemias).
- **Geriatrics:** Geriatrics, Community Medicine, Cardiology, Neurology (cerebrovascular disease), Dermatology (herpes zoster) and Psychiatry.
- **Women's Health:** Reproductive Health, Geriatrics (osteoporosis, incontinence), Psychiatry, Pediatric and Adolescent Medicine (eating disorders, female athletic triad), Surgery (breast cancer), and Community Medicine (domestic violence).
- **Maternity Care:** Reproductive Health (obstetrics), Psychiatry, and Community Medicine (domestic violence).
- **Emergent/Urgent Care:** Emergency/Urgent Care, Psychiatry, Surgery, Pediatric and Adolescent Medicine (common acute conditions), and Community Medicine (bioterrorism).
- **Hospital Medicine:** Cardiology, Pulmonary Medicine, Endocrinology (DKA, HHNS), Gastroenterology (GI bleeding, end-stage liver disease, diverticulitis, pancreatitis), Hematology and Oncology (oncology), Infectious Disease, Pulmonary (lower respiratory disease), Nephrology (acute renal failure), Neurology (cerebrovascular disease, seizure, syncope), Surgery, and Emergency/Urgent Care.
- **Sports Medicine:** Sports Medicine.

## Other High-Yield Areas

Focus on topic areas that are typically not emphasized during residency training but are board favorites. These include the following:

- Basic biostatistics (e.g., sensitivity, specificity, positive predictive value, negative predictive value).
- Adverse effects of drugs.

## TEST-TAKING ADVICE

By this point in your life, you have probably gained more test-taking expertise than you care to admit. Nevertheless, here are a few tips to keep in mind when taking the exam:

4

- For long vignette questions, read the question stem and scan the options, and **then** go back and read the case. You may get your answer without having to read through the whole case.
- There's no penalty for guessing, so you should **never** leave a question blank.
- Good pacing is key. You need to leave adequate time to get to all the questions. Even though you have one minute per question on average, you should aim for a pace of 45 seconds per question. If you don't know the answer within a short period of time, make an educated guess and move on. You can flag that question to come back to if you have time at the end.
- It's okay to **second-guess** yourself. Research shows that our "second hunches" tend to be better than our first guesses.
- Don't panic over "impossible" questions. These may be **experimental questions** that won't count in your score. Again, take your best guess and move on.
- Note the age and race of the patient in each clinical scenario. When race or ethnicity is given, it is often relevant. Know these well, especially for more common diagnoses.
- Questions often describe clinical findings instead of naming eponyms (e.g., they cite "tender, erythematous bumps in the pads of the finger" rather than "Osler's node" in a febrile adolescent).
- As described above, visit the Web site https://www.theabfm.org/cert/failsafe.pdf for study strategies specific to the ABFM certification/recertification exam.

*Never, ever leave a question blank! There is no penalty for guessing.*

## TESTING AND LICENSING AGENCIES

**American Board of Family Medicine**
2228 Young Drive
Lexington, KY 40505-4294
859-269-5626 or 888-995-5700
Fax: 859-335-7501 or 859-335-7509
www.theabfm.org

**Educational Commission for Foreign Medical Graduates (ECFMG)**
3624 Market Street, Fourth Floor
Philadelphia, PA 19104-2685
215-386-5900
Fax: 215-386-9196
www.ecfmg.org

**Federation of State Medical Boards (FSMB)**
P.O. Box 619850
Dallas, TX 75261-9850
817-868-4000
Fax: 817-868-4099
www.fsmb.org

# CHAPTER 2

# Community Medicine

Christina S. Chen, MD
Miranda D. Lu, MD

The following represent some basic definitions used in the context of preventive medicine. The sections that follow elaborate on key issues pertaining to preventive medicine.

- **1° prevention:** Defined as disease prevention measures taken before disease develops. Includes counseling for at-risk behaviors, immunizations, and chemoprevention.
- **2° prevention:** Early detection and treatment of asymptomatic disease, including risk assessment.
- **3° prevention:** Management of chronic diseases to **prevent or minimize complications.**
- Characteristics that make a disease appropriate for screening include the following:
    - The disease → **significant morbidity and mortality.**
    - **Effective treatment** is available.
    - The disease is **detectable** in the asymptomatic period.
    - Testing is accurate and simple.
    - Treatment administered during the asymptomatic period yields a better outcome than treatment in the symptomatic period.
- Characteristics of appropriate risk factors for screening are as follows:
    - There is a **high prevalence** of the risk factor in the population to be screened.
    - A large percentage of those with the risk factor are unidentified.
    - The associated **disease** should have a **high incidence** in the population to be screened.
    - The disease should have **serious consequences.**
    - Treatment that can modify the risk factor should be readily available.
    - **Risk modification should ↓ disease incidence.**

*A good screening test is **S**afe, **S**ensitive, **S**pecific, **S**imple, and cheap and is **S**upported by patients and practitioners.*

## Adult Immunizations

Table 2.1 outlines common adult immunizations and their indications. For information on immunization of pediatric populations, refer to the Pediatric and Adolescent Medicine chapter.

## Cancer Screening

The following guidelines are based on recommendations from the United States Preventive Services Task Force (USPSTF) and the American Academy of Family Physicians (AAFP).

### CERVICAL CANCER

- Routine screening for cervical cancer with a Pap smear is **strongly recommended** for all women who have been sexually active and have a cervix. Screening should begin **within three years of the onset of sexual activity or at age 21,** whichever is first, and should be repeated at least every three years.
- Routine screening is **not** recommended in the following:
    - Women **> 65 years of age** with a history of adequate ⊖ screening and who are otherwise **not at high risk.**
    - Women who have had a **hysterectomy for benign disease.**

**TABLE 2.1.** **Indications for Adult Immunizations**

| TETANUS AND DIPHTHERIA (Td) | MEASLES, MUMPS, RUBELLA (MMR) | INFLUENZA | PNEUMOCOCCAL | VARICELLA |
|---|---|---|---|---|
| Give the complete Td vaccine series if the patient has not received the 1° series. Give a booster every 10 years or at least at age 50.[a] | If the patient was born before 1957, consider immune. If the patient was born after 1957, two doses should be given at least one month apart. For rubella specifically, ensure that women of childbearing potential have immunity. | Administer yearly to all patients with cardiopulmonary disease, residents of long-term care facilities, adults ≥ 50 years of age, patients with chronic diseases (diabetes, HIV, renal diseases, immune compromise), and pregnant women who will be in their second or third trimester during influenza season. | Give to all patients > 65 years of age. Give to patients > 50 years of age who are immunocompromised or who have chronic diseases. Revaccinate patients ≥ 65 years of age if they received their 1° vaccine > 5 years ago or are at high risk. | If the patient has a history of chickenpox, consider immune. Otherwise, vaccinate with two doses given 1–2 months apart. |

[a]The CDC's Advisory Committee on Immunization Practices now recommends a single-dose Tdap (tetanus toxoid, reduced diphtheria toxoid, and acellular pertussis) rather than the Td booster for 19- to 65-year-olds.

## OVARIAN CANCER

Routine screening for ovarian cancer by ultrasound, measurement of tumor markers, and pelvic examination is **not** recommended. Although the specificity for screening strategies is high, the positive predictive value is low because of the low prevalence of ovarian cancer in the general population. Further, the invasive nature of testing that follows a positive screening test led the USPSTF to conclude that the potential risks outweigh the potential benefits.

## BREAST CANCER

A screening mammogram with or without a clinical breast exam is **recommended** every **1–2 years** for women **≥ 40 years of age.**

## PROSTATE CANCER

- Consider screening men ≥ 50 years of age if the patient is expected to live at least ten years. Begin screening at an earlier age if patients are at ↑ risk (e.g., African-American men or those with a first-degree relative with prostate cancer).
- The USPSTF found that there was **insufficient evidence** to recommend for or against routine screening by means of a DRE, serum PSA, or transrectal ultrasound.
- The AAFP recommends that **men 50–65 years of age be counseled** about the known risks and uncertain benefits of prostate cancer screening (e.g., early detection vs. false-⊕ results, biopsies, anxiety).

COMMUNITY MEDICINE

## COLON CANCER

- Routine screening in adults ≥ 50 years of age is **strongly recommended** and should include an annual fecal occult blood test and sigmoidoscopy every 3–5 years or colonoscopy every ten years.
- Screening should begin earlier if there is an ↑ risk for colorectal cancer—e.g., if the patient has a personal or strong family history of colorectal cancer or adenomatous polyps or a family history of a hereditary syndrome (familial adenomatous polyposis, hereditary nonpolyposis colon cancer).

A 40-year-old man comes to your office for a routine annual physical exam. He is a nonsmoker who is generally healthy and has no current medical complaints. In an average week, he exercises by jogging 30 minutes two times a week. However, he has a family history of high blood pressure, and his older brother recently had an MI at age 48. The patient asks if there is anything that can be done to prevent this from happening to him. What do you suggest? Recommend checking his BP today, ordering a lipid panel, and discussing the benefits of a healthy diet and aspirin therapy.

## Adult Health Maintenance

Adult health maintenance exams were first endorsed in the 1920s by the American Medical Association despite the fact that the science used to support this recommendation was flawed. Significant empirical evidence for the benefit of annual physical exams did not become available until the 1970s, when the Canadian Task Force on Preventive Health Care developed explicit criteria by which to judge the quality of evidence from published clinical research. The information in Tables 2.2 through 2.4 is based on the latest recommendations from the USPSTF and the AAFP.

## Dental Care

### PREVENTION OF DENTAL CARIES IN PRESCHOOLERS

As many as 19% of children 2–5 years of age and 52% of children 5–9 years of age experience dental caries. Ethnic minority and economically disadvantaged children are at ↑ risk compared with other groups. Although a first dental visit is recommended when a child is approximately one year of age, few preschool-aged children ever visit a dentist. Guidelines for the dental care preschool children are as follows:

- The USPSTF recommends that 1° care clinicians prescribe currently recommended doses of oral fluoride supplementation to preschool children > 6 months of age whose 1° water source is fluoride deficient.
- Professionally applied topical fluoride varnishes may serve as adjuncts to oral supplementation. These offer several advantages, including ease of use, ↓ potential for toxicity, and more widespread patient acceptance.
- The most common harm of any form of fluoride supplementation is dental fluorosis, which is usually mild and primarily of cosmetic significance.

**TABLE 2.2. Recommended Clinical Preventive Services for All Adults**

| AGE | CONDITION | RECOMMENDATION |
|---|---|---|
| ≥ 18 | Accidental injury | Counsel as appropriate for age. |
| | Alcohol misuse | Screen and counsel behavior to ↓ misuse. |
| | CAD | Counsel adults at ↑ risk regarding the benefits and risks of aspirin prophylaxis. |
| | Depression | Screen for depression. |
| | Hypertension | Screen for high blood pressure. |
| | Obesity | Screen for obesity by measuring height and weight. Offer counseling and behavioral interventions to promote sustained weight loss for obese adults. |
| | Physical activity | Recognize that physical activity is desirable, and provide advice accordingly. |
| | Secondhand smoke | Counsel parents who smoke regarding the harmful effects of smoking on children's health. |
| | STDs | Counsel patients regarding the risks for STDs and how to prevent them. |
| | Tobacco use | Screen for tobacco use and provide tobacco cessation interventions as appropriate. |
| ≥ 65 | Hearing difficulties | Screen and counsel. |
| | Visual difficulties | Screen with the Snellen acuity test. |

## ENDOCARDITIS PROPHYLAXIS

- **Dental procedures** for which bacterial endocarditis prophylaxis is recommended are as follows:
  - Dental extractions
  - Periodontal procedures (surgery, scaling, root planing, probing and recall maintenance)
  - Dental implant placement and reimplantation of avulsed teeth
  - Endodontic (root canal) instrumentation or surgery
  - Subgingival placement of antibiotic fibers or strips
  - Initial placement of orthodontic bands (but not brackets)
  - Intraligamentary local anesthetic injections
  - Prophylactic cleaning of teeth or implants where bleeding is anticipated

**TABLE 2.3. Recommended Clinical Preventive Services Specific for Adult Men**

| AGE | CONDITION | RECOMMENDATION |
|---|---|---|
| ≥ 35 | Lipid disorders | Screen with a fasting lipid profile or nonfasting total and HDL cholesterol. |
| ≥ 65 | Abdominal aortic aneurysm | Offer one-time screening by ultrasonography for individuals who have ever smoked. |

| AGE | CONDITION | RECOMMENDATION |
|---|---|---|
| ≥ 18 | Osteoporosis | Counsel patients to maintain adequate calcium intake. |
| 18–25 | Chlamydia | Screen sexually active women. |
| 18–50 | Congenital rubella syndrome | Screen by ensuring immunity via history, serology, or vaccination. |
| Pregnancy | Bacteriuria, symptomatic | Screen with urine culture at 12–16 weeks' gestation at the first prenatal visit. |
| | Chlamydia | Screen asymptomatic pregnant women. |
| | HBV | Screen at the first prenatal visit. |
| | HIV infection | Screen all pregnant women. |
| | Neural tube defects | For those with no history of a previous pregnancy affected by a neural tube defect, prescribe folic acid at a dosage of 0.4–0.8 mg/day from one month prior to conception through the first trimester of pregnancy. For those with a history of a previous pregnancy affected by a neural tube defect, the dose should be increased to 4 mg/day. Prescribe 0.4 mg/day of folate supplementation in women of childbearing potential. |
| | Rh(D) incompatibility | Order Rh(D) blood typing and antibody testing at the first prenatal visit; repeat antibody testing for all Rh(D)-⊖ women at 24–28 weeks' gestation. |
| | Syphilis | Screen all pregnant women. |
| | Tobacco use | Provide smoking cessation counseling for all pregnant smokers. |
| ≥ 45 | Lipid disorders | Screen with a fasting lipid profile or nonfasting total and HDL cholesterol. |
| 60–64 | Osteoporosis | Screen selected women at risk for fractures. |
| ≥ 65 | Osteoporosis | Screen all women for osteoporosis. |

- Endocarditis prophylaxis for these procedures is **highly recommended** for patients with the following:
  - Prosthetic cardiac valves
  - Previous bacterial endocarditis
  - Complex cyanotic congenital heart disease
  - Surgically constructed systemic pulmonary shunts or conduits
  - Acquired valvular dysfunction
  - Hypertrophic cardiomyopathy
  - Mitral valve prolapse **with** valvular regurgitation and/or thickened leaflets
- Conditions for which endocarditis prophylaxis is **not recommended** include the following:
  - Isolated secundum ASD
  - Surgical repair of ASD, PSD, or PDA
  - Previous coronary bypass graft surgery
  - Mitral valve prolapse without valvular regurgitation
  - Physiologic, functional, or innocent heart murmur
  - Previous Kawasaki disease without valvular dysfunction
  - Previous rheumatic fever without valvular dysfunction
  - Cardiac pacemakers and implanted defibrillators

**NUTRITION**

### Obesity

The prevalence of obesity among the adult population of the United States has ↑ from 13% to 27% over the past 40 years. One study has also found a 30% ↑ in the prevalence of childhood obesity from 1994 to the present. Awareness of the health consequences of obesity has also ↑, creating a renewed interest in developing effective interventions for this growing epidemic.

- Obesity is associated with an ↑ **risk of both cardiovascular and overall mortality.** In addition, there are clear associations between obesity and ↑ morbidity.
  - Obesity ↑ the risk of cardiovascular disease, hypertension, stroke, type 2 DM and insulin resistance, dyslipidemia, cancer (including those of the colon, kidney, and gallbladder), sleep apnea, gallbladder disease, GERD, and knee osteoarthritis.
  - Obesity is also associated with a ↓ quality of life, including ↓ mobility and social stigmatization.
- By contrast, a reduction of 5–7% of body weight is associated with a ↓ incidence of diabetes, ↓ BP, and improved dyslipidemia. In one study, intentional **weight loss of > 9.1 kg was associated with a 25% ↓ in cardiovascular disease, cancer, and overall mortality.**

In view of these findings, clinicians should screen all adult patients for obesity and should offer intensive counseling and behavioral interventions to promote sustained weight loss for obese adults. Outlined below are some fundamental concepts that can guide one's clinical approach to obesity treatment.

### BODY MASS INDEX (BMI)

BMI, a measure of body fat based on a patient's height and weight, is a means used to gauge obesity for clinical purposes (see Table 2.5). It is calculated as BMI = weight (kg) / height (m²). The limitations of using BMI for diagnostic purposes include the following:

- It does not account for body fat distribution, which is an independent risk factor (i.e., central obesity, as measured by the waist circumference or waist-to-hip ratio).
- It does not take into account the proportion of muscle weight as opposed to fat weight.

*A BMI of ≥ 30 is associated with an ↑ risk of both cardiovascular and overall mortality. Intentional weight loss of 25 pounds has been associated with a ↓ in cardiovascular disease, cancer, and overall mortality.*

**TABLE 2.5.** **BMI Measurements**

| Definition | BMI (kg/m²) |
|---|---|
| Overweight | 25–29 |
| Obese | 30–39 |
| Morbidly obese | 40–49 |
| Super-obese | 50–59 |

## Treatment Methods

The following modalities are used in the treatment of obesity:

- **Counseling and behavioral interventions:** The most effective interventions combine diet and exercise counseling with behavioral strategies to help patients **change eating patterns and become physically active.** These interventions → small to moderate degrees of weight loss (1–6 kg) that are typically sustained over at least one year.
- **Medications:** Weight loss resulting from medications (see Table 2.6) is modest (average 3–5 kg), and discontinuation of medications may → rapid weight gain. For this reason, medication should be considered when a patient's BMI is > 30, when diet and exercise attempts have failed, and when the patient has comorbidities. Use of weight loss medications in combination with lifestyle changes → greater weight reduction than use of medication alone.

*Medications for the treatment of obesity allow for sustained weight loss only if they are continued.*

**TABLE 2.6.** **Medications Used to Treat Obesity**

| Medication | Mechanism | Notes |
|---|---|---|
| Sibutramine | A norepinephrine and serotonin uptake inhibitor → early satiety. | Can be used on a long-term basis, with average weight loss approximating 10 kg at one year. Can ↑ BP. |
| Orlistat | Inhibits pancreatic lipase. | Can be used on a long-term basis, with average weight loss approximating 9 kg. Side effects include abdominal cramps, flatus, and oily spotting. |
| Phentermine and diethylpropion | Sympathomimetic agents. | Approved for use up to 12 weeks only, as these are Schedule IV drugs with abuse potential. |
| Fluoxetine | Acts as an appetite suppressant. | Not FDA approved for weight loss; must use 60 mg/day or greater. |
| Bupropion | Acts as a norepinephrine modulator. | Not FDA approved for weight loss. |

- **Surgery:**
  - Patients are eligible for **gastric bypass and vertical banded gastroplasty** if they have a BMI > 40 (> 35 with comorbidities), have failed to respond to previous nonsurgical weight loss attempts, and are well informed and motivated. The postoperative mortality rate of such surgery is 0.2%. Other complications include wound infection, reoperation, vitamin deficiency, diarrhea, and hemorrhage.
  - **Bariatric surgery** should be performed only at high-volume centers by experienced surgeons. Successful surgical weight loss occurs when patients are appropriately prepared and then supported. Psychological screening and a diet and exercise program are advisable.

## Malnutrition

Table 2.7 outlines the clinical manifestations and treatment of severe malnutrition.

## Vitamins and Minerals

*If neurologic deficits are present, diagnose and treat vitamin $B_{12}$ deficiency quickly to prevent irreversible symptoms.*

A 47-year-old homeless man presents to your clinic to establish care. His known medical conditions include diabetes, hypertension, and a recently ⊕ PPD, for which he is currently taking INH. The patient complains of some cough, diarrhea, and tingling in his feet. On exam, his BP is 156/97, and you note that he smells of alcohol. He has pale conjunctivae, a red tongue, and fissures at the corners of his mouth. He also appears to have some loss of sensation to light touch in his feet bilaterally. How do you proceed? You check a hematocrit, a peripheral blood smear, and $B_{12}$ and folate levels and treat him accordingly.

**TABLE 2.7. Presentation and Treatment of Severe Malnutrition**

|  | MARASMUS | KWASHIORKOR |
| --- | --- | --- |
| Definition | Total calorie malnutrition. | Protein malnutrition. |
| Etiologies (in developed countries) | COPD, CHF, cancer, AIDS. | Trauma, burns, sepsis. |
| Symptoms/exam | Weight loss/**wasting.** | Normal weight. Edema, ascites. |
| Treatment | Correct fluid and electrolyte abnormalities; treat infections; give vitamins and minerals. Start with 1 g protein/kg and 30 kcal/kg, preferably enterically. | Treatment is the same as that for marasmus. |
| Complications | Immunosuppression, poor wound healing, impaired growth and development, muscle atrophy → organ dysfunction. | Same as those for marasmus. |

## VITAMIN DEFICIENCIES

Vitamin deficiencies may be more common in developed countries than is generally believed. Vitamins are needed for basic metabolism, but since most of them cannot be synthesized, they must be present in our diets. The presentation and treatment of water- and fat-soluble vitamin deficiencies are summarized in Tables 2.8 and 2.9.

## VITAMINS AND DISEASE PREVENTION

There has been increasing interest in the prevention of chronic disease through vitamin supplementation. Vitamins generally recommended for this

*Breast-feeding babies should receive 200 IU of vitamin D supplementation per day beginning in the first two months of life.*

**TABLE 2.8.    Presentation and Treatment of Water-Soluble Vitamin Deficiencies**

| VITAMIN | ETIOLOGY | SYMPTOMS/EXAM | TREATMENT |
|---|---|---|---|
| $B_1$ (thiamine) | The most common cause is alcoholism. | Anorexia, muscle cramps, paresthesias. Dry beriberi → neuropathy and Wernicke-Korsakoff syndrome; wet beriberi → high-output heart failure. | Oral thiamine. |
| $B_2$ (riboflavin) | Usually occurs with other deficiencies. | Nonspecific symptoms (e.g., mouth soreness, glossitis, cheilosis, weakness, irritability) plus seborrheic dermatitis and anemia. | Oral vitamin $B_2$. |
| $B_3$ (niacin) | Associated with alcoholism. | Nonspecific symptoms (see above); **pellagra** (dermatitis, diarrhea, dementia). | Oral nicotinamide. |
| $B_6$ (pyridoxine) | Associated with medication interactions (INH, OCPs) or with alcoholism. Fat malabsorption syndromes may contribute. | Nonspecific symptoms (see above); peripheral neuropathy, anemia, and seizures. Levels can be measured (normal > 50 ng/mL). | Oral or intramuscular vitamin $B_6$. |
| $B_{12}$ (cyanocobalamin) | Found in vegans, gastrectomy patients, and those with pernicious anemia. | Megaloblastic anemia, glossitis, anorexia, diarrhea. Peripheral neuropathy, balance problems, dementia (reversible if treated within six months). | Vitamin $B_{12}$ administered intramuscularly. |
| C (ascorbic acid) | Found in the urban poor, the elderly, alcoholics, cancer patients, smokers, and those in renal failure. | **Scurvy:** Poor wound healing, easy bruising, bleeding gums, subperiosteal hemorrhage, and anemia → edema, oliguria, neuropathy, and intracerebral hemorrhage. | Oral vitamin C. |
| Biotin | Caused by eating large quantities of raw eggs. | Myalgias, dysesthesias, anorexia, and nausea → dermatitis and alopecia. | Oral biotin. |
| Folic acid | Caused by inadequate dietary intake. | Megaloblastic anemia, neural tube defects. | Oral folic acid. |

**TABLE 2.9.** **Presentation and Treatment of Fat-Soluble Vitamin Deficiencies**

| VITAMIN | ETIOLOGY | SYMPTOMS/EXAM | TREATMENT |
|---|---|---|---|
| A (retinol) | Found in the urban poor, the elderly, and those with fat malabsorption syndrome. | Night blindness, xerosis, Bitot's spots (white patches on the conjunctivae) → keratomalacia, endophthalmitis, and blindness. | High-dose vitamin A. |
| D | Found in the elderly, those with insufficient sun exposure, those suffering from malnutrition or malabsorption, breast-feeding infants, and anticonvulsant users. | **Children:** Rickets (restlessness, craniotabes, costochondral beading, bowlegs, kyphoscoliosis).<br>**Adults:** Osteomalacia. | High-dose oral vitamin D. |
| E | Associated with severe malabsorption. | Areflexia, peripheral neuropathy, gait abnormality, ophthalmoplegia, ↓ proprioception. | Oral vitamin E. |
| K | Caused by poor diet, malabsorption, antibiotic use. | Clotting factor deficiencies (II, VII, IX, X). | Vitamin K, administered subcutaneously. |

purpose are summarized in Table 2.10. Several vitamins, including A, C, and E, have antioxidant functions. However, studies examining the role of these vitamins in protecting against cancer, heart disease, and Alzheimer's disease have yielded equivocal results. In fact, several vitamins have been shown to have detrimental effects at high doses and should therefore be used with caution.

### Herbal Medicines

*Herbal remedies that interact with warfarin (Coumadin) include **g**arlic, **g**inger, **g**ingko, **g**inseng, feverfew, and CoQ10.*

Herbal remedies are readily available to the public, and their uses and purported health benefits have been widely publicized in recent years. Accordingly, > 40% of the U.S. population use some type of complementary or alternative medicine. While many such patients are reluctant to volunteer this information to health care providers, others may openly question their physicians about the effectiveness of herbal remedies in treating various disorders. Although claims regarding herbal supplements are difficult to evaluate 2° to problems in isolating the active component, some have been demonstrated to be both safe and effective (see Table 2.11). At the same time, many others have been found to have deleterious effects. Herbal remedies that should be used with caution include the following:

- **Black licorice:** → hypertension.
- **Chromium:** ↓ blood sugar.
- **Garlic, ginger, gingko, ginseng, feverfew, CoQ10:** Prolong INR.

**TABLE 2.10.** **Vitamin Supplements to Prevent Chronic Disease**

| VITAMIN | DOSE | PREVENTION |
|---|---|---|
| Folic acid | 400–1000 μg/day in women of childbearing age. | Neural tube defects. |
| D | 800 IU/day (with 1–2 g of calcium). | Fractures, osteoporosis. |

**TABLE 2.11.** **Safe and Effective Herbal Medications**

| HERBAL MEDICATION | DISEASE/CONDITION | NOTES |
|---|---|---|
| Garlic powder | High cholesterol | Has modest effect; prolongs INR. |
| Ginger root | Nausea, motion sickness | Prolongs INR. |
| Glucosamine | Osteoarthritis | Use with caution in the presence of seafood allergy. |
| Horse chestnut | Venous insufficiency | |
| Peppermint oil | IBS | |
| Saw palmetto | BPH | Give at a dose of 160 mg BID or 320 mg QD. |
| St John's wort | Depression | Use with caution in light of multiple drug interactions. |

A 30-year-old businessman presents to your office seeking advice about his upcoming job relocation to Calcutta. He is leaving in five weeks and will be staying in India for six months. The man has no significant past medical history and is generally in good health. He has his immunization record with him but is concerned that he may need some boosters or perhaps some additional vaccinations. His biggest concerns, however, are of contracting malaria and having his stay in India tainted by bouts of diarrhea. How do you address his concerns? Review his immunization records, looking specifically for the date of his last tetanus booster and whether or not he has been immunized against HAV and HBV; offer general travel advice regarding food, water, and insect repellant; and provide prescriptions for both malaria prophylaxis and traveler's diarrhea with strict and clear instructions on when and how they should be taken.

## TRAVEL MEDICINE

More individuals than ever before are traveling to international destinations for both business and leisure. Despite the ease of planning a trip, travel itself is associated with potential morbidity and even mortality arising from infectious sources, modes of transportation, environmental exposures, and adverse medical outcomes from illnesses independent of travel. The risk of adverse events, however, can be significantly ↓ with appropriate pretravel evaluation and travel-related medical advice. The following sections offer guidelines and recommendations that can be offered to those contemplating or planning such travel.

COMMUNITY MEDICINE

### Pretravel Assessment

- Determine the patient's health status (e.g., infants, elderly, pregnant women, or those with chronic illnesses or underlying medical conditions).
- Identify potential medical needs (e.g., allergy to vaccine components, medication use, immunosuppression).
- Evaluate the patient's travel itinerary (e.g., planned destinations, climate and altitude, rural vs. urban environment, duration of stay, accommodations, purpose of travel)

### General Guidelines

The following are some guidelines that can be used to counsel patients who plan to travel abroad.

*Guidelines for travelers with regard to food and water: "Boil it, cook it, peel it, or forget it!"*

- **Food:** Patients should be advised that **fruits are safe only when peeled** and that **vegetables need to be fully cooked** to prevent contamination from fecally passed organisms in the soil. Unpasteurized dairy products and inadequately cooked fish or meat should be avoided.
- **Water:** Patients should be counseled to **avoid ice cubes** and should be advised that water is safe only after it has been boiled. Chlorination will kill most viral and bacterial pathogens, but protozoal pathogens such as *Giardia lamblia* can survive. Carbonated drinks, beer, wine, and drinks made from boiled water are safe.
- **Insect repellents:** Travelers should be advised to use at least **20% DEET** on clothing and exposed skin to prevent mosquito-borne infections such as malaria, yellow fever, and dengue fever. Protection with DEET lasts for several hours but is mitigated by swimming, washing, sweating, wiping, and rain. Travelers may also choose to treat clothing and bed netting with **permethrin,** which can effectively repel mosquitoes for more than a week even with washing.
- **Medications:** Travelers should be advised to bring adequate supplies of regularly used medications, since equivalent drugs may not be available at their destinations. Medications should be stored in carry-on luggage in the event that checked baggage is lost in transit.
- **Other:**
  - Patients should be counseled to **avoid swimming in fresh water** in areas where schistosomiasis is prevalent. Swimming in chlorinated or salt water is safe.
  - Patients should be given safe-sex counseling and advice regarding sun protection.

### Recommended Vaccinations

There are **three categories of vaccinations** that must be addressed:

- **Routine or standard immunizations:** Childhood immunization programs and age-appropriate updates should be addressed regardless of travel (see Table 2.1).
- **Required immunizations:** The only vaccination required by international health regulations is the **yellow fever** vaccine for travel to certain parts of sub-Saharan Africa and tropical South America. The **meningococcal** vaccine is required by the Saudi Arabian government for travel during the Hajj.
- **Recommended immunizations:** Recommendations depend on the trip-related risk of exposure to diseases such as HAV, HBV, typhoid fever, meningococcal meningitis, Japanese encephalitis, rabies, and tick-borne encephalitis.

## Malaria Prophylaxis

Malaria is one of the most common infections worldwide, especially in tropical climates, and it must therefore be addressed for all patients planning travel to endemic regions. Malaria is transmitted by the bite of the female *Anopheles* mosquito and is most commonly caused by the organism *Plasmodium falciparum*; other species include *P. vivax*, *P. malariae*, and *P. ovale*. Symptoms can begin anywhere from eight days after the initial infection to several months following departure from the malarious region. The two most important components of malaria prevention are avoidance of mosquitoes and chemoprophylaxis (see Table 2.12).

*The mosquitoes that transmit malaria usually feed at night, so travelers should be advised to minimize exposure between dusk and dawn.*

## Traveler's Diarrhea

One of the most common fears of travelers visiting developing nations is that of developing diarrhea. In fact, 40–60% of travelers to these countries do develop diarrhea. Of these cases, 85% are caused by bacterial pathogens, the most common of which is **enterotoxigenic *E. coli* (ETEC)**. Parasites ac-

**TABLE 2.12. Drugs Used for Malaria Prophylaxis**

| DRUG NAME | INDICATION | ADMINISTRATION | SAFE FOR CHILDREN? | SAFE IN PREGNANCY? | SIDE EFFECTS |
|---|---|---|---|---|---|
| Atovaquone/ proguanil (Malarone) | Prophylaxis in areas with chloroquine-resistant or mefloquine-resistant *P. falciparum.* | Daily dosing. Begin 1–2 days before travel and continue for seven days after leaving the malarious area. | Yes, if weight is > 11 kg. | **No.** | Abdominal pain, nausea, vomiting, headache, rash. |
| Chloroquine phosphate (Aralen and generic) | Prophylaxis only in areas with chloroquine-sensitive *P. falciparum.* | Weekly dosing. Begin 1–2 weeks before travel and continue for four weeks after departure from the malarious area. | Yes. | Yes. | GI disturbance, dizziness, blurred vision, headache, insomnia, pruritus. |
| Doxycycline | Prophylaxis in areas with chloroquine-resistant or mefloquine-resistant *P. falciparum.* | Daily dosing. Begin 1–2 days before travel and continue for four weeks after departure from the malarious area. | Yes, if ≥ 8 years of age. | **No.** | Photosensitivity skin reactions. |
| Mefloquine (Lariam and generic) | Prophylaxis in areas with chloroquine-resistant *P. falciparum.* | Weekly dosing. Begin 1–2 weeks before travel and continue for four weeks after departure from the malarious area. | Yes. | Yes, in the second and third trimesters. | Nausea, dizziness, vertigo. Lightheadedness, bad dreams, paranoid ideation, seizures, psychosis in patients with significant psychopathology. |

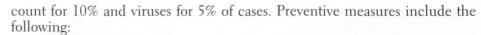

count for 10% and viruses for 5% of cases. Preventive measures include the following:

- Attention should be paid to food and beverage selection (see the guidelines listed above).
- **Bismuth subsalicylate**, the active ingredient in Pepto-Bismol, has been shown to ↓ **the incidence of traveler's diarrhea** from 40% to 14%. Side effects include blackening of the tongue and stool, nausea, constipation, and, rarely, tinnitus. **Avoid use in children** with viral infections because of the risk of Reye's syndrome.
- Prophylactic antibiotics are **not** recommended for most travelers.

### SYMPTOMS/EXAM

- Onset is between four and fourteen days after arrival, with symptoms lasting 1–5 days.
- Presents with malaise, anorexia, and abdominal cramps followed by sudden onset of watery diarrhea.
- Nausea and vomiting may also be seen.
- Typically does not present with symptoms of colitis such as blood or pus in the stool +/− low-grade fever.

### TREATMENT

- **Fluid replacement:** The 1° and most important treatment! Both fluid **volume** and **electrolytes** must be repleted. A simple solution of ½ teaspoon of salt, ½ teaspoon of baking soda, and 4 tablespoons of sugar in 1 L of water may be used.
- **Antibiotics:** Indicated for those who present with moderate to severe diarrhea characterized by > 4 unformed stools daily; fever; or blood, pus, or mucus in the stool. The usual choice is a fluoroquinolone such as **ciprofloxacin.** In areas of increasing resistance to fluoroquinolones, **azithromycin** is an effective alternative.
- **Antimotility agents:** Not usually indicated for mild to moderate cases; should be used only in severe cases in conjunction with antibiotics. Discontinue if abdominal pain worsens or if diarrhea persists after two days.
- **Bismuth subsalicylate:** Has antisecretory and antimicrobial properties. A dosage of 15 mL or two tablets every 30 minutes for up to eight doses has been shown to ↓ stool frequency and shorten the duration of illness.
- Medical care should be sought in the presence of high fever, severe abdominal pain, bloody diarrhea, or vomiting and when antibiotics have not been helpful.

## DOMESTIC VIOLENCE

### Child Abuse

Defined as any recent act or failure to act by a parent or caretaker that → the death, serious physical or emotional harm, sexual abuse, or exploitation of a child < 18 years of age. In the United States, the incidence of child abuse and neglect ranges from 15 to 42 per 1000 children. All 50 states have laws requiring physicians to report suspected child abuse to Child Protective Services. Table 2.13 outlines common risk factors for child abuse. Factors that **raise suspicion of child abuse** include the following:

- A history that is **inconsistent with the child's injuries.**
- A history that is **vague** or that changes in repeated versions.
- A history that is **inconsistent with the developmental stage** of the child.

*Avoid the use of bismuth subsalicylate in patients with aspirin allergy, renal insufficiency, and gout and in those taking anticoagulants, probenecid, or methotrexate.*

*Patients with diarrhea should be rehydrated with a solution of ½ teaspoon of salt, ½ teaspoon of baking soda, and 4 tablespoons of sugar in 1 L of water.*

**COMMUNITY MEDICINE**

TABLE 2.13. **Risk Factors for Child Abuse**

| PERPETRATORS | ENVIRONMENT | VICTIMS |
|---|---|---|
| Most commonly fathers, mothers' boyfriends, female babysitters, and mothers (in descending order of frequency) | Financial difficulties | Young age |
| | Divorce or interpersonal conflict | Past history of abuse or repeated injuries |
| | Illness | Speech and language disorders |
| | Professional problems | Learning disabilities |
| Young or single parents | Social isolation | Conduct disorders |
| Parents with lower levels of education | Distant or absent extended family | Congenital anomalies |
| Those with unstable family situations | Acceptability of violence as a means of problem solving | Mental retardation or other handicaps |
| Those with a history of abuse | | Chronic illnesses |
| Those with a history of substance abuse | | Hyperactivity |
| Those with psychiatric illness | | Adopted children |
| | | Stepchildren |
| | | Prematurity and low birth weight |

COMMUNITY MEDICINE

- An **implausible** history.
- Multiple injuries in various stages of healing, or different types of coexisting injuries.
- Evidence of poor caretaking.
- Behavioral disturbances in the child.
- Arguing, roughness, or observed **violence** in interaction with a parent.
- **Aloofness** or lack of emotional interaction between the parent and child.
- Inappropriate parental response to the severity of injury.
- A **delay** in seeking medical care.
- Partial confession by the parent.

*A history that is inconsistent with the patient's injuries is the hallmark of physical abuse.*

There are **four major types** of child abuse: **physical abuse** (inflicting physical pain or injury); **sexual abuse** (nonconsensual contact of any kind); **emotional or psychological abuse;** and **child neglect.** Hallmarks of **physical abuse** include the following:

- Nonaccidental injuries are commonly bilateral, symmetric, and seen on the buttocks, genitalia, back, and back of hands (vs. accidental injuries which are seen on the shins, forearms, and hips.)
- Highly suspicious for abuse are fractures to the metaphyses caused by pulling or wrenching (e.g., chip fractures where the corner of the metaphysis of a long bone is torn off with damage to the epiphysis).
- Characteristic burns caused by abuse are cigarette burns, immersion burns affecting the buttocks and perineum, clearly demarcated scald lines without evidence of splash marks, and stocking-glove burns on the hands or feet.
- Injury to the head is the most common cause of death from physical abuse. Children can present with convulsions, apnea, ↑ ICP, subdural hemorrhages, retinal hemorrhages, or coma.
- A complete skeletal survey is indicated in children < 2 years of age when physical abuse is suspected.
- Children with a history of "easy bruising" should receive a screen for a bleeding diathesis, including CBC, PT, PTT, and bleeding time.

Hallmarks of **sexual abuse** are as follows:

- Signs and symptoms such as vaginal, penile, or rectal pain as well as erythema, discharge, bleeding, chronic dysuria, enuresis, constipation, or encopresis.

■ Inappropriate behaviors such as sexualized activity with peers or objects or seductive behavior also suggest a history of sexual abuse.

### RECOMMENDATIONS FOR SCREENING

■ The AMA, the American Academy of Pediatrics (AAP), and the AAFP recommend that physicians remain alert for signs and symptoms of child physical and sexual abuse during routine examinations.

■ The USPSTF found insufficient evidence to recommend for or against the routine screening of parents or guardians for the abuse of children.

## Intimate-Partner Abuse

Intimate-partner abuse is defined as **intentional controlling by or violent behavior from** a person who was or is in an intimate relationships with the victim. This behavior may take the form of **physical abuse, sexual assault, emotional abuse, economic control, and/or social isolation.** Women are far more likely than men to be the victims of chronic physical abuse. Violence in gay and lesbian relationships appears to be just as common as in heterosexual relationships. Most states do not currently require mandatory reporting of domestic violence against competent adult women. Table 2.14 outlines risk factors for intimate-partner abuse.

### RECOMMENDATIONS FOR SCREENING

■ The AMA and the AAFP recommend that physicians conducting routine exams remain alert for signs and symptoms of intimate-partner violence.

■ The USPSTF found insufficient evidence to recommend for or against the routine screening of women for intimate-partner violence.

## Elder Abuse

Elder abuse can be divided into three categories: domestic, institutional, and self-neglect. **Domestic elder abuse** refers to the maltreatment of an el-

TABLE 2.14.    **Risk Factors for Intimate-Partner Abuse**

| RISK FACTORS | WHEN TO SUSPECT |
|---|---|
| Female gender | Inconsistent explanation of injuries |
| Young age | Delay in seeking treatment |
| Low socioeconomic status | Multiple somatic complaints |
| Pregnancy | Gynecologic conditions such as premenstrual syndrome, |
| Mental health problems | STDs, unintended pregnancy, or chronic pelvic pain |
| Substance abuse on the part of | Lateness for prenatal care visits |
| victims or perpetrators | Frequent ER visits |
| Separated or divorced status | Patient noncompliance |
| History of childhood abuse | Central distribution of injuries (breasts, abdomen, genitals) |

derly individual living at home or in the home of a caregiver. **Institutional elder abuse** involves the maltreatment of an elder living in a residential facility. **Self-neglect** refers to the behavior of an elderly individual living alone that threatens his or her own safety and health. All health care providers and administrators are mandated by law to report suspected elder mistreatment. The seven common types of elder abuse are as follows (see also Table 2.15):

- **Physical abuse:** Inflicting physical pain or injury.
- **Sexual abuse:** Nonconsensual sexual contact of any kind.
- **Psychological abuse:** Inflicting mental anguish (threatening, humiliating, intimidating).
- **Financial abuse:** Improper or illegal use of the resources of an elderly individual without his or her consent.
- **Neglect:** Failure of a caregiver to provide goods or services.
- **Abandonment:** Desertion of an elderly individual by someone who has assumed responsibility for his or her care.
- **Self-neglect:** Behavior of an elderly individual that threatens his or her own safety and health.

### RECOMMENDATIONS FOR SCREENING

- The AMA recommends that physicians routinely ask elderly patients direct and specific questions about abuse.
- The USPSTF concluded that there is insufficient evidence to recommend for or against the use of **specific screening instruments** for elder abuse but did recommend the inclusion of direct questions about abuse as part of a routine history.

TABLE 2.15.    **Risk Factors for Elder Abuse**

| RISK FACTORS | WHEN TO SUSPECT |
| --- | --- |
| Female gender | Multiple somatic complaints |
| Age > 80 | Frequent unexplained crying |
| Low income | Unexplained fear or suspicion of particular |
| Social isolation | person(s) in the living environment |
| Minority status | Multiple injuries in various stages of evolution |
| Low level of education | Unexplained injuries or implausible |
| Functional debility | explanations for injuries |
| Cognitive impairment | Malnutrition |
| Substance abuse by the caregiver or by | Dehydration |
| the elderly person | Gross inattention to hygiene |
| Caregiver burnout or frustration | |
| Psychological disorders or character | |
| pathology | |
| Previous history of family violence | |
| Dependence of the abuser on the victim | |

A 57-year-old smoker comes to see you complaining of feeling out of breath when he takes walks with his wife. He wonders if he is just getting old. He denies any chest pain or other cardiac symptoms. You discover that he has worked in shipbuilding for > 30 years, and on pulmonary exam you note some fine crackles. He also has clubbing of his fingernails. What are your next steps? Suspecting COPD as well as possible asbestosis, you obtain a CXR and PFTs.

## OCCUPATIONAL MEDICINE

Work-related injuries and illnesses are quite prevalent and are associated with significant morbidity, mortality, and cost both to the individual and to society. Without removal of the precipitating trigger or cause of illness that is embedded in the workplace, occupational illnesses will often persist or worsen despite other appropriate treatment. For this reason, a thorough history is critical.

### Evaluation of Illness

Although there are hundreds of occupational illnesses, pulmonary diseases predominate. Common nonpulmonary occupational illnesses include carpal tunnel syndrome, low back pain/injury, and contact dermatitis. The etiologies and presentation of common occupational pulmonary illnesses are outlined in Table 2.16. Listed below are guidelines for the evaluation of occupational illness in general.

- A brief history of possible work-related injuries or illnesses should include symptoms/review of systems; current and past jobs held; and the temporal relationship of the symptoms to jobs or work schedule.
- Further components of the history should include the following:
    - Evaluation of products used or manufactured at the workplace.
    - Examination of Material Safety Data Sheets (MSDSs).
    - Assessment of the degree of protective measures taken (e.g., protective clothing, appropriate ventilation).
- If on-site investigation is necessary, the following groups may be of aid:
    - **The Occupational Safety and Health Administration (OSHA):** Within the Department of Labor. Creates and enforces workplace safety and health regulations.
    - **The Environmental Protection Agency (EPA).**
    - **The National Institute for Occupational Safety and Health (NIOSH):** Part of the Centers for Disease Control and Prevention (CDC) and within the Department of Health and Human Services (HHS). Conducts research and makes recommendations for the prevention of work-related illnesses and injuries.
    - Private certified industrial hygienists.
- **Exam:** The physical exam should include evaluation of the lungs, skin, any painful musculoskeletal region as well as an examination of the extremities for clubbing.
- **Dx:** Diagnostic testing will often include a CXR and PFTs.

*Occupational exposures that can present with fever include toxic organic dust syndrome, hypersensitivity pneumonitis, and metal fume fever (zinc exposure).*

TABLE 2.16.   Common Occupational Pulmonary Disorders

| ILLNESS | AGENTS/POTENTIAL EXPOSURE | CLINICAL PRESENTATION |
|---|---|---|
| Asthma | Isocyanates, flour, dyes, metals, wood dust, latex. Rubber or plastic production, bakers. | Rhinoconjunctivitis, wheezing. |
| Silicosis | Crystalline silica mining, quarrying, sandblasting, masonry, foundry work, ceramics. | May be asymptomatic with an abnormal CXR (nodules or fibrosis), or may present with cough and dyspnea. |
| Asbestosis | Textiles, shipbuilding, cement, insulation, plumbing, pipefitting, renovation of asbestos-containing buildings. | After 20–30 years, presents with dyspnea on exertion. Fine bibasilar crackles and clubbing may also be seen. CXR shows interstitial fibrosis and pleural involvement. **Can → mesothelioma.** |
| Toxic organic dust syndrome | Moldy hay. | Fever, cough, wheezing, dyspnea. |
| Hypersensitivity pneumonitis (extrinsic allergic alveolitis) | Farmer's lung, hot tub lung, humidifiers, birds/poultry, grain processing, lumber milling/construction. | **Acute:** Fever, malaise, cough, dyspnea, chest tightness (no wheeze!) 4–6 hours after exposure. **Chronic:** Weight loss, fatigue, dyspnea, clubbing. Consider in the presence of recurrent "pneumonias." |

COMMUNITY MEDICINE

## Impairment vs. Disability

Impairment is distinguished from disability as follows:

■ **Impairment:** Defined as a specific failure in the function of a body part or organ system.
■ **Disability:** An impediment that prevents an individual from interacting with the environment, with the specific level determined by legal system. Defined by the Social Security Administration as "the inability to engage in any substantial gainful activity by reason of any medically determinable physical or mental impairment which can be expected to lead to death or which has lasted or can be expected to last for a continuous period of not less than 12 months."

## PUBLIC HEALTH

## Smoking Cessation

In 2003, the prevalence of cigarette smoking among adults in the United States was estimated to be 22%. This behavior → as many as 400,000 deaths per year and is the most common preventable cause of death. Most smokers tried their first cigarette before 18 years of age and have attempted to quit more than once. Some 35–40% of patients relapse within five years of quitting.

### HEALTH BENEFITS

Smoking cessation is known to confer the following health benefits:

*Three years after smoking cessation, the risk of recurrent MI ↓ to that of a nonsmoker.*

- **MI:** ↓ mortality risk. The risk of recurrent coronary events is progressively ↓ to near that of a nonsmoker by three years postcessation.
- **Stroke:** Associated with a ↓ risk over time.
- **Pulmonary disease:** ↓ progression in the decline of $FEV_1$ in patients with COPD. Also associated with a ↓ risk of pulmonary infections such as bacterial pneumonia and TB.
- **Malignancy:** ↓ risk of lung, kidney, bladder, stomach, and cervical cancers, among others.
- **PUD:** ↓ risk of developing PUD; accelerated rate of healing.
- **Osteoporosis:** ↓ risk of bone loss and fracture (begins ten years after quitting).

### CESSATION METHODS

- The first step is to evaluate the patient's cigarette use, assess his or her interest in quitting, and find out about previous attempts at quitting. Many behavioral methods have been advocated to encourage patients to work toward quitting.
- Once the patient is ready, strategies include setting a "quit day" and defining alternative oral behaviors to substitute for the cigarette (e.g., gum, throat lozenges).
- Methods for cessation (see Table 2.17) should be discussed and agreed upon in advance of the "quit day."

## Reportable Diseases

When a communicable disease is diagnosed, timely notification of public health authorities plays an important role in epidemiologic work as well as in infection control. Some of the more common diseases that generally require immediate notification are botulism, GI illnesses (cholera, *E. coli* O157:H7, HAV, *Salmonella*, *Shigella*), measles and rubella, meningococcal disease, and TB. STDs (including chlamydia, gonorrhea, syphilis, and HIV/AIDS) consti-

**TABLE 2.17.** Methods for Smoking Cessation

| METHOD | DESCRIPTION | EFFICACY |
|---|---|---|
| Group counseling | Lectures, groups, exercises, strategies. | Associated with a 20% one-year quit rate. |
| Hypnosis and acupuncture | | There is no evidence to support the efficacy of these procedures. |
| Nicotine replacement (gum, patch, nasal spray, inhaler) | Suppresses withdrawal symptoms: depressed mood, insomnia, irritability, restlessness, weight gain. | When used with a behavioral program, gum and patch methods double the quit rate. |
| Bupropion | Enhances central noradrenergic and dopaminergic function when administered at a dosage of 150 mg daily. | Has greater efficacy than nicotine replacement. |

tute another important category of reportable diseases. Measures for postexposure prophylaxis (PEP), which are also key to infection control, are as follows:

- **TB:** Close contacts of individuals with active TB should undergo tuberculin skin testing. A reaction ≥ 5 mm is considered ⊕. A ⊖ test should be repeated 10–12 weeks later. Those with a ⊕ test should be treated with isoniazid (INH) in the same manner as any other case of latent TB infection.
- **HAV:** This picornavirus is transmitted by fecal-oral spread. PEP consists of concurrent administration of immune globulin (IgG) and the first dose of the HAV vaccine. Consider PEP in the following individuals who have had close contact with an individual with serologic confirmation of infection:
    - Unvaccinated household and sexual contacts.
    - Those who have shared needles with the infected individual.
    - Staff, attendees, or residents of day care and nursing home facilities.
    - Food handlers.
- **HBV and HCV:** These two viruses are blood borne or transmitted sexually. An estimated 600,000–800,000 needlestick injuries occur annually in hospitals in the United States. Guidelines for prophylaxis are as follows.
    - Exposure of health care workers by needlestick or mucous membrane contact must → an OSHA-required evaluation. This must include identification of the source individual and testing of his/her blood for HBV, HCV, and HIV.
    - An unvaccinated individual who has been exposed to HBV should receive hepatitis B immune globulin (HBIG) and should start the vaccine series.
    - There is no proven effective PEP for HCV. Instead, liver enzymes, HCV-RNA, and serologic testing should be obtained at the time of exposure as well as four weeks later.
- **HIV:** Exposure to HIV can occur in health care settings as well as through sex, needle sharing, or blood transfusions. The seroconversion rate of health care workers after a needlestick injury is estimated to be < 1%. The risk of conversion is influenced by the type of exposure as well as by the viral load of the source. For sexual transmission, receptive anal intercourse confers the highest risk of infection. Guidelines are as follows:
    - For health care worker exposures, an OSHA-required evaluation similar to that described for the hepatitis viruses must be conducted.
    - PEP for HIV is more inconvenient and is associated with possible toxicity. Any decision that is made to administer PEP must therefore weigh its contraindications against the risk of infection. PEP in nonoccupational exposures is handled in a similar manner, although management of individuals with ongoing behavioral risk is difficult.
    - When deemed appropriate, PEP should be started as soon as possible (within 72 hours of exposure). The CDC recommends a four-week course of a dual nucleoside or nucleotide reverse transcriptase inhibitor (NRTI) regimen consisting of zidovudine (AZT) plus lamivudine (3TC) or emtricitabine (FTC) OR tenofovir (TDF) plus 3TC or FTC. A protease inhibitor is added for severe or high-risk exposures.
    - HIV serology testing is obtained at the time of exposure as well as at 6 weeks, 12 weeks, and 6 months.

*No proven effective postexposure prophylaxis is available for HCV.*

## Bioterrorism

Biological weapons have in recent years become a credible threat to the public. The most dangerous organisms and toxins are those that are sturdy, readily grown in large quantities, and easily disseminated over large areas. These higher-priority agents include anthrax, smallpox, plague, botulism, tularemia, Ebola/Marburg viruses, and Lassa/Junin viruses.

### ANTHRAX

*Bacillus anthracis,* a sporulating gram-⊕ rod, is transmitted to humans through direct contact with infected animals or with animal products through skin exposure, inhalation, or ingestion.

#### SYMPTOMS/EXAM

- **Cutaneous:** Small, painless papules enlarge to become vesicles that ulcerate with eschar formation within two days. Fever and hematologic abnormalities may also be seen.
- **Inhalational (woolsorters' disease):** Acquired from inhalation of spores that → hemorrhagic necrosis of thoracic lymph nodes and hemorrhagic mediastinitis. Initially presents with flulike symptoms and then progresses to severe respiratory distress and to bacteremia and meningitis. A widened mediastinum is seen on CXR.
- **Pharyngeal and GI:** Acquired from consumption of infected meat. Presents with fever, pharyngitis, neck swelling, and eschars in the oropharynx or with severe abdominal pain, hemorrhagic ascites, and melena.

#### DIAGNOSIS

Diagnosis is made through Gram stain and culture of lesions, PCR, or serologic testing.

#### TREATMENT

Treat with ciprofloxacin or doxycycline for cutaneous anthrax. A multidrug regimen should be used for inhalational anthrax.

### SMALLPOX

A highly contagious disease that is caused by the variola virus and once accounted for 10% of all deaths in the world. There have been no reported cases of smallpox since its global eradication in 1979. Smallpox was transmitted via inhalation and was generally not widespread owing to the severity of the disease. The incubation period was 7–19 days.

#### SYMPTOMS/EXAM

- Infection begins with 2–4 days of fever, headache, backache, and vomiting. The rash progresses as illustrated in Figure 2.1.
- The rash then spreads centrifugally, and as lesions evolve, they may become confluent or umbilicated (see Figure 2.2). Lesions then crust over by day 14.

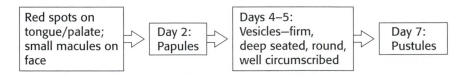

**FIGURE 2.1.** **Progression of smallpox infection.**

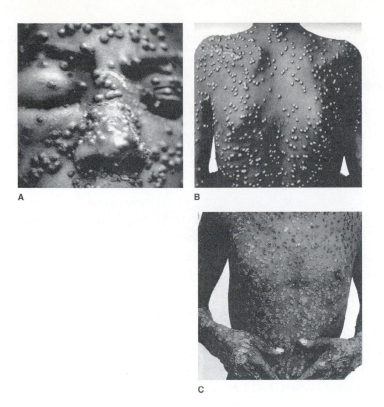

**FIGURE 2.2. Smallpox lesions.**

Multiple pustules becoming confluent on the face (A). Multiple pustules on the trunk, all in the same stage of development (B). Multiple crusted healing lesions on the trunk, arms, and hands (C). (Reproduced, with permission, from Wolff K et al. *Fitzpatrick's Color Atlas & Synopsis of Clinical Dermatology*, 5th ed. New York: McGraw-Hill, 2005: 771.) (Also see Color Insert.)

### *DIAGNOSIS*

Diagnosis is made clinically by the criteria described in Table 2.18. If all three major criteria are met, immediate reporting to local health authorities is warranted along with infectious disease consultation. Diagnosis is confirmed through culture of the virus from skin lesions and serologic tests.

### *TREATMENT*

There is no known effective treatment for smallpox. Individuals with suspected smallpox should be placed in respiratory and contact isolation. Vacci-

**TABLE 2.18. Diagnostic Criteria for Smallpox**

| MAJOR CRITERIA | MINOR CRITERIA |
| --- | --- |
| Febrile prodrome | Centrifugal distribution |
| Classic smallpox lesions | First lesions on oral mucosa/palate, face, or |
| Lesions in the same state of development | forearms |
| | The patient appears toxic or moribund |
| | Slow evolution (each stage lasting 1–2 days) |
| | Lesions on palms and soles |

nation of exposed individuals during the incubation period can prevent spread.

## COMPLICATIONS

The prognosis depends on the type of smallpox. Variola major strains had a mortality rate of approximately 20%, while minor strains had a mortality rate of < 1%. Death was usually related to toxic shock. Bacterial superinfection of rash was also a frequent complication.

A 43-year-old homeless man presents to your clinic to establish care. He has occasional wheezing but otherwise has no complaints. His medical problems include diabetes, hypertension, and tobacco use. He wonders if he should be tested for TB, since some of the men who lived at his previous shelter were recently diagnosed with active TB infection. He has had no fevers, night sweats, or cough. What do you advise? On the basis of his homeless status and diabetes, he should be screened annually for latent tuberculosis infection. Since he may have had contact with active TB, induration ≥ 5 mm would constitute a ⊕ test for him. He would then require a CXR to rule out active disease and need nine months of INH therapy to ↓ the risk of reactivation.

## Tuberculosis

### LATENT TUBERCULOSIS INFECTION (LTBI)

LTBI represents a large subset of infections caused by *Mycobacterium tuberculosis*, which infects between 19% and 43% of the world's population. The lifetime risk of acquiring reactivation TB with LTBI is roughly 10–20%, with 2–5% developing active TB in the first two years. If cases of LTBI are not detected and treated, new cases of TB will continually develop from this group.

### DIAGNOSIS

- Tuberculin skin testing via purified protein derivative (PPD) is the method used to detect LTBI. A delayed-type hypersensitivity reaction mediated by T lymphocytes → induration of the skin 48–72 hours after inoculation.
- An annual screening PPD (in asymptomatic individuals) is indicated for:
    - Those with HIV infection.
    - Health care workers, prison guards, and mycobacteriology laboratory personnel.
    - Those with a medical condition that ↑ the risk of active TB (e.g., diabetes, use of immunosuppressive medications, end-stage renal disease, alcoholism, conditions associated with rapid weight loss or chronic malnutrition).
    - Homeless and IV drug users.
    - Those who reside in a long-term care facility.
- A one-time screen is indicated for:
    - Those with a single potential exposure to TB (repeat PPD in 6–12 weeks if the exposure is recent).
    - Those with an incidentally discovered fibrotic lung lesion.
    - Immigrants and refugees from countries with a high prevalence of TB.

- False-⊖ skin tests may be seen in the following:
  - Anergic states such as HIV and malignancy.
  - Newly diagnosed pulmonary TB or severe extrapulmonary TB.
  - Corticosteroids or immunosuppressive therapy.
  - Concurrent viral infection.
  - Poor nutrition.
- Because different types of exposures and varying baseline immune status → a wide distribution of PPD reactions, criteria have been developed to minimize the number of false ⊕s. These are described in Table 2.19.
- In persons who have received the BCG vaccine as children, interpret on the basis of the criteria used for unvaccinated persons. Large PPD reactions in these individuals are still likely to represent TB infection.
- All individuals with a ⊕ PPD should undergo assessment to exclude active disease, including a CXR.

*Tuberculin skin test conversion occurs 2–12 weeks after 1° infection.*

### TREATMENT

- INH therapy is effective in reducing the risk of reactivation TB in individuals with a ⊕ PPD. Its protective effect lasts at least 20 years and probably lasts for life. Current guidelines recommend treatment of any individual who has a ⊕ PPD regardless of age.
- INH should be given for 6–12 months (nine months is ideal). Rifampin should be reserved for suspected INH-resistant strains in view of the ↑ incidence of rifampin-associated liver toxicity.
- Consider ordering initial and monthly liver panels in patients at an ↑ risk of hepatitis (e.g., alcoholics, those with chronic liver disease, HIV-⊕ patients, drug interaction).
- Warn patients of signs of hepatitis.
- Consider concurrent administration of pyridoxine (vitamin B$_6$, 25–50 mg/day) for patients at ↑ risk of peripheral neuropathy, paresthesias, and ataxia. This high-risk group includes the elderly, HIV-⊕ patients, children, diabetics, alcoholics, pregnant or breast-feeding women, those with chronic liver disease, and those in renal failure.

*INH therapy ↓ the risk of reactivation TB in LTBI by roughly 70% if taken for six months and by > 90% if taken for 12 months.*

### EXTRAPULMONARY TUBERCULOSIS

Includes miliary TB, tuberculous lymphadenitis, skeletal TB, and tuberculous meningitis. TB can also lead to ocular disease, renal disease, pericarditis, salpingitis, peritonitis, and intestinal TB. In the United States, 5.4% of all TB is extrapulmonary. Approximately one-third of these cases are lymphatic and

**TABLE 2.19.  Criteria for a Positive PPD**

| ≥ 5-MM INDURATION | ≥ 10-MM INDURATION | ≥ 15-MM INDURATION |
|---|---|---|
| Recent contact | Immigrants who have come from a high-prevalence country within the last five years | No risk factors |
| HIV | | |
| Chronic steroid use | IV drug users | |
| Organ transplant/immunosuppression | Residents/employees of high-risk facilities (hospitals, jails, nursing homes, shelters) | |
| Inactive TB on x-ray, untreated | Those < 4 years of age | |
| | Those < 18 years of age who have been exposed to a high-risk adult | |

up to one-third skeletal. TB can manifest in many different organ systems and should therefore be regularly considered when formulating a differential. HIV-infected patients are at particularly high risk, with as many as 60% developing extrapulmonary TB.

### DIAGNOSIS

If not already performed, tuberculin skin testing should be the first step in diagnosis, although a ⊖ PPD (especially in HIV-infected patients) does not exclude the diagnosis.

### TREATMENT

A six-month, four-drug regimen of the antitubercular agents used for pulmonary TB is sufficient for most manifestations of extrapulmonary TB. However, many experts recommend extension to 9–12 months in miliary, meningeal, or skeletal TB, as well as in immunocompromised hosts (see below).

## MILIARY TUBERCULOSIS

Defined as the disseminated hematogenous spread of *M. tuberculosis*. An ↑ risk is associated with older age and comorbidities that alter cellular immunity (e.g., diabetes, HIV, renal failure).

### SYMPTOMS/EXAM

Presentation is highly variable, ranging from fevers, night sweats, and failure to thrive/generalized malaise to specific organ system dysfunction (see Table 2.20).

### DIAGNOSIS

- CBC reveals hematologic derangements in either direction. An ↑ ESR and hyponatremia are also commonly seen.
- A miliary pattern is seen on CXR in more than two-thirds of cases.
- Obtain an AFB smear and culture of accessible and suspicious body fluids.

**TABLE 2.20.** **Organ System Involvement in Miliary Tuberculosis**

| ORGAN SYSTEM | CLINICAL MANIFESTATIONS |
| --- | --- |
| GI | Abnormal LFTs, hepatomegaly, cholestatic jaundice, pancreatitis, cholecystitis. |
| CNS | Meningitis, tuberculomas. |
| Skin | Tuberculosis cutis miliaris disseminata. |
| Cardiovascular | Pericarditis (rare). |
| Adrenal | Adrenal insufficiency (rare). |
| Renal | Sterile pyuria. |

### Tuberculous Lymphadenitis

- **Sx:** Commonly presents as a lone nontender lymph node (most often cervical—scrofula).
- **Dx:** Diagnosed by FNA or excisional biopsy. The latter is a necessary aspect of treatment as well.

### Skeletal Tuberculosis

#### Symptoms/Exam

- About one-half of cases involve the spine (Pott's disease), but other common manifestations include tuberculous arthritis and extraspinal tuberculous osteomyelitis.
- The most common presentation of Pott's disease is progressive localized pain over weeks to months, sometimes associated with muscle spasm and rigidity. Fewer than 40% have constitutional symptoms.

#### Diagnosis

- Vertebral plain films show osteolytic lesions.
- Further imaging with CT or MRI can be useful.
- CT-guided biopsy of infected lesions is recommended. For tuberculous arthritis, biopsy of the synovium or periarticular bone is necessary.

#### Treatment

Early surgical intervention can ↓ morbidity, although conservative medical management is often successful as well.

#### Complications

Cord compression during the active phase of the infection → paraplegia.

### Tuberculous Meningitis

- **Sx:** Headache, fevers, meningismus, vomiting, and other neurologic signs.
- **Dx:** AFB stain and culture of CSF. Hydrocephalus is noted in a minority of patients on CT scan.
- **Tx:** Corticosteroids for the first 6–8 weeks of therapy have been shown to ↓ mortality in both children and adults.

## EPIDEMIOLOGY AND BIOSTATISTICS

## Leading Causes of Death

Table 2.21 outlines the principal causes of mortality, grouped by age.

## Test Parameters

The following are common terms used in statistical methodology:

- **Incidence:** The number of **new cases** of a disease in a defined population over a specific period of time.
- **Prevalence:** The number of cases of existing disease in a given population at a specific period of time or a particular moment in time.

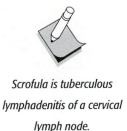

*Scrofula is tuberculous lymphadenitis of a cervical lymph node.*

**TABLE 2.21.**   **Leading Causes of Death by Age Group**

| AGES 1–24 | AGES 25–64 | AGES 65 AND OLDER |
|---|---|---|
| Unintentional injuries | Malignant neoplasms | Heart disease |
| Suicide and homicide | Heart disease | Malignant neoplasms |
| Malignant neoplasms | Unintentional injuries | Cerebrovascular disease |
| Heart disease | HIV | COPD |
| Congenital anomalies | Suicide and homicide | Pneumonia and influenza |

*Disease*

|  | + | – |
|---|---|---|
| Test  + | a | b |
|        – | c | d |

$Sn = a / a + c$

$Sp = d / b + d$

$PPV = a / a + b$

$NPV = d / d + c$

*Sensitivity and specificity are independent of disease prevalence in a tested population, whereas PPV and NPV are dependent on disease prevalence.*

*Screen-detected patients will always live longer than clinically detected patients even if early detection and treatment confer no benefit because of lead-time and length-time biases.*

■ **Sensitivity (Sn)—"PID" (Positive in Disease):** The probability that a test will be ⊕ in someone with the disease when compared to a gold standard—in other words, **the ability to correctly identify individuals who truly have the disease.**

■ **Specificity (Sp)—"NIH" (Negative in Health):** The probability that a test will be ⊖ in someone who truly does not have the disease when compared to a gold standard—in other words, the test's **ability to correctly identify individuals who truly do not have the disease.**

■ **Positive predictive value (PPV):** The proportion of persons testing ⊕ who have the condition—in other words, **of all the people who test ⊕, the probability that they truly have the disease.**

■ **Negative predictive value (NPV):** The proportion of persons testing ⊖ who do not have the disease—in other words, **of all the people who test ⊖, the probability that they truly do not have the disease.**

■ **Likelihood ratio (LR):** Calculated as LR = sensitivity / (1 − specificity) or true positives/false positives; defined as the proportion of patients **with** a disease who have a certain test result over the proportion of patients **without** the disease who have the given test result ("WOWO"—with over without). For example, a high-probability V/Q scan has an LR of 14. This means that a ⊕ V/Q scan is 14 times more likely to be seen in patients **with** pulmonary embolism than in those **without** pulmonary embolism.

■ **Lead-time bias:** Lead time is the time by which a screening test advances the date of diagnosis from the usually symptomatic phase to an earlier presymptomatic phase. The time between diagnosis and death will always ↑ by the amount of lead time (see Figure 2.3). To avoid lead-time bias, the lead time must be subtracted from the overall survival time of screened patients. Example: A new screening test for pancreatic cancer is able to detect disease in a presymptomatic stage. Unfortunately, because the poor overall prognosis for the disease remains the same, screened patients know about their disease sooner and live with the disease longer but will still die of pancreatic cancer.

■ **Length-time bias:** Because cases vary in the length of their asymptomatic phase, screening will overdetect cases of slowly progressing disease (longer asymptomatic phases) and miss rapidly progressive cases.

■ **Relative risk (risk ratio) and cohort studies, randomized controlled trials:** The incidence of a disease in exposed individuals divided by the incidence of disease in unexposed individuals. For example, those with and without colon cancer in a specific population are evaluated for dietary fiber intake to determine if it is a risk factor for colon cancer. Results may be a statement such as "Individuals who do not have a high-fiber diet have been shown to have a relative risk of 1.7 of developing colon cancer."

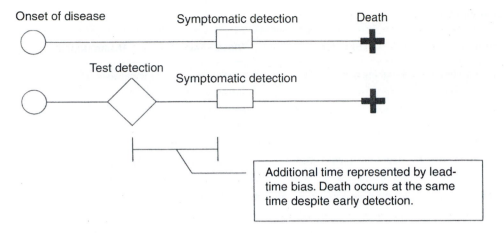

Additional time represented by lead-time bias. Death occurs at the same time despite early detection.

**FIGURE 2.3.    Lead-time bias.**

(Reproduced, with permission, from Le T et al. *First Aid for the Internal Medicine Boards*, 1st ed. New York: McGraw-Hill, 2006: 57.)

- **Odds ratio and case-control studies:** The odds that an individual with a specific condition has been exposed to a risk factor divided by the odds that a control has been exposed. For example, individuals with colon cancer would be compared with matched controls without colon cancer in terms of fiber intake. Results may be a statement such as "Individuals with colon cancer were *x* times less likely to have had a high-fiber diet than those without colon cancer."
- **Absolute risk:** Calculated by subtracting the incidence of a disease in nonexposed persons from the incidence of disease in exposed persons.
- **Number needed to treat (NNT):** the number of patients one needs to treat to prevent one additional bad outcome. NNT is the inverse of absolute risk.

|  | Disease | No Disease |
|---|---|---|
| *Exposed* | A | B |
| *Unexposed* | C | D |

*Relative risk:* $\dfrac{A/(A+B)}{C/(C+D)}$

*Odds ratio:* $\dfrac{AD}{CB}$

## Major Study Types

Table 2.22 outlines the types of studies conducted in epidemiologic and biostatistical analyses.

## Threats to Validity

- **Confounding factor:** A variable that is associated with both the predictor variable and the outcome variable but does not have a causal relationship with either.
- **Recall bias:** Self-reporting by subjects is often influenced by knowledge of the study hypothesis.
- **Misclassification bias:** Occurs when a person without disease is "misclassified" into the disease group or vice versa.
- **Random misclassification:** Occurs when subjects are randomly placed in the wrong group, biasing results to the null hypothesis.
- **Nonrandom misclassification:** Occurs when subjects are selectively placed in the wrong group, biasing results either toward or away from the null hypothesis.
- **Selection bias:** Occurs when subjects are selected into or drop out of a study in a way that falsely changes the degree of association.

**TABLE 2.22.** **Categories of Studies**

| Study Type | Definition | Example | Advantages | Disadvantages |
|---|---|---|---|---|
| Randomized controlled trial | Subjects are **assigned** to an exposure and disease outcomes are observed. | Assigning patients with hypertension to receive either a diuretic or an ACEI. | Assesses unforeseen confounders. | Expensive. |
| Cohort study | Exposed subjects are identified and then **followed** for disease outcomes. | Identifying obese children and then following them for the development of type 2 diabetes. | The most robust observational study type; can evaluate multiple exposures. | May take a long time to develop disease outcomes. |
| Case-control study | Cases and noncases of the disease are identified **before** defining the exposure. | Identifying children with certain birth defects and then looking for possible prenatal exposures. | Inexpensive; fast; ideal for rare diseases. | Prone to biases. |
| Cross-sectional study | Exposures and disease outcomes are **identified at the same time** within a **specific population** of subjects. | Checking for childhood diabetes while obtaining data on obesity in all children seen in specific community health clinics. | Survey data. | Cannot detect temporal relationship between exposure and outcome. |

COMMUNITY MEDICINE

### Hypothesis Testing

- **Null hypothesis:** The theory that the exposure or intervention being studied is not associated with the outcome of interest.
- **p-value:** A quantitative estimate of the probability that a study's outcome could occur by chance alone. A study with a $p < .05$ means that the probability of the results occurring by chance alone is < 1 in 20 and is thus "statistically significant."
- **Type I error ($\alpha$):** The probability of detecting a difference when none exists and thus rejecting the null hypothesis.
- **Type II error ($\beta$):** The probability of failing to detect a difference when one exists and thus failing to reject the null hypothesis.
- **Power:** The probability of avoiding a type II error in a study—in other words, the probability that a study will not accept the null hypothesis and conclude that there was no difference when there really was one.

### Evidence-Based Medicine

An approach to clinical medicine that provides practitioners with the tools for finding, understanding, and using the most up-to-date evidence from clinical research. The best evidence is then used to make a recommendation that is applicable to patient care. The criteria by which evidence is graded are listed in Table 2.23; grades of evidence are described in Table 2.24.

### Clinical Trials

Defined as studies in humans that answer specific health questions, including whether experimental treatments or new ways of using known treatments are

TABLE 2.23. **Levels of Evidence (Oxford Centre for Evidence-Based Medicine)**

| LEVEL | DESCRIPTION |
|---|---|
| 1a | Systematic review of randomized controlled trials. |
| 1b | Individual randomized controlled trial. |
| 1c | All-or-none. [a] |
| 2a | Systematic review of cohort studies. |
| 2b | Individual cohort study. |
| 2c | Outcomes research.[b] |
| 3a | Systematic review of case-control studies. |
| 3b | Individual case-control study. |
| 4 | Case series. |
| 5 | Expert opinion. |

[a] Met when all patients died before the treatment became available, but some now survive on it; or when some patients died before the treatment became available, but none now die on it.

[b] Looks at whether predicted outcomes (based on randomized controlled trials) are actually being observed in clinical practice.

safe and effective. Ideally conducted clinical trials provide one of the fastest and safest tools with which to change disease management and improve health in a population. Types of trials include the following:

- **Treatment trials:** Test experimental treatments, new combinations of drugs, or new approaches to surgery or radiation therapy.
- **Prevention trials:** Those that look for better ways to prevent disease in a disease-free population or to prevent recurrent disease.
- **Diagnostic trials:** Those that look for better tests or procedures for diagnosing a specific disease.
- **Screening trials:** Those that test the best way to detect disease and health conditions.

TABLE 2.24. **Grades of Recommendation (Oxford Centre for Evidence-Based Medicine)**

| GRADE | DESCRIPTION |
|---|---|
| A | Consistent level 1 studies. |
| B | Consistent level 2 or 3 studies or extrapolations from level 1 studies. |
| C | Level 4 studies or extrapolations from level 2 or 3 studies. |
| D | Level 5 evidence or troublingly inconsistent or inconclusive studies of any level. |

**TABLE 2.25. Phases of Clinical Trials**

| PHASE | DESCRIPTION |
| --- | --- |
| Phase I | The experimental drug or treatment is tested in a small group of people (20–80) for the first time to evaluate **safety**, to determine safe **dosage ranges**, and to identify **side effects.** |
| Phase II | The experimental drug or treatment is tested in a larger group of people (100–300) to evaluate **efficacy** and further evaluate **safety.** |
| Phase III | The experimental drug or treatment is given to large groups of people (1000–3000) to confirm **efficacy,** to monitor for **side effects,** and to **compare** it to treatments already in use. |
| Phase IV | Postmarketing studies to determine additional information, including risks, benefits, and optimal use. |

■ **Quality-of life-trials:** Those that look for ways to improve comfort and quality of life for individuals with chronic diseases or illnesses.

Table 2.25 describes the phases through which drugs and treatments must proceed in clinical trials.

## OTHER TOPICS

### Medicare and Medicaid

The United States has two major publicly funded health insurance plans: Medicare and Medicaid. These plans are compared in detail in Table 2.26.

### Disability Programs

The United States government publicly funds three major disability programs: Social Security Disability Insurance (SSDI), Supplemental Security Income (SSI), and Workers' Compensation.

■ **SSDI:** Like Medicare, SSDI is funded through payroll taxes. Once an individual meets both the definition of disabled (see the section on occupational medicine) and the eligibility criteria based on length of time employed and wages earned, he and his dependents qualify for benefits. After two years on SSDI, the individual becomes eligible for Medicare benefits.
■ **SSI:** Funded through general taxes rather than payroll or Social Security taxes. In order to be eligible, an individual must be > 65 years of age, blind, or disabled. In addition, only individuals with limited income and resources qualify.
■ **Workers' Compensation:** This program pays for medical expenses incurred from an injury or illnesses related to employment. A portion of the worker's wages is also paid out during the period of disability. Workers who are partially disabled can receive long-term payments of a portion of their salary.

### Health Insurance Portability and Accountability Act (HIPAA)

In April of 2003, the first-ever federal privacy standards to protect patients' medical records and other health information took effect. Developed by

TABLE 2.26. **Comparison of Medicare and Medicaid**

| | MEDICARE | MEDICAID |
|---|---|---|
| Funding source | Federal government. | Federal and state governments (the federal government reimburses each state 50–83% of costs). |
| Eligibility | Those > 65 years of age (who have worked and therefore have contributed to Medicare through payroll taxes). Those < 65 years of age who are receiving Social Security disability. Patients receiving dialysis. | Pregnant women plus women and their children < 6 years of age if their family income is < 133% of poverty level. Children 6–17 years of age if their family income is < 100% of poverty level. The elderly poor. The disabled poor. Other optional groups vary by state. |
| Benefits | **Part A:** Inpatient services, skilled nursing facility, home health and hospice. **Part B:** Outpatient care, x-rays, durable medical equipment, laboratory work. **Part C (Medicare Advantage):** Allows enrollment in Medicare-eligible HMOs or PPOs; includes additional services such as dentures, eyeglasses, and drugs. **Part D:** Prescription drug benefit. **Medigap:** Private supplemental insurance. | Physician services; laboratory, x-ray, inpatient hospital care, family planning, prenatal, and maternity services. Nursing home care services. **Optional benefits:** Rehabilitation services, dental care, physical therapy, eyeglasses, intermediate-care facilities, inpatient psychiatric care for individuals > 65 or < 21 years of age. |
| Physician reimbursement | **Medicare-Approved Amount (MAA):** Government-determined payment for any given service. The physician can bill only up to the MAA. Medicare pays 80% of the MAA and the patient pays 20%. | Providers receive reimbursement directly from Medicaid and must accept that amount as payment in full. |

COMMUNITY MEDICINE

HHS, these standards apply to health plans, doctors, hospitals, and other health care providers. In short, these new standards provide patients with access to their medical records and control over how their personal health information is used and disclosed. Patient protections include the following:

- **Access to medical records:** Patients should be able to see and obtain copies of their medical records and request that corrections be made.
- **Notice of privacy practices:** Covered health plans, doctors, and other health care providers must notify the patients of their rights and how their personal medical information may be used.
- Limits on use of personal medical information.
- **Prohibition of marketing:** Patient authorization must be obtained before specific information may be used for marketing purposes.
- Confidential communications.
- **Complaints:** Patients have the right to file formal complaints regarding the privacy practices of a health plan or provider.

COMMUNITY MEDICINE

# Cardiology

Umang Sharma, MD

## Physical Exam

Outlined below are key components of a cardiovascular exam along with guidelines for the interpretation of each.

### PULSES

- **Arterial pulses:**
    - Diminished in peripheral vascular disease and in low cardiac output.
    - Exaggerated in aortic regurgitation, PDA, hyperthyroidism, and any high-output state such as sepsis.
    - **Water-hammer pulses (Corrigan):** Rapid rise and fall of the radial pulse. Occurs in chronic aortic regurgitation.
    - **Pulsus paradoxus:** An SBP ↓ of > 10 mmHg during inspiration. Occurs with tamponade, constrictive pericarditis, asthma, and COPD.
- **Carotid pulses:**
    - **Delayed upstroke:** Aortic stenosis.
    - **Pulsus bisferiens:** Two discrete peaks; occurs with aortic stenosis and aortic regurgitation.
- **Normal jugular venous pulsations** (see Figure 3.1):
    - **a wave:** Atrial systole.
    - **c wave:** Closure of the tricuspid valve.
    - **x descent:** Atrial relaxation.
    - **v wave:** Ventricular systole with passive venous filling of the atrium.
    - **y descent:** Opening of the tricuspid valve with rapid emptying of the right atrium.

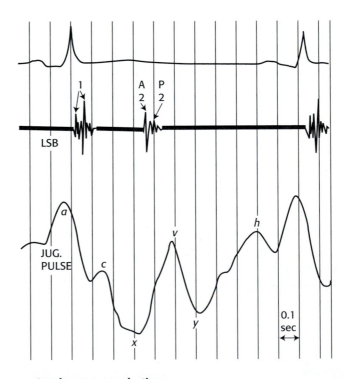

**FIGURE 3.1.** Jugular venous pulsations.

- **Abnormal venous pulsations:**
  - **Cannon a wave:** AV dissociation (the atrium contracts against a closed tricuspid).
  - **Large a wave:** Tricuspid stenosis, pulmonary hypertension, pulmonary stenosis.
  - **Absent a wave:** Atrial fibrillation (AF).
  - **Large cv wave:** Tricuspid regurgitation.
  - **Rapid y descent:** Constrictive pericarditis; restrictive cardiomyopathies.
  - **Blunted y descent:** Cardiac tamponade.

## HEART SOUNDS

- **S1:** Closure of the mitral and tricuspid valves. Diminished with LV systolic dysfunction, mitral regurgitation, and long PR interval.
- **S2:** Closure of the aortic and pulmonary valves. Normally, the aortic component (A2) precedes the pulmonic component (P2).
  - **Physiologic splitting: Widened time period between A2 and P2 with inspiration.** Normalizes when the breath is held.
  - **Paradoxical splitting:** ↑ **splitting with expiration.** Causes include aortic stenosis, left bundle branch block (LBBB), use of a pacemaker, and LV systolic dysfunction.
- **S3:** A low-pitched sound immediately after S2, best heard with the bell. Abnormal in older adults. Suggests ventricular enlargement and LV systolic dysfunction.
- **S4:** A low-pitched sound immediately preceding S1. Occurs with many conditions, most notably stiffening of the left ventricle.

## Cardiac Testing

### STRESS TESTING

Used to evaluate patients with suspected CAD as well as to predict future events in patients with known CAD. Modalities used, along with their relative advantages and disadvantages, are described in Table 3.1. Other parameters that are monitored during exercise include BP, heart rate, functional aerobic impairment, symptoms, and symptom duration. A higher risk of CAD is associated with a delayed decline in heart rate and BP, an impaired ↑ in heart rate, and poor exercise capacity.

### RESTING ECHOCARDIOGRAPHY

Used to identify **anatomic abnormalities;** to assess the size, thickness, and function (ejection fraction, or EF) of chambers; and to evaluate valvular function. Wall motion abnormalities are highly suggestive of CAD. Subtypes are as follows:

- **Doppler:** Characterizes blood flow and pressure gradients across valves. Useful for detecting stenotic or regurgitant blood flow.
- **Bubble study:** Agitated normal saline injected intravenously to diagnose shunts.
- **Transesophageal echocardiography (TEE):** An ultrasound probe in the esophagus that allows for better visualization of posterior cardiac structures.
  - **Indications:** Suspicion of left atrial thrombus, aortic dissection, or valvular vegetations.

TABLE 3.1.   **Stress-Testing Modalities**

| Mode | Method | Advantages | Disadvantages |
|---|---|---|---|
| Stress ECG | Exercise treadmill | **Widely available.** Downsloping ST segments have moderate sensitivity and specificity for CAD. | The patient must be able to exercise vigorously. Cannot be used if the resting ECG shows LBBB. **Less sensitive and specific than other modes.** |
| Stress echocardiography | Exercise, pharmacologic (dobutamine) | **Provides structural information.** Sensitivity and specificity are high; comparable to perfusion imaging. | Can be used only if resting echo is normal. Images may be nondiagnostic. Interpretation is somewhat subjective. |
| Perfusion imaging[a] | Exercise, pharmacologic (adenosine or dipyridamole) | Sensitivity and specificity are high. **Can assess tissue viability with restriction study** (reversible vs. fixed defects). Assesses the extent of lesions. | ↑ cost and time. Institution dependent. Involves radiation exposure. |

[a] A test in which radioactive isotopes show differential perfusion indicative of ischemia.

- The sensitivity of TEE in endocarditis is 95–100% (vs. 40–75% with transthoracic echocardiography [TTE]).

### CARDIAC CATHETERIZATION AND CORONARY ANGIOGRAPHY

- Indications:
  - Stable angina with persistent symptoms despite medical management.
  - Unstable angina and **acute coronary syndrome.**
  - Previous revascularization with recurrent symptoms to look for reocclusion.
  - Aortic disease with concurrent angina to determine if CABG might be performed at the time of valve replacement.
- Interventions:
  - Angioplasty.
  - Stents:
    - The standard of care for CAD.
    - Aspirin and clopidogrel must be taken for at least one month after the procedure for bare metal stents and for 3–6 months for drug-eluting stents.
    - Drug-eluting stents ↓ the incidence of restenosis.

### ELECTROCARDIOGRAPHY (ECG)

Definitions and guidelines pertinent to reading ECGs are as follows:

- **Dimensions:** With standard settings, one small box represents 1 mm, 40 msec (horizontally), or 0.1 mV (vertically).

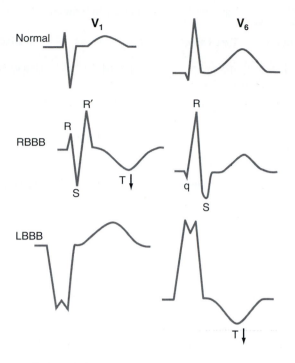

**FIGURE 3.2. Bundle branch blocks.**

(Reproduced, with permission, from Kasper DL et al. *Harrison's Principles of Internal Medicine*, 16th ed. New York: McGraw-Hill, 2005: 1315.)

- **Rate:** The normal rate is 60–100 bpm.
- **Axis:**
  - **Normal:** From −30 degrees to 90 degrees. QRS is net ⊕ in I and II.
  - **Left deviated:** Less than −30 degrees. QRS is net ⊕ in I and net ⊖ in II. Associated with left anterior fascicular block (LAFB), inferior MI, Wolff-Parkinson-White (WPW) syndrome with posteroseptal pathway, and COPD.
  - **Right deviated:** Greater than 90 degrees. QRS is net ⊖ in I and net ⊕ in II. Associated with RVH, lateral or anterolateral MI, WPW with left-lateral pathway, and left posterior fascicular block (LPFB).
- **Intervals:**
  - **PR:** Normal 0.12–0.20 sec.

**TABLE 3.2. ECG Changes in Intraventricular Blocks**

| TYPE | AXIS | ECG | QRS | MISCELLANEOUS |
|---|---|---|---|---|
| LAFB | Left | Upright QRS in I; ⊖ QRS in aVF. | Narrow | |
| LPFB | Right | ⊖ QRS in I; ⊕ QRS in aVF. | Narrow | |
| RBBB | Right or normal | rSR′ in $V_1$–$V_2$; **rabbit ears.** | Wide | Can still read ischemia. |
| LBBB | Left or normal | Tall, wide R in I, L; two peaks. | Wide | Difficult to read ischemia. |
| Bilateral block | | Third-degree heart block. | Wide and bizarre | |

**TABLE 3.3.**   **Electrocardiographic Patterns of Injury in Ischemia**

| ST-T CHANGES | TIME FRAME | CARDIAC MARKERS | DIAGNOSIS |
|---|---|---|---|
| ST depressions | Transient | Normal | Angina without infarction |
| ST elevations | Transient | Normal | Prinzmetal's angina |
| ST depressions, T-wave inversions, no Q waves | Prolonged | Elevated | **Non-ST-elevation MI** |
| ST elevations, T-wave inversions, Q waves eventually | Prolonged | Elevated | **ST-elevation MI** |

- **QRS:** Normal < 0.12 sec. The QRS interval is **widened in bundle branch blocks.**
    - **Right bundle branch block (RBBB):** rSR′ is seen in precordial leads, with R′ > r. A rabbit-ear appearance is seen in $V_1$–$V_2$ (see Figure 3.2).
    - **LBBB:** Broad R wave in I; broad S in $V_1$; RS in $V_6$.
    - The QRS interval is also widened with ventricular tachycardias, aberrantly conducted supraventricular tachycardias, WPW syndromes, and pacemakers.
- **QT:** Normal < 50% of RR.
- **QTc:** Abnormal > 0.44 sec. The interval is **prolonged** in congenital conditions, metabolic abnormalities, drug use (antiarrhythmics, antibiotics, psychotropic drugs), MI, and mitral valve prolapse.
- **ECG findings:**
    - **Hypertrophy:** ↑ LV mass associated with an ↑ incidence of poor outcomes, including systolic dysfunction, heart failure, CVA, and death.
        - **LVH:** Many different criteria. Characterized by ↑ QRS voltage and duration. One set of criteria: R in aVL is > 11 mm (1.1 mV) OR the sum of S in $V_1$ and R in $V_5$ or $V_6$ is > 35 mm (3.5 mV).
        - **RVH:** Right axis deviation. One criterion is R:S > 1 in $V_1$. Another criterion is $RV_1$ + $SV_6$ > 11 mm.

**TABLE 3.4.**   **Localization of Transmural Infarction**

| LEADS | LOCATION | ARTERY | MISCELLANEOUS |
|---|---|---|---|
| II, III, aVF | Inferior | Right coronary artery or left circumflex | Perform right-sided ECG. |
| $V_1$–$V_3$ | Anteroseptal | Left anterior descending (LAD) | See Figure 3-3. |
| $V_4$–$V_6$ | Apical | LAD | |
| $V_4$–$V_6$R | RV | | Place right-sided leads. |
| $V_7$–$V_9$, esophageal | Posterior | | |

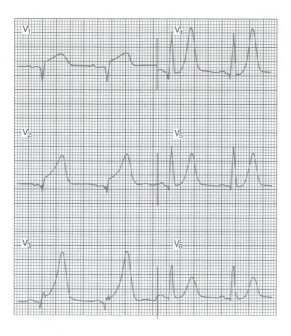

**FIGURE 3.3.** Anteroseptal transmural MI.

ST elevations, Q waves in $V_{1-3}$ with anteroseptal MI. (Reproduced, with permission, from Kasper DL et al. *Harrison's Principles of Internal Medicine*, 16th ed. New York: McGraw-Hill, 2005: 1316.)

- **Intraventricular blocks** (see Table 3.2): Occur with CAD, cardiomyopathies, and acute ischemia. Pacemakers should be considered in some situations.
- **Ischemia: ST depression or T-wave inversion.**
- **Infarction:** ST elevation is > 1 mm (0.1 mV) in two contiguous precordial leads or two adjacent limb leads (see Table 3.3).
  - **Hyperacute T waves:** High-amplitude T waves seen in early infarction.
- **Localization:** Transmural infarction can be localized by ST elevations (see Table 3.4).
- **J-point elevation:** Elevation at the point where the QRS meets the ST segment. Can be indicative of MI or can be a normal variant. This is determined by the appearance of the ST segment.
- **U wave:** Deflection immediately after the T wave in the same direction. Can be associated with hypokalemia or a normal finding.

## HYPERTENSION

**High blood pressure is defined as a systolic BP ≥ 140 or a diastolic BP > 90 on more than two occasions** (see Table 3.5). Hypertension is associated with MI, heart failure, stroke, and kidney disease and has a higher prevalence among ethnic minorities, in women, and with ↑ age. As a screening measure, **BP should be checked at least every two years starting at age 18.**

### SYMPTOMS/EXAM

- Perform a **funduscopic exam for retinopathy** to look for arteriolar narrowing or sclerosis, AV nicking, hemorrhages, and hard exudates.
- Palpate pulses and auscultate for renal artery bruit.

TABLE 3.5.  Classification of Blood Pressure

| BP CLASS | SYSTOLIC BP (mmHg) | DIASTOLIC BP (mmHg) | INITIAL DRUG THERAPY |
|---|---|---|---|
| Normal | < 120 | and < 80 | |
| Prehypertension | 120–139 | or 80–89 | No drug therapy, but ↑ risk of hypertension. |
| Stage 1 hypertension | 140–159 | or 90–99 | Thiazides for most; may consider ACEIs, angiotensin II (AT II) receptor blockers, β-blockers, calcium channel blockers, or a combination. |
| Stage 2 hypertension | ≥ 160 | or ≥ 100 | Two-drug combination for most (usually thiazide first; then ACEIs, AT II receptor blockers, β-blockers, or calcium channel blockers). |

Adapted, with permission, from The Seventh Report of the Joint National Committee on Prevention, Detection, Evaluation, and Treatment of High Blood Pressure. *JAMA* 2003: 290: 1314. Copyright © 2003 American Medical Association. All rights reserved.

### DIAGNOSIS

- **Elevated BP on three separate occasions.**
- Correct cuff size is important for an accurate reading. The cuff bladder should be at least 80% of arm circumference.
- Assess lifestyle and other cardiovascular risk factors (e.g., diabetes).
- Rule out 2° causes of hypertension (see below) and assess for end-organ damage.
- Lab studies should include hematocrit, UA, electrolytes, glucose, creatinine, calcium, and ECG.
- **Twenty-four-hour ambulatory BP monitoring** may be helpful to diagnose white-coat hypertension or to evaluate labile BPs or resistant hypertension.

### TREATMENT

- The goal is < 140/90, or < 130/80 in patients with **diabetes, renal disease, or cardiovascular disease.**
- Patients with prehypertension and stages 1 and 2 hypertension should be counseled about lifestyle modifications, including adherence to a low-sodium/DASH diet (rich in fruits, vegetables, and low-fat dairy), weight reduction, aerobic activity, and ↓ alcohol consumption.
- Assess factors that may modify treatment choices (see Table 3.6).

## 2° Hypertension

Should be considered in severe, treatment-refractory hypertension as well as for those in whom onset occurred before puberty. Some experts recommend screening those with onset before age 30 or after age 50 as well. The etiologies of 2° hypertension include intrinsic renal disease, renovascular hypertension, obesity, alcohol abuse, medications, hyperaldosteronism, Cushing's disease, sleep apnea, coarctation, polycythemia vera, hyperparathyroidism, hypothyroidism, and hyperthyroidism.

*The goal of hypertension treatment is a BP of < 140/90, or < 130/80 in patients with diabetes, renal disease, or cardiovascular disease.*

CARDIOLOGY

TABLE 3.6. **Antihypertensive Medications**

| | THIAZIDES | β-BLOCKERS | ACEIs | AT II RECEPTOR BLOCKERS | CALCIUM CHANNEL BLOCKERS |
|---|---|---|---|---|---|
| Drug examples | HCTZ, chlorthalidone. | Atenolol, metoprolol. | Captopril, enalapril, ramipril, lisinopril. | Irbesartan, losartan, valsartan. | Nondihydropyridines: diltiazem, verapamil; dihydropyridines: amlodipine, felodipine, nifedipine. |
| Side effects | Hypokalemia, ED, ↑ insulin resistance, hyperuricemia, ↑ TG. | Bronchospasm, depression, fatigue, impotence, ↑ insulin resistance. | Cough (10%), hyperkalemia, renal failure. | Less cough, hyperkalemia, renal failure. | Conduction defects (nondihydropyridines); lower extremity edema (dihydropyridines). |
| Indications for use as first-line drug | **Most patients** as mono- or combination therapy (stage 1 or 2 hypertension), including **isolated systolic hypertension in elderly, osteoporosis.** | **MI,** high CAD risk. | **DM with micro-albuminuria; MI** with systolic dysfunction or anterior infarct; mild chronic renal failure with non-DM-related **proteinuria.** | | |
| Other indications | Recurrent stroke prevention. | CHF. | CHF. | CHF, DM, chronic renal failure, ACEI-related cough. | Atrial arrhythmias (nondihydropyridines), isolated systolic hypertension in elderly (dihydropyridines). |
| Contra-indications | | Bronchospasm; high-degree (type II second- or third-degree) heart block. | **Pregnancy.** | **Pregnancy.** | High-degree heart block. |

Reproduced, with permission, from Le T et al. *First Aid for the Internal Medicine Boards,* 1st ed. New York: McGraw-Hill, 2006: 49.

**CARDIOLOGY**

### SYMPTOMS/EXAM

- Determine BP patterns and medication use. Screen for symptoms that typically accompany the conditions outlined above, including muscle weakness, thinned skin, and flank pain.
- Target the physical exam to the conditions listed above. Include weight, body habitus, auscultation of renal arteries, upper and lower extremity pulses, and BP.

### DIAGNOSIS

- Labs to obtain include electrolytes, creatinine, TSH, and UA.

- Additional labs and tests should be directed toward the conditions above on the basis of clinical suspicion.
- Obtain a renal ultrasound to rule out renal artery stenosis.

---

A 58-year-old woman with low back pain and urinary incontinence comes to your office for a yearly physical exam. She is a smoker and has no family history of premature heart disease. Her BP is 150/95 and has been elevated in the past. Her lipid panel includes an HDL-C of 38, an LDL-C of 170, and a triglyceride level of 150. The woman has no CAD equivalents but has three risk factors: tobacco use, low HDL-C, and hypertension. You calculate her 10-year Framingham risk at 24% and determine that her LDL-C goal is 130. What do you do? Counsel her about exercise and advise her to meet with a nutritionist. Six months later, her lipid profile is not significantly different. How do you proceed? Initiate a statin.

---

## HYPERLIPIDEMIA

Lipid abnormalities underlie a significant proportion of heart disease. The prevalence of hyperlipidemia is estimated to be about 20% in the adult population in the United States. Coronary risk increases proportionally with total cholesterol. Accordingly, the control of hyperlipidemia through meticulous screening is critical to decreasing the incidence of CAD. Mortality benefits have been noted both in patients without known CAD as well as in patients with established CAD.

### Screening Guidelines

Screening guidelines for hyperlipidemia are as follows:

- The United States Preventive Services Task Force (USPSTF) recommends screening men > 35 years of age and women > 45 years of age.
- Those > 20 years of age with CAD risk factors may also be screened.
- Screening is generally **not** recommended for patients > 75 years of age. Repeat screening of those > 65 is not thought to be necessary, as lipids usually remain stable in this age group.
- Measurement of fasting lipids is optimal, but measurement of nonfasting total cholesterol and HDL-C constitutes an acceptable alternative.
- The screening interval is generally five years but should be shorter for patients with borderline values.

### Risk Factors

Risk factors influencing cholesterol goals are as follows (see also Table 3.7):

- **CAD equivalents:** DM, symptomatic carotid disease, abdominal aortic aneurysm, peripheral arterial disease, and renal insufficiency (Cr > 1.5).
- **CAD risk factors:** Tobacco use, hypertension (> 140/90) or use of antihypertensives, HDL-C < 40, family history of premature CAD (male relative < 55 years of age, female relative < 65 years of age), and patient age (men > 45, women > 55). **HDL-C > 60 is a ⊖ risk factor.**

TABLE 3.7. **Risk Categories That Modify LDL Cholesterol Goals**

| Risk Category | LDL Goal | Level at Which to Initiate Therapeutic Lifestyle Changes | Level at Which to Consider Drug Therapy |
|---|---|---|---|
| CAD or CAD risk equivalents (10-year risk > 20%) | < 100 mg/dL | ≥ 100 mg/dL | ≥ 130 mg/dL (100–129 mg/dL: drug optional)[a] |
| 2+ risk factors (10-year risk ≥ 20%) | < 130 mg/dL | ≥ 130 mg/dL | 10-year risk 10–20%: ≥ 130 mg/dL<br>10-year risk < 10%: ≥ 160 mg/dL |
| 0–1 risk factor | < 160 mg/dL | ≥ 160 mg/dL | ≥ 190 mg/dL (160–189 mg/dL: LDL-lowering drug optional). |

[a] Some authorities recommend use of LDL-lowering drugs in this category if an LDL cholesterol < 100 mg/dL cannot be achieved by therapeutic lifestyle changes.

Adapted from the Third Report of the National Cholesterol Education Program, Panel on Detection, Evaluation, and Treatment of High Blood Cholesterol in Adults (Adult Treatment Panel III) Executive Summary. Washington, DC: National Institutes of Health, NIH Publication No. 01-3670, May 2001, www.nhlbi.nih.gov/guidelines/cholesterol/index.htm.

## Management

Table 3.8 outlines the drugs that are commonly used in conjunction with lifestyle modifications in the treatment of hyperlipidemia.

TABLE 3.8. **Classes of Drugs Used in the Treatment of Hyperlipidemia**

| Drug | LDL | HDL | TG | Side Effects | Best For | Monitor |
|---|---|---|---|---|---|---|
| Nicotinic acid (niacin) | ↓ | ↑ | ↓ | Flushing, gout, GI distress, elevated LFTs, pruritus, ↑ blood glucose. | Elevated LDL and TG; low HDL ("jack of all trades"). | LFTs |
| Statins (atorvastatin, simvastatin, pravastatin) | ↓ | ↑ | ↓ | GI distress, elevated LFTs, myositis. | Elevated LDL only; elevated LDL and TG. | LFTs, CK |
| Bile acid–binding resins (cholestyramine) | ↓ | ↑ | ↑ | GI distress, ↓ absorption of fat-soluble vitamins and other drugs, ↑ TG. | Elevated LDL only. | |
| Fibrates (gemfibrozil) | ↓ | ↑ | ↓ | GI distress, myositis (especially in combination with statins). | Elevated LDL and TG. | LFTs |

Reproduced, with permission, from Le T et al. *First Aid for the Internal Medicine Boards,* 1st ed. New York: McGraw-Hill, 2006: 23.

## Hypertriglyceridemia

Epidemiologic data suggest that hypertriglyceridemia is independently associated with CAD. Suggested management according to the Adult Treatment Panel III (ATP III) includes the following:

- **Triglycerides 150–199 (borderline):** Nonpharmacologic interventions (weight loss, increased activity); pharmacologic treatment to achieve the LDL goal.
- **Triglycerides 200–499 (high):** Consider pharmacologic therapy directed toward lowering triglycerides in high-risk patients or those with known CAD.
- **Triglycerides ≥ 500 (very high):** Pharmacologic treatment to lower triglycerides (fibrates, nicotinic acid) and to prevent pancreatitis.

> A 65-year-old man comes to see you at your office after having been hospitalized with a new diagnosis of heart failure following presentation with dyspnea and edema. His history is notable for hypertension and hyperlipidemia. An echocardiogram during his hospitalization showed an EF of 25%, LVH, and no wall motion abnormalities. His clinical presentation is most consistent with class II heart failure. He was discharged from the hospital on furosemide, an ACEI, a statin, and HCTZ, and his symptoms have improved since that time. What do you do? Add a β-blocker. The patient returns after a few months with ongoing dyspnea with exertion. His BP is well controlled. How do you proceed? You add digoxin in an attempt to improve his symptoms.

## CONGESTIVE HEART FAILURE (CHF)

CHF is defined as a condition in which the ability of the heart to maintain circulation is compromised. It is estimated that five million individuals in the United States suffer from heart failure, with the prevalence significantly higher in older individuals. The prevalence of diastolic heart failure is being increasingly recognized. CHF is most often chronic but may also be acute or subacute. Risk factors generally include ischemic heart disease, valvular disease, tobacco use, hypertension, obesity, and diabetes. CHF may be classified by symptom severity (see Table 3.9) or by stage of evolution:

- **Stage A:** High risk for heart failure due to comorbidities (hypertension, CAD, DM) without symptoms or structural disease.
- **Stage B:** Structural heart disease associated with the development of heart failure (LVH; enlarged, dilated ventricle; valvular disease; previous MI) without symptoms.

**TABLE 3.9. NYHA Classification of CHF by Symptom Severity**

| CLASS I | CLASS II | CLASS III | CLASS IV |
|---|---|---|---|
| Symptoms at levels identical to those of normal individuals. | Symptoms with moderate exertion. | Symptoms with mild exertion only. | Symptoms at rest. |

- **Stage C:** Structural heart disease with previous or current symptoms. This is the **largest group.**
- **Stage D:** Refractory heart failure despite medical therapy, requiring specialized interventions.

Systolic and diastolic function can be found in some patients with CHF, whose symptoms of heart failure may be explained by obesity, lung disease, or sleep apnea. Most patients with CHF have combined systolic and diastolic LV dysfunction.

- **Systolic dysfunction:** Defined as ↓ EF evidenced on echocardiogram in the setting of signs or symptoms of heart failure. Etiologies include CAD (present in 70% of patients with systolic dysfunction), dilated cardiomyopathy, hypertension, AF, and valvular disease.
- **Diastolic dysfunction: Abnormal LV filling** and normal systolic function. Etiologies are as follows:
    - Impaired myocardial relaxation due to ischemia, hypertrophy, cardiomyopathies, and aging.
    - ↑ myocardial stiffness due to fibrosis, scarring, hypertrophy, and infiltration.
    - Endocardial fibrosis.
    - Constrictive pericarditis, tamponade.

Most patients with CHF have combined systolic and diastolic dysfunction.

### SYMPTOMS

- **Subacute or acute:** Presents with dyspnea at rest or with exertion, orthopnea.
- **Chronic:** Fatigue, edema, and anorexia may be more prominent.
- Diastolic dysfunction is often asymptomatic.

### EXAM

- **Systolic:** Elevated JVP, lung crackles, leg edema, S3.
- **Diastolic:** The same as systolic except for the presence of an **S4.** An S3 should **not** be present in isolated diastolic dysfunction.

### DIFFERENTIAL

COPD, pneumonia, cirrhosis, nephrotic syndrome.

### DIAGNOSIS

- Labs to obtain include CBC, electrolytes and creatinine (for initiation of diuretics), TSH, fasting glucose, LFTs, CXR, and ECG (to rule out ischemia, arrhythmias).
- **Brain natriuretic peptide (BNP):** Released with myocyte stretch. Highly accurate in diagnosing heart failure and in distinguishing between cardiac and pulmonary causes of dyspnea.
- **Echocardiography:**
    - **Systolic dysfunction:** Demonstrates an **EF < 40%** with an enlarged, dilated left ventricle.
    - **Diastolic dysfunction:** EF is normal, but hypertrophy, RV enlargement, pericarditis, and infiltrative disease may be seen.

### TREATMENT

- **Systolic dysfunction:**
    - **Stepwise medication approach:**
        - **Diuretics:** Used acutely to relieve symptoms of pulmonary edema. Confers **no mortality benefit.**

- **ACEIs:** Confer a mortality benefit in **all classes of CHF.** If not tolerated, an angiotensin receptor blocker may be substituted.
- **β-blockers:** Mortality benefits in **classes II, III, and IV** have been shown with carvedilol, metoprolol, and bisoprolol. Avoid starting in decompensated heart failure.
- **Digoxin: May provide symptomatic relief, but confers no mortality benefit.** Helpful in achieving rate control in patients with AF.
- **Hydralazine with nitrates:** Has not been shown to have significant benefit but may have some benefit in African-Americans.
- **Spironolactone:** Confers a mortality benefit in **class III–IV heart failure.**
- **Recombinant BNP:** Acts primarily as a vasodilator. Consider in severe heart failure requiring ICU care.
- **Advanced treatments:**
  - **Mechanical therapy:** Consider a balloon pump for severe heart failure due to ischemia. Consider ventricular assist devices for very poor cardiac output as a bridge to transplantation.
  - **Cardiac resynchronization:** Pacers used with severe systolic heart failure and wide QRS. Improve ventricular synchrony and cardiac output.
  - **Cardiac transplantation:** Reserved for end-stage heart disease that either limits survival to < 2 years or severely limits daily quality of life.
- **Diastolic dysfunction:**
  - The goals are to improve ventricular relaxation, ↓ heart rate, maintain sinus rhythm, and treat hypertension to achieve LVH regression.
  - The mainstays are β-blockers and nondihydropyridine calcium channel blockers (verapamil, diltiazem). ACEIs and diuretics are also used.

*ACEIs, β-blockers, hydralazine, and spironolactone provide mortality benefit; diuretics and digoxin are used for symptomatic relief.*

An 81-year-old woman with a history of CAD, diabetes, hypertension, and hyperlipidemia comes to your office complaining of progressive fatigue, chest pain, dyspnea, and lightheadedness over the previous several years. She has had several episodes of syncope over the past few weeks without accompanying palpitations but with chest pain and dyspnea. Her BP is 170/90. She has a late-peaking systolic murmur at the left upper sternal border radiating to the carotids. PMI is displaced and sustained. Her ECG is normal, and her echocardiogram shows severe aortic stenosis with a valve area of 0.75 cm². How do you proceed? You continue to work with her toward improved BP and lipid control but also refer her to a cardiologist and a cardiothoracic surgeon for consideration of a valve replacement. You also advise her to receive endocarditis prophylaxis during surgical procedures.

## VALVULAR HEART DISEASE

### Aortic Stenosis

On a worldwide basis, aortic stenosis is most commonly caused by rheumatic heart disease, when it always occurs with mitral valve disease. In the United States, the most common causes are senile (age-related) calcific aortic stenosis and congenital bicuspid aortic valve. Of patients requiring an aortic valve replacement (AVR), one-third to half may have a bicuspid valve; this is much higher in younger patients requiring an AVR.

### Symptoms

- Although the classic triad is **angina, syncope,** and **heart failure,** the most common symptoms are ↓ exercise tolerance with ↑ dyspnea with exertion.
- Symptoms do not usually develop until the area is < 1 cm² (the normal valve area is 3–4 cm²), jet velocity is > 4 m/sec, and the pressure gradient is > 40 mmHg.

### Exam

- Presents with a late-peaking crescendo-decrescendo systolic murmur that is best heard at the heart base with radiation to the carotids.
- Carotid upstroke may be diminished and delayed (parvus et tardus).
- PMI may be sustained due to LVH. S2 is ↓ in intensity.
- A systolic ejection click can occur in patients with bicuspid aortic valve.

### Diagnosis

- **Echocardiography:** Calculations are used to derive pressure gradient and valve area.
- **Coronary angiography:** Used to exclude significant CAD in at-risk patients preoperatively. Left heart catheterization may also be used to confirm the severity of aortic stenosis with discrepant clinical and echocardiographic findings.

### Treatment

- There is no effective pharmacologic therapy for aortic stenosis.
- **AVR is the only therapy for symptomatic aortic stenosis and should be pursued as soon as symptoms develop.** Valve replacement is associated with ↓ symptoms and improved mortality. Many older patients tolerate the surgery well, and age should not be a disqualification. Patients unlikely to outlive a bioprosthesis may be better served by a bioprosthetic valve, which would obviate the need for lifelong coagulation (which is needed with a mechanical valve).
- Valvuloplasty may be effective in congenital aortic stenosis. It is less effective with degenerative aortic stenosis but may be used palliatively or as a bridge to surgery.
- **All patients should receive endocarditis prophylaxis with antibiotics.**

*The only therapy for symptomatic aortic stenosis is aortic valve replacement, which should be pursued as soon as symptoms develop.*

### Complications

- Sudden death is uncommon in patients with severe asymptomatic aortic stenosis.
- In symptomatic patients, survival is 2–5 years without treatment.

## Aortic Regurgitation

Also called aortic insufficiency. Symptoms in chronic aortic regurgitation usually evolve over a long period of time. Asymptomatic individuals with chronic aortic regurgitation generally have a good prognosis. Prognosis is determined by symptoms and LV size and function. This condition may also occur acutely. Etiologies are as follows:

- **Valve leaflet destruction or malfunction:** From infective endocarditis, bicuspid aortic valve, or rheumatic valve disease.
- **Marfan's syndrome and aortic dissection:** Dilatation of the aortic root such that leaflets do not coapt.

### SYMPTOMS

Symptomatic disease presents as follows:

- **Acute:** Rapid-onset cardiogenic shock.
- **Chronic:** Characterized by a long asymptomatic period in which the disease slowly evolves followed by progressive exertional dyspnea and heart failure.

### EXAM

- Soft S1; **decrescendo blowing diastolic murmur at the base;** wide pulse pressure and water-hammer pulses.
- Acute aortic regurgitation may present with only ↓ S1 intensity and a soft, blowing diastolic murmur.
- In severe aortic regurgitation, an apical diastolic rumble mimicking mitral stenosis (Austin Flint murmur) may be heard.

### DIAGNOSIS

- **TTE:** Essential for determining LV size and function as well as for characterizing aortic valve structure. Can be used to determine the severity of regurgitation. TEE may be necessary to rule out endocarditis in acute regurgitation.
- **Coronary angiography:** Aortography can estimate the degree of regurgitation more definitively.

### TREATMENT

*Afterload reduction is essential in asymptomatic patients with aortic stenosis.*

- **Asymptomatic: Afterload reduction is essential.** ACEIs and other vasodilators can reduce LV overload and slow progression to heart failure.
- **Aortic valve replacement:** Should be considered in **symptomatic patients** or in **those with worsening LV dilatation and systolic function.**
- **Acute aortic regurgitation:** Surgery is the definitive treatment. Vasodilators can be used as a bridge to surgery.
- **Endocarditis prophylaxis: Should be considered in all patients** based on the invasiveness of the procedure.

### COMPLICATIONS

Irreversible LV systolic dysfunction can occur with delay of valve replacement.

## Mitral Stenosis

Mitral stenosis is **almost always due to rheumatic heart disease.** Rarely, it may be caused by infective endocarditis, congenital lesions, or calcification of the mitral annulus.

### SYMPTOMS

- The mean interval to symptoms is 16 years.
- **Dyspnea is the most common complaint.**

- Hemoptysis and a subtle ↓ in exercise tolerance may also be seen and eventually → pulmonary hypertension and right heart failure.
- May also present with thromboembolism.

### EXAM

- Presents with diminished arterial pulses, a loud S1, and an opening snap of stenotic leaflets followed by an apical diastolic rumble.
- Signs of right heart failure (elevated JVP, edema, hepatic congestion) may be apparent in later stages.

### DIAGNOSIS

- **TTE:** Used to evaluate valve morphology, area, pressure gradient, and etiology. These characteristics indicate the appropriateness of valvotomy.
- **TEE:** Used to exclude left atrial thrombus in patients scheduled for valvotomy.
- **Catheterization:** Primarily used prior to valvotomy for more precise measurements of valve gradient and hemodynamic status.

### TREATMENT

- Exercise is encouraged but should be symptom-limited.
- **Acute rheumatic fever:** Treat with short-term anti-inflammatories and long-term prophylactic antibiotics to prevent recurrent carditis.
- **Endocarditis prophylaxis:** Antibiotics should be given during procedures causing bacteremia. Further episodes of rheumatic fever predispose to the progression of stenosis and should be prevented through use of antibiotics during suspected group A strep infections.
- **Percutaneous mitral balloon valvotomy:** Shown to be effective, but contraindicated in patients with concomitant mitral regurgitation, severe annular calcification, and atrial thrombus.
- **Mitral valve replacement:** Indicated for patients who have at least moderate disease and heart failure symptoms and are not candidates for valvotomy.

### COMPLICATIONS

Left atrial enlargement; AF → left atrial thrombus formation and risk of embolism.

## Mitral Valve Prolapse

Defined as abnormally thickened mitral valve leaflets that project across the mitral annulus into the left atrium during systole. Etiologies are as follows:

- 1°: Idiopathic, familial, Marfan's syndrome, connective tissue disease.
- 2°: CAD, rheumatic heart disease, "flail leaflet," reduced LV dimension.

### SYMPTOMS

Usually asymptomatic and found incidentally. Atypical chest pain, palpitations, or TIAs may be seen.

### EXAM

Exam reveals a nonejection midsystolic click and a murmur at the apex. The late systolic murmur of mitral regurgitation may be seen later in the disease.

### DIAGNOSIS

- **Echocardiography:**
  - Can be used to evaluate valve structure and function, the extent of regurgitation and prolapse, and LV function.
  - If the condition is symptomatic or associated with mitral regurgitation, echocardiography should be repeated every year; otherwise, it may be repeated every 2–3 years.
- Echocardiography should not be done in the absence of auscultatory features of mitral valve prolapse.

### TREATMENT

- **Aspirin:** If there is a history of TIA or lone AF.
- **Warfarin:** Appropriate for patients with chronic AF, a previous thromboembolic event, CVA, mitral regurgitation, or heart failure (target INR 2–3).
- No treatment is necessary if none of these complications are present.

## Mitral Regurgitation

Results from structural abnormalities in the mitral annulus, valve leaflets, chordae, and papillary muscles. Acutely and chronically, this may be caused by infective endocarditis, myocardial ischemia or infarction, trauma to the valve, mitral valve prolapse, myxomatous disease, or acute rheumatic fever.

### SYMPTOMS

- **Acute:** Can present with cardiogenic shock with pulmonary edema, hypotension, and poor tissue perfusion. Right heart failure may also be seen.
- **Chronic:** ↓ exercise tolerance, fatigue, dyspnea. May be asymptomatic.

### EXAM

- Soft S1; blowing, soft systolic murmur best heard at the left sternal border and base; S3.
- Acute mitral regurgitation will → symptoms of left heart failure.

### DIAGNOSIS

- Early detection of mitral regurgitation is essential because **treatment should be initiated before symptoms occur.**
- **Echocardiography:**
  - **TTE:** Used to detect and grade the severity of mitral regurgitation. Also used for surveillance once the diagnosis is established, with frequency depending on the severity of disease.
  - **TEE:** Used prior to surgical repair or replacement.
  - **Catheterization:** Used to exclude CAD prior to surgery; can evaluate the extent of mitral regurgitation.

### TREATMENT

- **Acute mitral regurgitation:**
  - **Emergent situations:** Surgical intervention is almost always required.
  - Prior to surgery, stabilization should aim to ↑ forward flow with vasodilators such as IV nitroprusside or an intra-aortic balloon pump.
- **Chronic mitral regurgitation:**
  - The fundamental approach to asymptomatic patients is as follows:
    - **Control any concurrent dysrhythmia;** often this is AF.

- Monitor LV function with an annual echocardiogram.
- Give **endocarditis prophylaxis.**
- **Medical management:** The role of medical management is controversial. ACEIs are often used for afterload reduction.
- **Surgery: Patients with symptoms should be considered for surgery.** Other indications are LV dysfunction, AF, and pulmonary hypertension. Surgery should be performed early in patients with progressive disease. Ideally, this is **when symptoms develop but EF is still preserved.**

## Prosthetic Valves

Bioprosthetic valves are preferable to mechanical valves for older patients with a life expectancy of < 10 years and for those who are unable to take long-term anticoagulants.

### ANTICOAGULATION

- **Bioprosthetic valves:** Give three months of warfarin after placement; then consider aspirin in high-risk patients.
- **Mechanical valves:** All patients should be anticoagulated in light of the higher risk of thrombus formation. The target INR depends on the type and location of the valve.

### COMPLICATIONS

- **Thrombosis is the most common problem.** Risk is ↑ with the mitral valve, AF, previous emboli, left atrial thrombus, and LV dysfunction.
  - The highest risk occurs with the mitral valve and inadequate anticoagulation.
  - Can present with heart failure, poor perfusion, and hemodynamic instability.
  - Diagnosed by echocardiogram.
  - Larger thrombi (> 5 mm) require fibrinolysis or valve replacement. Heparin may be used with smaller thrombi.
- **Endocarditis:**
  - With invasive procedures, patients should receive antibiotic prophylaxis.
  - **Early:** Occurs during the first 60 days after placement. Often fulminant with high mortality.
  - **Late:** A higher risk is associated with multiple valves or bioprosthetic valves.
- Other problems include hemolysis, perivalvular leak, valve failure, and dysrhythmias.

*Valves should be chosen on the basis of life expectancy and suitability for long-term anticoagulation.*

> A 65-year-old man with a history of MI and a three-vessel CABG ten years ago comes to your office to establish care. He is a nonsmoker who is active and feels well, and he is currently on aspirin, statins, and HCTZ. On exam, you note that he is obese, his BP is 160/80, and he has an S4. You check his lipids, and his LDL-C is 125. What further interventions are necessary? You

*Bioprosthetic valve < 10 yrs life expectancy.* (handwritten margin note)

add an ACEI and a β-blocker for BP control and for 2° prevention of CAD, and ↑ his statin dose to improve his LDL-C toward his goal of 70. You also encourage him to continue to exercise and abstain from tobacco, and you discuss nutritional strategies to improve his cardiac health.

## CORONARY ARTERY DISEASE (CAD)

CAD is the leading cause of mortality in women and men in the United States, with its highest prevalence seen in individuals > 65 years of age. Traditional risk factors have been identified and vary slightly between organizations. More innovative markers of CAD are being investigated and integrated into clinical practice. **Risk factors for CAD according to the Seventh Joint National Committee on the Prevention, Detection, Evaluation, and Treatment of Hypertension (JNC-7)** include the following:

- **Age:** There is an ↑ risk in women > 65 years of age, with premature menopause, and in men > 55 years of age.
- **Family history:** There is an ↑ risk with a family history of CAD in a first-degree female relative < 65 years of age or a male relative < 55 years of age.
- **Cigarette use.**
- **Hypertension** with a BP > 140/90 or use of an antihypertensive.
- **HDL-C < 40 on several occasions (an HDL-C > 60 is a ⊖ risk factor).**
- **Elevated LDL.**
- **Obesity** (BMI > 30) and **physical inactivity.**
- **Diabetes:** Patients with diabetes are at a level of risk equivalent to those with established CAD.

**More novel risk factors** include elevated CRP, elevated homocysteine, coronary artery calcification on cardiac CT, and LVH.

*Diabetes is a CAD equivalent.*

### Prevention

#### 1° PREVENTION

- **Risk factor reduction** includes the following:
    - **Smoking cessation:** Yields an immediate ↓ in risk that reverts to a normal level after several years.
    - **Diet:** Should include fiber, whole grains, fruits, vegetables, and omega-3 fatty acids. Saturated fats should be minimized.
    - **Hypertension:** The goal BP is < 140/90 or 130/85, depending on risk factors.
    - **Hyperlipidemia:** Target LDL-C cholesterol levels should be based on the patient's ten-year risk for heart disease.
    - **Diabetes:** Intensive control of diabetes ↓ coronary events. The American Diabetes Association recommends an $HbA_{1c}$ goal of 6.5.
    - **Other risk factors** that should be addressed include obesity and physical inactivity. Low to moderate alcohol intake (1–2 drinks a day) has been postulated to slightly ↓ the risk of CAD.
- **Pharmacologic therapy:** Consider **aspirin** therapy in patients with risk factors.

- **Risk factor reduction measures** are the same as those outlined above.
- **Pharmacologic therapy:**
  - **Aspirin:** ↓ mortality with daily use (75–325 mg). If contraindicated, clopidogrel may be used.
  - **Clopidogrel:** ↓ mortality in patients with recent acute coronary syndrome or in those with a stent.
  - **Statins:** ↓ mortality and the risk of acute cardiac events. **Current guidelines** set the goal for patients with a history of CAD as an **LDL < 100.** An LDL goal of < 70 is recommended by some groups.
  - **β-blockers:** ↓ mortality. All patients with CAD should be on a β-blocker unless an absolute contraindication exists. In patients with reactive airway disease, cardioselective β-blockers may be tried.
  - **ACEIs:** ↓ mortality and risk of MI and stroke. If not tolerated, an angiotensin receptor blocker may be used.

*β-blockers, ACEIs, statins, and aspirin ↓ CAD-related mortality.*

## Stable Angina

Thought to involve fixed artery stenosis limiting $O_2$ delivery in times of stress.

### SYMPTOMS/EXAM

Classically presents with chronic, reproducible, exercise-induced chest discomfort that is relieved by rest and nitroglycerin. Exam findings are nonspecific.

### DIAGNOSIS

Nuclear imaging and echocardiography are noninvasive, but **catheterization is the gold standard.**

### TREATMENT

- Essentially the same as 2° prevention of CAD. Antianginal medical therapy includes nitrates, β-blockers, and calcium channel blockers.
- **Indications for revascularization** are as follows:
  - Chronic stable angina with three-vessel disease.
  - Two-vessel disease with prominent LAD involvement.
  - One- or two-vessel disease with high-risk features such as LV dysfunction.
  - Significant left main artery disease (> 50% stenosis).
  - Refractory symptoms or chronic angina.

An 85-year-old woman is admitted to the ER after presenting with palpitations, dyspnea, and lightheadedness intermittently over the last month. Her medical problems include hypertension, diabetes, CAD with a previous stent, and hypothyroidism. Her BP is 145/80 and her pulse 120. An ECG shows AF. Review of her records shows a previous ECG with this finding three years ago with normal ECGs in the interim. In the ER, you determine that there is no urgent indication for cardioversion, and you lower her heart rate with β-blockers and start anticoagulation with heparin. During admission, she has no evidence of ischemia by biochemical markers. An echocardiogram shows LVH but no other structural abnormalities or thrombus, and it also reveals systolic heart failure with an EF of 30%. How do you proceed? Once you have determined that her heart failure is not decompensated, you control her heart rate with β-blockers and, given her relatively high risk for embolism, begin warfarin anticoagulation with a goal INR of 2–3.

### Atrial Fibrillation (AF)

The **most common dysrhythmia in the general population** (0.5–1.0%); prevalence ↑ with age. AF is most commonly found in the setting of structural heart disease with ventricular failure. The most frequent etiologies are **hypertension and CAD** with acute heart failure or MI. Also common are valvular heart disease and heart failure. Less common etiologies include pulmonary disease (COPD, pulmonary embolism), ischemia, rheumatic heart disease, hyperthyroidism, congenital heart disease, sepsis, alcoholism, WPW syndrome, and cardiac surgery. Categories are as follows:

- **Paroxysmal:** Episodes last < 7 days and usually < 24 hours.
- **Persistent:** Lasts > 7 days; responds to cardioversion but may recur afterward.
- **Permanent:** Present > 1 year; failed cardioversion.
- **Lone:** One episode of AF in the absence of structural heart disease.

#### SYMPTOMS/EXAM

Often asymptomatic. Palpitations, fatigue, dyspnea, dizziness, diaphoresis, heart failure, or ↓ exercise tolerance may be seen.

#### DIAGNOSIS

- **ECG:** The most common cause of irregularly irregular is AF. The absence of P waves is noted (see Figure 3.4).
- **Echocardiogram:** Used to predict stroke risk with structural abnormalities such as left atrial enlargement, valvular disease, LVH, and ↓ EF. TEE is more effective for visualizing left atrial thrombi.

#### TREATMENT

- Cardioversion:
  - Indicated if the patient is unstable or if the duration of AF is < 48 hours.
  - Perform TEE-guided cardioversion if the duration is > 48 hours or unknown. Therapeutic anticoagulation should be established first.
  - Anticoagulate for at least four weeks postcardioversion.
  - If AF recurs after cardioversion, treat with rate control and anticoagulation.
    - **Paroxysmal AF:** Patients should be anticoagulated if AF is present a substantial portion of the time.
    - **Lone AF:** Aspirin 325 mg daily will suffice.
- Anticoagulation:
  - To determine the need for anticoagulation, estimate stroke risk with the **CHADS2 score:**
    - CHF

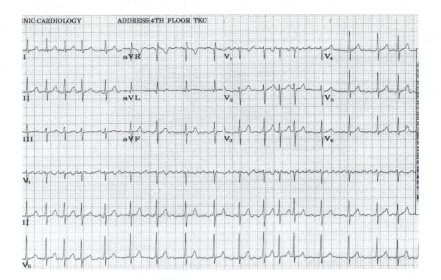

**FIGURE 3.4. Atrial fibrillation.**

Note irregular QRS complexes and lack of P waves. (Reproduced, with permission, from Fuster V et al. *Hurst's the Heart*, 11th ed. New York: McGraw-Hill, 2004: 826.)

- ▪ Hypertension
- ▪ Age > 75 years
- ▪ Diabetes
- ▪ Stroke/TIA (**two** points each)
- ▪ **Score 0:** Aspirin 325 mg daily.
- ▪ **Score 1–2:** Indeterminate; based on the individual patient.
- ▪ **Score 3+:** Warfarin; target INR of 2.5 (range 2–3) in most patients. Target INR is 3.0 (2.5–3.5) with valvular disease, previous thromboembolism, or mechanical valve.
- ▪ **Rate control:** β-blockers or nondihydropyridine calcium channel blockers (diltiazem, verapamil). With a ↓ EF, use digoxin or amiodarone.
- ▪ **Rhythm control:** Flecainide, propafenone, amiodarone, sotalol, ibutilide.

*Rhythm control and rate control with anticoagulation have similar mortality benefits.*

### Atrial Flutter

Uncommon in a structurally normal heart. Can occur with LV dysfunction and rheumatic heart disease. Other etiologies are similar to those associated with AF. The circuit can follow either a typical (see Figure 3.5) or an atypical route. **The typical route is isthmus-dependent and counterclockwise,** but other variations exist.

#### SYMPTOMS/EXAM

- ▪ Symptoms include palpitations, fatigue, and dyspnea. Chest pain and syncope are less commonly seen.
- ▪ The H&P should be targeted toward identifying coexisting heart disease.

#### DIAGNOSIS

Diagnosed by ECG; findings are as follows:

- ▪ **Typical isthmus-dependent flutter (counterclockwise):** Atrial rate of 250–350 (see Figure 3.6). Can present with or without typical flutter waves.

65

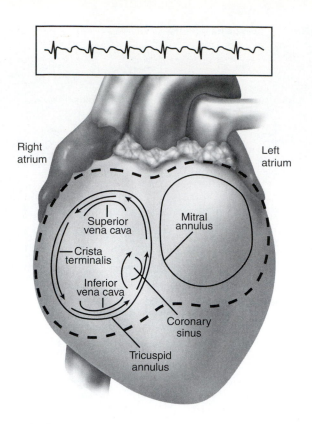

**FIGURE 3.5.**    **Atrial flutter.**

Typical isthmus-dependent flutter with counterclockwise conduction with the isthmus between the tricuspid annulus and IVC. (Reproduced, with permission, from Morady F: Drug therapy: Radio-frequency ablation and treatment for cardiac arrhythmias. *N Engl J Med* 1999; 340: 534–544. Copyright © 1999 Massachusetts Medical Society. All rights reserved.)

- **Clockwise flutter:** Presents with a sawtooth pattern in leads II, III, and aVF. Flutter rate should be around 300. Consider the diagnosis in patients with a ventricular rate of 150, as flutter usually presents with 2:1 conduction.

### TREATMENT

- **Lone atrial flutter** (without structural heart disease): Unclear; consider anticoagulation.
- **Unstable patients:** Cardioversion.
- **Stable patients:**
  - Watchful waiting is an option, since spontaneous reversion to normal sinus rhythm occurs.
  - The anticoagulation approach is similar to that of AF.
  - **Antiarrhythmics:** Ibutilide, flecainide, propafenone.
  - **Overdrive pacing:** A temporary pacemaker may be placed to terminate tachycardia.
  - **Cardioversion:** Management of anticoagulation around cardioversion similar to that of AF.
  - Rate control with calcium channel blockers, β-blockers, or digoxin.
- **Long-term control:**
  - Radiofrequency ablation is highly effective and is the preferred treatment.

CARDIOLOGY

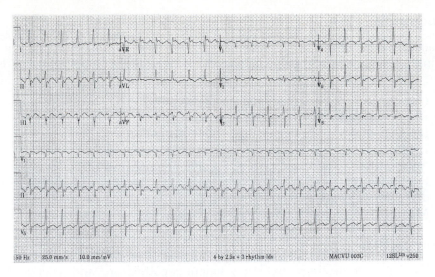

**FIGURE 3.6. Isthmus-dependent atrial flutter.**

Note typical flutter waves. (Reproduced, with permission, from Fuster V et al. *Hurst's the Heart*, 11th ed. New York: McGraw-Hill, 2004: 843.)

- Alternatives include antiarrhythmics or pacemakers, which require long-term anticoagulation.

### Supraventricular Tachycardia (SVT)

If wide QRS complexes are present with SVT, ventricular tachycardia should be differentiated from SVT with aberrant conduction (discussed below). Types of SVT with narrow QRS complexes are as follows:

- **Reentrant SVT.** The point of reentry can be:
  - **AV node:** Most common, accounting for 60% of cases of reentrant SVT.
  - The bypass tract or other site.
- Atrial tachycardia.
- Multifocal atrial tachycardia.
- AF/flutter.
- Junctional tachycardia.

#### SYMPTOMS/EXAM

May be asymptomatic or may present with palpitations, lightheadedness, presyncope, syncope, or chest pain. Exam should focus on auscultation for evidence of valvular disease or cardiomyopathy.

#### DIAGNOSIS

ECG shows regular rhythm. QRS is generally narrow, although it may be wide if aberrant conduction is present. Wide-complex tachycardia may also represent ventricular tachycardia. Varying morphologies of P waves may be seen in **multifocal atrial tachycardia.**

#### TREATMENT

Valsalva; carotid sinus massage. Adenosine may be given next if these maneuvers are unsuccessful. Cardioversion is indicated if the patient is unstable.

## Bradycardia

Bradycardia is defined as a heart rate < 55–60. However, some healthy individuals, particularly athletes, may have heart rates as low as the high 40s. Etiologies include the following:

- **Common:** Idiopathic degeneration, ischemic.
- **Rheumatologic:** SLE, RA, scleroderma.
- **Infectious.**
- **Infiltrative:** Sarcoidosis, amyloidosis, hemochromatosis.
- **Autonomic:** ↑ vagal tone (carotid sinus hypersensitivity).
- **Iatrogenic:** Heart transplant, β-blockers, calcium channel blockers, clonidine, digoxin, antiarrhythmics.
- **Metabolic:** Electrolyte abnormalities, hypothyroidism, hypothermia.

### SYMPTOMS/EXAM

- Presents with dizziness, weakness, fatigue, heart failure, and syncope. May be asymptomatic.
- Exam reveals ↓ pulse. Look for signs associated with the underlying cause of the bradycardia.

### DIAGNOSIS

- **ECG:** Heart rate < 60 bpm. Look for dropped beats or AV dissociation.
- Telemetry, event monitors, tilt-table testing, and electrophysiology studies can be helpful.

*Consider a permanent pacemaker for documented symptomatic bradycardia, third-degree heart block, > 3-second pause, or a pulse < 40.*

### TREATMENT

- For unstable patients, follow the ACLS protocol.
- **Medications:** Atropine, glucagon (for β-blocker overdose), calcium (for calcium channel blocker overdose).
- **Transcutaneous or transvenous pacing.**
- **Permanent pacemaker:** Consider for those with documented symptomatic bradycardia, third-degree heart block, > 3-second pause, or a pulse < 40.

## Ventricular Tachycardia (VT) and Ventricular Fibrillation (VF)

Causes include ischemia, infarction, cardiomyopathy, electrolyte abnormalities, and drug toxicities. Types of VT are as follows:

- **Monomorphic:** Uniform QRS pattern. Usually associated with myocardial scar.
- **Polymorphic:** Characterized by a bizarre and changing QRS. Often precipitated by ischemia. **Torsades de pointes** (in which the QRS complex oscillates around a baseline) is often associated with medications and electrolyte abnormalities that prolong the QT interval.

### SYMPTOMS/EXAM

Chest pain, dyspnea, syncope. **Often presents with sudden cardiac death.**

### DIAGNOSIS

*VT must be distinguished from SVT with aberrant conduction.*

- **Must be distinguished from SVT with aberrant conduction.**
- **Unstable patients:** Assume VT (see Figure 3.7).

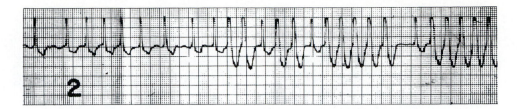

**FIGURE 3.7.** **Ventricular tachycardia.**

(Reproduced, with permission, from Tintinalli JE et al. *Emergency Medicine*, 6th ed. New York: McGraw-Hill, 2004: 189.)

- **Stable patients:** VT is evidenced by AV dissociation, complexes not typical of LBBB or RBBB, variation in QRS complexes, and fusion beats of simultaneously occurring ventricular and supraventricular beats.

### TREATMENT

- **Unstable patients:** Cardioversion.
- **Stable VT:** First-line treatment is IV amiodarone.
- **Polymorphic VT** (including torsades): Can be treated with magnesium infusion and overdrive pacing.
- A defibrillator should be placed if the cause is not transient or reversible.

## Wolff-Parkinson-White (WPW) Syndrome

Results when an accessory pathway between the atria and ventricles persists after fetal development. May be found incidentally, but even asymptomatic patients are at risk for tachyarrhythmias. Prevalence is around 0.25% in the general population and 0.5% in those with first-degree relatives with WPW.

### DIAGNOSIS

- **Antegrade accessory pathway conduction:** Impulses conduct from the atria to the accessory pathway to the ventricles. Characterized by ventricular preexcitation with **short PR and delta waves** (slurred upstroke of QRS; best seen in lead $V_4$). Delta waves with net-$\ominus$ deflection can resemble Q waves (see Figure 3.8).
- **Retrograde accessory pathway conduction:** Impulses conduct from the ventricles to the accessory pathway to the atria. Resting ECG is often normal; no delta wave is seen.

### TREATMENT

Electrophysiologic study; ablation of the bypass tracts.

### COMPLICATIONS

Primarily AF. Avoid AV nodal blockers in patients with a delta wave, as this can cause 1:1 conduction of AF $\rightarrow$ VF and cardiac arrest.

CARDIOLOGY

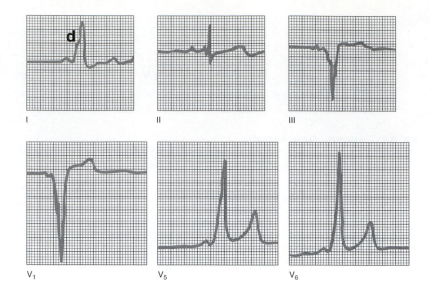

**FIGURE 3.8. Wolff-Parkinson-White syndrome.**

Note the delta wave (d), short PR, and wide QRS. (Reproduced, with permission, from Kasper DL et al. *Harrison's Principles of Internal Medicine*, 16th ed. New York: McGraw-Hill, 2005: 1350.)

## CARDIOMYOPATHIES

Diseases of the heart muscle that have a variety of causes. The clinical presentation is variable and related to the underlying etiology. Types of cardiomyopathy include hypertrophic, restrictive, dilated, ischemic, valvular, and hypertensive. Less common is arrhythmogenic right ventricle.

- **Hypertrophic:** A genetic disorder with autosomal-dominant inheritance but variable penetrance. First-degree family members of affected individuals should be screened with an ECG and an echocardiogram.
- **Restrictive:** Impaired diastolic filling with preserved systolic functioning. Can be idiopathic, infiltrative, or familial.
- **Dilated:** Causes may be ischemic, valvular, genetic, or idiopathic.

### SYMPTOMS/EXAM

- Usually presents with symptoms of heart failure, chest pain, and syncope.
  - **Hypertrophic:** Often asymptomatic and found on routine family screening. Can present with symptoms of heart failure or sudden cardiac death.
  - **Restrictive:** Presents with symptoms of heart failure.
  - **Dilated:** Can present with arrhythmias, heart failure, or sudden death.
- The type of cardiomyopathy is further distinguished through **echocardiography,** which shows features specifically associated with hypertrophic, restrictive, or dilated cardiomyopathies (see below).

### DIAGNOSIS

- **Hypertrophic:** Characterized by LV thickening on echo. May be asymmetric around the septum → a systolic pressure gradient.
- **Restrictive:** Ventricles do not appear dilated or hypertrophied on echocardiogram.
- **Dilated:** Dilation of ventricles affects systolic functioning, which can eventually → hypertrophy.

- **Hypertrophic:** Treatment with β-blockers or verapamil is directed toward improving diastolic filling in patients who are symptomatic.
- **Restrictive:** Treatment aims to ↓ elevated filling pressures and treat symptoms of heart failure. Diuretics may relieve symptoms; calcium channel blockers may improve diastolic relaxation. Consider amiodarone or a defibrillator for high-risk patients with previous dysrhythmias, LVH, syncope, or specific genetic mutations.
- **Dilated:** Treatment is influenced by the development of heart failure.

## PERICARDIAL DISEASE

Pericardial disease often results from systemic disease. Many patients with pericardial disease present with both pericarditis and an effusion. The extent to which either of these causes symptoms varies.

## Acute Pericarditis

Etiologies of acute pericarditis are as follows:

- **Idiopathic:** The most common cause.
- **Infectious:** Usually viral (including HIV), but may also be caused by TB.
- **Metabolic disorders:** Most commonly uremia.
- **Other: Previous radiation, postinfarction** (Dressler's syndrome), **inflammatory, neoplastic** (often lung or breast cancer), **degenerative, traumatic.**

*SYMPTOMS/EXAM*

- Presents with pleuritic chest pain that worsens when the patient is supine and improves when the patient leans forward. Angina-like symptoms may also be seen.
- Exam reveals pericardial friction rub.
- Diffuse ST elevations are found on ECG. Elevated cardiac markers may also be seen. Echo is often normal unless there is an associated effusion.
- **High-risk features** include high fever, gradual onset, evidence of tamponade, acute trauma, and failure to respond to medical therapy.

*DIAGNOSIS*

Diagnosed clinically based on the findings above.

*TREATMENT*

NSAIDs. Colchicine and steroids can also be used.

## Pericardial Effusion

**Often accompanies acute pericarditis.** Causes are similar to those of acute pericarditis, with the most common being idiopathic, infectious, and malignancy.

*SYMPTOMS/EXAM*

Similar to acute pericarditis; persistent fever may also be seen.

### DIAGNOSIS

- **Echocardiography:** Used to confirm the presence of effusion and determine the hemodynamic impact. Hemodynamic compromise is demonstrated by impaired ventricular filling.
- **Pericardiocentesis:** Most useful for cytology and cultures. Must weigh the risks and benefits.

### TREATMENT

Treatment is specific to the cause.

*Pericardial effusion may accompany acute pericarditis.*

## Tamponade

**Caused by an effusion under pressure** → impaired ventricular filling. May be acute or subacute. Etiologies are as follows:

- **Acute:** Usually traumatic (penetrating trauma, aortic rupture, procedures such as pacer placement).
- **Subacute:** Neoplasm, pericarditis.

### SYMPTOMS/EXAM

- **Acute:** Presents with chest pain and dyspnea. Classic exam findings include elevated JVP, muted heart sounds, and hypotension. Potentially life-threatening.
- **Subacute:** Presents with chest pain. On exam, hypotension, tachycardia, and a narrowed pulse pressure may be seen.

### DIAGNOSIS

- **ECG:** Low voltage; the QRS axis varies beat to beat ("electrical alternans") due to cardiac positional changes.
- **Echocardiography:** Shows right atrial collapse during diastole and equalization of RV and LV pressures.

*Cardiac tamponade is an effusion under pressure → impaired ventricular filling. Classic exam findings include elevated JVP, distant heart sounds, and hypotension.*

### TREATMENT

Drainage via either pericardiocentesis or an open procedure is required. Pericardiectomy may also be necessary.

## PERIPHERAL VASCULAR DISEASE

Almost always due to peripheral atherosclerosis. Prevalence ↑ with age and is estimated to be about 14% in those > 70 years of age. Prevalence is significantly higher in those with risk factors, which are the same as those in coronary atherosclerosis (hypertension, hyperlipidemia, diabetes, tobacco use).

### SYMPTOMS/EXAM

- Often asymptomatic. **The classic symptom is claudication,** or pain in a muscle group that is reproduced with exercise and relieved by rest. Severity varies.
- The calf is the most frequently affected area, but the buttocks, thighs, and feet may also be affected.
- Can → poor wound healing.

- Rest pain is a late finding that often occurs at night.
- Exam findings include diminished pulses, peripheral bruits, and cool, shiny extremities with ↓ hair.

### DIAGNOSIS

- The **ankle-brachial index** (ABI) is < 0.9. Highest systolic ankle pressure/systolic brachial pressure by Doppler. Performed at rest and after exercise. Calcified vessels can cause an abnormally high ABI (> 1.3).
- **Segmental limb pressures** are used to evaluate the extent of disease.
- Ultrasound with duplex scanning is another common modality. MRI and CT are less commonly used.

### TREATMENT

- **Risk factor reduction:** Tobacco cessation; treatment of hyperlipidemia; glucose and BP control. Rehabilitation and structured exercise programs are also effective.
- **Pharmacologic:**
  - **Aspirin:** Has only modest benefit. Ticlopidine and clopidogrel can also be used.
  - **Cilostazol:** Inhibits platelet aggregation and improves vasodilation.
  - **Pentoxifylline:** ↑ RBC deformity and ↓ serum viscosity.
  - **Ginkgo biloba:** Has been shown to be somewhat effective, although the mechanism is unclear.
- **Interventional procedures:**
  - Indicated for symptoms that limit activity as well as with rest pain or tissue loss.
  - Include percutaneous revascularization with percutaneous angioplasty or stents, generally for more focal lesions.
  - The risks of surgical revascularization must be weighed against its potential benefits.

*Peripheral vascular disease is characterized by an ankle-brachial index < 0.9.*

CARDIOLOGY

CARDIOLOGY

# CHAPTER 4

# Endocrinology

Amanda Price, MD

Diana Antoniucci, MD

Karen Earle, MD

An 81-year-old man comes to your clinic because he is concerned that he has diabetes. The patient recently had his blood sugar checked at a health fair and was told that it was around 200 mg/dL. He denies any symptoms of diabetes. You order a fasting blood glucose, which turns out to be 150 mg/dL. Further labs reveal an HbA$_{1c}$ of 8.2% and a creatinine level of 1.3. What further testing should you do before starting the patient on metformin? A second fasting glucose should be done to confirm the diagnosis, and creatinine clearance should be determined, since serum creatinine can be misleading in elderly individuals with low muscle mass.

DM is defined as impairment in carbohydrate metabolism → hyperglycemia. There are two main types of DM, distinguished as follows:

- **Type 1:** Destruction of pancreatic islet cells → absolute insulin deficiency. Type 1 DM is typically autoimmune but can be idiopathic.
- **Type 2:** Due to insulin resistance and variable degrees of relative insulin deficiency. Type 2 DM accounts for roughly 90% of DM cases in the United States.

Although type 1 DM was formerly known as juvenile diabetes, more children are currently being diagnosed with type 2 than with type 1 DM.

### SYMPTOMS/EXAM

- **May be asymptomatic (common in type 2 DM).**
- Presents with the **3 P's: polyuria, polydipsia,** and **polyphagia.**
- Weight loss, blurry vision, acanthosis nigricans (a sign of insulin resistance), dehydration, and neuropathy may also be seen.
- **Diabetic ketoacidosis (DKA)** and **hyperosmolar coma** are acute complications (see below).

### DIAGNOSIS

The American Diabetes Association (ADA) has established the following diagnostic criteria for the diagnosis of DM:

- Symptoms of diabetes plus a **random** glucose concentration of **≥ 200 mg/dL.**
- A **fasting** plasma glucose of **≥ 126 mg/dL** on **two** separate occasions.
- A serum glucose of ≥ 200 mg/dL two hours after a 75-g glucose load during an oral glucose tolerance test.

### TREATMENT

- **Routine diabetic care:** Table 4.1 outlines measures for the routine management of diabetes.
- **Glycemic control:**
  - **Nonpharmacologic:** Diet, exercise, weight loss, and stress management can all help control glucose levels and ↓ the need for other medications in type 2 DM.
  - **Pharmacologic:**
    - Table 4.2 outlines medications that are appropriate for the treatment of type 2 DM. First-line therapy consists of metformin and/or

*More children are being diagnosed with type 2 DM than type 1.*

*Metformin is the first-line agent in obese patients with a creatinine < 1.5 in men and < 1.4 in women because it promotes weight loss.*

*Hold metformin in surgery patients until renal function has normalized after surgery because of the ↑ risk of lactic acidosis.*

ENDOCRINOLOGY

TABLE 4.1. Routine Management of Diabetes

| CATEGORY | TREATMENT |
|---|---|
| Diet and exercise | Advocate that patients adhere to a low-calorie, low-fat diet with regular exercise. |
| Glucose control | Measurement of $HbA_{1c}$ monitors glucose levels over the past three months. Check at least biannually in stable patients. The goal $HbA_{1c}$ is < 6.5–7.0 (< 6.5 by American Endocrine Society and < 7 by ADA criteria). |
| BP control | The goal BP is < 130/80. |
| Lipid control | The goal LDL is < 100 mg/dL, and < 70 mg/dL in high-risk patients. |
| Aspirin therapy | Daily aspirin therapy is recommended for adults with DM and macrovascular disease or in those ≥ 40 years of age who have one or more additional risk factors. |
| Smoking cessation | Advise all patients to stop smoking. |
| Nephropathy screening | Annual microalbuminuria screening with spot urine protein/creatinine or albumin/creatinine ratio. Type 2 patients should be screened immediately and type 1 patients five years after diagnosis. Treat with ACEIs or ARBs. Tolerate up to a 15–20% ↑ in serum creatinine with the initiation of ACEIs/ARBs. Tight BP and glucose control also delays development. |
| Retinopathy screening | Schedule an annual ophthalmology exam immediately for patients with type 2 DM and five years after diagnosis for those with type 1. Maintain tight glucose and BP control for prevention. Laser therapy can slow diabetic retinopathy and ↓ the risk of vision loss. |
| Foot care | Recommend an annual complete foot exam with monofilament testing, visual inspection on each visit, and prophylactic foot care education for all diabetic patients. |
| Immunizations | Pneumococcal vaccine in adults; annual influenza vaccine. |
| Tuberculosis testing | High-risk populations should be tested in light of ↑ reactivation rates. |

sulfonylurea followed by combinations of the other classes of medications.

- **Insulin** is appropriate for type 1 and type 2 DM (see Table 4.3). Options include a "basal-bolus" regimen (basal coverage with intermediate- to long-acting insulin plus a short-acting bolus insulin before meals), insulin in combination with other agents, or continuous insulin infusion via an SQ catheter.

- **Experimental treatment:** Immunosuppression in type 1 DM; pancreatic/islet cell transplantation.

A 10-year-old boy presents to the ER with lethargy, nausea, and vomiting. Exam reveals that he is tachypneic and has a fruity odor to his breath. His urine shows 4+ glucose and ketones, and his bedside blood glucose level is > 500 mg/dL. Even before labs are obtained, what therapy can be initiated in this patient? The boy should be placed on NS and IV insulin. Labs are obtained

TABLE 4.2. **Medications Used in Type 2 DM**

| CLASS | DRUGS | ADVERSE EFFECTS | COMMENTS |
|---|---|---|---|
| Sulfonylureas | Glipizide, glyburide, glimepiride, tolazamide, tolbutamide | Hypoglycemia. | Often first-line treatment; can cause weight gain. |
| Biguanides | Metformin | GI side effects (nausea, diarrhea), lactic acidosis ($\uparrow$ risk in renal disease [Cr > 1.5]), CHF, respiratory disease, liver disease in the elderly. | Often first-line agents. Promote weight loss; hypoglycemia is rare. |
| Meglitinides | Repaglinide, nateglinide | Hypoglycemia. | Short acting; use for postprandial hyperglycemia. |
| Thiazolidinediones | Rosiglitazone, pioglitazone | Rare hypoglycemia; fluid retention, edema, liver disease. | Monitor LFTs; do not use in patients with CHF. |
| $\alpha$-glucosidase inhibitors | Miglitol, acarbose | Gas, bloating, diarrhea. | Start low and gradually $\uparrow$ dosage. |
| Amylin replacement | Pramlintide | Nausea. | Given SQ with meals in patients on basal-bolus insulin. |
| GLP-1 agents | Exenatide | Nausea, vomiting, diarrhea. | SQ: promotes weight loss. |
| DPP-4 inhibitors | Sitagliptin, vildagliptin | GI upset. | Oral agents, weight neutral. |

and show a K$^+$ level of 4.0, a blood glucose level of 550 mg/dL, a serum HCO$_3$ level of 15 mEq/L, and a pH of 7.29. What can now be added to his fluids? K$^+$ supplementation. Should bicarbonate be given? No; it is indicated only with severe acidosis (pH < 7.2 or HCO$_3$ < 15 mEq/L). Several hours later, the boy's labs show a blood glucose level of 210 mg/dL, a K$^+$ level of 4.2, and a serum HCO$_3$ level of 15 mEq/L. Should you switch to an SQ insulin regimen? Not yet; instead, add 5% dextrose to the boy's fluids and continue IV insulin until acidosis resolves.

### Acute Complications

Acute complications of DM include the following:

- **DKA:** Much more common in type 1 than in type 2 DM. Can be the initial manifestation of type 1 or may occur later in either type 1 or type 2. Usually precipitated by a stressor (e.g., infection, surgery, infarction, medical noncompliance).

TABLE 4.3. Insulin Types

| | INSULIN TYPE | ONSET | PEAK ACTION | DURATION |
|---|---|---|---|---|
| Ultra-short-acting | Lispro, insulin aspart, glulisine | 5–15 minutes | 1.0–1.5 hours | 3–4 hours |
| Short-acting | Regular | 15–30 minutes | 1–3 hours | 5–7 hours |
| Intermediate-acting | Lente, NPH | 2–4 hours | 8–10 hours | 18–24 hours |
| Long-acting | Ultralente, glargine, detemir | 4–5 hours | 8–14 hours (glargine has virtually no peak) | 25–36 hours |

- **Sx/Exam:** Abdominal pain, vomiting, Kussmaul respirations (rapid deep breaths), a fruity breath odor (from acetone), and lethargy. Can progress to coma.
- **Dx:** Lab findings include hyperglycemia, hyperosmolality, and a high anion-gap metabolic acidosis (serum $HCO_3$ < 15 mEq/L, pH < 7.3, serum ketones > 5 mmol/L).
- **Tx:**
  - **Insulin drip:** To close the anion gap and ↓ plasma glucose. Can switch to SQ insulin when the anion gap has closed.
  - **Fluids:** Glucose-induced osmotic diuresis → a fluid loss of approximately 3–6 L. Start with NS and then switch to ½ NS. Add D5 when glucose is < 250.
  - **Electrolytes: Potassium** is usually falsely elevated initially due to acidosis and will fall with treatment. Start potassium replacement with plasma levels in the 4.0–4.5 range. **Bicarbonate therapy is not usually indicated** unless there is severe acidosis (pH < 7.2 or $HCO_3$ < 10 mEq/L).

*In DKA or hyperosmolar coma, continue insulin drip until the anion gap closes even after glucose has normalized (add dextrose to IV to prevent hypoglycemia).*

- **Hyperosmolar coma (nonketotic hyperglycemia):** Defined as significant hyperglycemia, hyperosmolality, and dehydration without ketosis. Usually precipitated by a stressor (e.g., infection, infarction, intoxication, medical noncompliance).
  - **Sx/Exam:** Presents with **polyuria, polydipsia, polyphagia,** weakness, lethargy, confusion, and coma.
  - **Dx:** Serum glucose is often > 800 mg/dL. Serum $HCO_3$ is normal to slightly low; pH is > 7.3.
  - **Tx: Treat the underlying stressor;** give fluids, insulin drip, and electrolyte replacement. Similar to treatment for DKA. Often need 6–10 L of fluids in these patients. Watch for pulmonary edema and volume overload in elderly patients.
  - **Cx:** Mortality may be as high as 50%, likely due to the population affected.
- **Hypoglycemia:** A common occurrence in diabetics on insulin therapy. Can also occur with use of oral hypoglycemics.
  - **Sx/Exam:**
    - **Neuroglycopenic symptoms:** Include confusion, stupor, coma, and focal neurologic findings. Result from low glucose delivery to the brain.
    - **Autonomic symptoms:** Tachycardia, palpitations, sweating, tremulousness, nausea, hunger.

- **Tx:**
  - **Conscious patients:** Give glucose tablets, juice, and other high-glucose-containing drinks or snacks.
  - **Unconscious patients:** Administer glucagon 1 mg IM or 50% glucose IV.

## Chronic Complications

Most of the **chronic complications** of DM begin approximately five years after disease onset. Screening should begin five years after diagnosis for type 1 patients but should begin immediately for those with type 2 DM, since complications can be present even before formal diagnosis is made. Studies have shown that **tight glycemic control** can ↓ the incidence of chronic complications, especially microvascular disease. Complications and their associated treatment modalities are as follows:

- **Microvascular:**
  - **Retinopathy:** Schedule an annual eye exam by an ophthalmologist. Retinal neovascularization can be treated with photocoagulation therapy.
  - **Nephropathy:** Screen for microalbuminuria yearly. ACEIs or ARBs can slow progression in patients with microalbuminuria.
  - **Neuropathy:** Initially involves the distal feet and then affects the hands. Stress the importance of foot care and annual foot exams to prevent complications. Managed with improved glycemic control and pain management strategies. Avoid trauma.
- **Macrovascular complications:** Associated with an ↑ risk of MI and stroke. Control risk factors by instituting the following measures:
  - **Daily aspirin; smoking cessation.**
  - **BP control:** Goal BP is < 130/80.
  - **Lipids:** Goal LDL is < 100, or **< 70 in high-risk patients.**
  - **Diet and exercise.**

## Metabolic Syndrome

Also known as insulin resistance syndrome or "Syndrome X." Represents a compilation of traits associated with insulin resistance and an ↑ risk of type 2 DM.

### DIAGNOSIS

Diagnosis is based on any **three** of the following Adult Treatment Panel III criteria:

- Abdominal obesity (waist circumference > 40 inches in men, > 35 inches in women).
- TG ≥ 150 mg/dL.
- HDL < 40 mg/dL in men and < 50 mg/dL in women.
- BP ≥ 130/85.
- Fasting glucose ≥ 110 mg/dL.

### TREATMENT

Directed toward preventing the development of type 2 DM and coronary vascular disease. Includes lifestyle modifications (diet, weight loss, exercise) and even treatment of insulin resistance with medications.

The hypothalamus produces oxytocin and ADH, which are then stored and released by the posterior pituitary. The anterior pituitary produces six hormones: ACTH, TSH, FSH, LH, GH, and prolactin (see Table 4.4).

## Pituitary Tumors

Can arise from any cell. On the basis of size, they are classified as **microadenomas** (< 1 cm) and macroadenomas (> 1 cm). May → an ↑ in the hormone produced by that cell or a ↓ in other hormones by mass effect. Subtypes include the following:

*Prolactinomas are usually associated with a prolactin level > 200.*

- **Pituitary adenomas:**
    - Prolactinomas (the most common pituitary microadenoma)
    - GH-secreting
    - Nonfunctioning (comprise one-third of all pituitary tumors; the most common macroadenoma)
    - ACTH-secreting
    - TSH-secreting (rare)
- **Pituitary carcinomas**

**TABLE 4.4. Pituitary Hormones and Their Function**

| HORMONE | INCREASED BY | DECREASED BY | EXCESS | DEFICIENCY | NOTES |
|---------|--------------|--------------|--------|------------|-------|
| ADH | Thirst, high serum osmolality. | Low serum osmolality, low serum $K^+$. | SIADH. | DI. | |
| ACTH | CRH, stress. | High cortisol. | Cushing's syndrome. | Adrenal insufficiency. | Diurnal variation (peak at 3–4 A.M.). |
| TSH | TRH. | High $T_4$ and/or $T_3$. | Hyperthyroidism. | Hypothyroidism. | |
| LH/FSH | GnRH. | Gonadal sex steroids. | | Hypogonadism. | In men, inhibin inhibits FSH. |
| GH | GHRH, hypoglycemia, dopamine. | Somatostatin. | **Childhood:** gigantism. **Adulthood:** acromegaly. | **Childhood:** short stature. **Adulthood:** poor sense of well-being. | |
| Prolactin | Pregnancy, nursing, TRH, stress. | Dopamine. | Galactorrhea, hypogonadism. | Inability to lactate. | Under tonic inhibition by hypothalamic dopamine. |

Reproduced, with permission, from Le T et al. *First Aid for the Internal Medicine Boards,* 1st ed. New York: McGraw-Hill, 2006: 177.

**ENDOCRINOLOGY**

- Incidental discovery on MRI is very common; up to 10% of the general population have asymptomatic pituitary adenomas.
- Symptomatic cases may present as follows:
  - **Neurologic:** Headaches; visual field deficits.
  - **Hormonal excess/deficiency:** Hypothyroidism, hypogonadism, hyperprolactinemia (see specific sections for symptomatology).

### DIFFERENTIAL

The differential for sellar masses includes other benign masses (craniopharyngioma, meningioma), malignancies (1°—germ cell tumors and lymphomas; metastases—breast and lung cancer), cysts (Rathke's cleft, arachnoid, and dermoid cysts can cause sellar enlargement), and infections (abscesses, TB).

### DIAGNOSIS

- **Labs:** Check prolactin, insulin-like growth factor-1 (IGF-1), 24-hour urine for cortisol, ACTH, TSH, LH, FSH, and testosterone levels.
- **Imaging:** MRI of the pituitary/sella.

### TREATMENT

- If the tumor is < 20 mm and is not causing any signs or symptoms, observation may suffice.
- Treatment for symptomatic disease is as follows:
  - **Medical:** Treat hormone deficiency or excess as appropriate and discussed below.
  - **Surgical:** The transsphenoidal approach is successful in approximately 90% of microadenomas.
- **Radiation:** Conventional or stereotactic radiation. Side effects include panhypopituitarism (seen in up to 90% of cases).

## Diabetes Insipidus (DI)

Deficiency in ADH (also known as vasopressin) action → polyuria with very dilute urine (due to the inability to concentrate urine). Central and nephrogenic types are distinguished as follows:

- **Central DI:** ↓ release of ADH. May be caused by neurosurgery or trauma, tumors, ischemia, infiltrative diseases, or idiopathic DI.
- **Nephrogenic DI:** Resistance to the action to ADH. Causes include chronic renal disease, hereditary factors, hypercalcemia, hypokalemia, and **lithium toxicity.**

### SYMPTOMS/EXAM

- Presents with inappropriately **dilute** urine in the setting of ↑ **serum osmolality.**
- **Polyuria** and polydipsia are also seen.

### DIFFERENTIAL

**Osmotic diuresis** (e.g., elevated serum and urine osmolality); **psychogenic polydipsia** (low serum and urine osmolality).

### DIAGNOSIS

- High plasma and low urine osmolality.
- **Desmopressin (DDAVP) test** (synthetic vasopressin [ADH]).
- **Water deprivation test.**

### TREATMENT

- **Central DI: Treat any underlying lesion if present.** Administer intranasal DDAVP.
- **Nephrogenic DI:** Treat the underlying disorder. Thiazide diuretics and amiloride may be helpful (presumably act by inducing mild hypovolemia, thus increasing proximal reabsorption of sodium and water and decreasing overall urine output).

### COMPLICATIONS

Dehydration, hydronephrosis.

## Syndrome of Inappropriate Secretion of ADH (SIADH)

Involves excessive secretion of ADH. May be idiopathic. Additional etiologies are as follows:

- **CNS disturbances:** Any CNS pathology, including hemorrhage, stroke, or infection, that can enhance ADH secretion.
- **Tumors:** Ectopic production of ADH by tumors (the most common is small-cell lung carcinoma) can have the same effect.
- **Drugs:** Many drugs can ↑ the release of ADH or enhance its effects. These include carbamazepine, SSRIs, vincristine, haloperidol, amitriptyline, and amiodarone.

*If a patient is volume depleted with SIADH, he or she will have low urine sodium. These patients will respond to a saline load with an ↑ in urine sodium, and urine osmolality will remain high.*

### SYMPTOMS/EXAM

Initially, mild SIADH is often asymptomatic. Symptoms are usually associated with hyponatremia, with nausea and malaise progressing to headaches, lethargy, and eventually seizures and coma.

### DIAGNOSIS

Should be suspected in anyone with **hyponatremia, low plasma osmolality, a urine osmolality > 100 mOsm/kg, a urine sodium concentration** normally > 40 mEq/L, normal acid-base and potassium balance, and frequently a low plasma uric acid concentration.

### TREATMENT

- **Water restriction:** The mainstay of treatment. Avoid in SAH, as it may precipitate cerebral vasospasm or infarction.
- **Salt administration:** IV saline or hypertonic saline may be needed if hyponatremia is severe or symptomatic.
- **Loop diuretics:** Can enhance the effect of hypertonic saline.
- **Lithium and demeclocycline:** Act on collecting tubules to ↓ their response to ADH. Reserved for very severe cases.

## Hypopituitarism

Defined as ↓ secretion of one or more pituitary hormones. May be idiopathic. Additional etiologies are as follows:

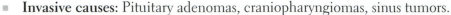

- **Invasive causes:** Pituitary adenomas, craniopharyngiomas, sinus tumors.
- **Infiltrative causes:** Sarcoidosis, hemochromatosis, histiocytosis X.
- **Infarction:**
    - **Sheehan's syndrome:** Infarction of the pituitary that occurs postpartum following substantial blood loss in childbirth. Presents with inability to lactate, lethargy, and amenorrhea.
    - **Pituitary apoplexy:** Sudden hemorrhage, often into a pituitary adenoma. Presents with severe headache, visual field defects, and hypotension. May resolve spontaneously or require high-dose steroids +/− decompression.
- **Injury:** Head trauma can → anterior pituitary dysfunction and vasopressin deficiency.
- **Immunologic causes:** Lymphocytic hypophysitis → lymphocytic infiltration. Can occur late in pregnancy or postpartum.
- **Iatrogenic:** Post–radiation therapy.
- **Infectious:** Rare. Etiologic agents include TB, syphilis, and fungi.
- **Empty sella syndrome:** Enlarged sella turcica not entirely filled with pituitary. May be 1° or 2°.
    - 1°: A defect in the diaphragm sella → infiltration with CSF fluid.
    - 2°: Enlargement of the sella by a mass that is then removed by surgery, radiation, or infarction.

*Remember the **8 I's** of hypopituitarism: Invasion, Infiltrative, Infarction, Injury, Immunologic, Iatrogenic, Infectious, Idiopathic.*

### SYMPTOMS/EXAM

May be asymptomatic or may present with symptoms ranging from mass effect to signs of hormone deficiency, with presentation depending on the hormone involved:

- **GH deficiency:** Presents as short stature in children. May → a variety of subtle effects in adults, including ↓ muscle mass, ↓ bone mineral density, and ↑ cardiovascular risk.
- **Prolactin deficiency:** Inability to lactate postpartum.
- **LH/FSH deficiency:** Hypogonadism. In women, presents with anovulation, infertility, and ↓ estrogen secretion. In men, infertility and ↓ testosterone are seen.
- **TSH deficiency:** Hypothyroidism.
- **ACTH deficiency:** ↓ cortisol secretion (hypotension, tachycardia, weakness, anorexia).

*ACTH deficiency differs from 1° adrenal insufficiency in that it does not cause salt wasting and hyperkalemia or hyperpigmentation.*

### DIAGNOSIS

Diagnosed by hormonal testing:

- **GH:** Low IGF-1.
- **Gonadotropins:** Low FSH/LH.
- **Thyroid:** Low free $T_4$ (TSH may be low or normal).
- **ACTH:** Abnormal ACTH and cortisol levels, and failure of synthetic corticotropin stimulation test.
- **Prolactin:** Low.

### TREATMENT

**Treat the underlying cause.** Correct hormone deficiencies as follows:

- **ACTH:** Steroids.
- **TSH:** Levothyroxine.
- **GnRH:** In men, treat with testosterone replacement in women, initiate estrogen replacement.

- **GH:** Human GH. Replacement of GH in adults is controversial.
- **ADH:** Intranasal DDAVP.
- **Prolactin:** No treatment

## Growth Hormone (GH) Excess

Etiologies are as follows:

- **Pituitary adenoma:** Accounts for > 99% of cases. Often has an insidious onset, causing the diagnosis to be delayed for > 10 years. Accounts for roughly one-third of all hormone-secreting tumors.
- **Iatrogenic:** Exogenous GH.
- **Ectopic GH or GHRH:** Very rare; can be seen with lung carcinoma, carcinoid, and pancreatic islet cell tumors.

### SYMPTOMS/EXAM

- **Childhood: Gigantism** from delayed epiphyseal closure → extremely tall stature.
- **Adulthood:**
  - Presents with **acromegaly.** Usually has an insidious onset.
  - Affects many different tissues and organs, with symptoms that may include **enlargement of the hands and feet,** glucose intolerance, hypertension, heat intolerance, weight gain, and fatigue.

### DIAGNOSIS

- **Labs:** IGF-1 levels must be assessed. Random GH is not helpful.
- **Imaging:** **MRI** of the pituitary.

### TREATMENT

- **Surgery:** Transsphenoidal resection is curative in 60–80% of cases but carries a risk of hypopituitarism or DI.
- **Medical:** Bromocriptine, octreotide, lanreotide, pegvisomant.

> A 31-year-old woman who is on OCPs presents to your office with bilateral galactorrhea of four months' duration and absent menses for the last year. Physical exam reveals a milky breast discharge and an otherwise normal breast exam. Her serum prolactin level, confirmed on two occasions, is > 200 ng/dL. What is the most likely diagnosis? With a prolactin level of > 200 ng/dL, a prolactinoma is the most likely etiology. While many drugs, including OCPs and antipsychotics, can ↑ prolactin levels, they would not do so to this level. Which diagnostic studies should you order? MRI of the pituitary with gadolinium enhancement. What treatment should you initiate? If a prolactinoma is found, start the woman on a dopamine agonist such as bromocriptine or cabergoline.

## Hyperprolactinemia

Elevated serum prolactin can be caused by a variety of physiologic conditions. **Prolactinomas,** the most common type of pituitary tumor, account for the majority of pathologic cases. Most are microadenomas (< 1 cm). Other etiologies are as follows:

- **Drugs:** Medications associated with hyperprolactinemia include dopaminergic drugs (e.g., antipsychotics, antihypertensives) as well as estrogen and SSRIs (typically clinically insignificant).
- ↓ **dopaminergic inhibition of prolactin.**
- **Pregnancy:** Prolactin can reach 200 ng/mL in the second trimester.
- **Hypothalamic lesions:** May → pituitary stalk compression or damage.
- **Hypothyroidism:** TRH stimulates prolactin secretion.

### SYMPTOMS/EXAM

- **Women: Galactorrhea;** anovulatory cycles with amenorrhea or oligomenorrhea.
- **Men:** Impotence, ↓ libido, galactorrhea (very rare).
- **Both:** Mass effect from large tumor (headache, visual field cuts, and hypopituitarism).

### DIAGNOSIS

- **Labs:** Show ↑ prolactin (typically > 200 ng/mL) with normal TSH; ⊖ pregnancy test.
- **Imaging:** Obtain an MRI in anyone with hyperprolactinemia in the absence of pregnancy or drugs known to cause elevation.

### TREATMENT

- **Pharmacologic:** Treat with a dopamine agonist such as **bromocriptine** or **cabergoline.**
- **Surgical:** Transsphenoidal resection is sometimes necessary if medical therapy is ineffective or the tumor is causing a mass effect.

*The most common cause of amenorrhea and galactorrhea in a premenopausal woman is pregnancy!*

## THYROID DISORDERS

### Hyperthyroidism

Most commonly caused by Graves' disease (60–90%). Etiologies, classified on the basis of findings on thyroid radioactive iodine (RAI) uptake and scan, are as follows (see also Table 4.5):

- ↑ **RAI uptake:**
  - **Graves' disease:** An autoimmune disorder in which **TSH receptor antibodies**—also known as **thyroid-stimulating immunoglobulin (TSI)**— stimulate the receptor to produce more thyroid hormone. The most common cause of hyperthyroidism. Females are affected more often than males (5:1).
  - **Solitary toxic hyperactive nodule.**
  - **Toxic multinodular goiter.**
- ↓ **RAI uptake:** Thyroiditis; exogenous thyroid hormone.

### SYMPTOMS/EXAM

- Presents with anxiety, weakness, palpitations, heat intolerance, diaphoresis, weight loss, and oligo- or amenorrhea.
- Exam reveals tachycardia, hyperreflexia, thin hair, and lid lag (exophthalmos and pretibial myxedema are seen in Graves' disease). May find a goiter.

TABLE 4.5. **Causes and Treatment of Hyperthyroidism**

| DISORDER | THYROID EXAM | UNIQUE FINDINGS | RAI UPTAKE AND SCAN | TREATMENT |
|---|---|---|---|---|
| Graves' disease | Diffusely enlarged thyroid; possibly bruit. | TSH receptor antibody (80–95% sensitive); TPO (50–85% sensitive; low specificity). | Diffusely ↑ uptake. | MMI, PTU; β-blockers; RAI. |
| Solitary toxic nodule | Single palpable nodule. | | Single-focus ↑ uptake. | Medications or RAI. |
| Multinodular goiter | "Lumpy-bumpy," enlarged thyroid. | | Multiple hot and/or cold nodules. | Medications or RAI. |
| Subacute thyroiditis (e.g., de Quervain's) | Tender, enlarged thyroid/painless. | Often postviral. ↑ ESR. | Diffusely ↓ uptake. | NSAIDs +/− steroids. |
| Exogenous hyperthyroidism | Normal. | Thyroglobulin levels are low. | Diffusely ↓ uptake. | Discontinue or ↓ thyroid hormone. |

### DIAGNOSIS

- **Labs:** TSH, free $T_4$, free $T_3$, thyroid antibodies in Graves' disease (thyroglobulin and TPO are present in 50–80% of patients; TSH receptor antibodies are found in 80–95%).
- **Imaging:** RAI uptake and scan.

### TREATMENT

- **Medications:**
  - **Antithyroid medications:** Block thyroid hormone production; can induce remission in 50% of Graves' patients.
    - **Propylthiouracil (PTU):** Blocks peripheral conversion of $T_4$ to $T_3$ at high doses; first choice during pregnancy.
    - **Methimazole (MMI):** Has a longer half-life, so can be used once per day.
  - **β-blockers:** Can be used to treat symptoms.
- **RAI:** Highly effective in treating toxic nodules and multinodular goiters; 90% effective in Graves' disease.
- **Surgery:** Used only in rare cases (e.g., for uncontrolled disease in pregnancy, very large goiters, goiters obstructing the airway, or patient preference).

### COMPLICATIONS

- **Cardiac:** Tachycardia, ↑ contractility, CHF, arrhythmias (including **atrial fibrillation,** the most common arrhythmia, occurring in 5–15% of patients), atrial flutter, paroxysmal atrial tachycardia.
- **Graves' ophthalmopathy:** Occurs in approximately 20% of patients. More common in **smokers.** Caused by accumulation of hydrophilic glycosaminoglycans, principally hyaluronic acid, in tissues. Can be worsened by RAI therapy. Treatment includes steroids and eye surgery.

- **Thyroid storm:** Presents with fever, tachycardia, delirium, diarrhea, vomiting, and CHF. Treat with high-dose propranolol, PTU, steroids, and iodide.

## Hypothyroidism

May be caused by a variety of conditions, including the following:

- **Hashimoto's thyroiditis:** An autoimmune thyroiditis that commonly leads to hypothyroidism but may initially present as hyperthyroidism. The most common cause of hypothyroidism in the United States.
- **Iodine deficiency:** Rare in the developed world, but the most common cause of hypothyroidism worldwide.
- **Drugs: Amiodarone, lithium,** interferon, drugs used to treat hyperthyroidism (iodide, PTU, MMI).
- **Iatrogenic:** Neck irradiation, thyroidectomy, RAI.
- **Subacute thyroiditis:** Typically transient.
- **Other:** 2° hypothyroidism (hypopituitarism); 3° hypothyroidism (hypothalamic dysfunction); peripheral resistance to thyroid hormone.

*Hypothyroidism can → galactorrhea because of its effect on prolactin secretion.*

### SYMPTOMS/EXAM

- Causes a generalized slowing of metabolic processes → a vague, nonspecific constellation of symptoms that includes **fatigue, weight gain, cold intolerance, dry skin, constipation,** and **menstrual irregularities.**
- Exam may reveal bradycardia and a delayed relaxation phase of DTRs. Accumulation of matrix glycosaminoglycans in many tissues can also → symptoms of coarse hair, enlargement of the tongue, hoarseness, and periorbital edema.

### DIAGNOSIS

- **Labs:** Generally show ↑ TSH and ↓ free $T_4$. ↑ TSH in the presence of a normal $T_4$ is considered subclinical hypothyroidism. If both TSH and free $T_4$ are low, think 2° or 3° hypothyroidism (occasionally can see mild depression of both TSH and $T_4$ with euthyroid sick syndrome). ⊕ antibodies may also be found (TPO, which is most sensitive, is found in 90–100% of patients with Hashimoto's thyroiditis).
- **Imaging:** Not generally indicated.

*Excess thyroid hormone replacement can → ↓ bone density.*

### TREATMENT

- **Thyroid hormone replacement:** Synthetic thyroxine ($T_4$). Titrate to normalize TSH.
- Pregnancy as well as the administration of some drugs (e.g., OCPs and other hormonal drugs) can affect the amount of thyroid-binding globulin (TBG) and may therefore ↑ the need for $T_4$.

### COMPLICATIONS

- Can precipitate depression and hyperlipidemia and may cause modest weight gain, so consider checking TSH in these settings.
- **Myxedema coma:** Severe hypothyroidism; constitutes a medical emergency. Characterized by ↓ mental status and hypothermia. Can progress to shock and death. Treatment is IV $T_3$ and/or $T_4$ along with supportive therapy, especially rewarming.

## Thyroiditis

Inflammation of the thyroid may present with hyper-, hypo-, or euthyroid states. Table 4.6 outlines the causes, presentation, and treatment of thyroiditis.

> A 62-year-old woman comes to your office for a routine visit. Exam reveals a 2-cm thyroid nodule. The exam is otherwise normal. What tests would you order? You order TSH, which is found to be within normal limits. What further workup is indicated? Fine-needle aspiration (FNA).

**TABLE 4.6.**  **Clinical Features and Differential Diagnosis of Thyroiditis**

| TYPE | ETIOLOGY | CLINICAL FINDINGS | TESTS | TREATMENT |
|---|---|---|---|---|
| Subacute thyroiditis (de Quervain's) | Viral. | Hyperthyroid early; then hypothyroid. Presents with a tender, enlarged thyroid and with fever. | ↑ ESR; ↓ RAI uptake. | NSAIDs; acetaminophen +/– steroids. |
| Hashimoto's thyroiditis | Autoimmune. | Usually hypothyroid; painless, +/– goiter. | Some 95% have ⊕ antibodies; anti-TPO antibodies are most sensitive. | Thyroid hormone. |
| Suppurative thyroiditis | Bacteria are more commonly implicated than other infectious agents. | Fever, neck pain, tender thyroid. | TFTs are normal. No uptake on RAI scan; ⊕ cultures. | Antibiotics and drainage. |
| Amiodarone use | Am**IOD**arone contains **IOD**ine. | 1. Asymptomatic TFT changes<br>2. Hypothyroidism<br>3. Hyperthyroidism | 1. ↑ free $T_4$ and total $T_4$; then low $T_3$ and high TSH.<br>2. High TSH; low $T_4$ and $T_3$.<br>3. Low TSH; high $T_4$ and $T_3$. | 1. Usually not necessary to stop medications; will normalize over time.<br>2. As for other hypothyroidism.<br>3. As for other hyperthyroidism +/– steroids. |
| Other medications | **Lithium,** α-interferon, interleukin-2. | | Lithium usually → hypothyroidism. | Stop medication if possible. |
| Postpartum thyroiditis | Lymphocytic infiltration; seen after up to 10% of pregnancies. | Small, nontender thyroid. Mild symptoms. | May see hyper- or hypothyroidism. Antibodies are often ⊕; RAI uptake is ↓. | β-blockers if needed. Otherwise, no treatment is necessary. |

## Thyroid Nodules and Cancer

The "90%" **mnemonic** applies to thyroid nodules: **90%** of nodules are benign; **90%** are cold on RAI uptake scan, with 15–20% of these malignant (hot nodules are rarely malignant); **90%** of thyroid malignancies present as a thyroid nodule or lump. Etiologies include the following:

- **Benign lesions:** Often regress spontaneously or with $T_4$ therapy.
- **1° thyroid cancer:**
  - **Papillary:** The **most common type.** Carries an excellent prognosis, with a 98% survival rate for stage I or II disease. Many tumors secrete thyroglobulin.
  - **Follicular:** A more aggressive form. Associated with metastasis to bone, lungs, and brain. Often retains the ability to form thyroglobulin and occasionally thyroid hormone (i.e., "functioning thyroid cancer").
  - **Medullary:** May secrete **calcitonin.** Can be associated with MEN 2A and 2B.
  - **Anaplastic:** Undifferentiated thyroid gland tumors. Very aggressive.
- **Other:** Lymphoma, metastasis to thyroid (breast, kidney, melanoma, lung).

### SYMPTOMS/EXAM

- Presents with a single, firm, palpable nodule. Otherwise, often asymptomatic unless associated with thyroid hormone abnormalities or advanced carcinoma.
- **Red flags** for thyroid carcinoma are **male** gender; age < 20 or > 65; a history of head/neck irradiation; a family history of thyroid cancer; a **hard, fixed nodule > 4 cm;** rapid growth of the nodule; and symptoms related to local invasion (**dysphagia, hoarseness**).

### DIAGNOSIS

Always start the evaluation by checking **TFTs.** In a patient with a **low TSH,** the next step is an RAI **uptake and scan.** If the nodule is hot, the evaluation ends there. If the nodule is cold or if TSH is normal or ↑, the nodule should be biopsied with **FNA** (see Figure 4.1).

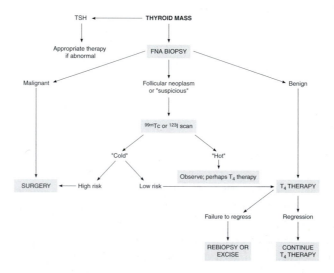

**FIGURE 4.1.** **Evaluation of a thyroid mass.**

(Reproduced, with permission, from Greenspan FS, Gardner DG. *Basic & Clinical Endocrinology,* 7th ed. New York: McGraw-Hill, 2004: 282.)

- **Benign nodules:** Observe if asymptomatic and confirmed to be benign. $T_4$ suppression therapy is only 50% effective. Surgical excision can be considered.
- **Malignancies:** Total thyroidectomy followed by **RAI ablation** therapy. Markers such as thyroglobulin and calcitonin (medullary carcinoma only) can be used to monitor for recurrence. For low-risk cases with very small nodules (< 1 cm), lobectomy can be considered.

A 26-year-old woman at a six-week postpartum visit is found to have weight loss, sweating, weakness, and heat intolerance. Exam shows a heart rate of 120, thyromegaly, and an upper eyelid 1 mm above the upper corneal limbus. In keeping with the fact that subacute thyrotoxicosis can occur in the postpartum period, what tests would you order? TSH and free $T_4$. If hyperthyroidism is confirmed, what treatment would you use? Propranolol.

## The Thyroid in Pregnancy

The following are treatment guidelines for thyroid changes that may arise in the course of pregnancy:

- **Normal changes in pregnancy:** An ↑ in TBG occurs in normal pregnancy and → an ↑ in total serum levels of $T_4$ and $T_3$. However, free thyroid hormone levels should remain normal.
- **Hyperthyroidism:**
  - **Dx:** TFTs. RAI is contraindicated in pregnancy.
  - **Tx:**
    - Antithyroid medications. All of these can cross the placenta and can therefore → hypothyroidism in the newborn (the effect is typically transient). **PTU is the recommended medication** during pregnancy. MMI is associated with rare congenital abnormalities.
    - Prolonged iodine therapy can → fetal goiter.
    - β-blockers may be used to control symptoms but can → fetal growth restriction, hypoglycemia, and bradycardia.
  - **Cx:** If hyperthyroidism goes **untreated,** the complication rate for the fetus is quite high and includes an ↑ risk for spontaneous **abortion, premature** delivery, and **low-birth-weight** newborns.
- **Hypothyroidism:**
  - **Dx:** New-onset hypothyroidism is rare. However, many women with preexisting hypothyroidism need higher doses of $T_4$ during pregnancy, so $FT_4$ levels should be monitored closely.
  - **Cx:** If hypothyroidism goes **untreated,** both fetal and maternal complications can result.
    - **Fetal complications:** Include congenital abnormalities, perinatal mortality, and impaired development.
    - **Maternal complications:** Anemia, preeclampsia, placental abruption, postpartum hemorrhage.

A 52-year-old man presents with nausea, constipation, lethargy, and impaired concentration and memory. His physical exam is essentially normal. His CBC and chemistry reveal ↑ calcium levels. What medications can cause hypercalcemia? Vitamins A and D, thiazide diuretics, calcium-containing antacids, and lithium. PTH is low. What is the likely etiology of this patient's hypercalcemia? Malignancy. How should you treat him? Institute aggressive fluids, loop diuretics, calcitonin, and bisphosphonate.

## Calcium Metabolism

Figure 4.2 illustrates the hormonal control loop that governs calcium metabolism and function.

## Hypercalcemia

High levels of calcium in the blood can stem from a variety of causes, but 1° **hyperparathyroidism** and **malignancy** account for 80–90% of cases. Pathophysiologic mechanisms are as follows:

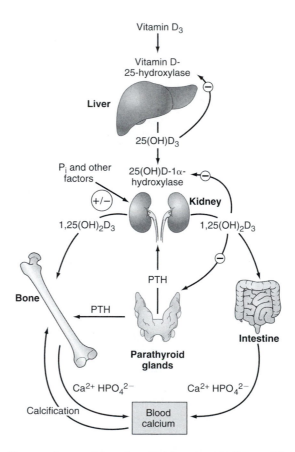

**FIGURE 4.2.** **Hormonal control loop for vitamin D metabolism and function.**

(Reproduced, with permission, from Kasper DL et al. *Harrison's Principles of Internal Medicine,* 16th ed. New York: McGraw Hill, 2005: 2246.)

- **1° hyperparathyroidism:** See the section below.
- **Malignancy-associated hypercalcemia:** Can occur in up to 10–15% of malignancies via several mechanisms:
  - **Tumor release of PTH-related peptide (PTHrP):** Most common. PTHrP is homologous to PTH but is not detected as PTH by serum assays and does not ↑ 1,25-dihydroxycholecalciferol (DHD) production. Seen in a variety of solid tumors (breast, lung, renal cell, ovarian, and bladder carcinoma).
  - **1,25-DHD production by tumor:** Associated with lymphomas.
  - **Local osteolysis from metastases or adjacent tumor mass:** Associated with multiple myeloma and breast cancer.
- **Granulomatous disorders:** Sarcoidosis in particular can → ↑ vitamin D production.
- **Endocrinopathies:**
  - **Thyrotoxicosis** can be associated with mild hypercalcemia.
  - **Adrenal insufficiency.**
- **↑ vitamin A and D:**
  - **Vitamin A:** Excess → bone resorption.
  - **Vitamin D:** Excess → ↑ 25-hydroxyvitamin D (25-HD) concentrations
- **Drug induced:** Thiazides, lithium, calcium-based antacids, estrogens, androgens.

### SYMPTOMS/EXAM

- Renal **stones.**
- **Bone pain.**
- **Abdominal pain,** often with constipation, nausea, vomiting, and anorexia.
- **Psychiatric symptoms:** Anxiety, depression, cognitive dysfunction

### DIAGNOSIS

- **Labs:** Repeat serum calcium, **PTH,** and phosphate. Consider protein electrophoresis to rule out multiple myeloma (see Table 4.7).
- **Imaging:** CXR to look for sarcoidosis or malignancy.

### TREATMENT

Treatment should be aimed at lowering the calcium level, especially if the patient is symptomatic, and at treating underlying cause.

- **↑ urinary excretion:**
  - **Fluids:** Begin with isotonic saline to expand volume and ↑ urinary excretion. Hydration with normal saline is the essential element in treating acute hypercalcemia.
  - **Loop diuretics.**
- **Inhibit bone reabsorption:**
  - **Calcitonin (SQ):** ↓ bony reabsorption by interfering with osteoclast function; also ↑ renal excretion. However, efficacy is lost after three days because tachyphylaxis develops.
  - **Bisphosphonates (IV):** Toxic to osteoclasts; more potent than calcitonin. Effects on serum calcium are seen 48–72 hours after initiation of therapy.
- **↓ intestinal absorption:**
  - **Glucocorticoids:** First-line treatment in patients with vitamin A- or D-mediated hypercalcemia.
  - **Phosphate:** Oral administration to bind calcium in the gut. Minimal effect on hypercalcemia.

*Hallmarks of hypercalcemia: Stones, bones, groans, and psychiatric overtones.*

TABLE 4.7.    Laboratory Findings Associated with Hypercalcemia

| | CALCIUM | PHOSPHORUS | PTH | PTHRP | OTHER |
|---|---|---|---|---|---|
| PTH mediated | ↑ | ↓ | ↑ | ↓ | |
| PTHrP mediated | ↑ | ↓ | ↓ | ↑ | |
| 1,25-DHD mediated | ↑ | ↑ | ↓ | ↓ | ↑ 1,25-DHD |
| Vitamin D intoxication | ↑ | ↑ | ↓ | ↓ | ↑ 25-HD |

Reproduced, with permission, from Le T et al. *First Aid for the Internal Medicine Boards,* 1st ed. New York: McGraw-Hill, 2006: 208.

- Chelation of ionized calcium with sodium EDTA or IV phosphate works quickly but is potentially toxic.
- Dialysis is used as a last resort.

### COMPLICATIONS

Long-standing or very high levels of hypercalcemia can → deposition of calcium in heart valves, coronary arteries, and myocardial fibers and can also → severe renal disease and neurologic deficits.

> A 50-year-old man comes to your office for a routine screening. Lab studies indicate that he has elevated serum calcium. What lab value do you check next? PTH. If elevated, what are the indications for parathyroidectomy? Age < 50, serum calcium > 1 mg/dL above normal, osteoporosis, unexplained ↓ creatinine clearance, and hypercalciuria (> 400 mg/dL).

## 1° Hyperparathyroidism

Eighty percent of cases of 1° hyperparathyroidism are due to a single parathyroid adenoma; the remainder are due to gland hyperplasia and cancer.

### SYMPTOMS/EXAM

- **Eighty-five percent are asymptomatic** and are diagnosed on screening labs.
- Hypercalcemia → "stones, bones, groans, and **psychiatric overtones.**"
- Osteoporosis is commonly seen.

### DIFFERENTIAL

- **Familial benign hypocalciuric hypercalcemia:** A hereditary, autosomal-dominant disorder that → lifelong asymptomatic mild hypercalcemia. Differentiated from 1° hyperparathyroidism by marked hypocalciuria. PTH can be normal or mildly elevated. No therapy is required.
- MEN syndromes.
- **Lithium therapy:** Lithium shifts the set point for PTH secretion → hypercalcemia.

- Labs show ↑ **PTH**, ↑ **Ca++**, and ↓ **phosphorus.**
- To investigate possible complications of 1° hyperparathyroidism, one should also check 24-hour urine calcium/creatinine, renal function, and bone mineral density.
- Imaging studies of the parathyroid glands are rarely indicated or necessary.

### TREATMENT

- **If surgery is not indicated, observe.**
- **Parathyroidectomy** is the only curative treatment. The cure rate is 95%, and the complication rate is low. Indications for surgery include age < 50, serum calcium > 1 mg/dL above normal, osteoporosis, hypercalciuria (calcium > 400 mg/day), and unexplained worsening in renal function.
- Treat osteoporosis with estrogen therapy or bisphosphonates.

### COMPLICATIONS

Nephrolithiasis, nephrocalcinosis with renal insufficiency, osteopenia, osteoporosis.

## Hypocalcemia

Serum calcium concentrations are regulated by DHD and PTH. Hypocalcemia can be caused by abnormalities in these regulatory mechanisms:

- **Hypoparathyroidism:** Usually postsurgical from thyroid or parathyroid surgery. Can also be autoimmune, familial, infiltrative, or idiopathic. Treatment is with chronic oral calcitriol (DHD) and calcium.
- **Pseudohypoparathyroidism:** Target organ resistance to PTH. Can be isolated or associated with Albright's hereditary osteodystrophy (short stature, round face, short neck, brachydactyly). Treatment is the same as that for hypoparathyroidism.
- **Vitamin D deficiency:**
    - Caused by malabsorptive states (e.g., IBD, celiac sprue), lack of sun exposure, and dark skin.
    - In children, the deficiency → **rickets** (bony deformities with rachitic rosary, bowing of the lower extremities, and frontal bossing).
    - In adults, it → osteomalacia with myopathy and poor bone mineralization.
    - Diagnosed by a **low 25-HD level** (< 20 ng/mL), hypocalcemia, hypophosphatemia, and 2° hyperparathyroidism.
    - Treatment is high-dose oral vitamin D replacement and calcium.
- **Acute deposition or complex formation of calcium:** Acute hyperphosphatemia (tumor lysis, excessive phosphate administration); acute pancreatitis; blood transfusion (citrate buffer in packed RBCs precipitates with calcium); hungry bone syndrome (relative hypoparathyroidism following parathyroidectomy or thyroidectomy).

### SYMPTOMS/EXAM

- **Neuromuscular manifestations:**
    - **Tetany:** Neuromuscular irritability → a mixture of spontaneous muscular and sensory nerve dysfunctions.

- **Chvostek's sign: Contraction of the facial muscles** in response to tapping of the facial nerve. About 25% of normal individuals have a ⊕ Chvostek's sign.
- **Trousseau's sign:** Induction of carpal spasm by inflation of a BP cuff to 20 mmHg above SBP for three minutes. ⊕ in 1–4% of normal individuals.
- **Paresthesias, especially of the fingertips and perioral area.**
- **Other:** Seizures, psychiatric symptoms.
  - **Cardiac:** The hallmark is a **prolonged QT interval.**
  - **Other:** Cataracts, skeletal abnormalities.

### DIAGNOSIS

Lab studies reveal a low calcium level, corrected for albumin; low-normal phosphorus; normal magnesium; and low PTH. If PTH is ↑ or normal, check 25-HD and renal function (see Table 4.8).

### TREATMENT

- **Acute:** In the presence of tetany, give a continuous IV calcium drip, start oral calcium, and add calcitriol if needed.
- **Chronic:** Oral calcium and calcitriol if needed.

*The most common fractures in Paget's disease are vertebral crush fractures.*

## Paget's Disease

A skeletal disease with **accelerated bone turnover** as its hallmark. Incidence is around 3–4% in patients > 40 years of age. More common among Caucasians.

### SYMPTOMS/EXAM

- **Two-thirds of patients are asymptomatic.** Symptoms can include **pain** (worsens with weight bearing and often occurs at night), **fractures,** and bony **deformity** most commonly affecting the sacrum, spine, femur, skull, and pelvis.
- Exam findings can include skull enlargement, frontal bossing, bowed legs, and often skin changes of the affected areas (erythema, warmth, tenderness).

### DIFFERENTIAL

Bony tumors, including malignancies.

TABLE 4.8. **Laboratory Findings Associated with Hypocalcemia**

|  | CALCIUM | PHOSPHORUS | PTH | OTHER |
|---|---|---|---|---|
| Hypoparathyroidism | ↓ | ↑ | ↓ | |
| PTH resistance | ↓ | ↑ | ↑ | |
| Vitamin D deficiency | ↓ | ↓ | ↑ | ↓ 25-HD |
| 1,25-DHD resistance | ↓ | ↓ | ↑ | ↑ 1,25-DHD |

Reproduced, with permission, from Le T et al. *First Aid for the Internal Medicine Boards,* 1st ed. New York: McGraw-Hill, 2006: 211.

- **Labs:** ↑ **alkaline phosphatase** and markers of bone turnover (osteocalcin, urinary hydroxyproline, N-telopeptide). Ca++ and phosphorus are usually normal.
- **Imaging:** Plain films of involved bones show ↑ density and size; erosions can be seen in the skull. Bone scan shows ↑ uptake in affected areas.

### TREATMENT

**Bisphosphonates** are the treatment of choice and often → remission.

### COMPLICATIONS

↑ risk of bone tumors. Immobilizing a patient with active Paget's disease can → hypercalcemia.

## ADRENAL DISORDERS

The adrenal gland is under the control of the hypothalamus and the pituitary. The hypothalamus secretes corticotropin-releasing hormone (CRH), which acts on the pituitary to produce ACTH. ACTH then acts on the adrenal gland to produce cortisol. The adrenal gland consists of the medulla and the cortex.

- **Medulla:** Produces catecholamines (epinephrine, norepinephrine, and dopamine).
- **Cortex:** Made up of three layers:
  - **Glomerulosa:** Produces mineralocorticoids (aldosterone).
  - **Fasciculata:** The 1° producer of cortisol and androgens.
  - **Reticularis:** Produces androgens and cortisol.

### Adrenal Insufficiency

1° adrenal insufficiency is known as **Addison's disease.** 2° adrenal insufficiency is much more common. Etiologies are as follows:

- **1° adrenal insufficiency:**
  - **Autoimmune:** Autoimmune destruction of the adrenal gland is the **most common** etiology. Can be accompanied by other autoimmune disorders.
  - **Metastatic tumors to the adrenals.**
  - **Hemorrhage:** Can occur in critical illness, pregnancy, and anticoagulated patients as well as those with antiphospholipid antibody syndrome.
  - **Infection:** Associated with **HIV,** TB, fungi, and CMV.
  - **Infiltrative disorders:** Include amyloid and hemochromatosis.
  - **Congenital adrenal hyperplasia.**
  - **Drugs:** Include ketoconazole, metyrapone, aminoglutethimide, trilostane, mitotane, and etomidate.
- **2° adrenal insufficiency:**
  - **Iatrogenic:** 2° to glucocorticoid and anabolic steroid administration.
  - Pituitary or hypothalamic tumors.

*The most common cause of adrenal insufficiency is exogenous glucocorticoid use.*

### SYMPTOMS/EXAM

- Presents with weakness, fatigue, anorexia, weight loss, nausea, vomiting, diarrhea, abdominal pain, and orthostatic hypotension, coma, and death.

ENDOCRINOLOGY

- **Hyperpigmentation** of the oral mucosa and palmar creases is found in 1° disease.

### DIAGNOSIS

- **Labs:** Hyponatremia and **hyperkalemia (in 1° disease).**
- **Confirm the diagnosis** as follows:
  - **Random cortisol:** A random level ≥ 18 µg/dL rules out adrenal insufficiency. **Early-morning cortisol < 5 µg/dL is strongly suggestive of adrenal insufficiency.**
  - **Cortrosyn stimulation test:**
    - Obtain baseline ACTH and cortisol levels.
    - Inject Cortrosyn (synthetic ACTH) 250 µg IM or IV.
    - Check cortisol level 45–60 minutes later.
    - A peak to ≥ 18–20 µg/dL excludes adrenal insufficiency. Can be falsely ⊖ in acute 2° adrenal insufficiency.
- **Distinguish 1° from 2° adrenal insufficiency:** An ↑ ACTH level in a patient with adrenal insufficiency is consistent with 1° adrenal insufficiency. In 2° disease, ACTH is low owing to the presence of ACTH-like hormones.
- **Evaluate the cause:** Exclude exogenous or iatrogenic steroids. In 1° adrenal insufficiency, a CT of the adrenal gland is usually indicated. In 2° disease, a pituitary MRI can be diagnostic.

### TREATMENT

- Hydrocortisone two-thirds in the morning and one-third in the evening or prednisone daily. Higher or "stress doses" of steroids should be used during illness or surgery in these patients.
- **In 1° adrenal insufficiency, fludrocortisone** is needed to replace mineralocorticoids.

### COMPLICATIONS

**Adrenal crisis,** an acute deficiency of cortisol, usually occurs 2° to abrupt discontinuation of exogenous steroids or major stress in the setting of adrenal insufficiency. Presents with headache, nausea, vomiting, confusion, fever, hypotension, and coma. Can be fatal if not treated immediately with steroids.

## Cushing's Syndrome

A syndrome due to excess endogenous or exogenous cortisol.

- **Exogenous corticosteroids:** The **most common** cause.
- **Cushing's disease:** Caused by ACTH hypersecretion from a **pituitary** microadenoma. Has a female-to-male ratio of 8:1.
- **Ectopic ACTH:** ACTH secretion from a nonpituitary neoplasm (**small cell lung carcinoma,** bronchial carcinoids).
- **Adrenal disease:** Adenoma, carcinoma, or nodular adrenal hyperplasia.

### SYMPTOMS/EXAM

Presents with centripetal obesity (with moon facies and buffalo hump), menstrual irregularities, hypertension, emotional lability, dermatologic manifestations (e.g., plethora, hirsutism, striae), and glucose intolerance.

### DIAGNOSIS

- Confirm excess cortisol production with an overnight dexamethasone suppression test.

- A.M. cortisol < 1.8 µg/dL is a negative test result and rules out excess cortisol.
- If ↑, check 24-hour urinary free cortisol.
- Check ACTH:
  - If < 5 pg/mL, the source is likely adrenal, warranting CT of the adrenal glands.
  - If > 10 pg/mL, the source is either pituitary or ectopic, warranting the following:
    - **MRI of the pituitary.**
    - **If MRI is negative, inferior petrosal sinus sampling (IPSS):** Measures levels of ACTH draining from the pituitary and periphery before and after CRH stimulation to see if the gradient is greater from the pituitary or the periphery.

### TREATMENT

- **Adrenal tumors:** Adrenalectomy.
- **Cushing's disease:** Transsphenoidal pituitary adenoma resection.
- **Ectopic ACTH:**
  - Treat the underlying neoplasm.
  - Blockade of steroid synthesis (ketoconazole, metyrapone, aminoglutethimide).
  - Potassium replacement (spironolactone can be helpful).
  - Bilateral adrenalectomy if needed.

### COMPLICATIONS

Complications may arise in association with long-term excess glucocorticoids (diabetes, hypertension, cardiovascular disease, obesity, osteoporosis). May also → ↑ susceptibility to infections.

## Hyperaldosteronism

Excess aldosterone can stem from a variety of sources and can be a cause of 2° hypertension. Common etiologies include the following:

- **Aldosterone-producing adenoma (Conn's disease):** More common in women than in men. Accounts for over half of 1° aldosteronism.
- **Idiopathic hyperaldosteronism:** Accounts for roughly one-third of cases.
- **Glucocorticoid-suppressible aldosteronism:** A rare autosomal-dominant disorder.
- **Angiotensin II–responsive adenoma.**
- **Aldosterone-producing adrenocortical carcinoma:** Rare. Hyperandrogenism occurs as well.

### SYMPTOMS/EXAM

**Most patients are asymptomatic. Hypertension** and **hypokalemia** are classic. Potassium can be normal.

### DIAGNOSIS

- **Plasma aldosterone concentration and plasma renin activity:** Measure after a high-salt diet or salt supplementation for a week.
- Twenty-four-hour urine **aldosterone level.**
- CT of the adrenal gland can differentiate Conn's disease from idiopathic hyperaldosteronism.

### TREATMENT

- **Spironolactone:** Give high-dose **spironolactone** or **eplerenone** mineralo-corticoid receptor and normalize potassium levels. Side effects include gynecomastia in men, rash, impotence, and epigastric discomfort.
- **Unilateral adrenalectomy** in patients with a single adenoma.

### COMPLICATIONS

Complications may arise 2° to hypertension or hypokalemia.

## Pheochromocytoma

Rare tumors of the cells of the adrenal medulla area of adrenal glands that produce **epinephrine and/or norepinephrine.** Approximately 90% arise in the adrenal gland itself. Others are in extra-adrenal locations.

### SYMPTOMS/EXAM

- Presents with episodic attacks of throbbing **headaches,** diaphoresis, and palpitations. Can also be associated with tremor, anxiety, nausea, vomiting, fatigue, weight loss, chest pain, and abdominal pain.
- The majority of patients have hypertension, but can be episodic. **Orthostasis** is commonly present.

### DIAGNOSIS

Pheochromocytoma is usually suggested by the history in a symptomatic patient or the family history in a patient with familial disease. Diagnosed as follows:

- First make a biochemical diagnosis with markedly elevated urinary metanephrines and catecholamines in a 24-hour urine collection or plasma metanephrines.
- Then localize the lesion with **imaging:**
    - MRI/CT scan of the adrenal glands to localize.
    - If the adrenals appear normal, [123]I-MIBG scan can be used to localize extra-adrenal pheochromocytomas and metastases.

### TREATMENT

- **Adrenergic blockade:** Phenoxybenzamine is the key first step.
- **β-blockers:** Used to control heart rate, but only after adrenergic blockade.
- **Surgical resection:** Has a 90% cure rate. It is important to hydrate patients and control symptoms before surgery.

*Do not use β-blockers in patients with pheochromocytoma before adequate adrenergic blockade is achieved, as they can cause worsening of hypertension and precipiatate a hypertensive crisis.*

### COMPLICATIONS

Hypertensive crises, MI, CVAs, arrhythmias, renal failure, dissecting aortic aneurysm.

## Adrenal Incidentalomas

Adrenal lesions are found incidentally in approximately 2% of patients undergoing abdominal CT scans for unrelated reasons. Autopsies indicate a prevalence of approximately 10%. Subtypes are as follows:

- **Functioning adenoma:** Cushing's syndrome, pheochromocytoma, Conn's disease.

- **Nonfunctioning adenoma:** Carcinoma, benign adenoma, metastatic lesion.

In patients with a history of malignancy, the probability that an adrenal lesion is metastatic is > 25%. In this case, biopsy is indicated once pheochromocytoma has been ruled out.

### Symptoms/Exam

Many are nonfunctioning. See above for functioning lesions.

### Diagnosis

- **Rule out functioning tumor:**
  - Plasma metanephrines or 24-hour urine for catecholamine and metanephrines to rule out pheochromocytoma.
  - Dexamethasone suppression test to rule out Cushing's disease.
  - If the patient is hypertensive, determine plasma renin activity and aldosterone level to rule out aldosteronoma.
- **CT/MRI:** Characteristics of a fine-cut CT or MRI can help define whether a lesion is likely benign or suspicious for a malignancy.

### Treatment

Treatment is based on the size and functional status of the lesion.

- **Lesions < 4 cm and nonfunctioning:** Repeat imaging in 3–6 months.
- **Lesions > 4 cm and nonfunctioning:** Resect.
- **Functioning lesions:** Treat as appropriate for the disorder (see previous sections).

# Gastroenterology

Brian Kim, MD

### Esophageal Dysphagia

Defined as a sensation of food sticking or obstruction in the esophagus (vs. **odynophagia,** or pain on swallowing). Due to disease in the body of the esophagus, the lower esophageal sphincter (LES), the cardia, or nearby structures. Patients typically complain of symptoms **seconds after swallowing** and identify the **suprasternal notch** or **retrosternal area** as the source of their discomfort. Etiologies include the following:

- **Gastroesophageal reflux.**
- **Anatomic abnormalities of the esophagus:** Zenker's diverticulum, cricopharyngeal bars, peptic strictures, radiation injury, esophageal webs/rings, and esophageal carcinoma.
- **Esophageal motility disorders:**
  - **Achalasia:** Failure of the LES due to idiopathic degeneration of neurons in the esophageal wall → failure of relaxation and distal peristalsis. Cases are largely 1° in the United States but can also be 2° to a variety of conditions (e.g., Chagas' disease).
  - **1° motility disorders:** A group of disorders with an unclear pathologic or pathophysiologic basis, each characterized by specific manometric findings. Features include diffuse esophageal spasm, nutcracker esophagus, and hypertensive LES. Chest pain is common.
- **Globus sensation:** A persistent or intermittent sensation of a lump or foreign body in the throat for > 12 weeks that is present **even when the patient is not swallowing.** More common in women, and usually worsens with emotional stress. An association with GERD has not been substantiated.
- **Autoimmune disorders:** Scleroderma; Sjögren's syndrome (dysphagia is independent of xerostomia but is worsened by it).
- **Cardiovascular abnormalities:** Can → dysphagia via compression of the esophagus (e.g., vascular rings, aneurysms, left atrial enlargement)
- **Xerostomia** (e.g., anticholinergics).
- **Functional dysphagia:** Dysphagia for > 12 weeks over one year with no identifiable cause.

#### DIFFERENTIAL

**Oropharyngeal dysphagia,** in which patients complain of food getting stuck **immediately upon swallowing** and identify the **cervical region** as the source of discomfort. Caused by a variety of neuromuscular disorders (e.g., CVA).

#### DIAGNOSIS

- **EGD:** Most commonly used for the diagnosis of esophageal dysphagia.
- **Barium swallow:** Less diagnostic but safer than EGD; the initial test of choice for suspected achalasia, revealing classic "bird's beak" narrowing.
- **Esophageal manometry:** Usually performed if the aforementioned studies are ⊖ to evaluate for a 1° esophageal dysmotility disorder. Also confirmatory for achalasia.
- **Videofluoroscopic swallow study:** Useful in the evaluation of oropharyngeal dysphagia.
- **Laryngoscopy:** Should be considered in patients with globus sensation to rule out malignancy.

#### TREATMENT

Directed at the underlying cause.

*Dysphagia only for solids suggests a mechanical obstruction (but can include liquids with severe obstruction). Dysphagia for solids and liquids equally suggests a motility disorder.*

*Immediate endoscopic evaluation is indicated in cases of dysphagia with rapid progression, unexplained weight loss, or unexplained anemia (to rule out malignancy with occult blood loss).*

*It is essential to rule out cardiac chest pain in a patient suspected of having a 1° esophageal dysmotility disorder.*

## Esophagitis

Inflammation of the esophagus with variable etiologies (see Table 5.1). Can be asymptomatic or present with symptoms such as odynophagia, dysphagia, and retrosternal chest pain.

## Gastroesophageal Reflux Disease (GERD)

Caused by **failure of antireflux mechanisms,** which consist of the LES, the crural diaphragm, and the portion of the gastroesophageal junction below the hiatus. Its prevalence is high, with 15% of those affected experiencing symptoms at least once a week and 7% having daily symptoms.

**TABLE 5.1.**   **Etiologies and Presentation of Esophagitis**

| SUBTYPE | CHARACTERISTICS | DIAGNOSIS | TREATMENT |
|---|---|---|---|
| HSV | Usually found in immunocompromised patients. Has an acute onset, and exam may reveal concomitant vesicles on the nose and lips. | EGD, biopsy, culture. | Acyclovir. |
| CMV | Usually found in immunocompromised patients. Presents with odynophagia, chest pain, hematemesis, nausea, and vomiting. | EGD, biopsy. | Ganciclovir. |
| HIV | May present in 1° infection. | HIV testing. | Usually self-limited. |
| Candida | Usually found in immunocompromised patients. Exam may reveal thrush, but **the absence of thrush does not preclude the diagnosis.** | EGD, biopsy; alternatively, therapeutic trial. | Fluconazole. |
| Radiation | A complication of therapy for head and neck tumors. May present as acute or chronic (from fibrosis and ischemia). | | Acutely, viscous lidocaine; indomethacin may ↓ chronic damage. |
| Corrosive | Caustic ingestion. | | Acutely, prednisone; strictures formed later require balloon dilation. |
| Pill | Relatively sudden onset; classically caused by taking an offending medication without water prior to sleep. Commonly implicated drugs include antibiotics (tetracycline, doxycycline, clindamycin), vitamin C, $FeSO_4$, KCl, NSAIDs, and bisphosphonates. | Usually clinical. | Prevention. The role of acid suppression is unsubstantiated in the absence of GERD. |
| Eosinophilic | Causes are idiopathic or allergic; usually → dysphagia and food impaction due to stricture and ring formation. | EGD, biopsy. | Esophageal dilation, swallowed aerosolized fluticasone, systemic steroids, elimination diet trial. |
| Reflux | See section on GERD. | | |

### SYMPTOMS/EXAM

- Presents with regurgitation of sour material in the mouth along with heartburn (usually postprandial), dysphagia, chest pain, and water brash (hypersalivation).
- In severe cases, laryngitis, chronic coughing, morning hoarseness, and pulmonary aspiration may be seen.
- Exam is usually normal.

*Asthma unresponsive to conventional therapy is highly suspicious for GERD.*

### DIFFERENTIAL

Infectious esophagitis, pill esophagitis, gastritis, PUD, functional dyspepsia, biliary tract disease, CAD, esophageal motility disorders.

### DIAGNOSIS

- Mild, low-risk cases (i.e., those with no dysphagia, odynophagia, anemia, or weight loss) are usually diagnosed clinically and supported by patients' response to empiric treatment.
- **EGD:** Can be used to evaluate for Barrett's esophagus, erosions, strictures, or ulcers. Barium swallow is less popular owing to its lower sensitivity in milder cases of GERD.
- **Wireless capsule endoscopy:** Has been approved by the FDA for evaluation of the esophagus in patients with heartburn. Sensitivities are nearly equal to those of EGD.
- **Twenty-four-hour pH probe monitoring:** Can be useful for confirming the disease in patients with persistent symptoms, especially if a trial of acid suppression has failed and/or EGD is $\ominus$.

### TREATMENT

- **Lifestyle modifications:**
    - **Elevation of the head of the bed:** Especially beneficial for nocturnal or laryngeal symptoms. Elevation should be approximately six inches.
    - **Dietary modifications:** Include avoidance of **reflux-inducing foods** (chocolate, peppermint, alcohol, fatty foods); avoidance of **acidic foods** (orange juice, coffee, colas, red wine); consumption of **smaller, more frequent meals;** and use of lozenges or chewing gum (promote salivation, which neutralizes gastric contents).
    - **Other:** Avoidance of tight-fitting garments; smoking and alcohol cessation.
- **Antacids:**
    - **H₂ blockers:** Good for mild cases, but not effective for more severe disease.
    - **PPIs:** More effective than H₂ blockers in healing and providing symptomatic relief.
    - Intermittent therapy with 2–4 weeks of H₂ blockers or PPIs is a reasonable approach for mild GERD.
    - Maintenance therapy is usually required, with doses titrated to the minimum needed to prevent recurrence.
- **Prokinetics:** Metoclopramide, bethanechol. Useful adjuncts, but not appropriate as monotherapy. Side effects limit their use.
- **Surgery:**
    - Generally reserved for patients in whom symptoms persist despite optimal medical therapy; those who are unable to tolerate or comply with medical management; and those with severe esophagitis, stricture, Barrett's metaplasia, or pulmonary complications.

*There is no clear relationship between H. pylori and GERD and no evidence that H. pylori eradication improves GERD symptoms.*

- The most common techniques (**Nissen fundoplication, Hill repair, Belsey Mark IV**) improve symptoms and heal the disease in about 85% of cases.

### COMPLICATIONS

Complications of GERD include the following:

- **Complications of prolonged acid suppression:** Include pneumonia and enteric infections (due to easier colonization of pathogens in the upper GI tract) as well as vitamin $B_{12}$ malabsorption (associated with prolonged omeprazole use).
- **Barrett's esophagus:**
  - Metaplastic process in which stratified squamous epithelium is replaced by **intestinal-type (columnar) epithelium** during the healing phases of esophagitis. Occurs in 4–10% of patients with significant heartburn.
  - The presence of Barrett's esophagus ↑ the risk of esophageal adenocarcinoma, with an annual cancer incidence of 0.2–2.0%. Treatment includes aggressive antireflux therapy.
  - There are no well-established guidelines for cancer surveillance; however, patients ≥ 50 years of age with persistent GERD symptoms are sometimes screened with EGD and biopsy.
- **Peptic stricture:** Suggested by progressive dysphagia and episodic obstruction. Barium swallows are helpful in diagnosis. The treatment of choice is endoscopic balloon dilation.
- **Asthma:** Caused by microaspiration and ↑ vagal tone from acid stimulation of the esophagus. Can occur in the absence of other reflux symptoms. Consider in asthmatics who fail to respond to conventional asthma therapy.
- **Others: Chronic cough,** periodontal disease, chronic sinusitis, recurrent pneumonitis, nocturnal choking, chronic hoarseness, pharyngitis, subglottic stenosis, laryngeal/tracheal stenosis (with prolonged intubation and concomitant reflux).

## DISORDERS OF THE STOMACH

### Gastritis/Gastropathy

Defined as injury to the mucosa of the stomach with epithelial cell damage and regeneration. Injury associated with inflammation is termed *gastritis*, and that unrelated to inflammation is termed *gastropathy*. The etiologies of gastropathy include drugs (**NSAIDs**), alcohol, bile reflux, severe illness, and portal hypertension. The etiologies of gastritis include the following:

- **Acute gastritis:** Typically caused by an acute **H. pylori infection,** although etiologic agents such as CMV have been implicated in immunocompromised and iatrogenic cases. Can progress to chronic gastritis if not treated.
- **Chronic (metaplastic) gastritis:** Categorized according to the site affected.
  - **Type A:** Primarily affects the fundus and body with antral sparing. Includes **autoimmune gastritis,** in which antibodies against parietal cells and intrinsic factor (IF) → pernicious anemia (cobalamin deficiency, megaloblastic anemia, subacute combined degeneration) and achlorhydria.

- **Type B:** Predominantly affects the antrum, progressing to the fundus. Caused by *H. pylori*. Can → multifocal atropic gastritis, gastric atrophy, and metaplasia, increasing the risk of developing gastric adenocarcinoma.

### SYMPTOMS

There is a **poor correlation** between symptoms (e.g., pain and dyspepsia) and endoscopic findings. However, acute *H. pylori* gastritis can → **sudden onset of epigastric pain, nausea, and vomiting,** while gastropathy caused by NSAID use, alcohol, or portal hypertension can present with **GI bleeding.**

### EXAM

- Exam is usually unremarkable, but abdominal tenderness may be seen.
- Signs of $B_{12}$ deficiency (anemia, neurologic signs) may also be noted.

### DIFFERENTIAL

See the differential for PUD below. Rarer causes include granulomatous disease (TB, fungal, sarcoid, Crohn's) and Ménétrier's disease (characterized by giant thickened folds of mucosa).

### DIAGNOSIS

- Diagnosis is largely clinical but can include noninvasive *H. pylori* testing (see Table 5.2), evaluation for suspected autoimmune gastritis via anti–parietal cell and IF antibodies, and analysis of the serum pepsinogen I-to-II ratio.
- **EGD** with biopsy can provide a pathologic diagnosis.

### TREATMENT

- Treatment generally consists of avoidance of causative factors (e.g., NSAIDs, alcohol) along with **prophylaxis** (IV ranitidine in critically ill patients; nonselective β-blockers for varices).
- *H. pylori* eradication; parenteral vitamin $B_{12}$ for pernicious anemia.

A 50-year-old man presents with one month of epigastric pain that seems to improve with meals and calcium carbonate. He has no family history of upper GI malignancies, weight loss, early satiety, vomiting, or dysphagia, and he has no signs of anemia. His only medication is naproxen, which he takes for low back pain. He does not smoke but enjoys having a glass of wine with each dinner. What do you tell the patient? You tell the patient that something may be wrong in his upper GI tract, and you recommend an EGD. He should stop taking naproxen and stop drinking wine. The patient's EGD demonstrates a duodenal ulcer, and his biopsy urease test is ⊕ for *H. pylori*. How will you treat him? You prescribe him triple therapy. Two months later, he reports some improvement but continues to have symptoms and remains on his PPI. Should you order a stool *H. pylori* antigen test to check for eradication? You defer this, as you know it won't be accurate while he is on a PPI. On closer questioning, you find that he actually never filled his prescription for the antibiotics because he felt that the drugs were "too expensive."

TABLE 5.2. Testing Methods for *H. pylori*

| TYPE | ADVANTAGES | DISADVANTAGES |
|---|---|---|
| **Invasive** | | |
| Biopsy urease test | The test of choice; sensitivity is 90–95% and specificity 95–100%. | False $\ominus$s occur with use of PPIs and $H_2$ blockers as well as with GI bleeding, antibiotics, and bismuth. |
| Histology | Useful in excluding gastritis, intestinal metaplasia, and MALT lymphoma. | Prone to sampling error and interobserver variability; has ↓ sensitivity if the patient is taking antisecretory therapy. |
| Brush cytology | Sensitivity and specificity are similar to those of the biopsy urease test. | Not commonly done unless the patient has a bleeding disorder. |
| Culture for *H. pylori* | | Not done routinely; mostly for suspected antibiotic resistance if sensitivities are needed. |
| **Noninvasive** | | |
| Urea breath test | The best nonendoscopic test. Uses urea with radiolabeled carbon, allowing liberated $CO_2$ to be detected. Has 88–95% sensitivity and 95–100% specificity. | The same factors causing false $\ominus$s with the biopsy urease test apply |
| Stool antigen testing | As good as the urea breath test. | Less accurate if the patient is on PPIs or bismuth. |
| *H. pylori* serology (IgG, IgA) | Inexpensive and has good sensitivity (90–100%). | Specificity is 76–96%; reliable if consistent with pretest probability. Not useful to confirm eradication, as it takes several months for patients to seroconvert. |

## Peptic Ulcer Disease (PUD)

The principal cause of PUD is ***H. pylori* infection,** which → 70–80% of duodenal and 60–70% of gastric ulcers. Most cases that are not associated with *H. pylori* are related to **NSAID** use. Zollinger-Ellison syndrome is another significant cause. Additional risk factors include tobacco, medications (e.g., aspirin, antiplatelet agents, KCl, mycophenolate), physiologic stress (i.e., ICU), and, less often, CMV, HSV-1, and chemoradiation. **Psychological stress is not a cause,** and corticosteroids are not a contributing factor unless they are used in association with NSAIDs.

### SYMPTOMS

- May be asymptomatic ("silent disease"; more common in the elderly and in NSAID users), or may present with dyspepsia or with severe, hunger-like epigastric pain accompanied by burning and gnawing.
- Symptoms are further distinguished as follows:
  - **Gastric ulcers:** Classically present with **severe pain soon after meals. Relief with antacid intake or food consumption is less frequent than with duodenal ulcers.**
  - **Duodenal ulcers:** Classically present as **pain 2–5 hours after meals** along with night symptoms occurring from 11 P.M. to 2 A.M. **Food and antacids tend to relieve symptoms.**

### EXAM

Exam may reveal epigastric tenderness.

### DIFFERENTIAL

Functional dyspepsia, gastric cancer, drug-induced dyspepsia (NSAIDs), sarcoidosis, Crohn's disease, infections (TB, strongyloidiasis, giardiasis), GERD, biliary tract disease, gastroparesis, pancreatitis, malabsorption.

### DIAGNOSIS

- **EGD:** The diagnostic **gold standard,** allowing for the **differentiation of benign ulcers from cancer.** Indicated to rule out malignancy if any **alarm signs** are present (e.g., if patients are > 45 years of age and have weight loss, anemia, bleeding, vomiting, dysphagia, a family history of gastric cancer, or previous gastric surgery).
- **Upper GI series:** Less favored owing to its variable sensitivity (50–90%).
- *H. pylori* **testing** (see Table 5.2).

*Many tests for* H. pylori *(except serology testing) will be falsely* ⊖ *if a patient is on acid suppression therapy.*

### TREATMENT

- **Lifestyle modifications:** Include **smoking cessation;** alcohol avoidance; caffeine avoidance; and avoidance of NSAIDs or aspirin.
- **Acid suppressors:** Include $H_2$ blockers, PPIs, and sucralfate. Maintenance acid suppression may be required to prevent recurrence or to treat complications.
- *H. pylori* **infection:** Eradicate *H. pylori* if indicated. Continued acid suppression is necessary to allow the ulcer to heal. In complex cases, *H. pylori* testing should be repeated roughly four weeks after healing to confirm disease resolution. Regimens include a combination of two antibiotics and a PPI or an $H_2$ blocker, +/– bismuth.
- **Surgical intervention:** Indications include failure of medical management; suspicion of cancer (e.g., a gastric ulcer that fails to heal after 12 weeks); perforation; outlet obstruction (failing to resolve after > 72 hours); and failure to arrest bleeding. Duodenal ulcers are typically treated with a highly selective vagotomy with either pyloroplasty or antrectomy (with a Billroth I or II anastomosis); gastric ulcers are treated with distal gastrectomy/antrectomy with a Billroth anastomosis, but vagotomies are not performed unless there is a coexisting duodenal ulcer.

*The prevalence of peptic ulcers in patients with dyspepsia who test positive for* H. pylori *is 15–30%. Therefore, if a patient is at* **low risk** *for malignancy,* H. pylori *eradication is considered acceptable without endoscopic evaluation.*

### COMPLICATIONS

- **Lack of response:** Causes of treatment failure include *H. pylori* resistance, noncompliance with medical therapy/supportive measures, giant ulcers (those > 2 cm have a lesser chance of healing), $H_2$ blocker/PPI resistance or tolerance, cancer, Crohn's disease, infection, and **Zollinger-Ellison syndrome** (pancreatic gastrinoma; ↑ **fasting serum gastrin**).
- Fibrotic scar, penetrating ulcers (more localized and intense pain radiating to the back), perforation (sudden diffuse abdominal pain and peritonitis), pyloric channel obstruction (early satiety, vomiting, nausea, weight loss, pain, and bloating), hemorrhage (nausea, hematemesis, melena, and dizziness).
- **Complications of surgery:** Ulcer recurrence, afferent loop syndrome (due to bacterial overgrowth or partial obstruction of loop), dumping syndrome (due to ↑ hyperosmolar loads to the small bowel), postvagotomy diarrhea, bile reflux gastropathy, maldigestion, malabsorption, and gastric cancer.

### Gastroparesis and Intestinal Pseudo-obstruction

Obstructive symptoms in the stomach/bowel in the **absence of an anatomic lesion.** May be idiopathic or 2° to diabetes, hypothyroidism, neurologic disorders, rheumatologic disease (scleroderma), amyloidosis, paraneoplastic disease, or drugs (e.g., anticholinergics, calcium channel blockers, $\alpha_2$-adrenergic agonists).

### SYMPTOMS/EXAM

- **Gastroparesis:** Presents with early satiety, nausea, and vomiting soon after meals.
- **Intestinal pseudo-obstruction:** Presents with bloating/distention, nausea, and vomiting.
- Exam may reveal abdominal distention and/or succussion splash (heard when shaking the abdomen by holding the pelvis, indicating free fluid).

### DIAGNOSIS

- **Plain films:** Occasionally show gaseous distention of the stomach or the bowel.
- **Upper GI series with small bowel follow-through:** Used to rule out mechanical obstruction.
- **Gastric scintigraphy:** Establishes delayed gastric emptying.

### TREATMENT

- **Acute episodes:** Treat with NPO, NG suction, and IV fluids.
- **Nutritional support:** Small, frequent meals with fewer fatty or gas-forming foods. Parenteral nutrition if necessary.
- **Prokinetics:** Metoclopramide, cisapride (has limited use in the United States because drug interactions ↑ the risk of fatal arrhythmias). **IV erythromycin** for acute episodes.
- **Strict glycemic control** in diabetic gastroparesis.
- Discontinue drugs that slow intestinal motility (e.g., anticholinergics, opioids).

## DISORDERS OF THE BOWEL

### Acute Diarrhea

Defined as diarrhea lasting **two weeks or less.** One of five leading causes of death worldwide. **Ninety percent** of cases are caused by **infectious agents.** Most of these agents are viral, but severe cases are more frequently caused by bacteria (1.5–5.6% of mild cases are due to bacterial infection, vs. 87% of severe cases). The remaining 10% are due to **medications, toxin ingestion, and ischemia.** Some chronic cases present acutely, as in **IBD** or **diverticulitis.** Risk factors for acute infection are as follows:

*Do not give antibiotics to patients with suspected enterohemorrhagic E. coli infection (bloody stools, abdominal pain/tenderness, little or no fever), as there is no evidence that antibiotics are of benefit, and there is a theoretical risk of causing hemolytic-uremic syndrome.*

- **Travel:** Forty percent of travelers to Asia, Latin America, or Africa get "traveler's diarrhea." The most common infectious agents are enterotoxigenic *E. coli, Campylobacter, Shigella,* and *Salmonella.* Campers, backpackers, and travelers to Russia are susceptible to *Giardia.*
- **Contaminated food ingestion:** Usually associated with food consumption at picnics, banquets, or restaurants. Commonly implicated foods include chicken, hamburger (enterohemorrhagic *E. coli*), fried rice, mayonnaise, eggs, and raw seafood.
- **High-risk populations:** Include immunocompromised patients, day care workers and their contacts, and health care workers.
- **Recent antibiotic use:** Can be related or unrelated to *C. difficile* infection.

## DIAGNOSIS

- Indications for evaluation include profuse diarrhea with dehydration, grossly bloody stools, fever ≥ 38.5°C, illness lasting > 48 hours without improvement, advanced age, severe abdominal pain in patients > 50 years of age, community outbreaks, > 6 stools in 24 hours, recent use of antibiotics, and hospitalization.
- Diagnostic modalities include the following:
  - **Fecal leukocytes:** Sensitivity and specificity for inflammation vary from 20% to 90%. Useful if preclinical suspicion for an inflammatory etiology is high.
  - **Bacterial stool culture:** Controversial because acute infectious diarrhea is often viral and bacterial cases are usually self-limited. However, stool cultures should be obtained in immunocompromised patients, those with significant comorbidities, and those with IBD (to differentiate flare from infection). Routine cultures will identify *Salmonella*, *Shigella*, and *Campylobacter* but not *Yersinia* or *Aeromonas*. The **false-⊖ rate is low** (i.e., repeat testing is not necessary).
  - **Viral stool culture and antigens.**
  - **Stool ova and parasites (O&P):** Usually obtained if diarrhea is persistent (> 2 weeks) or for patients who have traveled to the developing world, men who have sex with men (MSM), AIDS patients, those involved in waterborne outbreaks, and those with bloody diarrhea with few or no fecal leukocytes (suggestive of amebiasis). Send O&P on three consecutive days, each spaced > 24 hours apart.
  - **Endoscopy:** Appropriate if IBD or pseudomembranous/ischemic colitis is suspected.
  - **Other:** Toxin assays (e.g., *C. difficile*); stool *Giardia* antigen; *Entamoeba histolytica* antigen.
- Figure 5.1 shows an algorithm for the diagnosis of acute diarrhea.

## TREATMENT

- **Fluid and electrolyte replacement:** Consists of ½ teaspoon of salt, ½ teaspoon of baking soda, and 4 tablespoons of sugar in 1 L of water for oral rehydration. IV fluids may be needed.
- **Loperamide and diphenoxylate:** Generally safe for the alleviation of symptoms in afebrile and nonbloody cases, but may prolong disease in patients who are febrile.
- **Bismuth subsalicylate:** Can ↓ nausea and vomiting, but avoid in immunocompromised patients in light of the risk of bismuth encephalopathy.
- **Antibiotics** if indicated:
  - **Fluoroquinolones:** For suspected bacterial infection; give for 3–5 days. Administer a **macrolide** if resistance is suspected, especially in traveler's diarrhea.
  - **Metronidazole:** For cases suspected to be related to *Giardia* or *C. difficile*.
  - Always give antibiotics to elderly patients, immunocompromised patients, and those with heart or vascular grafts.
- **Probiotics:** Have been proven to aid recolonization in pediatric patients, but their efficacy has not been established in adults.

## Chronic Diarrhea

Defined as diarrhea **lasting > 4 weeks.** In the developing world, it is most often due to chronic infections, whereas in the developed world it is primarily caused by IBS, IBD, and malabsorption syndromes. Subtypes are as follows:

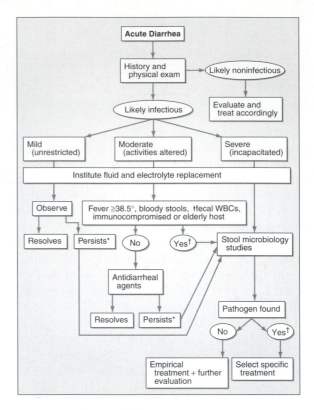

**FIGURE 5.1.** **Diagnosis of acute diarrhea.**

(Reproduced, with permission, from Kasper DL et al. *Harrison's Principles of Internal Medicine*, 16th ed. New York: McGraw-Hill, 2005: 227.)

*Nocturnal diarrhea is not characteristic of IBS and must be evaluated for another cause.*

- **Secretory:** Deranged transport of fluid and electrolytes across the mucosa. Usually presents with watery, large-volume diarrhea that persists with fasting. Causes include medications, laxatives, chronic alcohol consumption (enterocyte injury), toxins, cholerrheic diarrhea, partial obstruction/strictures/fecal impaction (→ paradoxical hypersecretion), carcinoid, and VIPoma.
- **Osmotic:** Due to a poorly absorbed osmotically active substance. Diarrhea is usually watery and ↑ with increasing solute load. Characterized by an ↑ **stool osmotic gap, calculated as 290 − [2 (Na + K)].** Causes include carbohydrate malabsorption (→ watery diarrhea) and fat malabsorption (→ greasy diarrhea).
- **Inflammatory:** Due to mucosal inflammation. Diarrhea is generally bloody and accompanied by fever and abdominal pain. Causes include infections, IBD, radiation enterocolitis, and eosinophilic gastroenteritis.
- **Dysmotile:** Associated with hyperthyroidism, diabetes, carcinoid, drugs, and IBS.
- **Factitious:** Associated with Munchausen's syndrome and bulimia.

### DIAGNOSIS

Figure 5.2 shows an algorithm to guide the diagnosis of chronic diarrhea.

### TREATMENT

- Treat the underlying cause.
- **Pharmacotherapy:**
  - **Loperamide and diphenoxylate:** Can be used for mild or moderate watery diarrhea.

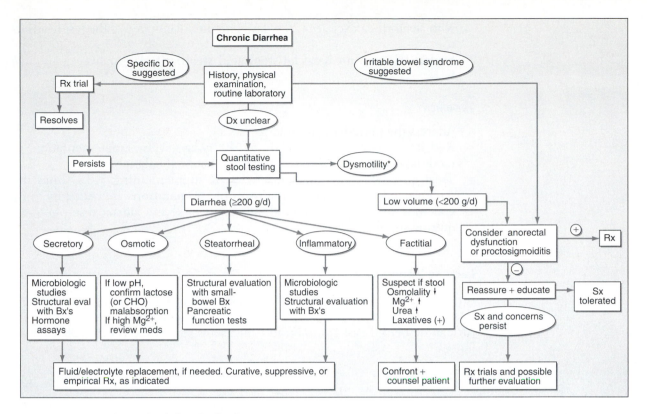

**FIGURE 5.2.** **Diagnosis of chronic diarrhea.**

(Reproduced, with permission, from Kasper DL et al. *Harrison's Principles of Internal Medicine*, 16th ed. New York: McGraw-Hill, 2005: 230.)

- **Codeine and tincture of opium:** Can be used for more severe diarrhea, but avoid in inflammatory diarrhea (can precipitate toxic megacolon in IBD).
- Fluid, electrolyte, and vitamin replacement as needed.

## Fat Malabsorption

Results from failure to digest, absorb, or transport fat or from a deficiency of bile with failed compensatory hepatic synthesis.

### SYMPTOMS/EXAM

- Presents with diarrhea, steatorrhea, and weight loss.
- Symptoms of fat-soluble vitamin deficiencies may be seen (associated blindness, osteopenia, and bleeding).

### DIFFERENTIAL

Lipolysis defects (i.e., chronic pancreatitis), ↓ bile acid synthesis (liver disease) or secretion (biliary disease), bile acid deconjugation (i.e., bacterial overgrowth) or loss (i.e., Crohn's, ileal resection), mucosal dysfunction (i.e., celiac disease), postabsorption defects (i.e., abetalipoproteinemia).

### DIAGNOSIS

- **Fecal fat collection** (72-hour stool collection): The gold standard. Fat malabsorption is defined as stool fat excretion > 6 g/day; however, patients

*Steatorrhea is not synonymous with cholerrheic diarrhea ("bile acid diarrhea"). In this disorder, excessive bile enters the colon and → a secretory diarrhea (via stimulation of chloride secretion), as seen in patients with ileal disease/resection.*

with steatorrhea excrete > 20 g/day. The inconvenience of the test limits its use.

- **Sudan III stain for fecal fat/stool acid steatocrit:** Alternative, qualitative tests.

### TREATMENT

- Address the underlying disorder.
- Restrict long-chain fatty acids to 40 g/day, with supplementation of medium-chain fatty acids to maintain nutritional balance.
- Treat fat-soluble vitamin deficiencies by supplementing **5–10 times** the recommended daily value. **Water-soluble preparations** are necessary.
- Calcium and magnesium bind fatty acids in severe fat malabsorption, requiring supplementation.

## Lactose Intolerance

**A prototypical carbohydrate malabsorption disorder.** Has a high prevalence in East Asians and Native Americans and a moderate prevalence in those of African descent. Least common in Caucasians (but still has up to 20% prevalence).

*Although lactose intolerance is commonly a 1° disorder, it may also be 2° to a number of conditions (e.g., celiac disease, bacterial overgrowth, gastroenteritis) because of the susceptible location of lactase on the distal villi.*

### SYMPTOMS/EXAM

- Presents with diarrhea, cramps, abdominal pain, and/or flatus following the ingestion of milk products. Symptom severity depends on the amount of lactose ingested and the fat content of the product (skim milk empties from the stomach faster → more symptoms).
- Exam may reveal abdominal distention and hyperactive bowel sounds.

### DIFFERENTIAL

See the differential for chronic diarrhea.

### DIAGNOSIS

- **Lactose tolerance test:** Measures serum glucose in blood 0, 60, and 120 minutes after the ingestion of 50 g of lactose. An ↑ in glucose of > 20 mg/dL in conjunction with symptoms is diagnostic.
- **Lactose breath hydrogen test:** Measures $H_2$ in the breath at 30-minute intervals following an oral challenge of 2 g/kg. An ↑ in breath hydrogen of > 20 ppm is diagnostic (the ↑ is due to bacterial fermentation of nonabsorbed lactose).
- **Other:** Nonspecific tests such as stool pH, stool-reducing substances, and stool osmotic gap (osmotic diarrhea) can aid in diagnosis.

*Loss of lactase does not happen until age five; an abnormal breath test in children under age five points to another mucosal problem.*

### TREATMENT

- Lactose restriction (milk and ice cream have more lactose than cheese).
- Lactase preparations can ↓ symptoms.
- Calcium and vitamin D supplementation if the patient ↓ milk products.

## Celiac Disease

An immune disorder that is triggered by the **gliadin component of gluten** and can affect any part of the intestine. Once considered a disease of infancy, it now presents more often between the ages of 10 and 40, presumably because of longer breast-feeding periods and later introduction of gluten into the diet. **Spontaneous remissions and exacerbations** are common. Associated with autoimmune disorders (type 1 DM, autoimmune thyroiditis, autoimmune hepatitis) as well as with dermatitis herpetiformis and IgA deficiency. More common among Caucasians.

*Iron deficiency anemia may be the only presenting sign of celiac disease in some patients.*

### SYMPTOMS/EXAM

- Can range from significant disease → diarrhea, steatorrhea, and weight loss to the absence of symptoms except those of a single nutrient deficiency (e.g., anemia, metabolic bone disease).
- Exam may reveal no abnormalities or only those due to a particular nutrient deficiency.

### DIAGNOSIS

- **Small intestinal biopsy:** The gold standard. Reveals suggestive (not diagnostic) changes that are confirmed by reversion to normal histology following initiation of a gluten-free diet.
- **Antiendomysial IgA** and **anti–tissue transglutaminase (anti-TTG) IgA:**
  - Excellent screening tests with 95% and 100% sensitivities, respectively. Can also be used to follow titers in order to gauge clinical improvement.
  - Screens should be followed by endoscopy with biopsy.
  - Antigliadin IgA is no longer favored owing to its lower sensitivity and specificity.
- Transaminases may be elevated.

### TREATMENT

- **Dietary modifications:**
  - Institute a **gluten-free diet** (avoidance of wheat, rye, and barley products) supplemented by nutritional counseling.
  - Avoid lactose, as 2° intolerance is common.
  - Specific dietary deficiencies, such as deficiencies of iron, folic acid, calcium, vitamin D, and, rarely, vitamin $B_{12}$, should be corrected.
- Educate patients about the relapsing and remitting nature of the disease.
- Consider pneumococcal vaccination, as celiac disease is associated with hyposplenism.

### COMPLICATIONS

**Refractory sprue.** May be due to other dietary agents. Associated with an ↑ risk of progressive malabsorption and death. Treatment consists largely of immunosuppression (steroids) and, increasingly, immunomodulator therapy.

## Short Gut Syndrome

A malabsorptive state following massive small bowel resection, usually for Crohn's disease, malignancy, mesenteric ischemia, or radiation.

### SYMPTOMS/EXAM

Presents with diarrhea and symptoms or signs of specific nutrient or vitamin deficiencies, depending on the nature of the resection. Common examples: resection of > 60 cm of ileum → malabsorpion of IF-bound $B_{12}$; > 100 cm of ileum → bile salt and, therefore, fat malabsorption; loss of ileocecal valve → bacterial overgrowth and ↓ intestinal transit time.

**DIAGNOSIS**

Usually clinical and suggested by the surgical history.

**TREATMENT**

- Treat with dietary adjustment to maximize nutrition while avoiding steatorrhea or osmotic diarrhea. Fiber can help adsorb water and also ↑ bacterial production of short-chain fatty acids to provide additional calories.
- Moderate use of **opiates** can ↑ transit time.
- **Cholestyramine** for cholerrheic diarrhea; **calcium supplementation** for hyperoxaluria.
- Monitor and replace vitamins and minerals (e.g., monthly vitamin $B_{12}$ IM).
- TPN may be necessary if alimentary feeds are insufficient.
- Intestinal transplantation if extensive resection has occurred and medical therapy fails.

## Bacterial Overgrowth

*Bacterial overgrowth should be suspected in any patient with a predisposing condition who presents with malabsorptive symptoms.*

There are relatively fewer bacteria in the upper GI tract than in the lower GI tract (especially the colon). In bacterial overgrowth, there is an ↑ in the number of bacteria in the more proximal GI tract. This can be caused by anything causing abnormal stasis (e.g., stricture, blind loops), ↓ motility, or abnormal communications between the proximal and distal GI tract (e.g., fistula, ileocecal valve resection). Bacterial overgrowth → **carbohydrate malabsorption** (due to bacterial consumption), **fat malabsorption** (through deconjugation of bile, which also has a direct toxic effect on the mucosa, aggravating carbohydrate malabsorption), and **vitamin $B_{12}$ deficiency** (as bacteria compete with the host for vitamin $B_{12}$). **Altered intestinal motility** is also seen.

**SYMPTOMS/EXAM**

- Presents with diarrhea, steatorrhea, bloating, flatulence, anemia, subacute combined degeneration, weight loss, and associated calcium and fat-soluble vitamin deficiencies.
- Exam may reveal a succussion splash or distention.

**DIAGNOSIS**

The gold standard is a **jejunal aspirate** showing a bacterial count of >$10^5$; breath hydrogen testing can also be done. Alternatively, an empiric trial of antibiotics can be attempted.

**TREATMENT**

- Treat the disorder predisposing to overgrowth.
- Correct vitamin deficiencies if present.
- **Antibiotics** to alter (not eliminate) flora include amoxicillin-clavulanate, cephalexin plus metronidazole, TMP-SMX plus metronidazole, norfloxacin, and oral gentamicin plus metronidazole. Usually given for 7–10 days, but it may be necessary to prolong treatment, offer repeat courses, and rotate antibiotics to prevent resistance.
- ↓ drugs that slow motility or gastric acidity.
- Periodic polyethylene glycol can help with overgrowth by transient reduction.

- A high-fat, low-carbohydrate diet is of benefit, as bacteria rely more on carbohydrates.
- Probiotics may be tried, but their efficacy is unclear.

## Inflammatory Bowel Disease (IBD)

Chronic inflammatory disease of the GI tract. The two main subtypes are Crohn's disease and ulcerative colitis (see Table 5.3).

A 35-year-old female human resource manager returns for her follow-up visit for six months of intermittent lower abdominal discomfort and bloating. The patient also has frequent diarrhea, which alleviates her discomfort to some degree. She is able to sleep well at night and has had no fever, weight loss, or bloody stools. She denies a family history of colorectal cancer. Initial tests, including a complete metabolic panel, CBC, TSH, fecal occult blood test (FOBT), and stool O&P, have all been ⊖, and two weeks of a food journal have revealed no dietary triggers. What is the most likely diagnosis? Irritable bowel syndrome. What treatments would you offer? Low-dose TCAs and loperamide as well as elimination trials of dairy, caffeine, and gas-causing foods.

## Irritable Bowel Syndrome (IBS)

A functional disorder characterized by **abdominal pain and discomfort** with associated **disturbed defecation.** Its etiology is believed to be multifactorial, involving altered gut motility/secretion, visceral hypersensitivity, and brain–gut axis dysregulation. IBS is the most commonly diagnosed GI condition and is the second most common cause of work absenteeism, exceeded only by the common cold. It is more prevalent in women and generally presents between the ages of 30 and 50.

### SYMPTOMS/EXAM

- **1° symptoms:** Abdominal discomfort, relief of discomfort with defecation, a change in frequency and/or form of stool (may be diarrhea- or constipation-predominant).
- **Other symptoms:** Straining, urgency, or a feeling of incomplete evacuation; passage of mucus; bloating.
- Exam typically yields no physical findings, but mild lower abdominal tenderness may be seen.

### DIFFERENTIAL

IBD, colon cancer, hyperthyroidism, hypothyroidism, chronic diarrhea (infectious, malabsorption), chronic constipation, celiac sprue.

### DIAGNOSIS

- Presumes the absence of a structural or biochemical explanation for the symptoms.
- The absence of alarm signs (e.g., fever, weight loss, blood in the stool, anemia, a family history of IBD or colon cancer, progressive symptoms, pain

**TABLE 5.3.** Crohn's Disease vs. Ulcerative Colitis

| | CROHN'S DISEASE | ULCERATIVE COLITIS |
|---|---|---|
| Disease characteristics | **Transmucosal inflammation** → ulceration, strictures, fistulas, and abscesses. | **Mucosal inflammation** → friability, erosions, and bleeding. |
| GI tract involvement | May affect any part of the GI tract from the mouth to the anus, but typically affects the **small bowel and colon.** Some 30% of disease occurs in the ileum; 20% occurs in the colon, and 50% occurs in both. | The **rectum** is invariably involved. Extends **proximally** in a **continuous** fashion to involve the colon. Some 50% of cases involve the rectosigmoid colon; 30% extend to the splenic flexure, and 20% extend proximal to the splenic flexure. |
| GI bleeding manifestations | Guaiac-⊕ stools are common; **grossly bloody stools are uncommon.** | **Bloody stools are common.** |
| Symptoms | Presents with chronic diarrhea, crampy abdominal pain, fever, weight loss, and fatigue. Strictures → obstructive symptoms. Fistulization → recurrent UTIs/pneumaturia, gas/feces from the vagina, psoas abscesses, and ureteral obstruction. | Presents with chronic bloody diarrhea, abdominal pain, cramps, tenesmus, and fecal urgency. |
| Exam | Exam may reveal pallor, weight loss, a palpable mass (in some cases of perforation and localized peritonitis), **aphthous ulcers, anal fissures, perirectal abscesses,** and **anorectal fistulas.** | Exam reveals abdominal tenderness and **gross blood on DRE.** |
| Extraintestinal manifestations | Uncommon, but those seen in ulcerative colitis may also be seen in Crohn's disease. | Uveitis, episcleritis, erythema nodosum, pyoderma gangrenosum, arthritis, ankylosing spondylitis, venous/arterial thromboembolism, sclerosing cholangitis. |
| Differential | Ulcerative colitis, acute infectious diarrhea (*Shigella, Salmonella, Campylobacter, E. coli* O157:H7), acute ileitis (*Yersinia* spp.), TB of the bowel, amebiasis, pseudomembranous colitis, CMV colitis (in the immunosuppressed), appendicitis, diverticulitis, ischemic colitis, lymphoma, carcinoma. | Crohn's disease, radiation proctitis, ischemic/pseudomembranous/infectious colitis, infectious proctitis (gonorrhea, chlamydia, herpes, syphilis), amebiasis, CMV/Kaposi's sarcoma in the immunosuppressed. |
| Endoscopic evaluation | **Colonoscopy** with intubation of the terminal ileum (reveals skip lesions, linear ulcers, and cobblestone mucosa) with biopsy. An upper GI series with small bowel follow-through or barium enema may also be needed to identify disease in the small bowel. | **Flexible sigmoidoscopy** is usually adequate (shows pseudopolyps, bleeding, petechiae, ulcers, and exudates) with biopsy. Colonoscopy may → perforation in severe disease but may be used to evaluate the extent of disease. |

TABLE 5.3. Crohn's Disease vs. Ulcerative Colitis (continued)

GASTROENTEROLOGY

|  | CROHN'S DISEASE | ULCERATIVE COLITIS |
|---|---|---|
| Autoantibodies (sent if diagnosis after endoscopy remains uncertain) | **ASCA** is present in 60–70% of cases; **p-ANCA** is present in 5–10%. **ASCA**-⊕/p-ANCA-⊖ findings are 90% specific for Crohn's disease. | **p-ANCA** is present in 50–70% of cases; **ASCA** is present in 10–15%. **p-ANCA**-⊕/ASCA-⊖ findings are 98% specific for ulcerative colitis. |
| Labs | Micro- or macrocytic anemia, leukocytosis, hypoalbuminemia. Stool studies are ⊖ for an infectious cause. | Same (but macrocytic anemia is less likely). |
| Diet recommendations | High-fiber diet with colonic involvement; conversely, low roughage if obstructive symptoms are present. A trial of lactose elimination may benefit those with 2° intolerance. | High-fiber diet; limit caffeine and gas-producing foods. A trial of lactose elimination may be beneficial. |
| Medical therapy | **Ileitis:** Mesalamine (sulfasalazine is activated in the colon, so it should not be used). **Ileocolitis/colitis:** Mesalamine or sulfasalazine. Steroids or antibiotics (ciprofloxacin for ileitis; metronidazole for ileocolitis/colitis) may be required. Refractory cases require azathioprine, 6-MP, or infliximab. **Surgery is not curative.** | **Proctitis:** 5-ASA suppositories (or steroid suppositories/foams); 5-ASA enemas (or steroid enemas) for left-sided colitis. **Extensive/pancolitis:** Combined oral/rectal ASA agents and/or steroid enemas, with oral corticosteroids for refractory cases (cyclosporine if steroid refractory). Treat severe/fulminant cases with bowel rest, IV steroids, and antibiotics if the patient appears septic. **Colectomy is curative.** |
| Complications | Localized perforation/peritonitis, abscess, fistulas, bowel obstruction, massive hemorrhage, toxic megacolon, colon cancer, short gut syndrome (after resection). | Massive hemorrhage, fulminant colitis, toxic megacolon, perforation, stricture, colon cancer. |

preventing sleeping or awakening the patient from sleep) is essential to diagnosis.

- Diagnostic tests may be used on a limited basis to exclude organic disease and include stool hemoccult, CBC, ESR (especially in younger patients), serum chemistry, albumin, stool O&P × 3, TSH, and antiendomysial/anti-TTG antibodies.

*IBS is a clinical diagnosis, so diagnostic testing should be limited.*

### TREATMENT

- **Establishment of a therapeutic alliance:** It is important to remain non-judgmental, to provide reassurance that the disease is benign, and to promote patient involvement in treatment decisions.
- **Dietary modification:** Limitation of dairy products, caffeine, and gas-producing foods (e.g., beans, onions) may be of benefit. A symptom diary to identify possible triggers may be useful as well.
- **Pain medications:**
  - **Antispasmodics:** Dicyclomine or hyoscyamine.

- **Antidepressants:** Low-dose TCAs or occasionally SSRIs, especially with comorbid depression, may be of use.
- For **constipation:**
  - ↑ dietary fiber unless bloating is a major factor.
- For **diarrhea:** Loperamide, diphenoxylate, atropine, alosetron.

## Constipation

*An anorectal exam is essential in evaluating neurologic causes of constipation. ↓ rectal tone and sensation suggests sacral nerve or cauda equina lesions, which → hypomobility, dilation, ↓ tone/sensation, stasis, and impaired defecation.*

Has variable causes, including IBS, medication side effects, and metabolic, neurologic, or obstructive intestinal disease (see Table 5.4). Chronic constipation is more common in women, nonwhites, and those > 60 years of age. Constipation can also be idiopathic, characterized by patterns seen on bowel function studies. For example, in **slow-transit constipation,** there is normal resting colonic motility but little or no ↑ after meals or with stimulants. With **dyssynergic defecation,** the pelvic floor muscles and external anal sphincter fail to relax during defecation, making evacuation difficult.

### DIAGNOSIS

- Diagnosis is largely clinical (see Figure 5.3). IBS should be excluded. Drugs should be reviewed for possible temporal relationships.
- Alarm signs for obstruction 2° to malignancy include weight loss, a family history of colon cancer or IBD, anemia, hematochezia, a ⊕ FOBT, or acute onset of symptoms. The presence of an alarm sign should prompt endoscopic evaluation.
- Laboratory tests include serum calcium and TSH for hypercalcemia and hypothyroidism, respectively.
- Barium enemas can detect structural changes, megacolon, and megarectum.

**TABLE 5.4. Causes of Constipation in Adults**

| TYPE OF CONSTIPATION | EXAMPLES |
| --- | --- |
| **Recent onset** | |
| Colonic obstruction | Neoplasm, stricture (ischemic, diverticular, inflammatory). |
| Anal sphincter spasm | Anal fissure, painful hemorrhoids. |
| Medications | Narcotics. |
| **Chronic** | |
| IBS | Constipation-predominant, alternating. |
| Medications | Narcotics, $Ca^{2+}$ blockers, antidepressants. |
| Colonic pseudo-obstruction | Slow-transit constipation, megacolon (rarely, Hirschsprung's and Chagas' disease). |
| Disorders of rectal evacuation | Pelvic floor dysfunction, anismus, descending perineum syndrome, rectal mucosal prolapse, rectocele. |
| Endocrinopathies | Hypothyroidism, hypercalcemia, pregnancy. |
| Psychiatric disorders | Depression, eating disorders, drugs. |
| Neurologic disease | Parkinsonism, MS, spinal cord injury. |
| Generalized muscle disease | Progressive systemic sclerosis. |

Reproduced, with permission, from Kasper DL et al. *Harrison's Principles of Internal Medicine,* 16th ed. New York: McGraw-Hill, 2005: 231.

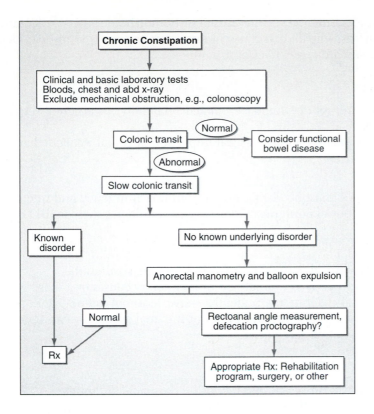

**FIGURE 5.3.** Diagnosis and treatment of constipation.

(Reproduced, with permission, from Kasper DL et al. *Harrison's Principles of Internal Medicine*, 16th ed. New York: McGraw-Hill, 2005: 232.)

- If idiopathic constipation is suspected, workup with marker studies, defecography, or anorectal manometry may prove useful.

### TREATMENT

- **Patient education:** Recommend that patients ↑ fluid and fiber intake, take advantage of ↑ colonic transit after meals (go to the bathroom after eating), and participate in regular physical activity (immobility worsens the condition).
- **Pharmacotherapy:** Fiber, stool surfactants (e.g., docusate), stimulant laxatives (e.g., bisacodyl, senna), osmotic laxatives (e.g., lactulose, polyethylene glycol).
- **Others:**
  - Enemas, biofeedback, digital rectal stimulation.
  - Slow-transit constipation requires aggressive medical treatment. Treatment failure or the presence of a megarectum or megacolon may suggest the need for surgery.

*There is little evidence to support the use of docusate in chronic constipation despite its widespread use.*

## Fecal Incontinence

Affects men and women equally (about 0.5–2.0% of the population), but tends to be more severe in women and the elderly. Usually multifactorial, but generally due to sphincter dysfunction, abnormal rectal compliance, ↓ rectal sensation, or abnormal puborectalis muscle function. Specific etiologies include anal sphincter tears or pudendal nerve trauma during vaginal childbirth, surgical trauma (during fistula or hemorrhoid repairs), ulcerative/radiation proctitis, impaired rectal sensation (e.g., neurologic disease, dementia), fecal impaction, or a cancer/obstructing mass.

### EXAM

- Anal wink reflex should be elicited bilaterally; its absence suggests nerve damage.
- DRE may show a mass or fecal impaction or reveal weakened anal tone.

### DIFFERENTIAL

Incontinence must be distinguished from bowel urgency and frequency **without loss of bowel contents,** which suggests etiologies such as IBD or IBS.

### DIAGNOSIS

- Mostly **clinical,** based on the history and physical exam.
- **Sigmoidoscopy** to evaluate for inflammatory causes or a mass.
- Anorectal manometry, pudendal nerve terminal latency, endorectal ultrasound, defecography, and EMG of the anal sphincter can be done if further evaluation is required.

### TREATMENT

- If present, diarrhea should be further evaluated and treated.
- **Stool disimpaction and bowel regimen:** If fecal impaction is the cause.
- **Regular defecation program:** Appropriate if the disorder is related to mental dysfunction or physical disability.
- **Biofeedback programs.**
- **Pharmacotherapy:**
  - **Bulk-forming laxatives:** Indicated with low-volume, loose stools.
  - **Loperamide:** ↓ stool frequency and ↑ internal anal sphincter tone.
  - **Anticholinergics** (hyoscyamine) may be helpful.
- **Topical phenylephrine gel:** ↑ anal sphincter tone (an $\alpha_1$-agonist).
- **Surgical repair:** Usually successful in patients with single anal sphincter tears following vaginal delivery or fistula surgery. Additional surgical options include plication of the posterior part of the sphincter, anal encirclement, and muscle transfer procedures.
- **Other modalities:** Novel treatments include implantable incontinence devices, silicone biomaterial injections (augmenting the internal anal sphincter), and sacral nerve stimulation.

## LIVER DISEASE

Table 5.5 outlines the differential diagnosis and treatment of common liver diseases. Viral hepatitis (HAV, HBV, and HCV) is not included in this table, as it is covered in detail in the Infectious Diseases chapter. The subtopics that follow discuss cirrhosis and related complications.

A 50-year-old woman presents to your office with fatigue, pruritus, and mild jaundice. Her electrolytes and CBC are normal, but a liver panel reveals an alkaline phosphatase level twice that of normal in the setting of a mildly elevated bilirubin and normal AST/ALT. What do you recommend? The setting is suspicious for 1° biliary cirrhosis, so you check for antimitochondrial antibodies and order an ultrasound. The patient's liver ultrasound is normal, and her antimitochondrial antibodies are $\oplus$. How should you proceed? In light of the high specificity and sensitivity of the antimitochondrial antibody test and the patient's normal ultrasound, the diagnosis of 1° biliary cirrhosis is likely but must be confirmed and staged by percutaneous liver biopsy. These confirm the diagnosis. What further procedures are necessary, and how should the patient be treated? The woman should have a DEXA scan to screen for osteoporosis. She can then be started on ursodeoxycholic acid to delay disease progression along with cholestyramine to relieve her itching.

## Cirrhosis

Generally irreversible scarring of the liver, with fibrosis and nodular regeneration. Represents the tenth leading cause of death in the United States.

### SYMPTOMS

- Weakness, fatigability, disturbed sleep, muscle cramps, and weight loss are common.
- Anorexia, nausea, vomiting, and abdominal pain may be seen.
- Men may develop impotence, loss of libido, sterility, and gynecomastia; women may develop amenorrhea.

### EXAM

- The liver is usually enlarged and firm. Splenomegaly, spider nevi, palmar erythema, Dupuytren's contractures, weight loss, and wasting may be seen.
- Late signs include jaundice, ascites, pleural effusions, ecchymoses, encephalopathy, asterixis, tremor, and GI bleeding.

### DIAGNOSIS

- **Liver biopsy:** The gold standard, but diagnosis is usually made with clinical, lab, and radiologic findings.
- **Labs:** Anemia, leukopenia, and thrombocytopenia may be seen. AST and alkaline phosphatase are mildly ↑, and albumin is low.
- **Imaging: Ultrasound** to assess the extent of disease and to detect nodules (which can be further evaluated by CT/MRI if suspicious for HCC); Doppler studies (to assess flow patterns in vasculature).

### TREATMENT

Rule out reversible causes (e.g., autoimmune hepatitis); stop alcohol; treat HBV and HCV if possible. Immunize against HAV and HBV; limit hepatotoxic drugs (e.g., acetaminophen < 2 g/day), manage complications, and consider transplantation referral.

## Ascites

Intra-abdominal fluid accumulation caused by transudative movement of fluid into the abdominal cavity as a result of portal hypertension. Table 5.6 lists causes of ascites.

**T A B L E  5 . 5 .    Common Liver Diseases**

| | CLINICAL CAVEATS | SYMPTOMS/EXAM |
|---|---|---|
| Drug/toxin-induced liver disease (always review meds in patients with liver disease) | Common offenders include **acetaminophen, INH, tetracyclines,** and some antiepileptics. | Variable. |
| Alcoholic liver disease | Includes (1) alcoholic fatty liver (develops in 90% of alcoholics), (2) alcoholic hepatitis (develops in 10–20%), and (3) alcoholic cirrhosis. Women are affected more than men; concomitant HCV is a risk factor. | **Fatty liver:** May be asymptomatic or present with hepatomegaly. **Alcoholic hepatitis:** Begins after a recent period of heavy drinking and presents with anorexia, nausea, hepatomegaly, and jaundice. |
| Nonalcoholic steatohepatitis | A condition in which **biopsy findings are indistinguishable from alcoholic hepatitis** in patients without significant alcohol consumption. Most commonly found in those 40–60 years of age; affects women more than men. Metabolic syndrome is a risk factor. | Usually asymptomatic, but may present with fatigue, malaise, RUQ discomfort, and hepatomegaly. |
| Ischemic hepatopathy (shock liver) | Liver disease due to an acute fall in cardiac output (e.g., MI, arrhythmia). | Variable; signs of fulminant failure may be present (e.g., encephalopathy, jaundice, coagulopathy). |
| Hemochromatosis | The **most common genetic disorder in Caucasians.** Characterized by inappropriately ↑ absorption of dietary iron → deposition in the liver, heart, pancreas, and pituitary (→ end-stage liver disease, hepatocellular carcinoma, dilated cardiomyopathy, DM, and hypogonadism). Associated with mutations of the **HFE gene on chromosome 6.** | Presents with weakness, fatigue, malaise, hepatomegaly, RUQ pain, arthralgias, impotence, amenorrhea, and slate-gray pigmentation of the skin (due to iron and melanin deposition; also known as "bronze diabetes"). |
| Wilson's disease | An **autosomal-recessive** disease (involving the **ATP7B gene**) → transmembrane transport (excretion) of copper in hepatocytes → copper accumulation in organs (liver, brain, kidneys, cornea). | Presents with symptoms of liver failure, Coombs-⊖ hemolytic anemia, ARF, **Kayser-Fleischer rings,** behavior change, cognitive decline, tremor, lack of motor coordination, drooling, dysarthria, dysphonia, spasticity, oropharyngeal dysphagia, depression, anxiety, and psychosis. |
| Autoimmune hepatitis | Unknown etiology; likely a heterogeneous group of liver disorders characterized by (1) **auto-antibodies** and (2) **high serum globulins.** Can be seen with other autoimmune diseases (hemolytic anemia, ITP, DM, ulcerative colitis, celiac disease, thyroiditis). Female predominance. | May be asymptomatic or fulminant (20–25%, with jaundice and coagulopathy). A subset of patients are **young, otherwise healthy women** with fatigue, malaise, spider nevi, anorexia, amenorrhea, acne, arthralgias, and jaundice. |
| 1° biliary cirrhosis | An **autoimmune disorder** → granulomatous destruction of the intrahepatic bile ducts and cholestasis. Ninety-five percent of patients are women, and onset is at 40–60 years of age. Osteopenia/osteoporosis develops in 25% of patients because of osteoblast dysfunction. Frequently associated with other autoimmune disorders such as Sjögren's and CREST. | **Usually asymptomatic** (60% are asymptomatic at the time of diagnosis), but fatigue and pruritus are common presenting symptoms. Jaundice, skin hyperpigmentation, xanthomas, hepatosplenomegaly, and other findings of end-stage liver disease may be present. **Osteoporosis** is seen. |
| 1° sclerosing cholangitis | An uncommon disease characterized by diffuse inflammation, fibrosis, and stricturing of the biliary tract as well as an ↑ risk of cholangiocarcinoma (associated with a 10–15% lifetime risk). **Two-thirds** of patients have **ulcerative colitis** (but only 5% of ulcerative colitis patients have 1° sclerosing cholangitis). Affects males more than females. | Presents with **progressive jaundice** with associated malaise, pruritus, anorexia, and indigestion. May have occasional bouts of acute cholangitis. Steatorrhea, fat-soluble vitamin deficiency, and osteopenia develop. |

**T A B L E  5 . 5 .  Common Liver Diseases (continued)**

| LFT Pattern | Other Findings | Treatment |
| --- | --- | --- |
| Variable. | | Stop the offending medication. For acetaminophen toxicity, give N-acetylcysteine if toxicity is likely based on nomogram (> 200 µg/mL at four hours). |
| Fatty liver: Modest elevation of aminotransferases (100–200s). Alcoholic hepatitis: AST usually > 300–400 and 2× ALT, alkaline phosphatase and bilirubin are generally elevated. | Fatty liver on ultrasound; biopsy shows macrovesicular fatty change; PMNs and Mallory bodies are seen. | Abstinence; alcohol rehabilitation (AA, family therapy); aggressive nutritional support (thiamine, folate); prednisolone if encephalopathic or discriminant function > 32 (PT − control × 4.6 + total bilirubin). Liver transplantation can be considered with abstinence > 6 months. |
| ↑ ALT and AST are seen in 90% of patients; unlike alcoholic hepatitis, the ALT-to-AST ratio is > 1. | Indistinguishable from that in alcoholic hepatitis (above). | Gradual weight loss (rapid loss can exacerbate NASH); dietary fat restriction, exercise. Can recur following liver transplantation. |
| A striking ↑ of transaminases (often > 5000); corrects quickly if reversed. ↑ PT may occur. | | Restore perfusion; aminotransferases usually correct quickly (within one week). |
| Variable (usually mild) elevation of AST and alkaline phosphatase is seen depending on the stage of the disease. | Fasting transferrin saturation > 45%; ↑ ferritin; genotype testing (performed if iron studies are ⊕ or there is a history of the disease in first-degree relatives). Liver biopsy should be offered to document the degree of fibrosis in homozygotes > 40 years of age with ↑ AST and ferritin > 1000 ng/mL. Hepatic iron index has fallen out of favor for diagnosis with genetic testing. | Phlebotomy therapy (remove one unit of blood 1–2 times per week). Deferoxamine is rarely needed. A normal diet is acceptable, but avoid iron supplements, vitamin C, shellfish (↑ susceptibility to Vibrio vulnificus and others). Liver transplant has relatively low survival due to concurrent cardiac disease and ↑ infection risk. |
| ↑ aminotransferases are seen. | Low copper and serum ceruloplasmin (< 5 mg/dL is strongly suggestive; low because of ↓ incorporation → ↓ half-life); ↑ 24-hour urinary copper excretion (> 40 µg is suggestive); hepatic copper content on biopsy (> 250 µg/g is the best biochemical evidence of disease; < 40–50 µg/g excludes the diagnosis); slit-lamp exam for Kayser-Fleischer rings (diagnostic with ceruloplasmin < 20 mg/dL); brain MRI to evaluate for neurologic complications. | D-penicillamine (binds copper and enhances urinary excretion); trientene is an alternative for those who cannot tolerate D-penicillamine. Oral zinc interferes with the absorption of copper in the GI tract. Reduction of copper-containing foods (shellfish, organs, legumes) is essential. Liver transplant for end-stage liver disease and fulminant failure. |
| Aminotransferases are ↑ (100–1000s). | ↑ gamma globulin (SPEP). Autoantibodies include ANA, ASMA (type I), and ALKM (type II). Liver biopsy may be nonspecific but aids in diagnosis, prognosis, and response to therapy. | Treatment is indicated if (1) aminotransferases are elevated tenfold, (2) aminotransferases are elevated fivefold AND serum globulin is elevated twofold, or (3) bridging or multiacinar necrosis is found on biopsy. Treat with prednisone with azathioprine or 6-MP. Disease can recur after liver transplantation (especially as immunosuppression is ↓). |
| Usually diagnosed in the presymptomatic phase, with alkaline phosphatase often more than twice normal (with elevations of GGT and 5-NT). Bilirubin ↑ with disease progression. AST and ALT may be normal. | Antimitochondrial antibodies are 95% sensitive and 98% specific for the disease. Liver biopsy is confirmatory. Other causes of cholestasis should be excluded (e.g., by ultrasound or cholangiography). DEXA scans to evaluate for concurrent osteoporosis. | Ursodeoxycholic acid delays progression, enhances survival, and is well tolerated. Cholestyramine improves pruritus (rifampin is second line). Liver transplantation is appropriate for treatment failure or severe osteoporosis. |
| Usually diagnosed in the presymptomatic phase with alkaline phosphatase elevation; aminotransferases may be ↑ to the 300s. | Diagnosis is established by ERCP (or MRCP) unless the disease is confined to small intrahepatic ducts, in which case a liver biopsy is needed to establish the diagnosis and staging. ANCA, ANA, anticardiolipin antibodies, anti-TPO antibodies, and RF may be ⊕. | Current medical therapy has failed to show consistent benefit in survival. However, ursodeoxycholic acid relieves pruritus, improves biochemical abnormalities, and stabilizes hepatic inflammation. Dominant biliary strictures should be biopsied to rule out carcinoma, with balloon dilation or stent placement to relieve obstruction. Liver transplantation significantly improves survival. |

**TABLE 5.6.** Causes of Ascites

| High Albumin Gradient (SAAG > 1.1 g/dL) | Low Albumin Gradient (SAAG < 1.1 g/dL) |
|---|---|
| Cirrhosis | Peritoneal carcinomatosis |
| Portal hypertension | Peritoneal tuberculosis |
| Alcoholic hepatitis | Pancreatitis |
| Nonalcoholic steatohepatitis (NASH) | Serositis |
| Chronic hepatitis C | Nephrotic syndrome |
| Congestive heart failure | Dialysis |
| Massive hepatic metastases | Chlamydial peritonitis |
| Hypothyroidism | |
| Budd-Chiari syndrome | |

### SYMPTOMS/EXAM

Presents with abdominal distention; exam may reveal flank dullness (e.g., shifting dullness), indicating at least 1500 cc of ascitic fluid.

### DIAGNOSIS

- Diagnosis is usually clinical but can be difficult in obese patients (for whom ultrasound can be useful).
- Usually occurs in the presence of portal hypertension (**serum-ascites albumin gradient [SAAG] > 1.1**).

### TREATMENT

- **Sodium restriction:** Restrict patients to 2 g (88 mmol) per day.
- **Spironolactone and furosemide:** If sodium restriction is inadequate, 90% of patients will respond to sodium restriction and spironolactone/ furosemide starting at 100 mg/40 mg, respectively (ensures normokalemia with normal renal function).
- **Repeated large-volume paracentesis:** Albumin replacement is controversial but should be considered if > 4–5 L is removed.
- **Transjugular intrahepatic portosystemic shunt (TIPS):** Controversial. Improves ascites (and a last resort for variceal hemorrhage), but can ↑ encephalopathy and has a high occlusion rate.
- **Liver transplantation:** For refractory cases.

A 57-year-old woman with a history of IV drug use is admitted to the inpatient service with a diagnosis of SBP. The admitting intern reports that he performed a diagnostic paracentesis in the ER and sent it for a cell count and culture prior to starting cefotaxime. What else would you recommend? You add an order to start an albumin infusion to prevent hepatorenal syndrome. In addition, you call the lab to add a total protein, glucose, and LDH to rule out 2° peritonitis. The patient's ascitic fluid glucose level is 30, her ascitic fluid LDH is twice the level of serum, and her total protein level is 2 g/dL. What should you do next? You order stat supine and upright films of the abdomen, which reveal free air. General surgery is called, and the patient is immediately taken to the operating room for bowel perforation. The ascites culture eventually grows multiple organisms.

### Spontaneous Bacterial Peritonitis (SBP)

Defined as infection of ascitic fluid caused by translocation of enteric bacteria across the gut wall or mesenteric lymphatics. Virtually all cases are monomicrobial, with *E. coli*, *Klebsiella*, *Enterococcus*, and *Pneumococcus* most frequently implicated.

#### SYMPTOMS/EXAM

Patients present with fever, ascites, and abdominal pain.

#### DIFFERENTIAL

- **Culture-⊖ neutrocytic ascites:** PMN > 250; ⊖ culture. Treat as SBP.
- **Monomicrobial non-neutrocytic bacterascites:** PMN < 250; ⊕ culture. Treat if the patient becomes symptomatic for SBP.
- **Alcoholic hepatitis:** If PMN > 250, treat as SBP. If < 250, treat as SBP for 48 hours and discontinue treatment if all cultures are ⊖.
- **Perforated viscus:** PMN > 250; multiple organisms found on culture. The presence of two of the following is suggestive of 2° bacterial peritonitis: total protein > 1 g, LDH higher than normal for serum, and glucose < 50.

#### DIAGNOSIS

Diagnosis is established by a PMN count > 250, a ⊕ **culture** of ascitic fluid obtained via paracentesis, and the exclusion of a surgical infection.

#### TREATMENT

- **Cefotaxime:** Administer intravenously with an **albumin** infusion (decreases the incidence of hepatorenal syndrome).
- **Prophylaxis:**
  - **Prior SBP:** Norfloxacin or TMP-SMX QD.
  - **GI bleeding in the setting of cirrhosis:** Norfloxacin or TMP-SMX × 7 days (there is an ↑ risk of SBP in these patients).
  - **Ascites and ascitic protein < 1 g/dL OR bilirubin > 2.5 mg/dL:** Norfloxacin or TMP-SMX QD.

### Hepatorenal Syndrome

- Characterized by **progressive renal failure** and **< 500 mg/dL of proteinuria** in the presence of **advanced liver failure** and **portal hypertension** with no other explainable cause.
- Believed to be caused by intense renal vasoconstriction, presumably resulting from failure of renal vasodilator synthesis. Also defined by lack of response to a fluid bolus or diuretic withdrawal. Can be rapidly progressive (type I) or insidious (type II).
- **Tx:**
  - **Supportive care:** IV albumin, with octreotide and midodrine to ↑ mean arterial pressure by 15 mmHg.

- **Liver transplantation:** Survival is essentially zero without liver transplantation.
- Hemodialysis alone does not improve patient outcome and is used only for patients awaiting transplantation.

## Hepatic Encephalopathy

Causes are multifactorial, but the **ammonia hypothesis** is still the predominant etiology. **Usually has a precipitating cause,** including GI bleeding ($\uparrow$ urea levels and ammonia levels), $\uparrow$ protein intake, hypokalemia ($\downarrow$ renal ammonia excretion), alkalosis (favors $NH_4^+ \rightarrow NH_3$, which crosses the blood-brain barrier), infection, or constipation ($\downarrow$ GI clearance of ammonia). Exacerbated by hypoxia and sedatives/tranquilizers.

### SYMPTOMS/EXAM/DIAGNOSIS

Initially presents as sleep disturbances but progresses to disorientation and confusion with asterixis and other neurologic signs. Usually diagnosed clinically; $\uparrow$ **ammonia** is common, but the level does not correlate to severity.

### TREATMENT

- **Correct the precipitating event**—e.g., NG lavage, potassium.
- **Pharmacotherapy: Lactulose;** a retention enema can be used if oral lactulose is not well tolerated. **Antibiotics** (e.g., neomycin, rifaximin) can be used; flumazenil can be considered if symptoms are worsened by benzodiazepines.
- Some institute **protein restriction,** although evidence does not support this.

 A 52-year-old man with recently diagnosed HBV with cirrhosis establishes care with you. He does not have ascites but did have an EGD showing esophageal varices. What do you recommend? Propranolol titrated to $\downarrow$ his heart rate by 25% or to 50–60 bpm.

## Esophageal Varices

*Fifty percent of cirrhotics have varices, and one-third of varices bleed. The mortality rate associated with bleed is 20%.*

Dilated submucosal veins due to portal hypertension that may bleed. Fifty percent of cirrhotics have varices, and one-third of all varices bleed. The mortality rate associated with variceal bleed is 20%; risk factors include size, the presence of "red color" markings, high Child's class, and active alcohol use. Gastric varices are also common.

### SYMPTOMS/EXAM/DIAGNOSIS

Asymptomatic unless there is acute hemorrhage (see the discussion of upper GI bleeding). Patients with cirrhosis should be screened with endoscopy.

### TREATMENT

- See the section on upper GI bleeding.
- **Banding and sclerotherapy:** Acute therapy for bleeding varices. Both arrest and prevent rebleeding, although their effect on in-hospital mortality is unclear.
- **Prophylaxis against SBP** or other serious infection (see above).

- **Somatostatin or octreotide drips:** ↓ splanchnic flow and portal pressures.
- **Balloon tube tamponade** (Minnesota, Sengstaken-Blakemore tubes): Have a high complication rate (esophageal ulceration, aspiration, perforation); used when bleeding cannot be controlled medically or endoscopically while awaiting TIPS/portosystemic shunt.
- **TIPS/portosystemic shunt:** Create a decompressive shunt between the portal and hepatic veins. Associated with high mortality rates.
- **1° prophylaxis for variceal hemorrhage:** Prophylaxis with nonselective β-blockers (propranolol, nadolol) is preferable to prophylactic banding therapy (offers a slightly better reduction in the risk of bleeding, but is more invasive). The goal for medical prophylaxis is generally to ↓ resting heart rate by 25% or to 50–60. Nitrates are **not** recommended.

## Hepatopulmonary Syndrome

Characterized by the triad of (1) chronic liver disease, (2) an ↑ alveolar-arterial (A-a) oxygen gradient on room air, and (3) intrapulmonary vascular dilatations → right-to-left intrapulmonary shunts. Thought to be caused by failure of the liver to clear pulmonary vasodilators.

### SYMPTOMS/EXAM

Usually characterized by dyspnea; **platypnea** and **orthodeoxia** (shortness of breath and deoxygenation in the upright position) are suggestive. There is a correlation between hepatopulmonary syndrome and the presence of **spider angiomata.**

### DIAGNOSIS

- **Contrast-enhanced echocardiography:** A useful screen for pulmonary vascular dilatations. **Macroaggregated albumin lung perfusion scanning** is more specific and is used to confirm the diagnosis.
- High-resolution CT scanning may also detect dilatations.

### TREATMENT

**Methylene blue** may improve oxygenation (inhibits nitric oxide–induced vasodilation). **Liver transplantation** may reverse the syndrome.

## BILIARY DISEASE

### Gallstones and Acute Cholecystitis

Caused by **aberrations in the solubilization of cholesterol.** More common in women and Native Americans. Risk factors include obesity, insulin resistance, rapid weight loss, and pregnancy. Cholecystitis is usually caused by an impaction of a gallstone (90% of cases).

### SYMPTOMS

- **Cholelithiasis:** May be asymptomatic or may → variable amounts of **RUQ or epigastric pain.**
- **Acute cholecystitis:** Presents with **fever** and **severe RUQ or epigastric pain** that may radiate to the infrascapular area. Symptoms are usually precipitated by a large or fatty meal and typically resolve after 12 hours. Vomiting is common.

### EXAM

- Usually normal or may reveal mild RUQ tenderness in cholelithiasis.
- In acute cholecystitis, exam reveals RUQ tenderness, a ⊕ **Murphy's sign,** guarding, and rebound pain. The gallbladder may be palpable, and jaundice may be present.

### DIFFERENTIAL

- **Precholecystectomy syndrome:** Biliary colic in the setting of ⊖ initial radiographic studies. Usually caused by undetected stenosis, adhesions, or kinking in the cystic duct. Diagnosed by ↓ gallbladder emptying on scintigraphy following cholecystokinin injection. Cholecystectomy is curative.
- **Acalculous cholecystitis:** Patients at high risk include those who have undergone major surgery and critically ill patients without enteral feeding for prolonged periods.
- **Infectious cholecystitis:** Found in HIV-⊕ patients, those with CMV, and those with crypto- or microsporidiosis.
- **Cholangitis:** Highly suspicious if jaundice is present (part of Charcot's triad, along with fever and RUQ pain)
- See the acute abdomen discussion in the Surgery chapter for a comprehensive differential.

### DIAGNOSIS

- **Labs:** Labs are usually normal in cholelithiasis. In acute cholecystitis, there may be leukocytosis along with ↑ serum bilirubin, aminotransferases, and alkaline phosphatase.
- **Imaging:**
    - **RUQ ultrasound:** Demonstrates the presence of stones in cholelithiasis. Not sensitive (67%) for cholecystitis but commonly used, and may show suggestive signs such as gallbladder wall thickening, pericholecystic fluid, and a sonographic Murphy's sign.
    - **HIDA scan:** Can demonstrate obstruction in the cystic duct, but reliable only if **bilirubin is < 5 mg/dL.**
    - **Cholangiography:** Usually performed intraoperatively to rule out choledocholithiasis or preoperatively by ERCP or MRCP.

### TREATMENT

- **Asymptomatic gallstones:** Cholecystectomy is indicated if the stone is > 2 cm or if the **gallbladder wall appears calcified.**
- **Symptomatic gallstones:** Laparoscopic cholecystectomy is indicated.
- Cheno- and ursodeoxycholic acids can dissolve some cholesterol stones in patients who refuse cholecystectomy or are poor surgical candidates.
- **Acute cholecystitis: NPO, IV fluids, pain control, antibiotics.** Laparoscopic cholecystectomy is indicated after acute illness resolves. Percutaneous cholecystostomy/ultrasound-guided aspiration may be considered in patients with a high operative risk.

### COMPLICATIONS

- **Gangrene:** Suggested by continuation or progression of symptoms beyond 24–48 hours. Cholecystectomy is mandatory.
- **Perforation:** Develops a picture of generalized peritonitis, although it usually remains anatomically localized. Cholecystectomy is mandatory.
- **Gallstone ileus:** Mechanical obstruction by a stone in the bowel (usually the ileocecal valve) caused by passage of a gallstone through a cholecystenteric fistula.

- Repeated episodes → chronic inflammation → choledocholithiasis, fistulization to the bowel, pancreatitis, and, rarely, carcinoma of the gallbladder.

## Choledocholithiasis and Cholangitis

Common duct stones occur in 15% of patients with gallstones.

### SYMPTOMS/EXAM

- Symptoms develop if **obstruction occurs** and → biliary colic and jaundice.
- **Pain, jaundice,** and **fever (Charcot's triad)** are classic findings in cholangitis.
- In acute suppurative cholangitis, patients may also present with **confusion and hypotension (Reynolds' pentad).**
- Exam reveals RUQ tenderness, icterus, and hepatomegaly.

### DIFFERENTIAL

Carcinoma, Mirizzi's syndrome (gallbladder neck stone compressing the common bile duct), benign biliary stricture, cholestatic liver disease (1° sclerosing cholangitis, 1° biliary sclerosis, drug-induced cholestasis), external obstruction, congenital disease (biliary atresia, choledochal cysts), parasites (*Ascaris lumbricoides, Echinococcus* spp.).

### DIAGNOSIS

- **Ultrasound:** The usual initial test looking for bile duct dilation.
- **ERCP:** Determines the cause, location, and extent of biliary obstruction; also preferred for interventions. **MRCP** for patients who cannot undergo ERCP.
- **Labs:** ↑ bilirubin, alkaline phosphatase, GGT, and PT/INR. Elevation of aminotransferases in the 1000s may be seen if acute necrosis of hepatocytes occurs.

### TREATMENT

- **Choledocholithiasis with cholelithiasis:** Endoscopic papillotomy and stone extraction followed by cholecystectomy.
- **Choledocholithasis with cholangitis:** Broad-spectrum antibiotics with ERCP, sphincterotomy, and stone extraction after acute illness resolves (or emergently if indicated)
- Vitamin K to correct coagulopathy may be required.

## PANCREATIC DISEASE

## Acute Pancreatitis

Disease ranges from edematous to necrotizing pancreatitis. The most common etiologies are **biliary disease** and **alcohol.** Other etiologies include drugs (2–5%), postoperative or post-ERCP, trauma, hypertriglyceridemia, viral infection (e.g., mumps), vasculitis, pancreas divisum, sphincter of Oddi dysfunction, and hypercalcemia. May also be idiopathic.

### SYMPTOMS

- Presents with a steady/boring abdominal pain with radiation to the back, chest, and lower abdomen.
- The pain worsens in a supine position and improves in a fetal position.
- Nausea, vomiting, distention due to GI hypomobility, and chemical peritonitis are common.

*In patients < 35 years of age with a strong family history and recurrent episodes of pancreatitis, consider genetic causes.*

**Causes of acute pancreatitis—**

**I GET SMASHED**

**I**diopathic
**G**allstones
**E**thanol
**T**rauma
**S**teroids
**M**umps
**A**utoimmune (PAN)
**S**corpion stings
**H**yperlipidemia/**H**yper-
 calcemia
**E**RCP
**D**rugs (including
 azathioprine and
 diuretics)

*Ranson's criteria:*

- *The presence of three or more of the following on admission is 60–80% sensitive for severe necrotizing pancreatitis: age > 55, WBC > 16,000, glucose > 200 mg/dL, LDH > 350 U/L, AST > 250 U/L.*

- *Development of the following in first 48 hours indicates a worse prognosis: hematocrit drop > 10%, BUN rise > 5 mg/dL, arterial $Po_2$ < 60 mmHg, Ca < 8 mg/dL, base deficit > 4 mEq/L, estimated fluid sequestration > 6 L.*

- *Mortality rates: 0–2 = 1%, 3–4 = 16%, 5–6 = 40%, 7–8 = 100%.*

## EXAM

- Patients appear distressed with fever, tachycardia, hypotension, and shock as well as with variable degrees of abdominal tenderness and rigidity.
- Diminished bowel sounds are noted.
- **Cullen's sign** (ecchymosis at the umbilicus) and **Grey Turner's sign** (ecchymosis of the flanks) point to severe necrotizing pancreatitis.
- Occasionally, left pulmonary rales and/or pleural effusion may be present.

## DIFFERENTIAL

Perforated viscus (peptic ulcer), acute cholecystitis, biliary colic, acute intestinal obstruction, mesenteric vascular occlusion, renal colic, MI, dissecting aortic aneurysm, vasculitis, pneumonia, DKA ($\rightarrow$ false elevation of amylase).

## DIAGNOSIS

- **Labs:**
  - **Serum amylase:** Values are usually three times normal and are pathognomonic if gut perforation/infarction have been excluded. However, values may also be normal, and there is **no correlation between level and disease severity.**
  - **Serum lipase:** Helpful in patients with nonpancreatic causes of hyperamylasemia. Specificity is 85–100%.
  - CBC may show leukocytosis and anemia (due to hemorrhage); chemistry may show hyperglycemia and hypocalcemia. LFTs may reveal transient elevation of AST, alkaline phosphatase, and bilirubin. An **ALT > 150** is 96% sensitive for gallstone-related pancreatitis. An albumin level < 3.0 suggests greater severity and higher mortality.
  - **ABGs:** Reveal hypoxemia in cases of impending ARDS.
- **Imaging:**
  - **AXR:** Important for excluding other diagnoses, especially gut perforation.
  - **Ultrasound:** Often used for initial investigation if pancreatitis is suspected. Efficacy is limited by obesity and intestinal gas.
  - **CT scan** (IV/PO contrast preferred): The best imaging study. Can confirm the diagnosis in the face of normal amylase levels; also indicates severity.
  - **Contrast-enhanced dynamic CT:** Indicated in the presence of > 2 Ranson's signs as well as for patients who are seriously ill or clinically deteriorating.
  - **MRI/MRCP:** Increasingly used. More effective at evaluating fluid collections; can detect milder cases. In addition, no nephrotoxicity results from the use of gadolinium-based contrast. MRCP rivals ERCP in detecting choledocholithiasis.

## TREATMENT

- Eighty-five to ninety percent of cases are self-limited.
- **NPO** and **IV fluids; NG tube** if needed.
- **Analgesics:** Typically morphine or fentanyl PCA.
- **Early refeeding** (with fat restriction): Increasingly supported by evidence.
- **Early enteral nutrition (distal jejunum).**
- **Antibiotics:** Broad-spectrum antibiotics for severe cases. **Fungicides** may also be needed with prolonged antibiotic use.
- For gallstone pancreatitis, urgent ERCP with papillotomy; planned cholecystectomy.

## COMPLICATIONS

- **Infected pancreatic necrosis** 1–2 weeks after onset.
- **Pancreatic abscess** 4–6 weeks after onset.
- **Pseudocysts** may develop over 1–4 weeks, diagnosed by sonography or CT; resolves in 25–40% of patients; drainage considered if complicated (i.e., infection) or if > 5 cm and persists for > 6 weeks.
- **Pancreatic ascites** is caused by an internal fistula between a duct or pseudocyst and the peritoneal cavity.
- **Pancreatic pleural effusions** are caused by a fistula between the duct and pleural space.

## Chronic Pancreatitis

The causes of chronic pancreatitis are outlined in the mnemonic **TIGAR-O**. The majority of cases are associated with alcoholism.

### SYMPTOMS/EXAM

May present with symptoms identical to those of acute pancreatitis; however, the pain pattern may be variable and located in the upper quadrants of the back or upper abdomen. Late symptoms and signs include weight loss, steatorrhea, and DM.

### DIFFERENTIAL

Same as acute pancreatitis (see above).

### DIAGNOSIS

- **Labs:**
  - **Amylase and lipase:** May be ↑ or **normal.**
  - ↑ alkaline phosphatase or bilirubin is seen if inflammation → ductal obstruction.
  - ↑ fasting glucose, ↑ fecal fat, and cobalamin malabsorption are seen in later stages.
  - **Classic triad: Pancreatic calcifications, steatorrhea,** and **DM** are pathognomonic.
  - **Secretion stimulation test:** Perform if the classic triad is not present (⊕ when 60% of exocrine function is lost).
  - Serum trypsinogen is low.
- **Imaging:** Sonography, CT, and ERCP (to delineate anatomy and to find a possible source amenable to intervention) are also used.

### TREATMENT

- **Treat pain:** Avoid alcohol and large fatty meals; narcotics may be needed for pain management (addiction is common).
- Pancreatic enzyme replacement; treat DM.
- Ductal decompression or pancreatic resection in selected cases.

### COMPLICATIONS

Associated with an ↑ risk of pancreatic carcinoma.

---

**Causes of chronic pancreatitis—**

**TIGAR-O**

**T**oxic/metabolic (alcohol, hypercalcemia, severe protein-calorie malnutrition)
**I**diopathic
**G**enetic
**A**utoimmune
**R**ecurrent severe/acute
**O**bstructive

*Seventy to eighty percent of cases of chronic pancreatitis are associated with alcoholism.*

## Esophageal Cancer

Most often affects patients between the ages of 50 and 70, with a male-to-female ratio of 3:1. **Squamous cell carcinoma** is strongly associated with chronic alcohol use and smoking and is more common in African-Americans. In the majority of cases, **adenocarcinoma** develops from Barrett's esophagus. A diet low in fruits and vegetables is a risk factor, as is obesity.

### SYMPTOMS/EXAM

- Presents with solid food dysphagia that progresses over weeks to months. Weight loss is common.
- Cough on swallowing, chest or back pain, and voice hoarseness are seen with invasive disease.

### DIAGNOSIS

- **Endoscopy with biopsy:** Disease is usually incurable at the time of diagnosis.
- **CT of the chest and liver:** For disease staging.
- If CT is ⊖, endoscopic ultrasound should be performed to evaluate wall involvement as well as local mediastinal and lymph node involvement (in conjunction with FNA). Bronchoscopy to evaluate airways for invasive disease.

### TREATMENT

- **Early-stage disease:** May be cured by **surgery alone** (transhiatal esophagectomy with anastomosis of the stomach with cervical esophagus). Radiation plus chemotherapy with cisplatin or 5-FU is more effective than radiation alone.
- **Advanced local spread or distant metastases:** Surgery is not warranted. Palliative treatment should be directed toward dysphagia and pain relief. Radiation and chemotherapy have significant side effects and may be considered in otherwise healthy patients with good functional status and minimal medical problems.

### PROGNOSIS

The prognosis is poor, with a five-year survival rate of 15%.

## Gastric Cancer

**Adenocarcinoma** is the most common form of gastric cancer. It has a mean age at diagnosis of 63 and is uncommon in patients < 40 years of age. The male-to-female ratio is 2:1. It is more common in Hispanics, African-Americans, and Asian-Americans. Additional risk factors include chronic *H. pylori* gastritis (responsible for 35–90% of distal cases), chronic atrophic gastritis, pernicious anemia, and a history of partial gastric resection.

### SYMPTOMS/EXAM

- Presents with dyspepsia, vague epigastric pain, anorexia, early satiety or vomiting, weight loss, occult fecal blood (and iron deficiency anemia), hematemesis, and melena. A gastric mass is palpable in 20% of cases.

- Metastatic spread may reveal palpable **left supraclavicular or umbilical nodes** (Virchow's and Sister Mary Joseph's nodes, respectively), a **rigid rectal shelf** (Blumer's shelf), or **ovarian metastases** (Krukenberg tumor).

### DIAGNOSIS

- **Endoscopy with brush cytology and biopsy:** Should be performed on any patient > 50 years of age with dyspepsia who does not respond to a short course of acid suppression.
- **Staging:** Performed with abdominal CT and endoscopic ultrasound.

### TREATMENT

- **Localized disease: Surgical resection** (depending on the location and extent of disease) can be curative. Chemotherapy and radiation confer no additional benefit.
- **Advanced disease:** Patients may have palliative tumor resection or, for unresectable tumors, a gastrojejunostomy (to prevent bleeding and obstruction by tumor). Chemotherapy may be used for palliation (single or multiagent with fluorouracil, doxorubicin, cisplatin, or mitomycin).

### PROGNOSIS

Has a 15% five-year survival rate. However, long-term survival is > 45% in patients who undergo curative resection.

---

A 44-year-old male construction worker comes to your office to establish care. He is generally healthy but tells you that he occasionally sees blood on the toilet paper following a bowel movement. When asked about a family history of colorectal cancer, he recalls that his father had in fact been diagnosed with "cancer in his rectum" when he was 52 years old. Anoscopy reveals internal hemorrhoids. What is the next appropriate step? The patient is at high risk for colorectal cancer, and screening should have begun at age 42. You refer your patient for colonoscopy, which is normal aside from revealing internal hemorrhoids. You advise the patient to use stool softeners and to avoid excessive straining at work, and his hemorrhoids subsequently improve. You remind him that he needs to be screened in another five years or sooner if he has any symptoms.

---

## Colorectal Cancer

Colorectal cancer is the **second leading cause of death due to cancer** in the United States, with a 6% lifetime risk. Almost all are **adenocarcinomas,** and slightly < 50% are distal to the splenic flexure. Colorectal cancer is believed to arise from transformation of adenomatous polyps. Risk factors include age > 45 (incidence ↑ sharply), IBD, a diet high in fats and red meat, African-American ethnicity, and a ⊕ family history (risk doubles if a first-degree relative has been diagnosed, quadruples if two family members have been diagnosed, and ↑ further if relatives were diagnosed at an early age). **Predisposing conditions** include the following:

- **Adenomatous polyps:** Present in 35% of those > 50 years of age. The risk of progression to cancer ranges from < 4% to > 10% depending on size and histologic features (larger size and villous features carry an ↑ risk). Commonly removed by colonoscopic polypectomy.
- **Familial adenomatous polyposis (FAP):** An autosomal-dominant syndrome characterized by > **100 colonic adenomatous polyps.** Polyps appear by age 15, adenomatous polyps by age 35, and **colorectal cancer by age 50.** Colectomy or proctocolectomy is indicated before age 20.
- **Hereditary nonpolyposis colorectal cancer (HNPCC):** An autosomal-dominant syndrome; also ↑ risk for endometrial and other cancers. Associated with a **70–80% lifetime risk of colorectal cancer.** Typically only a **few adenomas** develop, but these tend to be villous with high-grade dysplasia. If cancer is found, treatment is subtotal colectomy.

### SYMPTOMS/EXAM

- Presents with occult bleeding, hematochezia from the right colon, colicky abdominal pain, and altered bowel habits from obstruction in the left colon.
- Rectal cancers may present with tenesmus, urgency, and hematochezia. Weight loss is uncommon.
- Rectal exam may reveal a mass or fixation. Abdominal masses may be palpable, and the liver edge may be enlarged in the presence of metastases.

### DIAGNOSIS

- **Colonoscopy:** The procedure of choice, as it permits biopsy. If the cecum cannot be reached, CT colonography or barium enema may be considered.
- **CEA:** ↑; a level of > 5 ng/mL is predictive of a poorer prognosis.
- **Labs: Anemia with blood loss; liver enzymes may be** ↑ if metastases are present.
- **Staging:**
  - **Colon cancer:** CT of the abdomen and pelvis.
  - **Rectal cancer:** Pelvic MRI or endorectal ultrasound and chest CT.

### TREATMENT

- **Resection and regional lymph node dissection:** Even in advanced disease, a palliative resection can ↓ the likelihood of complications such as obstruction or bleeding. Transanal resections may be performed for some rectal cancers. Resection of isolated liver or lung metastases (1–3 sites) may improve survival.
- **Adjuvant chemotherapy and radiation:**
  - **Colon cancer:** Chemotherapy can be appropriate for node-⊕ disease. Radiation may be considered with locally advanced disease.
  - **Rectal cancer:** Treatment is more aggressive, involving **combination chemotherapy** and **radiation** with locally advanced disease.
- **Surveillance in survivors:**
  - **Colon cancer:** Evaluate every 3–6 months for 3–5 years with a history and exam, FOBT, LFTs, and CEA. Colonoscopy should be performed 6–12 months after surgery and every 3–5 years thereafter.
  - **Rectal cancer:** As with colon cancer, but sigmoidoscopy every 6–12 months for three years.
  - Any change in the clinical picture warrants a CXR and an abdominal CT to look for metastases.

### PREVENTION

Measures of **1° prevention** include the following:

- **Screening methods:** Annual FOBT; flexible sigmoidoscopy every five years; FOBT plus flexible sigmoidoscopy every five years; colonoscopy every ten years or barium enema every 5–10 years.
- Screen according to level of risk:
  - **Average risk:** No family history or one second- or third-degree relative with cancer. Begin screening at age 50.
  - **Elevated risk:** Refers to patients with a first-degree relative diagnosed with cancer/adenoma at > 60 years of age or two or more second-degree relatives with cancer only. Begin screening at age 40.
  - **High risk:** Describes patients with a first-degree relative diagnosed with cancer/adenoma at < 60 years of age or two first-degree relatives with cancer/adenoma. Begin at age 40 or when the patient is 10 years younger than the family member's age at diagnosis; repeat every five years.
  - **Adenomatous polyp on screening colonoscopy:** Repeat colonoscopy in three years.
  - **FAP:** Genetic testing offered to first-degree family members after age 10; if inconclusive, sigmoidoscopy performed beginning at age 12. Upper endoscopic evaluation of the duodenum/periampullary area every 1–3 years.
  - **HNPCC:** Offer genetic counseling and testing if the family history is suggestive. If testing is ⊕, screen with colonoscopy every 1–2 years starting at age 25 or when the patient is five years younger than the age of the family member at diagnosis. Also screen annually for endometrial cancer from 25 to 35 with endometrial aspirate or transvaginal ultrasound (or consider prophylactic TAH-BSO).
  - **IBD:** No consensus; the general recommendation is colonoscopy every 1–2 years beginning eight years after a diagnosis of IBD.

### PROGNOSIS

The long-term prognosis is 90% with early-stage cancer but is < 5% with metastatic disease. The prognosis for rectal cancer worsens with each stage.

## Hepatocellular Carcinoma (HCC)

Associated with cirrhosis in general, especially HBV/HCV and alcoholic liver disease. Other associations include aflatoxin exposure, hemochromatosis, $\alpha_1$-antitrypsin deficiency, and tyrosinemia.

### SYMPTOMS/EXAM

- Patients typically present in a deteriorated state with cirrhosis, cachexia, weakness, and weight loss.
- Bloody ascites may occur suddenly (suggesting portal or hepatic vein thrombosis or bleeding from tumor).
- Exam may show hepatomegaly or a palpable mass. A bruit may be audible over the tumor.

### DIAGNOSIS

- **α-fetoprotein (AFP)** is ↑ in 70% of cases but is **nonspecific.**
- **Arterial-phase CT scanning with and without contrast or MRI:** Preferred initial imaging studies.

*HCC usually develops in the setting of cirrhosis except in chronic HBV.*

*A ⊕ imaging test with ↑ AFP is adequate for the diagnosis of HCC.*

- **Liver biopsy:** Diagnostic, but imaging with ↑ AFP makes the diagnosis certain. Biopsy may be deferred if surgical resection is planned in light of possible seeding of the needle tract.

### TREATMENT

- **Surgical resection:** May result in cure, but not possible in advanced cirrhosis or when the tumor is multifocal. Chemotherapy has **not** been shown to prolong life.
- **Liver transplantation:** Associated with five-year survival in up to 75% of cases.
- **Palliative measures:** Include chemoembolization via the hepatic artery; small tumors may be amenable to ethanol injection, radiofrequency ablation, or cryotherapy.

### PREVENTION

- Screening for liver cancer is controversial.
  - **AFP:** Often ↑ in HCC, but levels do not correlate with size or stage. Also ↑ in pregnancy, gonadal tumors, and chronic liver disease (especially HCV). At low cutoff values, the test is nonspecific; at high cutoffs, the test loses sensitivity despite high specificity (> 500 µg/L in high-risk patients is virtually diagnostic).
  - **Ultrasound:** Noninvasive and widely available, but sensitivity ranges from 40% to 78%.
- Despite these limitations, many clinicians measure AFP and ultrasonography **every six months** in patients with Child-Pugh class A cirrhosis or chronic HBV who would be suitable candidates for partial hepatectomy, liver transplantation, or other percutaneous therapies.

### PROGNOSIS

For locally resectable disease, five-year survival is 56%. For unresectable disease, five-year survival is virtually zero.

## Pancreatic Cancer

Risk factors include age, obesity, tobacco use, prior abdominal radiation, and a ⊕ family history.

### SYMPTOMS/EXAM

- Presents with vague, diffuse pain in the epigastrium or LUQ (if the tail is involved) with occasional radiation to the back. Pain that is relieved by sitting or leaning forward suggests inoperable spread of disease.
- Diarrhea may be an early symptom; weight loss and depression are late signs.
- May also present with pancreatitis, and jaundice (sometimes painless) may be present with obstruction. A palpable gallbladder (**Courvoisier's sign**) may be present. A hard, fixed epigastric mass may be palpable.

### DIAGNOSIS

- **Multiphase thin-cut spiral CT or MRI:** Detects most tumors, demonstrates vessel invasion, delineates the extent of disease, and allows for FNA. **ERCP or MRCP** can aid in diagnosis if CT or MRI is ambiguous.
- **Endoscopic ultrasonography:** Also aids in diagnosis by demonstrating venous or gastric invasion.

- **Labs:**
  - **CA 19-9:** Has not proved sensitive enough (70%) for early detection. Specificity is 87%; ↑ values are also found in acute and chronic pancreatitis and cholangitis.
  - **Other:** Mild anemia, impaired glucose intolerance, and ↑ amylase/lipase may be seen. LFTs may suggest obstructive jaundice

### TREATMENT

- **Lesions limited to the head, periampullary zone, and duodenum:** Resection by a **Whipple procedure** (pancreaticoduodenectomy) is associated with a 20–25% five-year survival rate, increasing to 40% in the presence of ⊖ margins and lymph nodes. Adjuvant chemotherapy with fluorouracil or gemcitabine is beneficial.
- **Unresectable lesions:** Treatment is palliative. Treat jaundice with endoscopic stenting of the bile duct or cholecystojejunostomy; duodenal obstruction can be treated or prevented by gastrojejunostomy or endoscopic placement of a self-expandable duodenal stent. Combined irradiation and chemotherapy may be used for palliation of unresectable cancer confined to the pancreas.
- **Metastatic disease:** Chemotherapy has been disappointing in metastatic pancreatic cancer, although improved response rates have been reported with gemcitabine.
- Celiac plexus nerve block or thoracoscopic splanchnicectomy may improve pain control.

### PREVENTION

In patients with a ⊕ family history, consider screening with **spiral CT or endoscopic ultrasound** beginning 10 years earlier than the age of the family member at diagnosis.

### PROGNOSIS

The prognosis is poor, with a 2–5% five-year survival rate for masses in the body and tail and a 20–40% rate for ampullary lesions.

## GI BLEEDING

### Acute Upper GI Bleeding

More common after age 60. Associated with a mortality rate of 10%, but mortality is usually due to complications of underlying disease, not exsanguination. Etiologies include peptic ulcers, varices, Mallory-Weiss tears, erosive esophagitis, gastritis (e.g., NSAIDs, alcohol) and duodenitis, malignancy, vascular anomalies (ectasias, Dieulafoy's lesion), aortoenteric fistula, and hemobilia.

### SYMPTOMS/EXAM

- Commonly presents as **melena** or **hematemesis** (bright red or coffee-ground emesis). Melena develops with as little as 50–100 mL of bleeding.
- Ten percent of cases present with hematochezia, but this requires > 1000 mL of bleeding.
- Symptoms and signs of predisposing diseases may be present (e.g., a history of retching; stigmata of liver disease).

- *SBP > 100 and HR < 100 suggest minor hemorrhage.*
- *SBP > 100 and HR > 100 suggests moderate acute hemorrhage.*
- *SBP < 100 (irrespective of HR) suggests severe acute hemorrhage.*

DIAGNOSIS/TREATMENT

- **Initial resuscitation and stabilization:**
    - Patients should be **NPO; discontinue aspirin, NSAIDs,** and any **anti-coagulants.**
    - Place two 18-gauge IVs and initiate **aggressive fluid resuscitation** if there is hemodynamic compromise.
    - Place an **NG tube** for lavage. Aspiration of red blood or coffee-ground emesis confirms an upper GI source, but clear aspirate does not exclude it (e.g., duodenal bleed). An aspirate that clears with lavage suggests lower-risk bleeding, whereas failure to clear points to a high-risk bleed.
    - **Type and cross.**
    - The decision to transfuse should be based on the following:
        - **Hematocrit:** Consider transfusion if hematocrit is < 25–30% or if the patient is bleeding briskly regardless of hematocrit. Hematocrit takes 48–72 hours to equilibrate, so a normal value should not be considered reassuring in acute GI bleeding.
        - **Platelets:** Transfuse if the platelet count is < 50,000 or if bleeding is due to platelet dysfunction.
        - **INR:** Transfuse with FFP for values < 1.5. One unit of FFP is required for every five units of packed RBCs transfused.
    - Send laboratory studies based on suspicion for disease etiology (e.g., *H. pylori*, LFTs, INR, BUN, creatinine).
- **Triage:**
    - **Discharge:** Healthy patients with normal hemodynamics, an aspirate that clears with NG lavage, and normal labs may be discharged. Endoscopy should be scheduled as an outpatient procedure. The risk of rebleeding is low if the patient presents < 48 hours after the event.
    - **Admit to the hospital:** Everyone else must be admitted for observation and/or endoscopy.
    - **ICU admission:** Active bleeders, those with > 5 units of blood loss, and those with advanced liver disease or serious comorbidities must be admitted to the ICU.
- **Endoscopy:** All patients except those at low risk, as well as those with continued active bleeding, should have endoscopy within 12 hours after resuscitation and stabilization. Endoscopy is **diagnostic, prognostic,** and **therapeutic** (cautery, injection, or endoclips; injection of a sclerosant or application of a rubber band to the bleeding varix). Surgical intervention may be necessary if endoscopic interventions fail.
- **Other medical therapy:**
    - **IV PPIs:** ↓ the risk of rebleeding in peptic ulcers with high-risk features following endoscopic treatment. High doses of oral PPIs may also be effective.
    - **Octreotide infusion:** ↓ splanchnic blood flow and portal BP; effective in the initial control of variceal bleeding.
    - **Desmopressin (DDAVP):** Administer to uremic patients (those with dysfunctional platelets) with active bleeding.
- **Refractory bleeding: Surgical intervention;** intra-arterial embolizations/ vasopressin; **TIPS** for acute variceal hemorrhage.


## Acute Lower GI Bleeding

Defined as bleeding occurring below the ligament of Treitz. Approximately 95% of cases arise from the colon. Lower GI bleeds tend to have a **more be-**

nign course than upper GI bleeds, largely because there is less likelihood of hemodynamic compromise. Etiologies correlate with age:

- **Patients < 50 years of age:** Associated with infectious colitis, hemorrhoids, fissures, and IBD.
- **Patients > 50 years of age:** Associated with diverticulosis, vascular ectasias, neoplasm/malignancy, ischemia, and recent polypectomy (generally two weeks postprocedure).

### SYMPTOMS/EXAM

- Black stools (melena) indicate bleeding proximal to the ligament of Treitz; maroon stools point to the right colon or small intestine. Brown stools mixed or streaked with blood indicate a source in the rectosigmoid or anus.
- In 20% of acute bleeding episodes, no source of bleeding can be identified.

### DIAGNOSIS/TREATMENT

- **Initial resuscitation and stabilization:** Measures are the same as those for upper GI bleeding. An upper tract source should be excluded by NG lavage and possibly by EGD, especially if the patient is hemodynamically unstable.
- **Triage:**
  - For patients > 45 years of age or those with recurrent/persistent bleeding, colonoscopy is required.
  - For patients < 45 years of age with an isolated episode, anoscopy and sigmoidoscopy are sufficient if a cause is found; otherwise, colonoscopy.
- **Diagnostic and treatment options:**
  - **Colonoscopy:** Diagnostic, prognostic, and therapeutic (epinephrine injection, cautery, or application of metallic endoclips). Diagnostic accuracy is ↓ with inadequate prep (e.g., with severe, active bleeding).
  - **Nuclear bleeding scan** (technetium-labeled RBC scan) or **angiography:** Can identify the bleeding site for arterial embolization or bowel resection, but has poor diagnostic accuracy unless bleeding is brisk.
  - **Small intestine push enteroscopy** (a small-diameter endoscope that can reach the distal jejunum)/**wireless capsule imaging:** May help identify a source of persistent recurrent bleeding.
  - **Surgery:** Indicated with ongoing bleeding that requires > 4–6 units of blood within 24 hours or > 10 units in total. May also be indicated in patients with two or more hospitalizations for diverticular hemorrhage.

*Ten percent of cases of hematochezia are due to a brisk upper GI bleed and usually have concomitant hypotension and shock.*

**NOTES**

# CHAPTER 6

# Infectious Diseases

Craig M. Hileman, MD
Corrilynn O. Hileman, MD

A 45-year-old woman is seen in the ER for a five-day history of fever, cough, pleuritic chest pain, and purulent sputum. Her family brought her to the hospital today because earlier this morning she began complaining about a headache and neck pain. The family also notes that she has been acting strangely and seems confused. On physical exam, you note a temperature of 40.4°C and nuchal rigidity. The patient is oriented only to self. What would you do first? Perform a noncontrast head CT, order an LP, and then start empiric antibiotics (ceftriaxone and vancomycin)—all within the first 60 minutes of presentation. Also consider steroids prior to the first dose of antibiotics.

## Acute Bacterial Meningitis

A purulent infection of the leptomeninges that is usually associated with a profound inflammatory response. Early recognition, correct decision making, and early treatment have a significant effect on mortality. Typical bacterial pathogens include *Streptococcus pneumoniae*, *Neisseria meningitidis*, group B streptococci, and *Listeria monocytogenes*. Age and other characteristics predispose patients to different bacteria (see Table 6.1).

### SYMPTOMS/EXAM

- Commonly presents with fever, altered mental status, nuchal rigidity, headache, photophobia, and nausea/vomiting.

TABLE 6.1. **Causes and Treatment of Bacterial Meningitis**

| AGE GROUP | COMMON MICROORGANISMS | EMPIRIC ANTIBIOTICS—FIRST CHOICE | SEVERE PENICILLIN ALLERGY |
|---|---|---|---|
| < 1 month | Group B strep, *E. coli*, *L. monocytogenes*. | Ampicillin and cefotaxime /gentamicin + vancomycin. | N/A. |
| 1 month to 50 years of age | *S. pneumoniae*, *N. meningitides*. | Ceftriaxone/cefotaxime + vancomycin. | Chloramphenicol + vancomycin. |
| Adults > 50 years of age | *S. pneumoniae*, *L. monocytogenes*, gram-negative bacilli. | Ceftriaxone/cefotaxime + ampicillin + vancomycin. | Chloramphenicol (*N. meningitidis*) + TMP-SMX (*Listeria*) + vancomycin. |
| Impaired cellular immunity (or alcohol abuse) | *S. pneumoniae*, *L. monocytogenes*, gram-negative bacilli (*Pseudomonas*). | Ceftazidime + ampicillin + vancomycin. | TMP-SMX + vancomycin. |
| Postneurosurgery or post–head trauma | *S. pneumoniae*, *S. aureus*, gram-negative bacilli (including *Pseudomonas*). | Ceftazidime + vancomycin (for possible MRSA). | Aztreonam or ciprofloxacin + vancomycin. |

Adapted, with permission, from Tierney LM et al. *Current Medical Diagnosis and Treatment,* 44th ed. New York: McGraw-Hill, 2005: 1251.

**Meningeal signs:**

**K** is for **K**ernig's and **K**nee.
Remember, you move the **K**nee to test for **K**ernig's.

*The classic triad of bacterial meningitis consists of fever, altered mental status, and nuchal rigidity. Virtually all patients have at least one of these findings.*

*Consider neuroimaging before performing an LP if there is concern about ↑ ICP (i.e., mass effect with shift)!*

- Less common presentations are rash (petechiae and palpable purpura in meningococcal meningitis); cranial nerve palsies; cerebral involvement in the form of seizures, aphasia, or focal neurologic deficits (e.g., **syphilitic meningitis**); and coma.
- Traditional signs thought to correlate with meningeal irritation include **Kernig's sign** (with the thigh and knee flexed, passive leg extension → pain) and **Brudzinski's sign** (passive flexion of the neck → spontaneous flexion of the hip and knees). However, these signs are not sensitive for the diagnosis of bacterial meningitis.
- Atypical presentations are common in neonates, infants, and the elderly and immunocompromised.

### DIFFERENTIAL

- Other forms of meningitis, such as viral, fungal (*Cryptococcus neoformans*), tuberculous, and aseptic (absence of bacteria on routine examination and culture, e.g., medication-induced meningitis).
- Viral encephalitis or bacterial encephalitis (e.g., Rocky Mountain spotted fever, Lyme disease).
- A parameningeal focus such as epidural, subdural, or intraparenchymal abscess. **Epidural abscess** may present in varied ways, including headache, back pain, and neurologic deficits 2° to cord compression. Consider in patients with a history of IV drug abuse.
- Noninfectious causes include SAH, vasculitis, and connective tissue disease.

### DIAGNOSIS

- History and physical examination.
- **Labs:** CBC may show leukocytosis with PMN predominance or leukopenia (associated with severe infection). Thrombocytopenia may be seen if the patient develops DIC (think of meningococcemia).
- **CSF:**
  - Opening pressure will typically be ↑. CSF should routinely be sent for cell count and differential, total glucose, protein, Gram stain, and bacterial culture (see Table 6.2).
  - In the right clinical setting, consider sending CSF for viral PCR (HSV), viral culture, cryptococcal antigen, AFB stain and culture, fungal culture, or VDRL (syphilis).
- **Blood cultures:** Bacteremia is common and is seen in 40–90% of patients.

### TREATMENT

- Untreated bacterial meningitis is generally fatal. The goal is to begin antimicrobial therapy as early as possible, preferably within the first 60 minutes of presentation. Empiric therapy should be initiated while awaiting the results of CSF examination (see Table 6.1).
- All patients should receive a third-generation cephalosporin. In patients > 1 month of age, vancomycin should be added to cover possible penicillin-resistant *S. pneumoniae* infection. Ampicillin should be added in very young, elderly, or immunocompromised patients to cover *L. monocytogenes*.
- Consider corticosteroids as adjunctive therapy, as they have been shown to ↓ mortality when given 20 minutes prior to or with the first dose of antibiotics. In addition, corticosteroids reduce the risk of hearing loss in children with *H. influenzae* meningitis.

TABLE 6.2. CSF Profiles in Common CNS Diseases

| DIAGNOSIS | RBC (PER μL) | WBC (PER μL) | GLUCOSE (mg/dL) | PROTEIN (mg/dL) | OPENING PRESSURE (cm H₂O) | APPEARANCE |
|---|---|---|---|---|---|---|
| Normal[a] | < 10 | < 5 | About 2/3 of serum level | 15–45 | 10–20 | Clear |
| Bacterial meningitis | Normal | ↑ (PMNs) | ↓ | ↑ | ↑ | Cloudy |
| Aseptic/viral meningitis, encephalitis | Normal | ↑ (lymphs)[b] | Normal | Normal or ↑ | Normal or ↑ | Usually clear |
| Chronic meningtitis (TB, fungal) | Normal | ↑ (lymphs)[b] | ↓ | ↑ | ↑ | Clear or cloudy |
| Spirochetal meningitis (syphilis, Lyme disease) | Normal | ↑ (lymphs)[b] | Normal | ↑ | Normal or ↑ | Clear or cloudy |
| Neighborhood reaction[c] | Normal | Variable | Normal | Normal or ↑ | Normal or ↑ | Usually clear |
| SAH, cerebral contusion | ↑↑ | ↑ | Normal | ↑↑ | Normal or ↑ | Yellow or red |

[a] With traumatic tap, usually have 1 WBC/800 RBCs and 1 mg protein/1000 RBCs.

[b] May have PMN predominance in early stages.

[c] May be seen with brain abscess, epidural abscess, vertebral osteomyelitis, sinusitis/mastoiditis, septic thrombus, and brain tumor.

Reproduced, with permission, from Le T et al. *First Aid for the Internal Medicine Boards,* 1st ed. New York: McGraw-Hill, 2006: 411.

## COMPLICATIONS

- Mortality ranges from 1% to 20%.
- Systemic complications result primarily from bacteremia and include septic shock, DIC, ARDS, and septic or reactive arthritis.
- Neurologic complications include cerebral edema and ↑ ICP, hydrocephalus, seizures, cognitive impairment, hearing loss and other cranial neuropathies, subdural effusion, empyema, epidural abscess, and SIADH. Permanent neurologic morbidity may occur.

## Viral Meningitis and Encephalitis

Viruses can infiltrate the CNS in various ways, including hematogenous and axonal spread. They may also cause a range of disease processes, including meningitis and encephalitis (see Tables 6.3 and 6.4) as well as postinfectious autoimmune demyelination.

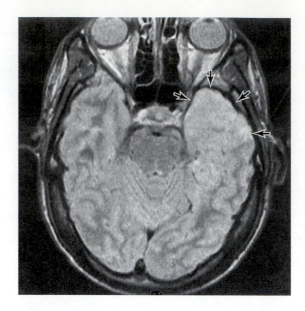

**FIGURE 6.1.** **MRI in HSV encephalitis.**

(Reproduced, with permission, from Aminoff MJ et al. *Clinical Neurology*, 6th ed. New York: McGraw-Hill, 2005: 30.)

### *SYMPTOMS/EXAM*

- A patient with encephalitis presents with altered mental status, motor/sensory deficits, and speech/movement abnormalities. Overlap may occur.
- Both meningitis and encephalitis can have rash (Rocky Mountain spotted fever, Lyme disease, VZV), fever, headache, nausea/vomiting, seizures, or focal neurologic deficits (flaccid paralysis in West Nile virus). However, photophobia and stiff neck are less common findings in pure encephalitis.
- HSV encephalitis can cause bizarre behavior such as olfactory hallucination and aphasia. This is due to the predilection for involvement of the **medial temporal lobes** (see Figure 6.1).

**TABLE 6.3.** **Etiologic Agents in Viral Meningitis**

| VIRUS | INCIDENCE | SEASONAL VARIATION | SOURCE | SUSCEPTIBLE POPULATION | SYSTEMIC INVOLVEMENT | LABORATORY FINDINGS |
|---|---|---|---|---|---|---|
| Echoviruses | 30% | Summer, fall | Fecal-oral | Children, members of affected families | Maculopapular, vesicular, or petechial skin rash; gastro-enteritis | — |
| Coxsackievirus A | 10% | Summer, fall | Fecal-oral | Children, members of affected families | Maculopapular, vesicular, or petechial skin rash; herpangina; gastroenteritis | — |

TABLE 6.3. Etiologic Agents in Viral Meningitis (continued)

| VIRUS | INCIDENCE | SEASONAL VARIATION | SOURCE | SUSCEPTIBLE POPULATION | SYSTEMIC INVOLVEMENT | LABORATORY FINDINGS |
|---|---|---|---|---|---|---|
| Coxsackievirus B | 40% | Summer, fall | Fecal-oral | Children, members of affected families | Maculopapular, vesicular, or petechial skin rash; pleuritis, pericarditis, myocarditis, orchitis; gastro-enteritis | — |
| Mumps virus | 15% | Late winter, spring | Inhalation | Children, male more than female | Parotitis, orchitis, oophoritis, pancreatitis | Amylase ↑; CSF glucose may be ↑ or ↓ |
| Herpes simplex virus (type 2) | Uncommon | — | Genital infection | Neonates with affected mothers | Vesicular genital lesions | — |
| Adenovirus | Uncommon | — | Inhalation | Infants, children | Pharyngitis, pneumonitis | — |
| Lymphocytic choriomeningitis virus | Uncommon | Late fall, winter | Mouse | Laboratory workers | Pharyngitis, pneumonitis | Marked CSF pleocytosis (1000–10,000 WBC/μL) |
| Hepatitis viruses | Uncommon | — | Fecal-oral, venereal, transfusion | Intravenous drug users, men who have sex with men, blood recipients | Jaundice, arthritis | Liver function abnormalities |
| Epstein-Barr virus (infectious mononucleosis) | Uncommon | — | Oral contact | Teenagers, young adults | Lymphadeno-pathy, pharyngitis, maculopapular skin rash, palatal petechiae, splenomegaly | Atypical lymphocytes, positive heterophil, liver function abnormalities |

Reproduced, with permission, from Aminoff MJ et al. *Clinical Neurology,* 6th ed. New York: McGraw-Hill, 2005: 27.

*DIFFERENTIAL*

See the differential for bacterial meningitis above as well as other common causes of altered mental status.

**TABLE 6.4.** Etiologic Agents in Viral Encephalitis

| Type of Encephalitis | Vector | Geographic Distribution | Comments |
|---|---|---|---|
| **Childhood exanthems** | | | |
| Measles, varicella, mumps, rubella | Human | Worldwide | Uncommon in the United States because of vaccination. |
| **Arthropod-borne viruses (arboviruses)** | | | |
| *Alphaviruses* | | | |
| Eastern equine | Mosquito | United States (Atlantic and Gulf coasts), Caribbean, South America | Children are usually affected; mortality is 50–75%; neurologic sequelae are common. |
| Western equine | Mosquito | Western and central United States, South America | Infants and adults > 50 years of age are usually affected; mortality is 5–15%; neurologic sequelae are uncommon except in infants. |
| Venezuelan equine | Mosquito | Florida, southwestern United States, Central and South America | Adults are usually affected; mortality is 1%; neurologic sequelae are rare. |
| *Flaviviruses* | | | |
| Japanese B | Mosquito | China, Southeast Asia, India, Japan | A vaccine is available. |
| St. Louis | Mosquito | United States (rural west and midwest, New Jersey, Florida, Texas), Caribbean, Central and South America | Adults > 50 years of age are most often affected; mortality is 2–20%; neurologic sequelae occur in about 20% of cases. |
| Murray Valley | Mosquito | Australia, New Guinea | |
| West Nile | Mosquito | Middle East, Africa, Europe, Central Asia, northeastern United States | |
| Rocio | Mosquito | Brazil | |
| Kyasanur Forest | Tick | India | |
| Powassan | Tick | New York, Ontario | |
| Russian spring-summer | Tick | Northern Europe, Siberia | |
| Louping-ill | Tick | United Kingdom | |
| *Bunyaviruses* | | | |
| California (including LaCrosse) | Mosquito | North America | Children are usually affected; mortality is < 1%; neurologic sequelae are uncommon. |
| Rift Valley | Mosquito | Africa | |
| *Orbiviruses* | | | |
| Colorado tick fever | Tick | Western and Rocky Mountain states of the United States | |
| **Other** | | | |
| Herpes simplex (type 1) | Human | Worldwide | Focal neurologic signs are common; responds to treatment with acyclovir. |
| Herpes simplex (type 2) | Human | Worldwide | Encephalitis usually affects neonates; causes meningitis in older children and adults. |

**TABLE 6.4.** Etiologic Agents in Viral Encephalitis (continued)

| TYPE OF ENCEPHALITIS | VECTOR | GEOGRAPHIC DISTRIBUTION | COMMENTS |
|---|---|---|---|
| Rabies | Wild and domestic mammals | Worldwide | Invariably fatal unless vaccine and antiserum are administered before symptoms occur following a bite by an affected animal. |

Reproduced, with permission, from Aminoff MJ et al. *Clinical Neurology*, 6th ed. New York: McGraw-Hill, 2005: 28.

### DIAGNOSIS

- The 1° goal is to **distinguish HSV from other causes.**
- A thorough history is essential and should include season, sexual activity, travel, and tick bites.
- Consider CT/MRI, especially in the setting of altered mental status.
- CSF profile (see Table 6.2) may reveal **RBCs** in HSV encephalitis.

### TREATMENT

- Untreated HSV encephalitis is associated with high morbidity and mortality. Therefore, in suspected cases of encephalitis without an obvious source, **empiric IV acyclovir** should be used until this is ruled out.
- Otherwise, no specific therapy exists for most viral meningitis and encephalitis. Supportive measures are the mainstay of treatment.
- Failure to improve within **48 hours** should prompt reevaluation of the diagnosis.

### COMPLICATIONS

- Survival from viral encephalitis is usually 100% with few sequelae.
- Complications from encephalitis vary by virus but range from no complications to chronic neurologic deficits or death.

*HSV is currently the only treatable type of viral encephalitis. IV acyclovir is the drug of choice.*

## HEAD AND NECK DISORDERS

## Eye Disease

### CONJUNCTIVITIS

The most common cause of a red eye. Infectious etiologies include both viruses and bacteria. These infections are usually self-limiting but may need treatment (see Table 6.5).

> A 15-year-old boy is being seen in urgent care for a one-day history of right eye pain and swelling. On exam, you note significant erythema and periorbital and eyelid swelling. What is the next step in this patient's management? Perform a CT scan of the orbits, obtain blood cultures, and admit to the hospital for IV antibiotics.

INFECTIOUS DISEASES

**TABLE 6.5.** **Manifestations and Treatment of Infectious Conjunctivitis**

| | **VIRAL** | **BACTERIAL** |
|---|---|---|
| Etiologies | Adenovirus, HSV. | *Staphylococcus* spp., *Streptococcus* spp., *Haemophilus influenzae, Neisseria gonorrhoeae* (GC), *Chlamydia trachomatis* (CT). |
| Symptoms/exam | Erythema, watery discharge, photophobia. Frequently bilateral. Concomitant URI. "Pink eye." | Erythema, mucopurulent discharge, "morning crustiness." Usually unilateral. |
| Treatment | Symptomatic; cold compresses. | Topical erythromycin, bacitracin-polymyxin, trimethoprim, fluoroquinolone. For GC, ceftriaxone IM/IV × 1. For CT, erythromycin syrup PO. |
| Prevention | Frequent hand washing (highly contagious). | Frequent hand washing. |
| Complications | Corneal abrasion 2° to rubbing. | Untreated *C. trachomatis* conjunctivitis is a common cause of **blindness** worldwide. |

## ORBITAL/PERIORBITAL CELLULITIS

A serious bacterial infection that can follow a URI, sinusitis, dental infection, or trauma. Common causative agents include *Staphylococcus* spp., *Streptococcus* spp., and *H. influenzae.*

### SYMPTOMS/EXAM

- **Periorbital (preseptal) cellulitis:** Presents with swelling and erythema of the eyelids, minimal pain, and fever. Conjunctivitis, proptosis, and restricted eye movements are not generally present.
- **Orbital cellulitis:** Presents with very painful, erythematous swelling of the eyelid, **conjunctivitis,** proptosis with **ophthalmoplegia,** and fever. Patients may also have ↓ visual acuity and an afferent pupillary defect.

### DIAGNOSIS/TREATMENT

- Consider CT scan of the orbit to evaluate for **abscess** (imperative in the presence of symptoms or signs of orbital cellulitis).
- Consider blood cultures, although these are generally ⊖.
- Most cases require hospital admission and IV antibiotics (broad-spectrum antistaphylococcal and antistreptococcal coverage).
- Prompt drainage of an abscess or the paranasal sinuses is indicated if vision deteriorates despite antibiotic therapy.

### COMPLICATIONS

Abscess, blindness, or extension into CNS causing meningitis or septic cavernous sinus thrombosis.

## Nose and Sinus Disorders

### COMMON COLD

- Usually caused by **rhinoviruses.** Other viruses implicated include coronavirus, parainfluenza virus, RSV, influenza virus, and adenoviruses.
- **Tx: Generally** treat with supportive measures. OTC cold preparations are not recommended in patients < 2 years of age.

### BACTERIAL SINUSITIS

Sinusitis results from impaired mucociliary clearance and obstruction of the osteomeatal complex. Viral or allergic rhinitis predisposes patients to acute sinusitis. The majority of acute sinusitis cases are due to viruses, with only about 20% due to bacteria. However, infections lasting > 1 week are more likely to have a bacterial etiology. When bacterial infection is suspected, the most common causative agents are S. *pneumoniae,* H. *influenzae,* and occasionally S. *aureus* and *Moraxella catarrhalis. Pseudomonas aeruginosa* and anaerobes are implicated in cases of **chronic** sinusitis.

#### SYMPTOMS/EXAM

- Frequently presents with unilateral or bilateral pain over the maxillary sinuses or teeth as well as with fever and nasal discharge (at times purulent).
- Acute sinusitis can last 1–4 weeks; sinusitis of > 4 weeks' duration is considered chronic.
- Transillumination of the sinuses may be attempted but is an insensitive test.

#### DIFFERENTIAL

- **Zygomycosis:** A rare but dangerous fungal infection that occurs in immunocompromised patients—e.g., those with diabetes, end-stage renal disease, bone marrow transplants, lymphoma, and AIDS.
  - Presents as **extreme facial pain** with a necrotic eschar of the nasal mucosa and subsequently with cranial nerve palsies.
  - Early diagnosis is paramount because the infection can spread rapidly. Treat emergently with antifungal therapy (traditionally amphotericin B; possibly posaconazole) and surgical debridement.
- **Other:** In chronic or resistant sinusitis, consider anatomic obstruction, common variable immunodeficiency, a CF variant, Wegener's granulomatosis, or periodontal or dental infection.

#### DIAGNOSIS

- Usually made by the history and physical exam.
- Routine imaging is **not indicated** in uncomplicated acute sinusitis. However, in chronic, resistant, or complicated sinusitis, a CT scan is more sensitive and cost-effective than plain film x-rays and may identify air-fluid levels or bony abnormalities.

#### TREATMENT

- **General:** Oral and/or nasal decongestants (e.g., oral pseudoephedrine, intranasal oxymetazoline).
- **Acute bacterial sinusitis:** Amoxicillin or macrolide × 10 days (although shorter courses may also be effective); amoxicillin-clavulanate or a 3rd generation cephalosporin in the presence of risk factors for anaerobes or

β-lactamase-producing organisms (some *H. influenzae* and *M. catarrhalis*). Risk factors include DM, other immunocompromised states, and recent antibiotic use.

- **Chronic sinusitis:** Amoxicillin-clavulanate for at least 3–4 weeks along with intranasal glucocorticoids.

### COMPLICATIONS

Complications are rare but include extension into the CNS and orbital or periorbital cellulitis.

## Throat Disorders

### PHARYNGITIS

Defined as an infection or irritation of the pharynx and/or tonsils. Etiologies include the following:

- **Bacterial:** The most important bacterial etiology is group A streptococcus (*Streptococcus pyogenes*), or "strep throat." Other bacterial agents include groups C and G streptococcus, *N. gonorrhoeae, Mycoplasma pneumoniae, Chlamydia pneumoniae,* and, rarely, *Corynebacterium diphtheriae.*
- **Viral:** Viruses are the most common etiology of pharyngitis. These include rhinovirus, coronavirus, adenovirus, and many others. Pharyngitis may also occur 2° to systemic viral infections such as mononucleosis (EBV), herpangina (coxsackievirus), and acute retroviral syndrome (HIV).
- **Other:** Allergy, gastroesophageal reflux, trauma, toxins, malignancy.

### SYMPTOMS/EXAM

- **Bacterial pharyngitis:**
    - *S. pyogenes* ("**strep throat**"):
        - When patients present with symptoms and signs of pharyngitis, it is important to identify those who may have *S. pyogenes,* as appropriate antibiotic treatment of this type of pharyngitis may ↓ potential complications.
        - According to the **Centor criteria,** the four classic features of streptococcal pharyngitis are a temperature > 38°C, tender anterior cervical lymphadenopathy, the absence of cough, and the presence of pharyngotonsillar exudates.
        - The presence of any concomitant URI symptoms makes the diagnosis of "strep throat" less likely and points instead to a viral etiology.
    - **Diphtheria:** Rare in the United States. Presents as malaise with gray pseudomembranes on the tonsils. More common in alcoholics.
- **Viral pharyngitis:** As above, suggested by upper respiratory symptoms and the absence of tonsillar exudates. Pharyngitis 2° to systemic viral infections presents as follows:
    - **Mononucleosis:** Characterized by the triad of **lymphadenopathy, fever,** and **tonsillitis.** Symptoms also include severe fatigue, headache, and malaise. More common in young adults. Transmitted in saliva and may persist for up to 18 months after 1° infection.
    - **Herpangina:** Presents with fever, sore throat, myalgias, and a vesicular exanthem on the soft palate.
    - **Acute retroviral syndrome:** Nonexudative pharyngitis and fever are common symptoms of this syndrome, which develops several weeks after infection with HIV.

- **Bacterial pharyngitis:**
  - The **test of choice** for group A streptococcus is the rapid antigen test, which has > 90% sensitivity for diagnosing the presence of this bacterium.
  - A routine bacterial culture is not indicated unless the rapid test is ⊖ or if suspicion for a different bacterial infection (not group A strep) is high.
- **Mononucleosis:** Diagnosed with a ⊕ heterophil antibody (Monospot) test or a high anti-EBV titer.
- In the right clinical setting, consider HIV or other viral testing.

### TREATMENT

- **Streptococcal pharyngitis:** Treatment is based on results of rapid testing and the Centor criteria.
  - In the presence of the Centor criteria:
    - **4 of 4:** Treat empirically without a rapid test.
    - **2–3 of 4:** Test and treat only if the rapid test is ⊕.
    - **0–1 of 4:** No test, no antibiotics.
  - Give a single dose of IM benzathine penicillin or a 10-day course of oral penicillin VK or erythromycin (for penicillin-allergic patients). Other antistreptococcal antibiotics (e.g., cefuroxime or amoxicillin) may be used, but the efficacy of these drugs in the prevention of rheumatic fever has not been adequately studied.
  - Patients may return to work or school 24 hours after initiation of therapy.
- **Viral pharyngitis:** Patients may return to work or school when fever resolves and when they are well enough to participate in normal activities.
- **All cases (bacterial or viral):** Acetaminophen or NSAIDs and salt-water gargling for symptomatic relief. Oral steroids may occasionally be needed for very severe pharyngitis.

### COMPLICATIONS

- **Streptococcal pharyngitis:**
  - Complications include rheumatic fever, glomerulonephritis, myocarditis, and peritonsillar abscess.
  - **Rheumatic fever** develops in only a few cases and is less common than in the past. The Jones criteria are used for diagnosis (see Table 6.6).
- **Mononucleosis:** Complications include hepatitis, a morbilliform rash following antibiotic administration, and splenomegaly occurring within the first three weeks. To ↓ the risk of **splenic rupture,** noncontact sports must be avoided for 3–4 weeks and contact sports for 4–6 weeks after the onset of symptoms.

## Dental/Periodontal Disease

### DENTAL CARIES

- The most common chronic childhood disease.
- For a patient to develop caries, three factors must be present: a **host,** a **substrate (sucrose),** and **bacteria.** The most common bacterial agent is *Streptococcus mutans.*
- **Prevention:** Fluoridated water and good oral hygiene combined with regular dental appointments are effective in reducing dental caries.

**TABLE 6.6.** The Jones Criteria for Rheumatic Fever

| MAJOR CRITERIA | MINOR CRITERIA |
|---|---|
| Carditis | **Clinical:** |
| Migratory polyarthritis | Fever |
| Sydenham's chorea | Arthralgia |
| Subcutaneous nodules | **Laboratory:** |
| Erythema marginatum | Elevated acute-phase reactants |
|  | Prolonged PR interval |
| *plus* | |
| Supporting evidence of a recent group A streptococcal infection (e.g., a ⊕ throat culture or rapid antigen detection test and/or an elevated or increasing streptococcal antibody test). | |

Reproduced, with permission, from Kasper DL et al. *Harrison's Principles of Internal Medicine,* 16th ed. New York: McGraw-Hill, 2005: 1978. Based on data from the Special Writing Group of the American Heart Association: *JAMA* 268: 2069–2073: 1992.

■ **Cx:** Complications of untreated caries include acute pulpitis, periapical abscess, granuloma, or cyst. Abscesses may track and → serious infections.

■ **Ludwig's angina:** A life-threatening infection of the sublingual and submandibular spaces that causes brawny sublingual edema potentially → airway obstruction. Treat with ampicillin/sulbactam or high-dose penicillin plus metronidazole.

■ **Lemierre's syndrome:** A suppurative thrombophlebitis of the internal jugular vein located in the posterior compartment of the lateral pharyn-

**TABLE 6.7.** Differential of Common Mouth Ulcers

| | APHTHOUS ULCER (CANKER SORE) | HERPES STOMATITIS |
|---|---|---|
| Cause | Common; unknown cause (possible association with HHV-6). | Common; HSV. |
| Symptoms | Pain up to one week; heals within a few weeks. | Initial burning followed by small vesicles and then scabs. |
| Exam | Small ulcerations with yellow centers surrounded by red halos on **nonkeratinized** mucosa (buccal and lip mucosa). | Vesicles, scabs. |
| Treatment | Anti-inflammatory: topical steroids. | No need for treatment, but oral **acyclovir** × 7–14 days may shorten the course and postherpetic pain. |
| Prognosis | Recurrent. | Resolves quickly; frequent reactivation in immunocompromised patients. |
| Differential diagnosis | If large or persistent, consider erythema multiforme, HSV, pemphigus, Behçet's disease, IBD, or SCC. | Aphthous ulcer, erythema multiforme, syphilis, cancer. |

Reproduced, with permission, from Le T et al. *First Aid for the Internal Medicine Boards,* 1st ed. New York: McGraw-Hill, 2006: 39.

geal space caused by *Fusobacterium necrophorum*. Leads to bacteremia and abscess in the lung and liver 2° to septic emboli.

## ORAL LESIONS

Table 6.7 outlines the differential diagnosis of common mouth ulcers.

**CARDIOVASCULAR DISORDERS**

A 33-year-old man is brought to the ER complaining of URI symptoms of three days' duration. On exam, the only pertinent findings are warm skin and some track marks in the left antecubital fossa. The nurse tells you that his current temperature is 39.5°C. You order a CXR, a UA, and blood cultures. Six hours later, the patient's blood cultures are ⊕ for Gram-positive cocci. On reexamination, you note a II/VI systolic ejection murmur. Which antibiotics would be the most appropriate empiric choice? Start vancomycin and gentamicin. Order an echocardiogram.

## Endocarditis

An infection of the endothelium of the heart that most frequently involves the valves. A vegetation consists of bacteria, platelets, fibrin, and inflammatory cells. Endocarditis is classified as acute vs. subacute and **native-valve endocarditis (NVE)** vs. **prosthetic-valve endocarditis (PVE)**. IV drug users are a special population at risk, particularly for tricuspid valve endocarditis (see Table 6.8).

TABLE 6.8. **Etiologies of Endocarditis**

| TYPE | ETIOLOGY |
| --- | --- |
| NVE | Viridans streptococci, other streptococci, *S. aureus*, enterococci. |
| PVE | *S. epidermidis*, *S. aureus*. |
| IV drug use | *S. aureus*. |
| "Culture-negative" endocarditis | Recent antibiotic use. <br> **HACEK** organisms (*Haemophilus*, *Actinobacillus*, *Cardiobacterium*, *Eikenella*, *Kingella*). <br> *Candida* and *Aspergillus* (IV drug users, long-term indwelling catheters, immunosuppressed). <br> Rare causes: *Chlamydia psittaci*, the "ellas" (*Bartonella*, *Legionella*, *Brucella*, *Coxiella*), and Whipple's disease. |

Reproduced, with permission, from Le T et al. *First Aid for the Internal Medicine Boards*, 1st ed. New York: McGraw-Hill, 2006: 390.

### SYMPTOMS

- **Acute bacterial endocarditis:** Presents with high fever (80%), chills, embolic phenomena, and, at times, symptoms of CHF.
- **Subacute endocarditis:** Presents with low-grade fever, weight loss, and poor appetite; has an indolent course. May also have signs or symptoms of CHF.

### EXAM

*Osler's nodes are **painful** nodules. Think **OUCH**ler's nodes.*

- Fever and a heart murmur are most commonly seen (although not all cases will have a murmur).
- Other symptoms and signs are as follows:
  - **Osler's nodes:** Tender nodules on the finger and toe pads.
  - **Janeway lesions:** Nontender hemorrhagic macules on the palms and soles.
  - **Splinter hemorrhages:** Reddish-brown streaks in the proximal nail beds (see Figure 6.2).
  - **Roth's spots:** Retinal hemorrhages seen with an ophthalmoscope (see Figure 6.3).
  - Petechiae, especially conjunctival and mucosal.
- Signs of right or left heart failure or CVA may also be seen.

### DIFFERENTIAL

Atrial myxoma, marantic endocarditis (nonbacterial thrombotic endocarditis, seen in cancer and chronic wasting diseases), **Libman-Sacks Endocarditis** (autoantibodies to heart valve, seen in **SLE**), acute rheumatic fever, suppurative thrombophelibitis, catheter-related sepsis, renal cell carcinoma, carcinoid syndrome.

### DIAGNOSIS

- **Labs:** Leukocytosis with left shift, mild anemia, and ↑ ESR.

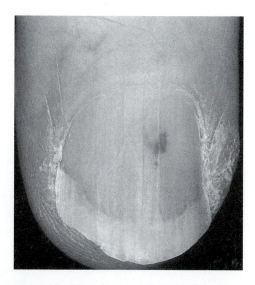

**FIGURE 6.2. Splinter hemorrhage.**

(Reproduced, with permission, from Wolff K et al. *Fitzpatrick's Color Atlas & Synopsis of Clinical Dermatology*, 5th ed. New York: McGraw-Hill, 2005: 1010.)

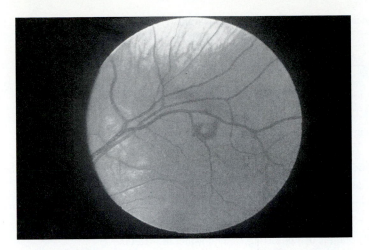

**FIGURE 6.3.   Roth's spots.**

This retinal image shows a lesion with central clear areas surrounded by hemorrhage. (Reproduced, with permission, from Le T et al. *First Aid for the Internal Medicine Boards*, 1st ed. New York: McGraw-Hill, 2006: 391.)

- **Blood cultures:** Critical in establishing the diagnosis; ⊕ in 85–95% of cases. It is recommended that **three** sets of blood cultures be taken at least **one hour** apart before antibiotics if subacute endocarditis is suspected.
- **Echocardiogram:** Transthoracic echo is 60–75% sensitive, whereas transesophageal echo is 95% sensitive. Both are 95% specific.
- **Duke criteria:** Definite endocarditis must meet two major, one major and three minor, or five minor criteria (see Table 6.9). The sensitivity of the Duke criteria is 95%.
- **ECG:** May show varying degrees of **heart block** if the conduction system is involved.
- **CXR:** May show multiple peripheral infiltrates with cavitation or effusions in patients with right-sided heart valve involvement.

### TREATMENT

- In general, therapy must be bactericidal, given intravenously, and administered for prolonged periods of time. The choice of antibiotic should be guided by clinical and epidemiologic clues in the absence of culture data or before culture data are available.
    - **NVE (empiric):** Start with nafcillin or vancomycin plus gentamicin. Gentamicin should be given every eight hours for synergistic killing. Adjust antibiotics on the basis of culture results and treat for 4–6 weeks. Uncomplicated right-sided, methicillin-sensitive staphylococcal endocarditis (with no embolic disease) can be treated with nafcillin and gentamicin for two weeks.
    - **PVE (empiric):** Vancomycin plus rifampin plus gentamicin initially. Adjust antibiotics in accordance with culture results and treat for six weeks.
- **Persistent fever** after one week suggests a septic embolic focus or inadequate antibiotic coverage.
- Reappearance of fever **after initial defervescence** suggests septic emboli, drug fever, or, less commonly, the emergence of antimicrobial resistance.
- **Indications for surgery** are individualized. Common indications include refractory CHF, valvular obstruction, myocardial abscess, perivalvular extension (new conduction abnormalities), persistent bacteremia, fungal endocarditis, and most cases of PVE.

161

**TABLE 6.9.** Duke Criteria for the Clinical Diagnosis of Infective Endocarditis

**MAJOR CRITERIA**

1. A $\oplus$ blood culture:
   - A typical microorganism consistent with infective endocarditis from two separate blood cultures, as follows:
     - Viridans streptococci, *S. bovis,* HACEK group, *S. aureus* **OR**
     - Community-acquired enterococci in the absence of a 1° focus

   **OR**

   - A persistently $\oplus$ blood culture, defined as recovery of a microorganism consistent with infective endocarditis from:
     - Blood cultures drawn > 12 hours apart; **OR**
     - All of three or a majority of four or more separate blood cultures, with the first and last drawn at least 1 hour apart

   **OR**

   - A single $\oplus$ blood culture for *Coxiella burnetii* or a phase I IgG antibody titer of > 1:800.
2. Evidence of endocardial involvement:
   - A $\oplus$ echocardiogram, defined as follows:
     - An oscillating intracardiac mass on the valve or supporting structures, in the path of regurgitant jets, or in implanted material in the absence of an alternative anatomic explanation, **OR**
     - Abscess, **OR**
     - New partial dehiscence of a prosthetic valve

   **OR**

   - New valvular regurgitation (an $\uparrow$ or change in a preexisting murmur is not sufficient).

**MINOR CRITERIA**

1. **Predisposition:** A predisposing heart condition or IV drug use.
2. **Fever:** ≥ 38.0°C (≥ 100.4°F).
3. **Vascular phenomena:** Major arterial emboli, septic pulmonary infarcts, mycotic aneurysm, intracranial hemorrhage, conjunctival hemorrhages, Janeway lesions.
4. **Immunologic phenomena:** Glomerulonephritis, Osler's nodes, Roth's spots, RF.
5. **Microbiologic evidence:** A $\oplus$ blood culture but not meeting major criteria as noted previously;[a] or serologic evidence of active infection with an organism consistent with infective endocarditis.

[a] Excluding single $\oplus$ cultures for coagulase-$\ominus$ staphylococci and diphtheroids, which are common culture contaminants, and organisms that do not cause endocarditis frequently, such as gram-$\ominus$ bacilli.

Reproduced, with permission, from Kasper DL et al. *Harrison's Principles of Internal Medicine,* 16th ed. New York: McGraw-Hill, 2005: 735.

***PREVENTION***

- **Antibiotic prophylaxis:** Recommended for known valvular disease (except mitral valve prolapse without murmur or only thickened leaflet), most congenital heart defects, hypertrophic cardiomyopathy, prosthetic valves, and prior endocarditis.
- **Procedures requiring prophylaxis:** Any procedure that could disrupt the GI or GU mucosa.
- Antibiotics are as follows:
  - **Procedures above the diaphragm:** PO amoxicillin, IV ampicillin, or PO/IV clindamycin 30–60 minutes prior to the procedure.
  - **Procedures below the diaphragm:** IV ampicillin plus gentamicin 30 minutes prior to the procedure and PO amoxicillin or IV ampicillin six hours after the procedure. An alternative regimen is IV vancomycin and gentamicin 30 minutes prior to the procedure.

- **CHF:** Caused by valvular destruction or myocarditis. The **most common cause of death** due to endocarditis.
- **Embolic phenomena:** Mycotic aneurysms, infarction, or abscesses in the CNS, kidney, coronary arteries, or spleen. Right-sided disease can → pulmonary emboli, but if a patent foramen ovale is present, it can also → systemic emboli.
- **Conduction abnormalities:** Include arrhythmia and heart block.
- **Myocardial or perivalvular abscess:** May extend to → pericarditis and tamponade. Most common with S. *aureus*.

## Myocarditis

Defined as inflammation of the myocardium; postulated to be a common cause of "idiopathic" dilated cardiomyopathy. The typical patient is young and healthy and may have had a recent viral URI. Can be a cause of sudden cardiac death. Etiologies include the following:

- **Infectious:** Usually **viral** (e.g., coxsackievirus, HIV, influenza), but may also be caused by other pathogens, including bacteria such as *Borrelia burgdorferi* in Lyme disease and parasites such as *Trypanosoma cruzi* in Chagas' disease.
- **Immune mediated:** Medication allergy, sarcoidosis, scleroderma, SLE, and others.
- **Toxin related:** Medications (anthracyclines), EtOH, heavy metals, and others.

### SYMPTOMS/EXAM

- Nonspecific. Flulike symptoms, fever, arthralgias, and malaise may be seen. In severe cases, patients may present with chest pain, dyspnea, and symptoms of heart failure.
- Physical exam may be normal or may exhibit findings consistent with heart failure.

### DIFFERENTIAL

**CAD/MI,** aortic dissection, pericarditis, pulmonary embolism, other pulmonary and GI processes.

### DIAGNOSIS

- **Endomyocardial biopsy:** The **gold standard.** However, the test is insensitive owing to the patchy involvement of the myocardium. Also, by the time most patients seek care, fibrosis is the only notable finding.
- **ECG:** Can be abnormal but is neither sensitive nor specific.
- **Cardiac enzymes:** May be ↑ in the acute phase.
- **Echocardiogram:** May reveal focal wall motion abnormalities and ↓ ejection fraction, but findings are nonspecific.
- **Cardiac catheterization:** To exclude CAD.

### TREATMENT

- No specific therapy. Treatment can be focused if there is a known cause (e.g., a parasite). Steroids have not been shown to be of use.
- Treat heart failure.
- Consider cardiac transplant in severe cases.

### COMPLICATIONS

Dilated cardiomyopathy, CHF, arrhythmias, death.

## Pericarditis

Defined as inflammation of the pericardium that → chest pain, pericardial friction rub, and typical ECG changes. It is commonly due to **viral,** connective tissue, post-MI, or idiopathic causes. Infectious etiologies include the following:

- **Viral:** Coxsackievirus A and B, echovirus, mumps, adenovirus, hepatitis, HIV, EBV, VZV, HSV.
- **Bacterial:** *S. pneumoniae* and other streptococci, *S. aureus*, *Neisseria* spp., *Legionella* spp., *Mycobacterium tuberculosis*, *Treponema pallidum*.
- **Fungal:** Histoplasmosis, coccidioidomycosis, *Candida* spp., blastomycosis.

### SYMPTOMS/EXAM

- Classically described as sharp, **pleuritic** chest discomfort that worsens when patients are supine and **eases when they lean forward.**
- On exam, a pericardial **friction rub** is the hallmark. The rub is classically described as having three components: atrial contraction, ventricular contraction, and ventricular filling.

### DIFFERENTIAL

The same as that of myocarditis, along with pneumothorax and costochondritis.

### DIAGNOSIS

- Look for a history of chest pain that is typical of acute pericarditis.
- Look for the presence of friction rub.
- Typical ECG changes (diffuse ST-segment elevation, PR-segment depression) are **not** compatible with a single coronary distribution (see Figure 6.4).
- Echocardiography is useful to exclude a large pericardial effusion, but many patients will have only a small effusion or a normal echocardiogram.

### TREATMENT

- Usually supportive, although treatment should be directed to the likely etiology.
- NSAIDs or colchicine (especially for patients with recurrent episodes).
- Steroids are often used as a last resort when patients do not respond to other therapies.
- Monitor for sign of enlarging pericardial effusion and/or tamponade (hypotension and elevated JVP).

## CATHETER-RELATED INFECTIONS

*In hemodialysis patients S. aureus is the most common etiology for catheter-related infections.*

A category of infections that includes catheter-related bloodstream infections as well as exit-site, tunnel, and pocket infections. The most commonly isolated etiologic agents are coagulase-⊖ staphylococci, *S. aureus*, *Enterococcus* spp., and *Candida* spp.

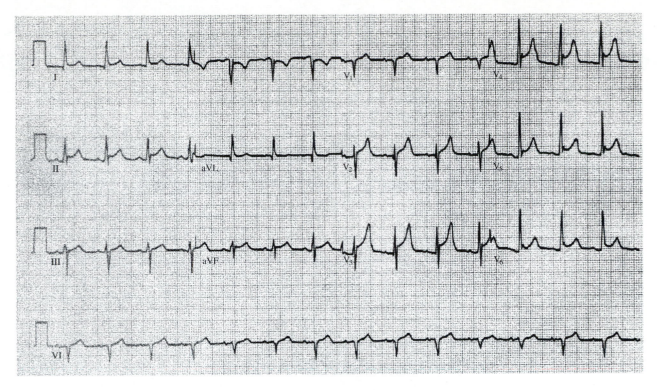

**FIGURE 6.4.** **Acute pericarditis on ECG.**

(Reproduced, with permission, from Crawford MH et al [eds]. *Current Diagnosis & Treatment in Cardiology*, 2nd ed. New York: McGraw-Hill, 2003: 210.)

### SYMPTOMS/EXAM

- Clinical findings are **unreliable.**
- Fever and chills are sensitive but not specific.
- Inflammation and purulence around the catheter are specific but not sensitive.

### DIAGNOSIS

- **Blood cultures:** Obtain two sets of cultures, at least one set drawn percutaneously.
- **Catheter tip culture:** Should be performed if line sepsis is suspected. The semiquantitative (roll plate) method is most commonly used. After the catheter has been removed from the patient, the tip is rolled across an agar plate. A colony count of > 15 after overnight incubation suggests catheter-related infection when blood cultures are also ⊕.

### TREATMENT

- **Catheter removal:** Used in most cases of nontunneled catheters. For tunneled catheters and implantable devices, removal should be considered in the presence of severe illness or documented infection (especially *S. aureus*, gram-⊖ rods, or *Candida* spp.) or if complications occur.
- **Initial antibiotic choice:** Empiric treatment should include vancomycin to cover methicillin-resistant *S. aureus* (MRSA) until culture data are available.
- **Duration of therapy:** Patients with uncomplicated bacteremia should be treated for 10–14 days. Those with complicated infections (e.g., those with

persistent ⊕ blood cultures after catheter removal, endocarditis, septic thrombophlebitis, or osteomyelitis) should be treated for 4–6 weeks.

### COMPLICATIONS

Septic thrombophlebitis, infective endocarditis, septic pulmonary emboli, osteomyelitis, or other complications due to septic emboli.

## Acute Bronchitis

A nonspecific term used to describe patients with or without underlying lung disease who develop an acute productive cough without evidence of pneumonia. By definition, the inflammation is limited to the trachea and to large and medium-sized bronchi. The most common causative organisms are respiratory viruses (RSV; rhino-, corona-, and adenoviruses; influenza and parainfluenza viruses) and, to a lesser extent, atypical bacteria (*M. pneumoniae, C. pneumoniae, Bordetella pertussis*).

### SYMPTOMS/EXAM

- Cough (productive or not) may persist for 1–3 weeks, often with initial URI symptoms (rhinorrhea or sore throat).
- Lung exam findings range from clear to wheezes (from bronchospasm) or rhonchi.

### DIFFERENTIAL

- It is important to rule out community-acquired pneumonia.
- Consider *B. pertussis* in children with a "whooping" cough and in adults with a severe paroxysmal cough.
- Other conditions that may → chronic cough include GERD, asthma, postnasal drip, foreign body, malignancy, CHF, and TB. Chronic cough may also be a side effect of ACEI use.

### DIAGNOSIS

Diagnosis is made clinically. CXR is not routinely indicated except, possibly, to rule out pneumonia.

### TREATMENT

- Given that the most common etiologies are viral, antibiotics are **not generally indicated** and should be reserved for the elderly, those with underlying cardiopulmonary disease, or immunocompromised patients.
- Expectorants can be used for symptomatic treatment.
- Bronchodilators may be used if there is a reactive airway component.

## Influenza

An acute viral respiratory infection caused by influenza A and B, members of the Orthomyxoviridae family. Winter is the predominant season for infection and influenza-related mortality. Transmission via aerosolized droplets is highly effective. Influenza is responsible for many local epidemics as well as for historical pandemics.

*Antigenic Shift occurs in Swine/Pigs and is the type of virus mutation responsible for Pandemics of influenza.*

### Symptoms/Exam

- Has a broad range of presentations, but usually presents with **abrupt onset** of fever (up to five days), chills, headache, myalgias, fatigue, anorexia, dry cough, sore throat, and/or clear rhinorrhea. Abdominal pain and diarrhea may be seen as well.
- Physical findings are few but may include hyperemic mucous membranes of the pharynx without exudates, lymphadenopathy, and scattered rhonchi or rales on auscultation of the lungs.

### Differential

Other respiratory viruses, atypical bacteria (*M. pneumoniae*, *Chlamydia pneumoniae*), bacterial pneumonia or pharyngitis, exacerbation of underlying co-morbidities such as COPD.

### Diagnosis

- **Viral testing:** If desired, rapid tests can be collected from the nasopharynx to detect viral particles within 30 minutes. In general, these tests are more specific than sensitive. Viral cultures, which can take up to 2–3 days, should be available even if rapid testing is not. Testing should be done within three days of onset of illness. Serologic techniques can also be used.
- **Blood tests:** WBC counts can vary from mild leukopenia to mild leukocytosis. Significant leukocytosis should prompt consideration of a bacterial etiology.

### Treatment

- **Symptomatic treatment:** Treat fever, headache, and myalgias with acetaminophen. Avoid salicylates in patients < 18 years of age in light of the risk of **Reye's syndrome**. Antitussives can be used sparingly. Encourage rest and hydration.
- **Antiviral therapy:** When used within the first 48 hours of illness, amantadine and rimantadine may ↓ the duration and severity of symptoms by up to 50%. However, these agents treat only influenza A (which is already developing resistance). Zanamivir and oseltamivir (neuraminidase inhibitors) can be used for influenza A and B. Consider ribavirin for severely ill patients.
- Consider hospitalization if there is concern about hydration and oxygenation or if the patient has significant comorbidities. Oseltamivir is generally used for hospitalized patients.

### Prevention

Yearly vaccination for at-risk patients (see Table 6.10). Because the vaccine is produced in eggs, it is contraindicated in patients with **egg allergy**. A newer (live attenuated) intranasal vaccine has been approved for children and healthy young adults who are not pregnant. Chemoprophylaxis with amantadine, rimantadine, or neuraminidase inhibitors should be considered in very high risk individuals during an influenza epidemic as susceptibilities allow.

### Complications

Most common in the very young, patients > 65 years of age with comorbid conditions, and during the second or third trimester of pregnancy.

*Reye's syndrome is a complication of influenza with concurrent aspirin use in children. Fatty liver and encephalopathy → a mortality rate of 30%.*

**TABLE 6.10.** **Recommendations for Influenza Vaccination**

**Those at ↑ risk for complications:**

- Those ≥ 65 years of age.
- Residents of nursing homes and other chronic care facilities that house persons of any age with chronic medical conditions.
- Adults and children (≥ 6 months of age) who have chronic disorders of the pulmonary or cardiovascular systems, including asthma.
- Adults and children (≥ 6 months of age) who have required regular medical follow-up or hospitalization during the preceding year because of chronic metabolic diseases (including DM), renal dysfunction, hemoglobinopathies, or immunosuppression (including immunosuppression caused by medications or by HIV).
- Children and adolescents (6 months to 18 years of age) who are receiving long-term aspirin therapy and therefore may be at risk for developing Reye's syndrome following influenza infection.
- Women who will be in the second or third trimester of pregnancy during the influenza season.

**Those 50–64 years of age:** Included because of the ↑ prevalence of high-risk conditions in this age group.

**Those who can transmit influenza to individuals at high risk:**

- Physicians, nurses, and other personnel in both hospital and outpatient care settings, including medical emergency response workers (e.g., paramedics and EMTs).
- Employees of nursing homes and chronic care facilities who have contact with patients or residents.
- Employees of assisted living and other residences for persons in groups at high risk.
- Those who provide home care to individuals in groups at high risk.
- Household members (including children) of those in groups at high risk.

Reproduced, with permission, from Kasper DL et al. *Harrison's Principles of Internal Medicine,* 16th ed. New York: McGraw-Hill, 2005: 1070.

- **Pneumonia:** 1° influenza viral pneumonia, 2° bacterial pneumonia, or mixed. Think of staphylococcal pneumonia as a cause of severe bacterial pneumonia in the postinfluenza setting, although pneumococcus probably remains more common.
- **Reye's syndrome:** Children present with nausea and vomiting followed by CNS changes several days after a viral illness. Currently, Reye's syndrome is uncommon due to ↓ aspirin use in children.
- **Musculoskeletal:** Myositis, rhabdomyolysis, and myoglobinuria are rare.
- **Cardiopulmonary:** Myocarditis (especially in younger patients), pericarditis, and exacerbations of COPD, asthma, or CHF.
- **Neurologic:** Encephalitis, transverse myelitis, Guillain-Barré syndrome.

## Community-Acquired Pneumonia (CAP)

The sixth leading cause of death in the United States. Four million cases are diagnosed annually, and one-fifth of these are admitted to the hospital for treatment.

### SYMPTOMS/EXAM

- Fever, dyspnea, and cough productive of purulent sputum are the most common symptoms.
- Pleuritic chest pain and rigors may occur.
- Patients who are immunocompromised, reside in an institution, have recently been hospitalized, or are at risk for aspiration should be considered separately from patients with suspected CAP.

## DIFFERENTIAL

- **Infectious:** Health care–associated, viral, or fungal pneumonia (including *Pneumocystis jiroveci*, formerly known as *Pneumocystis carinii*); TB, post-obstructive pneumonia, septic emboli from right-sided endocarditis.
- **Noninfectious:** Malignancy, foreign body, pulmonary infarct from emboli, collagen vascular disease with vasculitis → hemorrhage and hypersensitivity, radiation, chemical pneumonitis, aspiration pneumonitis.

## DIAGNOSIS

- **CXR:** Recommended for diagnosis; may characterize pneumonia severity, extent, and whether or not the pneumonia is complicated. May be nondiagnostic in the initial phase of illness.
- **Sputum Gram stain and culture:** Controversial because utility is limited, but **recommended for inpatients;** usually not necessary in outpatients. Must have < 10 squamous cells and > 25 neutrophils to be considered an adequate sample.
- **Blood cultures:** Should be taken in all hospitalized patients. Provide reliable data and allow for the tailoring of antimicrobial therapy if cultures are ⊕. However, cultures are ⊕ in only 10% of cases.
- **Tests for specific etiologies:** If there is a high clinical suspicion for a specific etiologic organism, seek appropriate available testing (see Table 6.11).

## TREATMENT

- Outpatient therapy is appropriate in low-risk patients. By assigning risk categories, the Fine index (or pneumonia severity index [PSI]) can help de-

**TABLE 6.11. Causative Organisms and Historical Features of Community-Acquired Pneumonia**

| ORGANISM | CAUSE (%) | SUGGESTIVE HISTORICAL FEATURES |
|---|---|---|
| *Streptococcus pneumoniae* | 20–60 | Acute onset; often follows URI; underlying COPD. |
| *Haemophilus influenzae* | 3–10 | Often follows URI; COPD. |
| *S. aureus* | 3–5 | May follow influenza infection; cavitary disease. |
| *Legionella* spp. | 2–8 | Exposure to humidifier, hot tub, or air-conditioning cooling towers; pleuritic chest pain and pleural effusion are common; diarrhea; hyponatremia. |
| *Klebsiella*, other gram-negative rods | 3–10 | Ethanol abuse, DM, residence in nursing home, aspiration. |
| *Mycoplasma pneumoniae* | 1–6 | Young adults in summer and fall; associated rash and bullous myringitis. |
| *Chlamydia pneumoniae* | 4–10 | Young adults; often follows prolonged sore throat. |
| Q fever (*Coxiella burnetii*) | Rare | Exposure to livestock (cattle, goats, sheep); elevated LFTs. |
| *Chlamydia psittaci* | Rare | Exposure to birds, including parrots, pigeons, and chickens; headache; temperature-pulse dissociation. |

Reproduced, with permission, from Le T et al. *First Aid for the Internal Medicine Boards,* 1st ed. New York: McGraw-Hill, 2006: 372.

termine which patients are appropriate for outpatient care and which should be hospitalized (see Tables 6.12 and 6.13).

- Antibiotic treatment is largely **empirical,** covering typical and atypical organisms. Appropriate choices for inpatient therapy include the following:
  - Extended-spectrum fluoroquinolones (e.g., moxifloxacin, levofloxacin).

**TABLE 6.12.** **Scoring System for Risk Class Assignment of Community-Acquired Pneumonia (PSI)**

| Patient Characteristic | Points Assigned[a] |
|---|:---:|
| **Demographic factor:** | |
| Age: men | Number of years |
| Age: women | Number of years minus 10 |
| Nursing home resident | 10 |
| **Comorbid illnesses:** | |
| Neoplastic disease[b] | 30 |
| Liver disease[c] | 20 |
| CHF[d] | 10 |
| Cerebrovascular disease[e] | 10 |
| Renal disease[f] | 10 |
| **Physical examination finding:** | |
| Altered mental status[g] | 20 |
| Respiratory rate $\geq$ 30 breaths/min | 20 |
| Systolic BP < 90 mmHg | |
| Temperature $\leq$ 35°C or $\geq$ 40°C | 15 |
| Pulse $\geq$ 125 bpm | 10 |
| **Laboratory or radiographic finding:** | |
| Arterial pH < 7.35 | 30 |
| BUN $\geq$ 30 mg/dL | 20 |
| Sodium < 130 meq/L | 20 |
| Glucose > 250 mg/dL | 10 |
| Hematocrit < 30% | 10 |
| Arterial $Po_2$ < 60 mmHg | 10 |
| Pleural effusion | 10 |

Reproduced, with permission, from Le T et al. *First Aid for the Internal Medicine Boards,* 1st ed. New York: McGraw-Hill, 2006: 373.

[a] A total point score for a given patient is obtained by summing the patient's age in years (age minus 10 for women) and the points for each applicable characteristic.

[b] Any cancer except basal or squamous cell carcinoma of the skin that was active at the time of presentation or diagnosed within one year before presentation.

[c] Clinical or histologic diagnosis of cirrhosis or another form of chronic liver disease.

[d] Systolic or diastolic dysfunction documented by history, physical examination and CXR, echocardiogram, multigated angiogram (MUGA) scan, or left ventriculogram.

[e] Clinical diagnosis of stroke or TIA or stroke documented by MRI or CT scan.

[f] History of chronic renal disease or abnormal BUN and creatinine concentration documented in the medical record.

[g] Disorientation (to person, place, or time, not known to be chronic), stupor, or coma.

TABLE 6.13. Recommendations for Site of Care for Community-Acquired Pneumonia by Point Score

| POINT SCORE | RECOMMENDED TREATMENT SETTING |
|---|---|
| ≤ 70 | Outpatient |
| 71–90 | Outpatient or brief inpatient |
| > 90 | Inpatient |

- A third-generation cephalosporin plus a macrolide or doxycycline.
- A β-lactam/β-lactamase inhibitor combination (amoxicillin-clavulanate) plus a macrolide.
- In severe CAP, consider **broader coverage** to include *Pseudomonas* and community-acquired MRSA.
- Antimicrobial therapy that is initiated within the **first 4–8 hours** has a significant association with improved outcomes.
- **Early conversion** from parenteral to oral therapy is appropriate once a patient has improved clinically, is hemodynamically stable, and is able to take oral medication.
- Patients may be discharged without delay at the time of conversion to oral therapy if they meet the discharge criteria (see Table 6.14).
- **Duration of treatment** varies, but many clinicians prescribe 10–14 days of therapy for inpatients and 5–7 days for outpatients, reserving longer courses (**at least** two weeks) for infections thought to be due to *S. aureus*, *Legionella*, *Mycoplasma*, and *Chlamydia* spp.
- A repeat CXR is **not** indicated during hospitalization except when complications are suspected (e.g., ongoing fever, hypoxia, clinical deterioration). A follow-up film in 4–8 weeks should be ordered to ensure that the infiltrate has cleared. This is especially important in smokers and older patients.

TABLE 6.14. Criteria for Discharge in Community-Acquired Pneumonia

- Clinical stability:
  - Improvement in cough/dyspnea
  - Adequate $O_2$ saturation (> 90%)
  - Afebrile (temperature < 37.8°C)
  - Resolution of tachycardia (< 100 bpm)
  - Resolution of tachypnea (RR < 24)
  - Resolution of hypotension (SBP > 90 mmHg)
- No evidence of complicated infection (e.g., extrapulmonary or pleural involvement)
- Ability to tolerate oral medications

Reproduced, with permission, from Le T et al. *First Aid for the Internal Medicine Boards*, 1st ed. New York: McGraw-Hill, 2006: 374.

### PREVENTION

Administer the pneumococcal vaccine to patients > 65 years of age and to adults with diabetes, cardiopulmonary disease, or asplenism.

### COMPLICATIONS

- **Pleural effusion/empyema:** Nearly 40% of patients with CAP will develop a radiographically evident effusion. Thoracentesis should be performed if the effusion is > 1 cm on a **lateral decubitus** film, if the patient is septic, or if the patient is not responding to antimicrobial therapy. For empyema or complicated parapneumonic effusions, a chest tube should be placed for drainage.
- **Recurrent pneumonia:** Recurrent CAP in the same anatomic location within two years may be due to an obstruction (i.e., mass or foreign body). If recurrence is in a new location, consider an immunodeficiency workup and a chest CT to rule out bronchiectasis.

---

An 82-year-old man is brought to the ICU following a cardiac arrest outside of the hospital. He is sedated and on a ventilator. On hospital day 5, the respiratory therapist notes a copious amount of brown sputum that persists with suctioning. Later that day, the patient has a temperature of 38.9°C and begins to show a decline in his systolic blood pressure. Which organisms should be empirically treated? Consider antibiotics that will cover *S. aureus* and *P. aeruginosa*.

---

## Health Care–Associated Pneumonia (HAP)

The second most common nosocomial infection (the most common is UTI). Most cases are due to aspiration of oral and hospital-acquired flora, with the highest incidence found in mechanically ventilated patients. Additional risk factors for HAP include recent antibiotic use, ↓ gastric acidity, use of an NG tube, ↓ level of consciousness, and comorbidities such as COPD, malnutrition, and old age. Infection is polymicrobial in up to 40% of cases, and common pathogens are *S. aureus*, *P. aeruginosa*, *Enterobacter* spp., *Klebsiella pneumoniae*, and *Acinetobacter* spp.

### SYMPTOMS/EXAM

Signs may include fever, cough, purulent sputum, chest pain, and shortness of breath. In the very old or young, altered mental status may be the only symptom.

### DIFFERENTIAL

ARDS, aspiration pneumonitis, and pulmonary embolism with pulmonary infarcts.

### DIAGNOSIS

- The distinction between CAP and HAP is somewhat arbitrary. Some experts state that symptoms must occur > 48 hours after hospital admission in order for HAP to be diagnosed, but others designate a longer period of time.
- Diagnosis requires new or progressive infiltrates on CXR with at least two of the following: fever > 37.8°C, WBC > 10,000/μL, or purulent sputum.

- Ventilator-associated pneumonia (VAP), a subset of HAP, must occur > 48 hours **after mechanical ventilation** and cannot have been developing prior to intubation.
- Try to obtain **endotracheal aspiration** prior to antibiotic administration. Obtaining specimens from the lower airway (via bronchoalveolar lavage [BAL]), mini-BAL, or bronchial brushing) and performing quantitative culture provides more specific information.

### TREATMENT

The initial empiric antimicrobial choices should be based on severity of infection and patient risk factors. Subsequent choices should be based on culture data. Some experts recommend two antipseudomonal antimicrobials (piperacillin-tazobactam, cefepime, ciprofloxacin, imipenem/meropenem) in patients with *P. aeruginosa* risk factors, but this is still controversial. MRSA should be covered as well.

### PREVENTION

- Prevention is paramount, as the mortality rate for HAP ranges from 40% to 70%. All providers must adhere to basic infection control principles (e.g., frequent hand hygiene and sterilization of ventilation equipment).
- Attempts should also be made to modify patient risk factors, including aspiration precautions, avoidance of gastric acid blocking agents unless clearly indicated, and judicious use of antibiotics.

### COMPLICATIONS

Respiratory failure, ARDS, complicated effusions, death.

## GASTROINTESTINAL DISORDERS

### Hepatic Disease

#### HEPATITIS A (HAV)

Most common in developing countries. The infection occurs sporadically or in epidemics associated with **seafood, especially shellfish.** HAV is transmitted via the fecal-oral route and causes only acute hepatitis. Symptoms and mortality vary with patient age.

*Hepatitis A and E are transmitted by the fecal-oral route.*

#### SYMPTOMS/EXAM

- Adults present with flulike illness, RUQ pain, jaundice, and pruritus. Children may be asymptomatic.
- Physical exam reveals jaundice and RUQ tenderness.

#### DIFFERENTIAL

- **Viral infections:** HAV, HCV, mononucleosis (EBV), CMV, HSV.
- **Nonviral infections:** Spirochetal disease (leptospirosis, syphilis), rickettsial disease (Q fever), acute bacterial gastroenteritis.
- **Noninfectious causes:** Autoimmune hepatitis, alcoholic hepatitis, fatty liver, hemochromatosis, Wilson's disease, gallbladder disease.

#### DIAGNOSIS

Anti-HAV IgM will be ⊕ in acute infection, while IgG will be ⊕ in prior infection or immunization.

### TREATMENT/PREVENTION

- Treatment is supportive.
- Vaccination (a series of two) should be given to travelers going to endemic regions, men who have sex with men (MSM), IV drug users, patients with chronic liver disease, food handlers, and day care center workers. HAV vaccine is a formalin-killed vaccine.
- Immune serum globulin should be given to household contacts of infected patients and to those who have eaten uncooked food prepared by an infected individual.

### HEPATITIS B (HBV)

Chronic infection with HBV is present in more than 400 million people worldwide. Transmission occurs via exposure to infected body fluids—i.e., blood and semen. Although most individuals clear the infection, 5–10% of infected individuals will become chronic HBV carriers. Of all patients with chronic HBV, 15–20% will develop cirrhosis and 10–15% will develop hepatocellular carcinoma (HCC). In mothers with acute HBV or those who carry HBsAg and HBeAg, the rate of virus acquisition by the infant is about 90%. Almost all of these infants will become chronic carriers unless passive immunization is given. Coinfection with hepatitis D virus is associated with a worse prognosis.

### SYMPTOMS

- **Acute HBV:** Flulike symptoms—e.g., malaise, anorexia, weakness, low-grade fever, nausea, and vomiting. RUQ pain and jaundice will also be present.
- **Chronic HBV:** Usually asymptomatic.
- **Extrahepatic manifestations:** Serum sickness–like rash, polyarteritis nodosa, glomerulonephritis.

### EXAM

- **Acute HBV:** Scleral icterus, jaundice, RUQ tenderness, arthralgias.
- **Chronic HBV:** Stigmata of cirrhosis—e.g., spider angiomata, palmar erythema, gynecomastia, caput medusae, and ascites.

### DIFFERENTIAL

See the HAV differential above.

### DIAGNOSIS

- ↑ liver enzymes, bilirubin, and PT.
- Serologic markers are the gold standard (see also Figure 6.5 and Table 6.15):
  - **HBsAg:** Surface antigen. Indicates **acute** or chronic HBV infection.
  - **Anti-HBs:** Antibody to surface antigen. Serves as the **protective** antibody and indicates past viral infection or immunization.
  - **Anti-HBc:** Antibody to core antigen. IgG indicates **prior HBV infection.** IgM indicates acute infection.
  - **HBeAg:** Envelope antigen. Proportional to the quantity of intact virus and therefore infectivity.
- HBV DNA can be used to measure active replication.

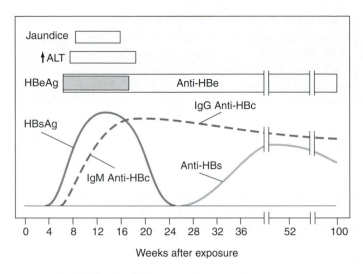

**FIGURE 6.5.** **Typical clinical and laboratory features of acute HBV.**

(Reproduced, with permission, from Braunwald E et al (eds). *Harrison's Principles of Internal Medicine*, 16th ed. New York: McGraw-Hill, 2005: 1825.)

- Liver biopsy is not routinely needed but should be considered if the diagnosis is in question or to rule out other processes.

### TREATMENT

- **Acute exposure/postexposure prophylaxis:** The CDC recommends that hepatitis B immune globulin (HBIG) be given in the first 24 hours along

**TABLE 6.15.** **Commonly Encountered Serologic Patterns of HBV**

| HBsAg | ANTI-HBs | ANTI-HBc | HBeAg | ANTI-HBe | INTERPRETATION |
|-------|----------|----------|-------|----------|----------------|
| + | – | IgM | + | – | Acute hepatitis B. |
| + | – | IgG[a] | + | – | Chronic hepatitis B with active viral replication. |
| + | – | IgG | – | + | Chronic hepatitis B with low viral replication. |
| + | + | IgG | + or – | + or – | Chronic hepatitis B with heterotypic anti-HBs (about 10% of cases). |
| – | – | IgM | + or – | – | Acute hepatitis B. |
| – | + | – | – | – | Vaccination (immunity). |
| – | – | IgG | – | – | False positive; less commonly, infection in remote past. |

[a] Low levels of IgM anti-HBc may also be detected.

Reproduced, with permission, from Le T et al. *First Aid for the Internal Medicine Boards,* 1st ed. New York: McGraw-Hill, 2006: 260.

INFECTIOUS DISEASES

with the first dose of vaccine if the patient was not previously immunized. Babies born to infected women should receive HBIG in the delivery room followed by three doses of the vaccine starting 24 hours after birth (prevents infection in 85–95% of infants exposed).

- **Corticosteroids:** Not indicated for viral hepatitis.
- **Interferon-α:** Given SQ for 4–6 months. Confers long-term benefit in 33% of cases, but has many side effects and is contraindicated in patients with cirrhosis.
- **Antiviral agents:** Lamivudine given PO is well tolerated, but resistance may develop. Adefovir and entecavir are alternatives for 1° therapy and for lamivudine-resistant virus.
- **Liver transplant:** In eligible patients with decompensated cirrhosis.
- **Chronic carriers should be encouraged to avoid hepatotoxic agents, including EtOH and high-dose acetaminophen.**

### PREVENTION

- 1° prevention is accomplished by the HBV vaccine, a recombinant vaccine. A series of three vaccines provides detectable HBsAb levels in > 95% of individuals.
- Patients with known HBV should be vaccinated against HAV.

### COMPLICATIONS

- HCC can develop **prior to** cirrhosis in HBV patients (this is not the case in HCV).
- Roughly 0.1% of patients develop fulminant hepatic failure.

## HEPATITIS C (HCV)

Generally transmitted via blood. Prior to screening, HCV was the most common cause of post-transfusion hepatitis, accounting for 90% of all such cases. Today, most infections occur 2° to IV drug use, but occupational exposure as well as sexual and vertical transmission may also be seen. Chronic HCV infection occurs in about 75% of those exposed; the remaining patients clear the virus without sequelae. Approximately 20% of carriers will develop cirrhosis within 20 years. HCC risk is 1–4% per year of cirrhosis.

### SYMPTOMS

- **Acute HCV:** Generally asymptomatic or very mild.
- **Chronic HCV:** Mostly asymptomatic as well, but may include renal failure, vasculitic skin rash and arthralgias, all 2° to cryoglobulinemia, and sicca syndrome.
- Symptoms of cirrhosis may also be seen.

### EXAM

See the HBV exam findings above.

### DIFFERENTIAL

See the HAV differential above.

### DIAGNOSIS

- Diagnosis is usually made after ↑ liver enzymes are noted on routine blood testing.

- **HCV antibody** will be present 4–6 weeks after infection. If qualitative PCR is used, antibody may appear as soon as two weeks postinfection. Recombinant immunoblot assay (RBA) can be used to rule out false ⊕ results.
- Liver biopsy is used to determine both prognosis and when to initiate therapy.

### TREATMENT

- **Acute exposure/postexposure prophylaxis:** Not recommended. Early treatment may be indicated if acute infection develops, as it appears to ↓ the risk of chronic carriage.
- **First-line treatment:**
  - Pegylated interferon-α SQ + ribavirin PO × 6–12 months. Treatment response varies from 40% to 80% depending on viral genotype (types 2 and 3 are considered favorable).
  - Up to 90% of virologic response occurs within the first 12 weeks of therapy. Side effects can be limiting and include flulike symptoms and depression.
- **Contraindications:** Psychiatric disease, CAD/CVD, decompensated cirrhosis, seizure disorders, bone marrow disease, autoimmune diseases, pregnancy (or inability to use birth control).

### HEPATIC ABSCESS

The liver is the most common organ for abscess development aside from the skin. Pyogenic liver abscesses can develop through bacterial invasion from the biliary tree (most common), portal vein, or hepatic artery as well as through direct trauma or adjacent bacterial infection. Approximately 15–40% of abscesses have no known cause and are termed cryptogenic. Predisposing conditions include advanced age, male gender, DM, malignancy, IBD, and a history of diverticulitis or cirrhosis. Abscesses are polymicrobial in > 50% of cases. Common organisms include *E. coli*, *Klebsiella pneumoniae*, *Proteus vulgaris*, *Enterobacter aerogenes*, and other gram-⊖ and anaerobic organisms. It is important to consider other etiologies as well—e.g., *Entamoeba histolytica* in immigrants and travelers and *Candida* spp. in neutropenic hosts.

### SYMPTOMS

- Onset is generally insidious. **Fever** is the most common presenting symptom.
- RUQ/epigastric pain, chills, nausea/vomiting, and weight loss are additional symptoms. Referred right shoulder pain occurs as well.

### EXAM

Fever, jaundice, RUQ tenderness.

### DIFFERENTIAL

Cholelithiasis, cholecystitis, cholangitis, hepatitis, gastritis, pancreatitis.

### DIAGNOSIS

- **Labs:** CBC, LFTs (nonspecific elevations, but alkaline phosphatase will be ↑ in 70% of patients), and blood cultures (⊕ in 33–100% of cases).
- **Imaging:** Abdominal CT with contrast is the imaging modality of choice, but ultrasound, MRI, and/or tagged WBC scan can detect hepatic abscesses as well.

### TREATMENT

- **Antibiotics:**
  - Aim to cover gram-⊖ organisms and anaerobes—i.e., use a third-generation cephalosporin and metronidazole. Treatment should be initiated intravenously, and total course duration should range from 6 to 12 weeks.
  - Use amphotericin if *Candida* spp. are suspected.
  - If amebic abscess is suspected, continue metronidazole until it has been ruled out by serology.
  - Additional empiric choices are available, and therapy should be tailored to culture results.
- **Interventions:** Drain if the abscess is ≥ 5 cm or is slow to respond to antibiotics. Drainage can be percutaneous or may require surgery.

### COMPLICATIONS

Mortality approaches 15% in some patients with complicated infection—e.g., abscess ruptures into the peritoneum, pleural space, or pericardium.

## Intestinal Disorders

A 39-year-old woman calls you at home complaining of 18 hours of intense abdominal pain, nausea, vomiting, and profuse, nonbloody, watery diarrhea. On further questioning, she states that she just returned from a trip to the Bahamas and adds that her sister has been experiencing similar symptoms. You instruct the patient to take her pulse, and she states that it is 120 bpm. After recommending that the patient go to the ER for IV fluids, you call the ER attending. What do you tell her is your leading diagnosis? Traveler's diarrhea caused by enterotoxigenic *E. coli.*

### INFECTIOUS DIARRHEA

Globally, diarrheal illnesses are the second leading cause of death behind cardiovascular disease and are the leading cause of death in children. However, most cases are mild and self-limited. Enteric pathogens are transmitted via the fecal-oral route, and risk factors for acquisition include travel, AIDS/immunocompromise, institutional care, and recent antibiotic use. Historical clues and diarrhea descriptions can be helpful in determining the etiologic agent. The most common bacterial causes of inflammatory enteritis in the United States are *Campylobacter jejuni*, *Salmonella* spp., and *Shigella* spp. Additional etiologies are as outlined in Table 6.16.

*There is an increasing incidence of **community-acquired** Clostridium difficile diarrhea.*

### SYMPTOMS

- **Noninflammatory diarrhea:** Pathogens act primarily in the **small intestine** to induce fluid secretion. Patients present with **large-volume, watery diarrhea** as well as with nausea, vomiting, cramping, and minimal fever.
- **Inflammatory diarrhea:** Pathogens induce inflammation in the **colon** via invasion or cytotoxins. Patients present with fever, **small-volume stools containing blood or mucus,** tenesmus, and lower abdominal cramping.

*The most common cause of infectious diarrhea in U.S. children is rotavirus.*

**TABLE 6.16. Microbiology of Infectious Diarrhea**

| INFLAMMATORY DIARRHEA | NONINFLAMMATORY DIARRHEA | GROSSLY BLOODY DIARRHEA | DIARRHEA IN HIV/AIDS PATIENTS | TRAVELER'S DIARRHEA |
|---|---|---|---|---|
| **Bacteria:** | **Bacteria:** | **Bacteria:** | **Bacteria:** | **Major causes:** |
| ▪ Campylobacter jejuni | ▪ S. aureus | ▪ Enterohemorrhagic E. coli | ▪ Campylobacter jejuni | ▪ Enterotoxigenic E. coli |
| ▪ Shigella spp. | ▪ Bacillus cereus | ▪ Shigella spp. | ▪ Shigella spp. | **Less common causes:** |
| ▪ Enterohemorrhagic | ▪ Clostridium perfringens | ▪ Campylobacter jejuni | ▪ Salmonella spp. | ▪ Campylobacter jejuni |
| E. coli | ▪ Enterotoxigenic E. coli | **Protozoa:** | ▪ C. difficile | ▪ Shigella spp. |
| ▪ C. difficile | ▪ Vibrio cholerae | ▪ Entamoeba histolytica | ▪ Enteroaggregative E. coli | ▪ Salmonella spp. |
| ▪ Vibrio parahaemolyticus[b] | ▪ Mycobacterium avium | | ▪ Mycobacterium avium | ▪ Rotavirus |
| ▪ Listeria monocytogenes | complex | | complex | ▪ Norwalk virus |
| ▪ Yersinia enterocolitica | ▪ Aeromonas hydrophila | | **Viruses:** | ▪ Vibrio parahaemolyticus |
| ▪ Enteroinvasive E. coli | ▪ Plesiomonas shigelloides | | ▪ CMV | ▪ Entamoeba histolytica |
| ▪ Enteroaggregative E. coli | **Viruses:** | | ▪ Enteric adenovirus | ▪ Giardia lamblia |
| **Viruses:** | ▪ Rotavirus | | ▪ Caliciviruses | ▪ Cryptosporidium parvum |
| ▪ CMV | ▪ Enteric adenovirus | | ▪ HIV enteropathy | ▪ Cyclospora cayetanensis |
| **Protozoa:** | ▪ Caliciviruses | | **Protozoa:** | |
| ▪ Entamoeba histolytica | ▪ Norwalk virus | | ▪ Cryptosporidium parvum | |
| | ▪ CMV | | ▪ Isospora belli | |
| | **Protozoa:** | | ▪ Cyclospora cayetanensis | |
| | ▪ Cryptosporidium parvum | | ▪ Microsporidia spp. | |
| | ▪ Giardia lamblia | | | |
| | ▪ Cyclospora cayetanensis | | | |
| | ▪ Isospora belli | | | |
| | ▪ Microsporidia spp. | | | |

[a] Cases can have no fever or focal leukocytes.

[b] May also cause a noninflammatory syndrome.

Reproduced, with permission, from Wilson WR. *Current Diagnosis & Treatment in Infectious Diseases*, 1st ed. New York: McGraw-Hill, 2001: 261.

INFECTIOUS DISEASES

179

### EXAM

Signs of dehydration, abdominal tenderness, and distention are commonly seen.

### DIFFERENTIAL

Noninfectious causes include drugs, food allergies, IBD, malabsorption, and motility disorders.

### DIAGNOSIS

- The history and physical are paramount.
- Further evaluation is indicated in the setting of fever > 38.5°C, severe abdominal pain, bloody diarrhea, immunocompromised hosts, age > 70 years, or severe dehydration.
- Specific testing is not needed in patients without the above warning signs.
- **Blood tests:** CBC, electrolytes, ameba serologies.
- **Stool tests:** Leukocytes (when present, suggest colonic inflammation and inflammatory diarrhea), lactoferrin (another marker of colonic inflammation), travelers or O&P (in recent transfers on immunocompressed hosts), *Giardia* antigen, *C. difficile* toxin, bacterial culture. Let the lab know suspected causative bacteria, as different media are required for the various possibilities.
- **Endoscopy:** Flexible sigmoidoscopy or colonoscopy with biopsy for chronic diarrhea.

### TREATMENT

- **Mild diarrhea:**
  - Oral rehydration therapy with oral glucose-electrolyte solutions.
  - A BRAT diet (bananas, rice, applesauce, toast) is recommended but is not evidence based.
  - **Antidiarrheals:** Loperamide. Use caution in infectious diarrhea, as it may prolong the duration of symptoms, may → toxic megacolon, and may also ↑ the risk of hemolytic-uremic syndrome (HUS).
- **Severe diarrhea:** Oral or IV rehydration. Consider hospital admission.
- **Antibiotics:**
  - Use only in the presence of fever, tenesmus, bloody stool (unless enterohemorrhagic *E. coli* [EHEC] is suspected), fecal leukocytes, or cultures showing bacteria or protozoa.
  - Empiric treatment consists of ciprofloxacin 500 mg PO or 400 mg IV BID × 3–5 days.
  - Antibiotics are **not** recommended for nontyphoidal *Salmonella* (may prolong shedding), *Aeromonas*, *Yersinia*, or *E. coli* O157:H7 infections. Antibiotics **are** recommended for *Campylobacter* infection, shigellosis, cholera, extraintestinal salmonellosis, severe traveler's diarrhea, *C. difficile* colitis (stop other antibiotics if possible and start metronidazole or vancomycin PO), giardiasis (metronidazole), amebiasis (metronidazole), and AIDS-related infectious diarrhea.

### COMPLICATIONS

- Volume depletion and electrolyte abnormalities are common.
- **HUS** is seen with **EHEC.** Patients present with renal failure, microangiopathic hemolytic anemia, and thrombocytopenia. Antibiotics and antimotility agents may ↑ the risk.
- **Guillain-Barré syndrome** is a potential complication of *C. jejuni* and presents with ascending paralysis.

*To prevent traveler's diarrhea, remind your patients to use the 5 P's when choosing food to eat:*

*Make sure it is **P**eeled, **P**iping hot, **P**ackaged, **P**urified, or **P**asteurized.*

A 24-year-old woman comes into your clinic with fever and nausea with mild dysuria. The patient states that she has had two UTIs in the past, but she adds this feels "a little different." On exam, she has mild epigastric pain and moderate CVA tenderness on the right side. UA shows ⊕ leukocyte esterase, 20–50 WBCs, and 3+ bacteria. What would be the most appropriate choice of antibiotic for this patient? Use ciprofloxacin/levofloxacin or TMP-SMX depending on local resistance patterns. Be sure to give the patient return instructions if she does not improve.

### Urinary Tract Infection (UTI)

An infection anywhere along the urinary tract; also known as cystitis. Generally more common in women. A UTI in a man should prompt consideration for a urologic workup. UTIs can be classified as complicated or uncomplicated:

- **Uncomplicated:** UTI in a young, healthy, nonpregnant woman. The most common organisms are *E. coli* and *Staphylococcus saprophyticus*. Less common are *Proteus mirabilis*, *Klebsiella* spp., and *Enterococcus* spp.
- **Complicated:** Defined as UTI in anyone else—e.g., male, elderly, hospitalized, and pregnant patients. This may also include those with an indwelling catheter, recent catheterization, anatomic abnormalities, recent antibiotics, symptoms > 1 week, immunosuppression, DM, recurrent UTI, or a history of resistant UTI. Culture data will be important for treatment, and duration of therapy should be longer.

#### SYMPTOMS

Commonly presents with dysuria, frequency, and urgency. Gross hematuria, fever, or suprapubic pain may also be present.

#### EXAM

- Suprapubic tenderness may be present; fever is uncommon.
- Consider a pelvic exam in sexually active women if STIs are being considered in the differential.
- A rectal exam should be done in men to rule out prostatitis; however, vigorous prostate massage can → bacteremia and should be avoided.

#### DIFFERENTIAL

- **Prostatitis:** In acute prostatitis, men present with fever, chills, dysuria, frequency, and perineal and low back pain. Exam will reveal an exquisitely tender prostate. Although it is most often caused by *E. coli*, other Enterobacteriaceae are common as well. Treatment should continue for four weeks.
- **Other:** Pyelonephritis, epididymitis, STIs, vaginitis (including atrophic), nephrolithiasis, interstitial cystitis, "bubble-bath" urethritis, and bladder tumors.

#### DIAGNOSIS

UA, focused STI testing, wet mount and KOH if there is a concern for vaginitis, and urine culture for complicated UTIs.

## TREATMENT

- **Uncomplicated:** Three days of TMP-SMX or ciprofloxacin. Nitrofurantoin or cephalexin may also be used and should be given for seven days. **Phenazopyridine** can be used for symptomatic treatment of severe dysuria for up to two days.
- **Complicated:** Should be treated with a broader-spectrum antibiotic, such as a fluoroquinolone, for a longer course (10–14 days). Culture data should be used to guide therapy.
- **Recurrence:**
  - Any patient with new symptoms of a UTI > 2 weeks after resolution of a prior UTI has a recurrence. Patients with two or more recurrences in a six-month period may need suppression. There are several antibiotics of choice for recurrent UTI, including daily nitrofurantoin, trimethoprim, or TMP-SMX.
  - In patients with recurrent complicated UTIs, consider imaging with IVP, renal ultrasound, or CT to rule out anatomic abnormalities or nephrolithiasis, which may act as a nidus for infection. Struvite stones (staghorn calculi) are associated with recurrent UTIs owing to urease-producing bacteria (*Proteus*, *Pseudomonas*, and *Klebsiella*).

## PREVENTION

Data are limited, but patients with recurrent UTIs are commonly instructed to clean themselves away from the urethra, to void immediately after intercourse, and to ↑ cranberry juice intake, which may ↓ bacterial adherence to the uroepithelium. Diaphragm use and use of spermicides should be avoided. Topical estrogen can be considered in postmenopausal women. There is an ↑ frequency of UTIs in uncircumcised infant males.

## Pyelonephritis

Caused by the same bacteria responsible for uncomplicated UTI. Ascending infection from the lower urinary tract → most cases of pyelonephritis; however, *S. aureus* is frequently hematogenous.

### SYMPTOMS

Presents with flank or back pain and fever. Patients often have concurrent lower urinary tract symptoms that occur 1–2 days before the other symptoms. Patients may also have nausea, vomiting, abdominal pain, and/or diarrhea.

### EXAM

Fever, CVA tenderness, mild to severe abdominal tenderness.

### DIFFERENTIAL

The same as that for UTIs above; also includes cholecystitis, appendicitis, and diverticulitis.

### DIAGNOSIS

- **CBC:** In ill-appearing patients, CBC may reveal leukocytosis with left shift.
- **UA:** Pyuria and bacteriuria are invariably present. Hematuria or WBC casts may also be seen.
- **Culture:** Urine culture is usually ⊕, and blood cultures may be ⊕ as well.

- **Outpatient:** Fluoroquinolone × 7–14 days. Second-line therapy consists of either amoxicillin-clavulanate or TMP-SMX for the same duration.
- **Inpatient:** Patients may require hospitalization if they are unable to tolerate PO, if signs of urosepsis are present, or if the patient is pregnant.
  - IV ceftriaxone for most patients.
  - Ampicillin plus IV gentamicin if **enterococcus** is suspected.
- Radiologic evaluation for complications may be necessary in patients who are severely ill, immunocompromised, or not responding to treatment, as well as for patients in whom complications are likely (e.g., pregnant patients, diabetics, and those with nephrolithiasis, reflux, transplant surgery, or other GU surgery).
  - Plain films can detect radiopaque stones (uric acid and indinavir stones are radiolucent), mass, and abnormal gas collections.
  - Ultrasound can examine the ureters and kidneys for fluid collections and stones. Ultrasound and voiding cystoureterography are recommended in patients suspected of having reflux disease.
  - CT with and without contrast is most sensitive but may be contraindicated in those with impaired renal function.

### COMPLICATIONS

- Perinephric abscess should be considered in patients who remain febrile 2–3 days after appropriate antibiotics. Patients with large abscesses or those who have failed antibiotics alone are treated by percutaneous or surgical drainage.
- Intrarenal abscess (e.g., infection of a renal cyst) < 5 cm in size usually responds to antibiotics alone.
- Diabetics may develop emphysematous pyelonephritis. This condition once required urgent nephrectomy because of its high mortality rate, but now it may often be treated medically with percutaneous drainage. In pregnant patients, pyelonephritis is associated with ↑ risk of preterm delivery and maternal complications.

## ORTHOPEDIC DISORDERS

### Septic Arthritis

An infection of the joint space that is usually spread by hematogenous seeding from another site. Risk factors for infection include trauma, DM, rheumatoid arthritis (RA), malignancy, frequent glucocorticoid injections, prior joint surgery, and IV drug use. The most common organism is S. *aureus*, but other etiologic agents include H. *influenzae*, gram-⊖ bacilli, S. *pneumoniae*, β-hemolytic streptococci, and N. *gonorrhoeae*.

### SYMPTOMS

Presents with acute onset of a painful, warm, swollen joint. Fever, chills, ↓ ROM, and skin rash may be seen.

### EXAM

- May be polyarticular. Most commonly involves the knee and hip; less commonly involves the shoulder, elbow, and small joints. If the sacroiliac or sternoclavicular joints are involved, screen the patient for IV drug use (the most common risk factor for these sites).

*If a young, sexually active adult presents with acute monoarticular joint pain, think about disseminated gonococcal disease (see Figure 6.6).*

**INFECTIOUS DISEASES**

- Findings include fever, warmth, intraarticular effusion, ↓ ROM, tenderness to palpation, and rash (see Figure 6.6).

### DIFFERENTIAL

- **Infectious:** Osteomyelitis, cellulitis, Lyme disease, fungal infection, rheumatic fever.
- **Rheumatologic:** Gout, pseudogout, SLE, RA, psoriatic arthritis.
- **Other:** Degenerative joint disease, internal derangement, reactive arthritis with serum sickness, Reiter's syndrome or poststreptococcal infection.

### DIAGNOSIS

- **Labs:** CBC; consider ESR and CRP (serial monitoring of CRP provides evidence of response to treatment); obtain blood cultures (⊕ in < 30% of cases).
- **Arthrocentesis:** Send synovial fluid for cell count, Gram stain (typically ⊖ in GC septic arthritis), culture, uric acid crystals, and calcium pyrophosphate dehydrate crystals (see Table 6.17).
- **Imaging:** Plain films may show soft tissue swelling but are otherwise unhelpful except in excluding other diagnoses. Consider bone scan, CT, or MRI if there is concern for osteomyelitis.
- **Other:** Urethral/cervical testing for GC.

### TREATMENT

- **Joint infection:**
  - Drainage by arthrocentesis. Usually necessary only once, but repeated "washouts" may be needed.
  - Start empiric antibiotics after cultures have been sent. Ideally, treat parenterally for 2–4 weeks.

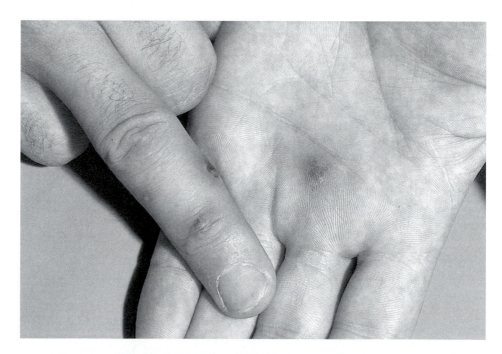

**FIGURE 6.6. Disseminated gonococcal infection.**

(Reproduced, with permission, from Wolff K et al. *Fitzpatrick's Color Atlas & Synopsis of Clinical Dermatology*, 5th ed. New York: McGraw-Hill, 2005: 910.)

TABLE 6.17. Examination of Synovial Fluid

| | NORMAL | NONINFLAMMATORY | INFLAMMATORY | SEPTIC |
|---|---|---|---|---|
| Clarity | Transparent | Transparent | Cloudy | Cloudy |
| Color | Clear | Yellow | Yellow | Yellow |
| WBC/μL | < 200 | < 200–2000 | 200–50,000 | > 50,000 |
| PMNs (%)[a] | < 25 | < 25 | > 50 | > 50 |
| Culture | Negative | Negative | Negative | > 50% positive |
| Crystals | None | None | Multiple or none | None |
| Associated conditions | | Osteoarthritis, trauma, rheumatic fever | Gout, pseudogout, spondyloarthropathies, RA, Lyme disease, SLE | Nongonococcal or gonococcal septic arthritis |

[a] WBC count and percent PMNs are affected by a number of factors, including disease progression, affecting organism, and host immune status. The joint aspirate WBC and PMNs should be considered part of a continuum for each disease, particularly septic arthritis, and should be correlated with other clinical information.

Reproduced, with permission, from Tintinalli JE et al. *Emergency Medicine: A Comprehensive Study Guide,* 6th ed. New York: Mc-Graw-Hill, 2004: 1795.

- Empiric antimicrobial choice is dependent on the age of the patient, whether or not the patient is sexually active, and Gram stain results.
- A third-generation IV cephalosporin is an appropriate first-line agent.
- If gram-⊕ cocci are seen on Gram stain, add vancomycin (for MRSA).
- For gonococcal disease, use IV/IM ceftriaxone. May switch to PO ciprofloxacin after 72 hours of IV antibiotics if the organism is susceptible.
- **Special situations:** Patients with **prosthetic joints** usually require orthopedic intervention.

## Acute Osteomyelitis

An infection of the bone or bone marrow. In adults, 80% of osteomyelitis cases result from contiguous spread. This is seen in patients with DM, prosthetic joints, decubitus ulcers, trauma, and recent neurosurgery. In 20% of cases, the infection is hematogenous in origin. Risk factors include IV drug use, endocarditis, sickle cell disease, and advanced age. Etiologies are as follows:

- **Common organisms:** *S. aureus* (most common), coagulase-⊖ staphylococci (prosthetic joints or postoperative infections), streptococci and anaerobes (bites, diabetic foot infections, decubitus ulcers), *Pasteurella* spp. (animal bites), *Eikenella corrodens* (human bites), *P. aeruginosa* (IV drug use and nail punctures).
- **Other causes:** *Salmonella* spp. (sickle cell patients), *Mycobacterium tuberculosis* (foreign immigrants, HIV), *Bartonella* spp. (HIV), *Brucella* spp. (unpasteurized dairy products).
- **By location:** *P. aeruginosa* affects the sternoclavicular joint and symphysis pubis (in IV drug use); *Brucella* spp. affect the sacroiliac joint, knee, and hip; and TB affects the lower thoracic vertebrae (Pott's disease).

### SYMPTOMS

Fever; localized pain and swelling of the affected extremity or area.

### EXAM

Fever, tenderness, erythema, and swelling over the affected bone. May present as a chronic draining wound that tracks to bone.

### DIFFERENTIAL

Cellulitis, RA, osteoarthritis, discitis, bone cyst/tumor, septic arthritis, simple skin ulcer.

### DIAGNOSIS

- **Labs:** CBC, ESR and CRP (serial monitoring of CRP may provide evidence of response to treatment), and blood cultures ($\oplus$ in 10–50% of cases where hematogenous spread in suspected). Serology for atypical causes can be ordered on an individual case basis.
- **Imaging: Plain films** are frequently normal but may reveal periosteal elevation or bony erosions. Three- or four-phase **bone scans** are helpful to distinguish bone from soft tissue inflammation. **MRI** is quickly becoming the preferred modality, especially for vertebral osteomyelitis.
- **Surgery:** Bone biopsy and culture is the gold standard and will in some cases reveal an etiologic agent. Very helpful if positive, but frequently negative. Swabs of exposed bone are generally not helpful, as they are frequently contaminated with flora and environmental organisms. May be used to determine if S. *aureus* is present.

### TREATMENT

- Empiric antibiotics such as nafcillin or vancomycin plus a third-generation cephalosporin should be started **after** all cultures have been obtained. The regimen should be directed toward the most likely organism(s). After culture results are received, therapy may be narrowed.
- IV antibiotics should be given for 4–6 weeks, although PO fluoroquinolones may be equally effective.
- Surgery is indicated for spinal cord decompression, bony stabilization, removal of necrotic bone, and reestablishment of vascular supply.
- Complications include epidural abscess and discitis (with vertebral osteomyelitis) and chronic osteomyelitis.

While finishing nursing home rounds, a nurse asks you to inspect a male patient's foot. As you approach the man, you note that he is one of your colleague's elderly diabetic patients. Exam reveals an erythematous, 1.5-cm foot ulcer. The ulcer is draining yellow, foul-smelling material. Pulses in the foot are palpable, but monofilament testing reveals peripheral neuropathy. The patient has been afebrile. What is the most appropriate management of this patient's infection? Obtain a radiographic study to rule out osteomyelitis. If no osteomyelitis is found, start a first-generation cephalosporin and metronidazole or amoxicillin-clavulanate. The patient should be serially examined, and if no improvement is seen, admission to the hospital for debridement and IV antibiotic therapy would be the next step.

## Diabetic Foot Infections

Because of neuropathy, abnormal blood flow, and poor biomechanics of the feet, diabetic patients are prone to foot ulcers and infections, including osteomyelitis. With these infections come significant morbidity and mortality. While most infections are polymicrobial, common organisms include S. *aureus*, streptococci (often group B), gram-$\ominus$ aerobes, and anaerobic bacteria.

### SYMPTOMS

May be asymptomatic due to neuropathy or may present with significant pain. Ulcer with eschar is frequently present.

### EXAM

Exam reveals an ulcer on the foot that may have indurated edges, erythema, swelling, and/or drainage (see Figure 6.7). The plantar surface of the foot is the most common site of infection. Fever is possible.

### DIFFERENTIAL

Cellulitis, noninfected ulcer, peripheral artery disease, venous stasis ulcer.

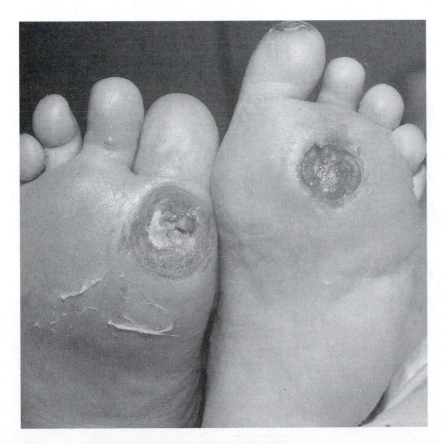

**FIGURE 6.7. Diabetic neuropathic ulcers on the soles.**

(Reproduced, with permission, from Wolff K et al. *Fitzpatrick's Color Atlas & Synopsis of Clinical Dermatology*, 5th ed. New York: McGraw-Hill, 2005: 436.)

### DIAGNOSIS

- **Labs:** CBC, ESR, CRP, $HbA_{1c}$.
- **Specimen:** Culture taken from a debrided ulcer or bone is most helpful.
- **Imaging:** Plain films are of some use, but a three-phase bone scan, a tagged WBC scan, and MRI are more helpful. Arterial flow to the foot should also be assessed.

### TREATMENT

- **Wound care:** Can range from daily dressing changes to bedside or intraoperative debridement.
- **Antibiotics:** Mild infections can be treated on an outpatient basis with first-generation cephalosporins PO and close follow-up. More extensive infections may need IV antibiotics such as cefepime, piperacillin/ tazobactam, or imipenem. Severe or unresponsive infections require coverage to include MRSA and *Pseudomonas*.

### PREVENTION

In addition to tight glycemic control, frequent foot exams, proper footwear, routine monofilament neuropathy screening.

### COMPLICATIONS

Osteomyelitis, sepsis, need for amputation.

---

## HEMATOLOGIC DISORDERS

> A 35-year-old man with a six-year history of known HIV comes into your clinic for a routine follow-up. He states that in the last two months he has had worsening dysphagia with both solids and liquids. On exam, you notice a moderate amount of thrush on his tongue and oropharynx. In addition to treating his candidal infection, you check a CD4 cell count, which has ↓ to 150. Which chemoprophylactic agents should be started today? TMP-SMX for PCP prophylaxis.

### Human Immunodeficiency Virus (HIV)

Since the initial cases in 1981, more than 50 million people have been infected with HIV. HIV targets and destroys CD4 T lymphocytes → AIDS. Transmission is via exposure to contaminated body fluids. Risk factors include unprotected sexual intercourse, IV drug use, maternal infection, and accidental needlesticks. Also at risk are patients who received blood products before 1985. Today, the fastest-rising demographic groups becoming infected are heterosexual women and African-Americans. Markers used to measure progression are CD4 count and HIV RNA viral load. The CD4 count measures the degree of immune compromise and predicts the risk of opportunistic infections. Viral load measures HIV replication rate, gauges the efficacy of antiretrovirals, and predicts long-term progression (see Figure 6.8 for the clinical course of HIV).

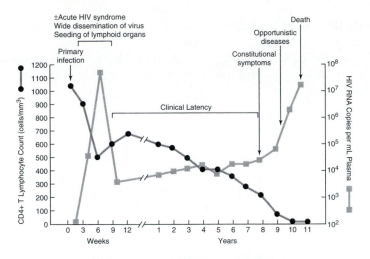

**FIGURE 6.8.** **Clinical course of HIV infection and disease in adults.**

(Reproduced, with permission, from Le T et al. *First Aid for the Internal Medicine Boards,* 1st ed. New York: McGraw-Hill, 2006: 404.)

## SYMPTOMS/EXAM

- **1° HIV infection:**
  - Often asymptomatic, or may present with **acute retroviral syndrome,** which consists of fever, sore throat, lymphadenopathy, and a truncal maculopapular rash or mucocutaneous ulceration occurring 2–6 weeks after initial infection.
  - Other signs and symptoms include myalgias, arthralgias, diarrhea, headache, nausea, vomiting, weight loss, and thrush.
- **Chronic HIV infection:**
  - Suspect and test for in patients with thrush, oral hairy leukoplakia, herpes zoster, seborrheic dermatitis, oral aphthous ulcers, or recurrent vaginal candidiasis.
  - Other symptoms may be vague and may include fatigue, fevers, night sweats, diarrhea, dysphagia, dyspnea, persistent lymphadenopathy, weight loss, and altered mental status.

## DIFFERENTIAL

- Acute retroviral syndrome resembles viral URI, influenza, infectious mononucleosis, acute CMV infection, aseptic meningitis, and syphilis.
- Chronic HIV infection may resemble malignancy, subacute bacterial endocarditis, connective tissue disease, depression, eating disorders, IBD, or malabsorption syndromes.

## DIAGNOSIS

- **ELISA/enzyme immunoassay (EIA):** Used to diagnose HIV by detecting antibodies to the virus in serum. In most cases, ELISA will be ⊕ three months after infection. Roughly 95% of infected patients will be ⊕ by six months. ⊕ tests must be confirmed by **Western blot.**
- **Other tests:**
  - There are rapid detection tests that provide results in 20–30 minutes. Such tests should be confirmed with traditional methods.
  - CD4 cell count should **not** be used for screening.

- **HIV RNA viral load** determination may be used when Western blot is indeterminate. False ⊕s do occur.
- Testing for **p24 core antigen** is approved by the FDA for diagnosis in the first few weeks after infection but is less readily available.

### TREATMENT

- The main goal is to suppress viremia and prevent immunosuppression. Four classes of antiretrovirals are available for this purpose:
  - **Nucleoside reverse transcriptase inhibitors (NRTIs):** Nucleoside analogs that interfere with viral DNA formation by inhibiting HIV reverse transcriptase. Include zidovudine (AZT), lamivudine, didanosine, stavudine, abacavir, and emtricitabine. There are several NRTI combinations available. Tenofovir is a **nucleotide** reverse transcriptase inhibitor.
  - **Non-nucleoside reverse transcriptase inhibitors (NNRTIs):** Use a different mechanism to inhibit reverse transcriptase. Include delavirdine, efavirenz, and nevirapine.
  - **Protease inhibitors (PIs):** Interfere with viral maturation by preventing cleavage of viral protein precursors. Include indinavir, nelfinavir, ritonavir (used for boosting other PIs), saquinavir, fosamprenavir, atazanavir, tipranavir, and lopinavir + ritonavir (Kaletra).
  - **Fusion inhibitors:** Prevent fusion of the virus to CD4 cell membrane. An example is enfuvirtide (Fuzeon).
- **Treatment initiation:**
  - The current recommendation is to start antiretroviral treatment in all patients who are **symptomatic.** Treatment of asymptomatic patients should be started when the CD4 count is 200–350 cells/mm$^3$.
  - Prior guidelines also recommend starting HIV treatment in patients with a viral load of > 55,000 copies/mL. Consider initiating antiretrovirals in patients with **severe** acute retroviral syndrome.
- **Treatment guidelines:**
  - Typical regimens use three drugs, generally consisting of two NRTIs plus one PI or NNRTI.
  - **Opportunistic infections:** Prophylactic medications should be initiated depending on CD4 cell count. Recommendations are outlined in Table 6.18.
  - **Strict adherence** to antiretroviral treatment is necessary for the success and longevity of a specific regimen. Patients should be counseled regarding the need for adherence, and antiretrovirals should not be initiated if the patient is not psychologically ready.
  - During **pregnancy,** women should be offered standard therapy in the form of two NRTIs (including AZT) plus nevirapine or a PI. Consider starting after 10–14 weeks of gestation to minimize the risk of teratogenicity. Efavirenz is contraindicated during pregnancy.
  - A multidisciplinary approach to care is recommended.
- **Side effects:** Antiretroviral medications have several expected side effects, including metabolic alterations. Common or notable side effects are as follows:
  - **NRTIs:**
    - **Zidovudine:** Anemia, neutropenia, myopathy.
    - **Lamivudine, didanosine, stavudine:** Pancreatitis.
    - **Abacavir:** If a patient develops a hypersensitivity reaction, rechallenge may be fatal.
    - **Peripheral neuropathy** is a common side effect of several of the NRTIs.

TABLE 6.18. **Prophylaxis Against AIDS-Related Opportunistic Infections**

| PATHOGEN | INDICATION FOR PROPHYLAXIS | MEDICATION | COMMENTS |
|---|---|---|---|
| *Pneumocystis jiroveci* cystic pneumonia (PCP) | CD4 count < 200/mm³ or a history of oral thrush. Prophylaxis may be stopped if CD4 > 200 for ≥ 3 months on HAART. | TMP-SMX or dapsone +/− pyrimethamine or pentamidine nebulizers or atovaquone. | Single-strength tablets of TMP-SMX are effective and may be less toxic than double-strength tablets. |
| *Mycobacterium avium* complex (MAC) | CD4 count < 50/mm³. Prophylaxis may be stopped if CD4 > 100 for ≥ 3 months on HAART. | Azithromycin or clarithromycin or rifabutin. | Azithromycin can be given once weekly; rifabutin can ↑ hepatic metabolism of other drugs. |
| *Toxoplasma* | CD4 count < 100/mm³ and *Toxoplasma* IgG ⊕. Prophylaxis may be stopped if CD4 > 100–200 for ≥ 3 months on HAART. | TMP-SMX or dapsone +/− pyrimethamine or atovaquone. | Covered by all PCP regimens except pentamidine. |
| *Mycobacterium tuberculosis* | PPD > 5 mm; history of ⊕ PPD that was inadequately treated; close contact to a person with active TB. | INH-sensitive: INH × 9 months (include pyridoxine). | For INH-resistant strains, use rifampin or rifabutin +/− pyrazinamide. |
| *Candida* | Frequent or severe recurrences. | Fluconazole or itraconazole. | |
| Herpes simplex virus (HSV) | Frequent or severe recurrences. | Acyclovir or famciclovir or valacyclovir. | |
| Pneumococcus | All patients. | Pneumococcal vaccine. | Some disease may be prevented with TMP-SMX, clarithromycin, and azithromycin. Repeat when CD4 > 200. |
| Influenza | All patients. | Influenza vaccine. | |
| HBV | All susceptible patients (i.e., hepatitis B core antibody ⊖). | Hepatitis B vaccine (three doses). | |
| HAV | All susceptible patients at ↑ risk for HAV infection or with chronic liver disease (e.g., chronic HBV or HCV). | Hepatitis A vaccine (two doses). | IV drug users, MSM, and hemophiliacs are at ↑ risk. |

Reproduced, with permission, from Le T et al. *First Aid for the Internal Medicine Boards,* 1st ed. New York: McGraw-Hill, 2006: 405.

- **NNRTIs:**
  - **Efavirenz:** Bizarre dreams.
  - **Nevirapine:** Hepatotoxicity.
- **PIs:**
  - **Indinavir:** Kidney stones.
  - **Tipranavir:** ↑ LFTs, hyperlipidemia.
  - **Atazanavir:** Hyperbilirubinemia.
  - **Fosamprenavir:** Rash.
  - Metabolic abnormalities and GI side effects, including diarrhea, are common with PIs.

### PREVENTION

- **Prevention counseling:** Needle exchange programs for IV drug users; safe sex practices; HIV testing in pregnant women; universal precautions for health care workers.
- **Postexposure prophylaxis (PEP):** Rapid initiation of PEP and nonoccupational postexposure prophylaxis (nPEP) is paramount in decreasing the risk of infection. A common regimen for PEP and nPEP is Combivir (zidovudine plus lamivudine). Individualized treatment should be formulated for high-risk exposures to highly resistant viruses. Consult with your local infection control officer.

---

## SPECIAL TOPICS

### The Splenectomized Patient

Patients who have undergone a splenectomy are at ↑ risk of serious bacterial infections, especially with encapsulated organisms such as *S. pneumoniae, N. meningitidis,* and *H. influenzae.* The highest risk is in the first three years after splenectomy. The most feared complication is overwhelming **postsplenectomy sepsis.** Patients present after a short viral-like prodrome that is followed by abrupt decompensation and shock. Vaccination against pneumococcus, *H. influenzae,* and *N. meningitidis* should be given two weeks prior to elective splenectomy or at hospital discharge for emergent cases.

All splenectomized patients should be counseled that new fever is a medical emergency and that they should seek attention immediately. Penicillin prophylaxis is not routinely recommended in adults. In children and adolescents, penicillin prophylaxis should be given for three years after splenectomy. These patients are also at ↑ risk of parasitic infections, specifically babesiosis.

*To remember the appearance of* Blastomyces *under the microscope, think* **B**lastomyces = **B**road-**B**ased, **B**udding yeast.

### Common Fungal Infections

Table 6.19 lists the presentation and treatment of common fungal infections.

### Tick-Borne Diseases

Table 6.20 outlines the presentation of tick-borne zoonoses.

TABLE 6.19. **Clinical Presentation and Treatment of Selected Fungal Infections**

| FUNGUS | GEOGRAPHY | MANIFESTATION | TREATMENT | NOTES |
|---|---|---|---|---|
| *Candida* spp. | Common yeast on the skin worldwide. | Thrush, esophagitis, intertrigo, vaginitis, candiduria, hepatosplenic candidiasis (in postneutropenic chemo patients), disseminated candidiasis. | Topical antifungals for mucosal disease. Oral fluconazole for esophagitis; IV or PO fluconazole, amphotericin formulation, or echinocandin for disseminated disease. Remove vascular catheters. | *Candida glabrata* is frequently resistant to azole therapy. |
| *Aspergillus* spp. | Widespread in soil, water, compost, potted plants, and ventilation ducts. | Allergic bronchopulmonary aspergillosis; aspergilloma of the lung or sinuses; invasive aspergillosis. | Voriconazole, echinocandin, or amphotericin for invasive disease (combination therapy is sometimes used); surgical excision of aspergilloma in the setting of hemoptysis. | A common infection in neutropenic patients or post-transplant. |
| *Cryptococcus* | Worldwide in bird droppings (especially pigeons). | Meningitis, especially in HIV patients with CD4 counts < 100 and in atypical pneumonia. | For meningitis, amphotericin and 5-flucytosine or fluconazole; fluconazole for mild lung disease. | Order India ink on CSF if available or cryptococcus antigen on CSF. |
| *Coccidioides* | Soil of the southwestern United States and the San Joaquin Valley. | "Valley fever," flulike syndrome, pneumonia. Disseminated disease in 1–5%. | Supportive therapy for "valley fever"; fluconazole or amphotericin for disseminated disease. | Check for *Coccidioides* antibody titer. |
| *Histoplasma* | Bird and bat droppings in the Mississippi and Ohio River valleys. | Pulmonary infection, disseminated disease. | Supportive therapy for lung disease; itraconazole or amphotericin for disseminated disease. | Risk factors include spelunking and contact with chicken coops. |
| *Blastomyces* | Upper Midwest and Great Lakes region. | Most commonly pneumonia; occasionally skin infections, osteomyelitis, and epididymitis/prostatitis. | Itraconazole or amphotericin. | Risk factors are exposure to forests and streams. |
| *Sporothrix* | Found in soil, especially rose bushes. | Most commonly skin and soft tissue infection. Can also → disseminated disease. | Itraconazole for mild disease; amphotericin for severe disease. | |

INFECTIOUS DISEASES

**TABLE 6.20.** **Tick-Borne Zoonotic Infections**

| Disease | Vector | Animal Reservoir | Clinical Features | Antibiotic Treatment | Geographic Distribution |
|---|---|---|---|---|---|
| Babesiosis | *Ixodes dammini, I. scapularis,* and *I. pacificus* | Cattle, horses, dogs, cats, rodents, deer | Fatigue, malaise, anorexia, nausea, headache, sweats, rigors, abdominal pain, emotional lability, depression, dark urine, hepatomegaly, fever, petechiae, ecchymosis, occasional rash, and occasionally pulmonary edema | For the seriously ill, atovaquone and azithromycin, or quinine plus clindamycin | Coastal areas of Massachusetts, Rhode Island, and New York; also in Maryland, Virginia, Minnesota, Wisconsin, Georgia, Washington, and Mexico |
| Colorado tick fever | *Dermacentor andersoni* | Deer, marmots, porcupines | Fever, chills, headache, myalgias, nausea, vomiting, photophobia, abdominal pain, and occasional sore throat; also may have conjunctivitis, lymphadenopathy, hepatosplenomegaly, stiff neck, retroorbital pain, weakness, and lethargy | Supportive care | Western and northwestern United States and southwestern Canada |
| Human granulocytic ehrlichiosis | *Ixodes scapularis* | Dogs, deer, other mammals | Fevers, chills, malaise, headache, nausea, muscle aches, cough, sore throat, and pulmonary infiltrates (especially in children) | Doxycycline or tetracycline | Japan, Malaysia, and the eastern, northeastern, and north central United States |
| Human monocytic ehrlichiosis | *Amblyomma americanum* (Lone Star tick) and *D. variabilis* | Dogs, deer, other mammals | Fevers, chills, malaise, headache, nausea, muscle aches, cough, sore throat, and pulmonary infiltrates (especially in children) | Doxycycline or tetracycline | Japan, Malaysia, and southern United States |
| Lyme disease (*Borrelia burgdorferi*) | *Ixodes dammini* | Deer, sheep, deer mice | Erythema migrans, meningitis, encephalitis, neuropathy, and joint and heart symptoms | Doxycycline, amoxicillin, cefuroxime, erythromycin, ceftriaxone, or cefotaxime | Atlantic central and north central United States |
| Rocky Mountain spotted fever (*Rickettsia rickettsii*) | *Dermacentor andersoni* (wood tick) and *D. variabilis* (dog tick) | North American mammals | Petechiae, purpura, pulmonary infiltrates, jaundice, myocarditis, hepatosplenomegaly, meningitis, encephalitis, and lymphadenopathy | Doxycycline or chloramphenicol | Most of the continental United States, although more prevalent in the southeast and south central United States |

INFECTIOUS DISEASES

TABLE 6.20. Tick-Borne Zoonotic Infections (continued)

| DISEASE | VECTOR | ANIMAL RESERVOIR | CLINICAL FEATURES | ANTIBIOTIC TREATMENT | GEOGRAPHIC DISTRIBUTION |
|---------|--------|------------------|-------------------|---------------------|------------------------|
| Relapsing fever (*Borrelia* spp.) | *Ornithodoros* spp. | Human body lice, wild rodents, humans | Fever, chills, headache, myalgias, and arthralgias; pain, nausea, vomiting, and hypotension | Erythromycin or doxycycline | Worldwide |
| Tularemia (*Francisella tularensis*) | *Dermacentor* spp. and *Amblyomma* spp. | Rabbits, deer, dogs | Pneumonia, regional lymphadenopathy and headache, cough, myalgias, arthralgias, nausea, vomiting, ulceration at inoculation site, and ocular findings | Tobramycin or gentamycin; chloramphenicol for meningitis | United States (except Hawaii) and Canada |

Reproduced, with permission, from Tintinalli JE et al. *Emergency Medicine: A Comprehensive Study Guide,* 6th ed. New York: Mc-Graw-Hill, 2004: 372.

## Fever of Unknown Origin (FUO)

Defined as a temperature > 38.3°C for ≥ 3 weeks that remains undiagnosed despite evaluation over three outpatient visits or three hospital days. Common etiologies include infection (25–40%), cancer (25–40%), and autoimmune disease (10–15%). Infection is more likely if the patient is older or from a developing country, as well as in cases of nosocomial, neutropenic, or HIV-associated FUO. In roughly 10–15% of cases, no diagnosis will be discovered, and the fever will resolve spontaneously.

### SYMPTOMS

Fever; otherwise variable, but a careful history should be taken on serial visits to elucidate any clues to a diagnosis.

### EXAM

Repeated physical exams may yield subtle findings in the fundi, conjunctivae, sinuses, temporal arteries, and lymph nodes. Heart murmurs, splenomegaly, and perirectal or prostatic fluctuance/tenderness should be assessed.

### DIFFERENTIAL

- **Infectious: TB, endocarditis,** and **occult abscesses** are the most common infectious causes of FUO in immunocompetent patients. Consider 1° HIV infection or opportunistic infections due to unrecognized HIV. In rare cases, the cause is babesiosis or other tick-borne diseases.
- **Neoplastic: Lymphoma** and **leukemia** are the most common cancers causing FUO. Other causes include hepatoma, renal cell carcinoma, and atrial myxoma.
- **Autoimmune:** Adult Still's disease, SLE, cryoglobulinemia, polyarteritis nodosa, and temporal arteritis (especially in the elderly).
- **Other:** Drug fever, thyroiditis, granulomatous hepatitis, sarcoidosis, Crohn's disease, Whipple's disease, familial Mediterranean fever, recurrent pulmonary embolism, retroperitoneal hematoma, factitious fever.

INFECTIOUS DISEASES

### DIAGNOSIS

- Ask about HIV risk factors, cardiac valve disorders, drug use, travel, exposure to animals/insects, occupational history, recent medications, sick contacts, and a family history of fever.
- Obtain routine labs and CXR. Blood cultures should be drawn off antibiotics and held for two weeks. Place a PPD. If indicated, obtain cultures of other body fluids (sputum, urine, stool, CSF). If travel history is present, obtain a blood smear (malaria, babesiosis). Do an HIV test.
- Perform echocardiography to look for vegetations. If neoplasm or abscesses are suspected, order a CT/MRI.
- Use more specific tests selectively (ANA, RF, viral cultures, antibody/antigen tests for viral and fungal infections).
- Invasive procedures are generally low yield except for temporal artery biopsy in the elderly, liver biopsy in patients with LFT abnormalities, and bone marrow biopsy in HIV.

### TREATMENT

- If there are no other symptoms, treatment may be deferred until a definitive diagnosis is made.
- Give broad-spectrum antibiotics if the patient is severely ill or neutropenic.
- Again, 10–15% of cases will spontaneously resolve.

## Methicillin-Resistant *S. aureus*

In light of the increasing incidence of community-acquired MRSA, clinicians should consider this diagnosis when skin and soft tissue infection treatment failures occur. The following antibiotics may be used depending on local resistance profiles: clindamycin, TMP-SMX, ciprofloxacin + rifampin, tetracycline derivatives, linezolid, vancomycin, and daptomycin.

Carriage of MRSA occurs in the nares and other skin sites. Therefore, in patients with recurrent MRSA infections, decolonization may be attempted with intranasal mupirocin and chlorhexidine-containing body washes. Although skin and soft tissue infections are the most common manifestation of community-acquired MRSA, severe life-threatening pneumonia has been increasingly reported.

# CHAPTER 7

# Hematology/Oncology

Andrea Taylor, MD

HEMATOLOGY/ONCOLOGY

## Approach to Anemia

Defined as low oxygen-carrying capacity of blood, represented by a low quantity of hemoglobin or volume percentage of red blood cells (hematocrit) in blood. General symptoms include **fatigue, dyspnea, pallor, postural lightheadedness,** and **tachycardia.** Workup is best accomplished by dividing the causes into categories based on typical MCV and reticulocyte count (whether they are hypo- or hyperproliferative). The etiology is often multifactorial, which can complicate the basic algorithm (see Figure 7.1 and Table 7.1). Treatment is dependent on etiology.

## Microcytic Anemia

### IRON DEFICIENCY ANEMIA

Etiologies include chronic blood loss, ↓ iron absorption due to celiac sprue or Crohn's, and ↑ demand during pregnancy.

### SYMPTOMS/EXAM

Symptoms associated with severe iron deficiency anemia include the following (most patients are asymptomatic unless deficiency is severe):

- **Angular cheilosis:** Fissures at the corners of the mouth.
- **Atrophic glossitis.**
- **Pica:** Craving for nonnutritive substances
- **Koilonychia:** Spooning of the fingernails.
- **Plummer-Vinson syndrome:** Esophageal webs and atrophic glossitis → dysphagia.

### DIAGNOSIS

- Peripheral smear may show microcytic, hypochromic RBCs and marked anisocytosis (the presence of cells of widely differing sizes).
- A serum ferritin < 12 is highly suggestive. Low serum iron and high TIBC and transferrin are also seen.
- An empiric trial of iron with a resultant ↑ in reticulocytes after 3–5 days.

> *Causes of microcytic anemia—*
>
> **TICS**
>
> **T**halassemia
> **I**ron deficiency
> **C**hronic disease
> **S**ideroblastic anemia

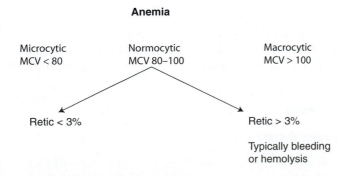

**FIGURE 7.1. Algorithm for categorizing anemia.**

TABLE 7.1. Classification of Anemia by MCV

| MICROCYTIC (MCV < 80) | NORMOCYTIC (MCV 80–100) | MACROCYTIC (MCV >100) |
|---|---|---|
| Iron deficiency anemia | **Hypoproliferative:** | **Megaloblastic:** |
| Anemia of chronic disease | Anemia of chronic disease | $B_{12}$ or folate deficiency |
| Sideroblastic anemia | Bone marrow disease | Drug-induced bone marrow suppression |
| Thalassemia | Renal failure | (methotrexate, phenytoin, phenobarbital) |
| Lead poisoning | Hypersplenism | **Nonmegaloblastic:** |
| INH | Infection: HIV, *Mycoplasma*, EBV | Liver disease |
| Chloramphenicol | Any early or mixed process of anemia | Alcoholism |
| | **Hyperproliferative:** | Hypothyroidism |
| | Hemolysis | Reticulocytosis |
| | Acute blood loss | Some bone marrow diseases (aplastic anemia, |
| | | myelodysplastic syndrome, myeloma) |

### TREATMENT

- If possible, take steps to correct the underlying cause
- Oral iron replacement should correct the anemia in about six weeks and should replete the body's iron stores in about six months. Parenteral iron can be used if anemia is refractory to oral replacement or if there is a problem with iron absorption.

### SIDEROBLASTIC ANEMIA

A group of diseases characterized by **defective heme biosynthesis** within RBC precursors. This leads to **impaired erythropoiesis** and **accumulation of iron** in mitochondria, producing the characteristic "ringed sideroblasts." May be hereditary, acquired, idiopathic, or reversible. Reversible causes include alcoholism, copper deficiency, INH, and chloramphenicol.

### DIAGNOSIS

- MCV may be low, normal or high.
- ↑ iron, transferrin saturation, and ferritin; ↓ transferrin.
- **Siderocytes on peripheral smear:** Hypochromic RBCs with **basophilic stippling** that stains ⊕ for iron (i.e., **Pappenheimer bodies**).
- Bone marrow with **ringed sideroblasts** and **erythroid hyperplasia**.

### TREATMENT

- Treat any reversible causes.
- Give periodic transfusions for severe anemia.
- **Pyridoxine** supplementation improves anemia in some hereditary forms.
- Iron chelation therapy or therapeutic phlebotomy for iron overload.

*ACD is commonly associated*

*with the following:*

- *Chronic infection*
- *Chronic inflammation*
- *Neoplasms*
- *Liver disease*

## Normocytic Anemia

### ANEMIA OF CHRONIC DISEASE (ACD)

Caused by a ↓ in RBC production 2° to a combination of factors, including trapping of iron in macrophages, ↓ erythropoietin (EPO) production, and ↓ ability of the bone marrow to respond to anemia by increasing erythropoiesis.

TABLE 7.2. ACD vs. Iron Deficiency Anemia

| | MCV | RDW | Fe | TIBC | FERRITIN | Fe/TIBC | TRANSFERRIN |
|---|---|---|---|---|---|---|---|
| Iron deficiency | Low/ normal | ↑ | ↓ | ↑ | Low | < 18% | ↑ |
| ACD | Low/ normal | Normal | ↓ | ↓ | Normal/high | > 18% | Normal |

Table 7.2 outlines the manner in which ACD is distinguished from iron deficiency anemia.

### TREATMENT

- Treat the underlying cause.
- EPO injections may be tried if the patient has low serum EPO levels.

*ACD is typically normocytic but can be microcytic if severe.*

### HEMOLYTIC ANEMIA

Hemolytic anemia may be classified as extravascular or intravascular based on the site of RBC destruction (see Table 7.3). Etiologies are as follows:

- **Autoimmune hemolytic anemias (AIHAs):** Acquired disorders in which RBCs are destroyed by autoantibodies. Associated with autoimmune disease, infection with *Mycoplasma* or EBV, and lymphoproliferative disorders.
- **Microangiopathic hemolytic anemia:** Etiologies include **DIC, thrombotic thrombocytopenic purpura,** malignant hypertension, HELLP syndrome, and prosthetic cardiac valves. Diagnosed by the presence of **schistocytes** and a ⊖ Coombs' test.
- **Glucose-6-phosphate dehydrogenase (G6PD) deficiency:** An X-linked defect that → ↑ susceptibility of RBCs to oxidative stress. Oxidative stressors include drugs (dapsone, sulfonamides, antimalarials, nitrofurantoin), infection, or foods (fava beans). A peripheral smear may show **Heinz bodies** and **bite cells.**

TABLE 7.3. Extravascular vs. Intravascular Hemolytic Anemia

| | EXTRAVASCULAR | INTRAVASCULAR |
|---|---|---|
| Site of RBC destruction | Spleen | Blood vessels, liver |
| Peripheral smear | Spherocytes | Schistocytes |
| Serum haptoglobin | Normal or mildly ↓ | Markedly ↓ |
| Urine hemosiderin | Normal | ↑ |
| Etiologies | Warm AIHA, hypersplenism, delayed hemolytic transfusion reaction | Cold AIHA, acute hemolytic transfusion reaction, microangiopathic hemolysis, G6PD deficiency, PNH, hemoglobinopathies |

Reproduced, with permission, from Le T et al. *First Aid for the Internal Medicine Boards,* 1st ed. New York: McGraw-Hill, 2006: 309.

- **Paroxysmal nocturnal hemoglobinuria (PNH):** Characterized by ↑ RBC sensitivity to complement and episodes of intravascular hemolytic anemia.
- **Sickle cell anemia:** See the discussion of hemoglobinopathies below.

### Macrocytic, Megaloblastic Anemia

Results from impaired DNA synthesis 2° to $B_{12}$ or folate deficiency or drug-induced bone marrow suppression (see Table 7.1).

#### DIAGNOSIS

- Anemia and ↑ MCV are usually found but are not required for diagnosis. Pancytopenia may be seen in the presence of severe disease.
- ↑ LDH and indirect bilirubin 2° to ineffective erythropoiesis.
- ↑ levels of homocysteine (in both $B_{12}$ and folate deficiency) and methylmalonic acid ($B_{12}$ deficiency only) occur 2° to a ↓ rate of metabolism.
- Peripheral smear shows **hypersegmented neutrophils,** macro-ovalocytes, and megaloblasts (see Figure 7.2).

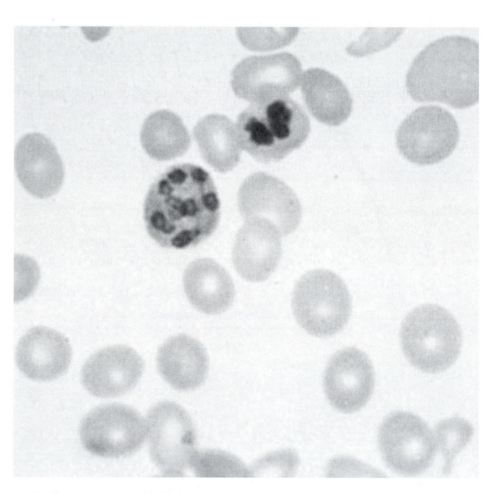

**FIGURE 7.2. Megaloblastic anemia.**

Note macro-ovalocytes and prominent hypersegmented neutrophil. (Reproduced, with permission, from Kasper DL et al [eds]. *Harrison's Principles of Internal Medicine*, 16th ed. New York: McGraw-Hill, 2005: 605.) (Also see Color Insert.)

## Vitamin B₁₂ Deficiency

Vitamin $B_{12}$ is found in animal products. It binds to intrinsic factor (IF) that is secreted by gastric parietal cells and is then absorbed in the terminal ileum. **Pernicious anemia** is the most common cause of $B_{12}$ deficiency and is an autoimmune disease characterized by autoantibodies against IF and gastric parietal cells. This → chronic atrophic gastritis and to a ↓ in both the production and function of IF. Patients have an ↑ **risk of gastric cancer and gastric carcinoid tumors.** Other etiologies are as follows:

- **Malnutrition** in strict **vegans.**
- ↓ **absorption** in the setting of an abnormal GI tract, metformin use, and PPI use.
- ↑ competition for $B_{12}$, as occurs with **fish tapeworm infestation** or bacterial overgrowth of the terminal ileum.

### Symptoms/Exam

- **Symmetric peripheral neuropathy** with paresthesias, **ataxia,** and eventually severe weakness, spasticity, and clonus.
- Memory loss, **personality changes,** and **dementia.**
- **Glossitis,** vaginal atrophy, and malabsorption.

### Diagnosis

- ↓ serum cobalamin (vitamin $B_{12}$).
- Pernicious anemia may be diagnosed by the presence of **anti-IF antibodies** or through a **Schilling test.**

*Neurologic symptoms of vitamin $B_{12}$ deficiency may precede the anemia.*

### Treatment

- IM or oral $B_{12}$ (IM $B_{12}$ is required if the deficiency is 2° to pernicious anemia).
- Neurologic abnormalities may not be reversible if they have been present for > 6 months.

## Folate Deficiency

Folate is found in animal products and in leafy green vegetables. Etiologies of folate deficiency include the following:

- **Malnutrition:** Especially common in **alcoholism.**
- **Malabsorption:** Sprue, IBD.
- **Drugs:** Methotrexate, trimethoprim, phenytoin.
- ↑ **requirements:** Occurs in **pregnancy, lactation, chronic hemolysis,** and **psoriasis.**

### Diagnosis

↓ serum folate.

### Treatment

- Give oral folate for 1–4 months or until the underlying condition resolves.
- Evaluate patients for vitamin $B_{12}$ deficiency before beginning folate, as folate replacement may mask the hematologic manifestations of $B_{12}$ deficiency.

### Thalassemias

Disorders caused by ↓ **production of either the α- or β-globin chains** of hemoglobin. Normal adult hemoglobin (HbA) consists of one pair of α chains and one pair of β chains ($\alpha_2\beta_2$).

- **α-chain disorders:** Most common in patients from **Southeast Asia** and **China** and sometimes people of African descent (see Table 7.4).
- **β-chain disorders:** Most common in those of **Mediterranean** origin and sometimes Asians and people of African descent(see Table 7.5).

### Sickle Cell Disease

*Factors that promote sickling:*

- *Cold*
- *Dehydration*
- *Hypoxia*
- *Infection*
- *Stress*
- *Menses*
- *Alcohol consumption*

An autosomal-recessive disease due to a defect in the β-chain gene that → an unstable form of hemoglobin called hemoglobin S (HbS). Deoxygenation of HbS → ↓ solubility, causing it to aggregate into long strands that give the RBC the appearance of a sickle. The sickled RBCs are less deformable and therefore less able to pass through microvasculature.

#### SYMPTOMS/EXAM

The following are common clinical manifestations of sickle cell disease (see also Table 7.6):

- **Sickle cell crisis:**
  - The most common symptom after age two.
  - Most commonly affects the back and long bones of the extremities and lasts for days.
  - Often accompanied by fever, swelling, tenderness, hypertension, tachypnea, and nausea/vomiting.
  - Cannot be diagnosed by labs.
- **Acute chest syndrome:**
  - Characterized by the presence of a **new pulmonary infiltrate** involving at least one whole lung segment, as well as by **chest pain, fever, and tachypnea, wheezing, or cough.**
  - Usually 2° to vaso-occlusion, but may be caused by infarction, embolism, or bacterial pneumonia.

**TABLE 7.4.** α-**Chain Disorders**

| ALLELES | DISEASE | CLINICAL RESULT |
| --- | --- | --- |
| (–/–) | Hydrops fetalis | Incompatible with life outside the uterus. |
| (a-/–) | Hemoglobin H disease | Moderate to severe hemolytic anemia; splenomegaly. May require occasional transfusions. |
| (a-/a-)(aa/–) | Thalassemia minor or α-thalassemia-1 trait | Mild microcytic anemia with a normal life expectancy. |
| (aa/a-) | Carrier/α-thalassemia-2 trait | Patients are clinically normal. |

TABLE 7.5. β-Chain Disorders

| β-CHAIN SYNTHESIS | DISEASE | CLINICAL RESULT |
|---|---|---|
| Near absence | β-thalassemia major | Severe anemia dependent on **lifelong transfusions.** **Bony changes** 2° to bone marrow expansion. Hepatosplenomegaly. Manifests during the first year of life as hemoglobin F (HbF) declines. Patients typically die in the third or fourth decade due to sequelae of **iron overload.** |
| Moderate ↓ | β-thalassemia intermedia | Mild bony changes and hepatosplenomegaly. May require transfusions. |
| Near normal | β-thalassemia minor | Mild anemia but overall asymptomatic. |

- Pulmonary complications are the most common cause of death in sickle cell disease.
- **Splenic sequestration crisis:**
  - Caused by vaso-occlusion within the spleen and a resultant pooling of RBCs and ↓ in peripheral hemoglobin concentration.
  - Associated with massive splenomegaly.
  - Patients are at risk for hypovolemic shock.
  - Usually occurs in younger patients because their spleens have not yet fibrosed.
  - Associated with a **10–15% mortality rate** and a **high rate of recurrence,** so splenectomy is usually recommended after the first episode.

*Patients with sickle cell disease have functional asplenia and are at ↑ risk for infection, especially from encapsulated organisms.*

### DIAGNOSIS

- Diagnosed by hemoglobin electrophoresis.
- Normocytic anemia and reticulocytosis are seen.
- Peripheral smear may show sickle cells, Howell-Jolly bodies, and target cells.
- **Fish-mouth vertebrae** may be seen on L-spine films.

TABLE 7.6. Complications of Sickle Cell Disease by Etiology

| ACUTE VASO-OCCLUSIVE COMPLICATIONS | CHRONIC VASO-OCCLUSIVE COMPLICATIONS | CHRONIC HEMOLYTIC ANEMIA COMPLICATIONS |
|---|---|---|
| Acute pain crisis | Retinopathy | Cholelithiasis |
| Acute chest syndrome | Splenic infarction | **Aplastic crisis** (precipitated |
| Splenic sequestration | Avascular necrosis of the | by **parvovirus B19** |
| Priapism | femoral or humeral head | infection) |
| Stroke | Chronic renal failure | |
| **Dactylitis** (the most common initial symptom) | | |
| Acute hepatic crisis | | |

**TREATMENT**

- **Chronic treatment:**
  - Pneumococcal vaccine.
  - Annual screening for retinopathy.
  - Folic acid 1 mg PO QD.
  - Consider chronic **hydroxyurea** therapy to ↓ the frequency of crises in patients with > 3 crises per year requiring hospitalization. It ↑ the production of HbF.
- **Acute treatment:**
  - Hydration, $O_2$, and analgesia.
  - Transfusion for aplastic or splenic sequestration crisis, acute chest, stroke, or recurrent priapism. Transfuse until HbS < 30%. Exchange transfuse to keep hematocrit > 40%.

**COMPLICATIONS**

Patients have a ↓ life expectancy, with the median age of death in the fifth decade. The most common causes of death include infection, stroke, and splenic sequestration.

## PLATELET DISORDERS

### Thrombotic Thrombocytopenic Purpura (TTP)/Hemolytic-Uremic Syndrome (HUS)

Acute, idiopathic diseases characterized by platelet aggregation and formation of platelet microthrombi that deposit in the microvasculature. Likely two variants of the same disease, with TTP more strongly associated with CNS involvement and HUS more strongly associated with renal involvement. Both are associated with the following conditions:

- **Pregnancy** and the postpartum state.
- **HIV.**
- **Medications: Estrogens,** quinine, ticlopidine, clopidogrel, bleomycin, cisplatin, cyclosporine, tacrolimus.
- **Autoimmune disorders:** SLE, antiphospholipid antibody syndrome (APS), scleroderma.
- **Enterohemorrhagic _E. coli_ (O157:H7).**

**SYMPTOMS/EXAM**

Characterized by **five classic features,** although these are not commonly found in the same patient.

- **Microangiopathic hemolytic anemia** with resultant **schistocytes** and **elevations in LDH and indirect bilirubin** (see Figure 7.3).
- **Thrombocytopenia** with resultant **purpura/petechiae** and bleeding.
- **Fever.**
- **Neurologic abnormalities:** Usually confusion or headache but occasionally seizures, aphasia, or hemiparesis.
- **Acute renal insufficiency.**

**DIFFERENTIAL**

Other causes of thrombocytopenia include idiopathic thrombocytopenic purpura (ITP), HIV, SLE, heparin-induced thrombocytopenia, microangiopathies, mechanical destruction, hypersplenism, bone marrow suppression, drug-induced thrombocytopenia, and platelet clumping.

---

**Features of TTP—**

**FAT RN**

**F**ever
**A**nemia
**T**hrombocytopenia
**R**enal insufficiency
**N**eurologic abnormality

_Drugs associated with thrombocytopenia:_

- *Heparin*
- *Acetaminophen*
- *$H_2$ blockers*
- *Sulfa drugs*
- *Furosemide*
- *Captopril*
- *Digoxin*
- *β-lactams*
- *Gold*
- *Quinine*

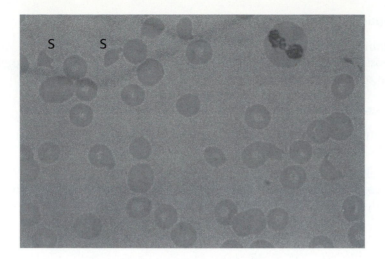

**FIGURE 7.3. Thrombotic thrombocytopenic purpura.**

Note the schistocytes (S) and paucity of platelets. TTP is characterized by microangiopathic hemolytic anemia, thrombocytopenia, fever, neurologic abnormalities, and renal failure. (Courtesy of Dr. Peter McPhedran, Yale Department of Hematology.) (Also see Color Insert.)

### DIAGNOSIS

Diagnosis is usually made clinically in the setting of the classic features mentioned above. Renal biopsy may be helpful if the diagnosis is unclear.

### TREATMENT

- Urgent **plasma exchange** to reverse platelet consumption.
- **Corticosteroids** for inadequate response to plasmapheresis.
- **Splenectomy** may be considered for recurrent cases.

### COMPLICATIONS

Survival with plasma exchange is about 80% at six months. There is a high rate of relapse after remission, especially within the first year. Some 25% of patients develop chronic renal failure. Complications of therapy include local infection, bacteremia, hypotension, and urticaria.

A 27-year-old woman presents with a complaint of frequent nosebleeds over the past week. She denies any gingival or GI bleeding. Her last period may have been slightly heavier than normal. She has no history of easy bleeding or bruising and denies any family history. On physical exam, you note petechiae over her bilateral lower legs. There is no splenomegaly. Her platelet count is 9000, but the rest of her CBC is within normal limits. Her peripheral smear shows an isolated thrombocytopenia and occasional megathrombocytes. What is the most likely diagnosis? In the absence of a history and exam suggesting another alternative, the probable diagnosis is ITP.

### Idiopathic Thrombocytopenic Purpura (ITP)

An autoimmune platelet disorder characterized by isolated thrombocytopenia. ITP most commonly affects patients < 40 years of age. Women are affected twice as often as men.

#### SYMPTOMS/EXAM

Symptoms and signs are related to bleeding 2° to thrombocytopenia and include the following:

- **Petechiae, purpura,** and ecchymoses.
- **Mucosal bleeding,** including epistaxis, gingival bleeding, and menorrhagia.
- Rarely, GI bleeding and gross hematuria may be seen.

#### DIAGNOSIS

- A diagnosis of exclusion that is made if no other etiologies are suggested by the history, physical exam, and CBC with smear.
- CBC and peripheral smear show **isolated thrombocytopenia** and **large platelets.**
- An HIV test should be done in patients with risk factors.
- A bone marrow biopsy should be obtained in patients > 60 years of age to rule out myelodysplasia.

#### TREATMENT

- **Acute treatment:**
    - **Corticosteroids.**
    - **IVIG** may be tried if refractory to steroids or for life-threatening bleeding. Platelet transfusions may also be tried for life-threatening bleeding.
    - **Splenectomy** for patients with more serious manifestations that are refractory to treatment.
- **Chronic treatment:** For cases that last > 3 months and are refractory to splenectomy, give danazol, rituximab, cyclophosphamide, azathioprine, or vincristine/vinblastine.

#### COMPLICATIONS

Fatalities are rare. Most patients achieve remission with corticosteroids. Cerebral hemorrhage is the most serious complication but is a rare occurrence.

### Heparin-Induced Thrombocytopenia (HIT)

Has **two forms:**

- **Nonimmune HIT:** Likely 2° to the effect of heparin on platelet aggregation.
- **Immune-mediated HIT:** Caused by antibodies against the platelet-heparin complex.

#### SYMPTOMS/EXAM

- **Nonimmune:** Onset occurs within 1–4 days of the initiation of treatment and → a mild thrombocytopenia. **Not associated with thrombotic events.**
- **Immune-mediated:**
    - Usually occurs within **4–10 days** of initiation of treatment.
    - Has a lower incidence with the use of low-molecular-weight heparin (LMWH) than with unfractionated heparin.

- Platelet count is usually < 60,000 but rarely falls below 20,000, so bleeding complications are uncommon.
- **Venous and arterial thrombosis,** especially DVT, is a common complication.

### DIAGNOSIS

- **Nonimmune:** Diagnosed clinically.
- **Immune-mediated:** Diagnosed via the clinical picture and HIT antibody confirmed by a functional platelet aggregation assay (> 90% specific) or an ELISA immunoassay (90% sensitive).

### TREATMENT

- **Nonimmune:** Can simply be observed for resolution.
- **Immune-mediated:**
  - Immediately stop all heparin, including flushes and LMWH.
  - Start **lepirudin** or **argatroban** for anticoagulation.
  - Warfarin should not be initiated until the patient is anticoagulated on a thrombin-specific inhibitor and the platelet count is > 100,000. This is because of the inherent danger in the combination of reduction in protein C and persistent generation of thrombin. Premature initiation of warfarin is associated with a high risk of venous limb gangrene.

## BLEEDING DISORDERS

### Hemophilia A and B

X-linked recessive disorders that → excessive bleeding due to clotting factor deficiencies, with the severity based on the extent of the deficiency. **Hemophilia A is a factor VIII deficiency. Hemophilia B,** or **Christmas disease,** is a factor IX deficiency.

> **Hemophilia clotting factor deficiencies—**
>
> **A8** (factor **VIII**)
> **B9** (factor **IX**)

### SYMPTOMS/EXAM

- Patients typically become symptomatic by age two.
- Many patients are diagnosed by excessive bleeding following a circumcision.
- The most common sites of spontaneous bleeding are the joints (80% of hemorrhages), muscles, and GI tract.
- **Spontaneous hemarthrosis** manifests as stiffness, warmth, pain, and swelling, often in the knees or ankles.
- Excessive bleeding that occurs following invasive procedures or injuries may be the initial manifestation in patients with mild or moderate factor deficiency.

### DIAGNOSIS

- The majority of patients are diagnosed on the basis of family history, but **one-third of patients have no family history.**
- Patients have a normal platelet count, a normal PT, and a **prolonged PTT.**
- **PTT should be corrected by a 1:1 mix of patient and normal plasma** unless inhibitors are present.
- Specific assays for factor deficiency typically reveal activity levels of 0–10%.

### TREATMENT

- Administer purified or recombinant **factor VIII or factor IX concentrate** during acute bleeding or prophylactically prior to invasive procedures (or fresh frozen plasma [FFP] if specific factor concentrates are unavailable).

- Consider **desmopressin** for mild hemophilia A. It → the release of factor VIII from endothelial storage sites and can therefore ↑ circulating levels prior to invasive procedures or during episodes of active bleeding.
- **Antifibrinolytic therapy such as ε-aminocaproic acid** can be used to stabilize clots in patients with mucosal bleeding that is difficult to control.
- **Chronic treatment:** Avoid high-impact activities or significant risks for trauma. Screen for hepatitis and HIV. Advise vigilant preventive dental care.

### COMPLICATIONS

Factor concentrates have → a relatively good prognosis, but there are three late complications:

- **Hemophiliac arthropathy:** Synovitis and joint destruction with resultant chronic pain and ↓ range of motion.
- Blood-borne infections from factor concentrates.
- Development of antibodies that inhibit the deficient factor (**inhibitors**), which subsequently ↓ the response to factor concentrates

A 24-year-old woman comes to your office with a complaint of easy bruising. She had a history of frequent epistaxis as a child that resolved in adolescence. She describes her periods as moderately heavy, and her dentist has told her that she bleeds somewhat more than his typical patient. Her father and aunt have both told her that they have a similar problem with easy bleeding. Initial laboratory work is significant for a slightly ↑ PTT and a prolonged bleeding time. Her platelet count and INR are normal. What is the most likely diagnosis? The most common inherited bleeding disorder is von Willebrand's disease. The diagnosis can be confirmed by checking plasma von Willebrand factor antigen and factor VIII activity.

### von Willebrand's Disease (vWD)

The **most common inherited bleeding disorder.** Characterized by ↓ production or activity of von Willebrand factor (vWF), which is produced by megakaryocytes and endothelial cells. vWF forms a platelet plug and acts as a carrier protein for factor VIII, prolonging the half-life of factor VIII. It is the only clotting factor that is not synthesized by the liver. vWD is usually inherited but may be acquired. There are three major types of inherited vWD. The most common type is a quantitative deficiency of vWF that is inherited in an autosomal-dominant pattern and → mild to moderate disease.

### SYMPTOMS/EXAM

- Bleeding patterns are similar to those seen in platelet disorders and include **easy bruising, mucosal bleeding,** heavy menses, and excessive bleeding after trauma or dental or surgical procedures.
- **Bleeding following aspirin or NSAID use** is common.

### DIAGNOSIS

- **Five screening tests:** ↓ plasma vWF antigen, ↓ plasma vWF activity, ↓ factor VIII activity, ↑ or normal PTT, and ↑ bleeding time.

- If screening tests are ⊕, then vWF multimers and ristocetin-induced platelet aggregation are checked to determine subtype.

### TREATMENT

- **Desmopressin (DDAVP)** indirectly ↑ the release of vWF from endothelial storage and can be used prophylactically before invasive procedures or during acute bleeding episodes. The effect is variable depending on disease type and subtype.
- **vWF replacement therapy** via **recombinant vWF** or **factor VIII concentrates** rich in vWF can be used in patients with more severe disease.

### PROGNOSIS

The prognosis is excellent. Severe disease is rare and can be managed with replacement therapy.

## Disseminated Intravascular Coagulation (DIC)

Consumptive coagulopathy that occurs as a complication of an underlying illness and → **bleeding AND thrombosis.** Common underlying illnesses include sepsis, transfusion reaction, neoplasia, trauma, and obstetric complications.

### SYMPTOMS/EXAM

- **Bleeding:** Petechiae, ecchymoses, oozing from wounds and IV sites, and mucosal bleeding.
- **Thrombosis:** DVT, migratory thrombophlebitis, digital ischemia, renal cortical necrosis.
- **End-organ damage:** Acute renal failure (ARF), hepatic dysfunction, and CNS dysfunction can occur 2° to microthrombi, hypotension, and sepsis.

### DIAGNOSIS

- ↑ fibrin split products, D-dimer, and PT/PTT.
- ↓ fibrinogen, platelets, and hematocrit.
- **Schistocytes** are found on blood smear.

### TREATMENT

- Correct the underlying disease.
- If no serious bleeding or thrombosis is present or anticipated, no specific coagulopathy treatment is required.
- **Transfuse platelets** for platelet counts < 20,000 or < 50,000 with serious bleeding.
- **Cryoprecipitate** to maintain a fibrinogen concentration > 100 mg/dL.
- Give **FFP** if antithrombin III levels are low.
- **Activated protein C (APC)** is appropriate for patients with severe sepsis.
- In patients with thrombotic manifestations, **heparin** can be used to achieve a goal PTT of about 45 seconds.

### PROGNOSIS

Prognosis varies widely depending on the ability to correct the underlying disease.

## Approach to Thrombophilia

The differential diagnosis of clotting disorders is outlined in Table 7.7. Consider screening for inherited coagulopathies in patients with the following:

- Idiopathic venous thrombosis at < 50 years of age.
- Recurrent thrombosis.
- A first-degree relative with idiopathic thromboembolism at < 50 years of age.
- Thrombosis associated with pregnancy or OCPs.
- Thrombosis in an unusual location.

### DIAGNOSIS

- **CBC with peripheral smear** to evaluate for myeloproliferative syndrome and thrombotic microangiopathies.
- **PTT** to screen for antiphospholipid antibody syndrome.
- Age-appropriate malignancy screening.
- **Screening for inherited coagulopathies:**
  - **APC resistance assay:** If abnormal, then genotype for **factor V Leiden** mutation.
  - **Homocysteine level** for hyperhomocysteinemia.
  - **Antiphospholipid antibody tests,** including anticardiolipin antibody test and lupus anticoagulant antibody assays.
  - **Prothrombin 20210 mutation** for deficiency.
  - If an inherited thrombophilia is strongly suspected, include **functional assays for protein C, protein S, and antithrombin III activity** as well. These tests should be done **two weeks after completion of anticoagulation therapy.**

## Factor V Leiden Deficiency

Results from a mutation in the gene for clotting factor V that → a gene product called factor V Leiden that is not susceptible to cleavage by APC and is therefore inactivated more slowly. It is the **most common cause of inherited thrombophilia,** with a prevalence of **5% among Caucasians.** Heterozygotes have a sevenfold ↑ risk of thrombosis, and homozygotes have a 50- to 80-fold ↑ risk.

**TABLE 7.7.** **Differential Diagnosis of Clotting Disorders**

| ARTERIAL AND VENOUS | VENOUS ONLY | ARTERIAL ONLY |
| --- | --- | --- |
| Malignancy | Factor V Leiden | Atherosclerosis |
| HIT syndrome | Prothrombin 20210 mutation | Vasculitis |
| Hyperhomocysteinemia | Protein C or S deficiency | |
| Paroxysmal nocturnal | Antithrombin III deficiency | |
|   hemoglobinemia | Hormonal | |
| Myeloproliferative disease | Postsurgical, pregnancy, | |
| APS |   immobilization | |

Reproduced, with permission, from Le T et al. *First Aid for the Internal Medicine Boards,* 1st ed. New York: McGraw-Hill, 2006: 339.

### SYMPTOMS/EXAM

DVT, pulmonary embolism, cerebral vein thrombosis, and unexplained pregnancy loss.

### DIAGNOSIS

APC resistance assay followed by genotyping for **factor V Leiden mutation.**

### TREATMENT

- Avoid smoking and OCPs.
- Anticoagulation after a first thrombotic event:
  - Heterozygotes should be treated like any other patient.
  - Homozygotes should have extended anticoagulation.

### PROGNOSIS

Despite the ↑ risk of thromboembolic events, there is no evidence of ↑ mortality.

## Antiphospholipid Antibody Syndrome (APS)

Characterized by thrombosis and/or pregnancy morbidity in association with antibodies to plasma proteins that are bound to phospholipids. May be associated with SLE or other rheumatic diseases.

### SYMPTOMS/EXAM

- May present with arterial and venous thrombosis, thrombocytopenia, recurrent spontaneous abortions, livedo reticularis, and hemolytic anemia.
- Catastrophic APS presents with widespread thrombotic disease with multiorgan failure.

### DIAGNOSIS

**Diagnostic criteria** are as follows:

- **Thrombosis OR pregnancy morbidity AND**
- **Anticardiolipin antibody OR lupus anticoagulant** present in serum on two or more occasions at least six weeks apart.

### TREATMENT

- Initial anticoagulation should be done with **LMWH,** since PTT cannot be used to titrate unfractionated heparin.
- After the first thrombotic event, patients should receive a minimum of six months of **warfarin** anticoagulation. Consider lifelong therapy, and use aspirin if warfarin is discontinued.
- Patients with a recurrent thrombotic event should receive lifelong anticoagulation with warfarin.
- The **goal INR** is controversial and is either **2–3 or > 3.**
- For asymptomatic, nonpregnant, non-aspirin-allergic patients, **prophylactic aspirin therapy** (81 mg/day) should be initiated, particularly in the presence of concomitant SLE or a history of miscarriage.

### PROGNOSIS

APS is associated with premature death from thromboembolic disease as well as from associated comorbidities.

A 46-year-old male patient becomes febrile 14 hours after a transfusion of two units of packed red blood cells. He then develops chills, flank pain, and hypotension. His urine appears brown but is ⊖ for nitrites and leukocyte esterase, and no bacteria are seen. What is the appropriate treatment? This clinical history is consistent with an acute hemolytic transfusion reaction. Aggressive hydration should be initiated to prevent acute tubular necrosis (ATN).

## Blood Products

Table 7.8 outlines and compares the categories of blood products used in transfusion medicine.

## Pretransfusion Testing

- Type and cross:
    - Use when transfusion is **probable**.

**TABLE 7.8. Types of Blood Products**

| PRODUCT AND DESCRIPTION | COMMENTS |
|---|---|
| Whole blood | Provides volume expansion. Used in patients with **acute massive blood loss.** |
| Packed RBCs | Concentrated. Each unit should ↑ hematocrit by 3–4%. |
| Washed RBCs | Removes the small amount of residual plasma from packed RBCs. Used for the following:<br>- Patients with a history of severe or recurrent allergic **transfusion reactions**.<br>- Patients with IgA deficiency if RBCs from IgA-deficient donors is unavailable.<br>- Patients with complement-dependent AIHA. |
| Irradiated RBCs | Prevents donor T lymphocytes from dividing in the recipient. Used in **immunodeficient or immunosuppressed patients at risk for graft-versus-host disease (GVHD).** |
| Leukocyte-depleted RBCs | Used because WBCs → **HLA** alloimmunization and cytokine release and carry **CMV.** Used for the following:<br>- Patients who are **chronically transfused.**<br>- Potential **transplant recipients.**<br>- Patients with a history of febrile nonhemolytic transfusion reactions.<br>- Patients in whom CMV-seronegative components are desirable but not available. |
| Pooled random donor platelets | Used for the following:<br>- Prophylactic transfusion for platelet counts < 10,000.<br>- Transfusions for platelet counts < 50,000 in bleeding patients or those undergoing major surgery.<br>Six units should ↑ the platelet count by 44,000 in a 68-kg patient. |
| Single-donor platelets | Used in patients refractory to random donor platelets 2° to alloimmunization. |

TABLE 7.8. Types of Blood Products (continued)

| PRODUCT AND DESCRIPTION | COMMENTS |
| --- | --- |
| FFP | Contains all coagulation factors. Used for the following:<br>▪ Patients with documented **coagulation factor deficiencies** who are actively bleeding or are scheduled for an invasive procedure.<br>▪ **Reversal of warfarin** anticoagulation if significant bleeding or risk of bleeding is present.<br>▪ Treatment of **TTP.** |
| Cryoprecipitate | Prepared from plasma and containing fibrinogen, vWF, factor VIII, factor XIII, and fibronectin. Used for the following:<br>▪ Patients with significant **hypofibrinogenemia** (< 100 mg/dL) who are actively bleeding or are scheduled for an invasive procedure.<br>▪ Replacement of factor VIII or vWF when specific factor concentrates are unavailable. |

- Obtain an indirect Coombs' test on **donor RBCs** to test for reactivity from recipient plasma.
- **Type and screen** (aka "type and hold"):
  - Use when transfusion is **possible.**
  - Obtain an indirect Coombs' test on a **standardized reference RBC panel** to test for reactivity from recipient plasma.
- Weigh the need for transfusion against the risks:
  - Transfusion reactions (see Table 7.9).
  - **Risk of infection:** Specific concerns in decreasing order of risk include CMV, HBV, HCV, and HIV.

## Transfusion Reactions

Management of transfusion reactions should proceed as follows (see also Table 7.9):

- Immediately discontinue the transfusion.
- Alert the blood bank and check for clerical errors.
- From the **other arm, draw blood** for CBC, direct antiglobulin test, plasma free hemoglobin, LDH, haptoglobin, indirect bilirubin, and PT/PTT. Repeat type and cross-match and blood culture.
- Save a **urine sample** for UA and urine hemoglobin.
- Send all untransfused blood with attached tubing back to the blood bank.

## MYELOPROLIFERATIVE DISORDERS

A 64-year-old man presents with a complaint of erythema and burning in his hands and feet. On review of systems, he is also found to have generalized pruritus, especially after a warm shower. He denies any history of tobacco use. You note plethoric facies and a palpable spleen on exam. His hematocrit is 62, WBC count 14, and platelet count 520,000. The peripheral smear is unremarkable. What is the most likely diagnosis? The patient's presentation is consistent with polycythemia vera. If his oxygen saturation is > 92% (in addition to the above laboratory values), he meets the diagnostic criteria.

**TABLE 7.9.** **Types of Transfusion Reactions**

| TYPE | RISK | CLINICAL FEATURES | TREATMENT | CAUSE | COMMENTS |
|---|---|---|---|---|---|
| Febrile nonhemolytic reactions | 1 in 100 | Fever, chills, mild dyspnea within six hours of transfusion. | Antipyretics +/− meperidine. | Antibodies against donor WBCs and cytokine buildup. | The **most common reaction.** |
| Allergic reactions<br>Urticaria<br><br>Anaphylaxis | 1 in 100 | Hives.<br><br>Bronchospasm, angioedema, hypotension. Occurs within seconds to minutes. | Diphenhydramine.<br><br>Epinephrine. | Allergic reaction to plasma proteins. Anti-IgA antibodies in **IgA-deficient patients.** | |
| Delayed hemolytic transfusion reaction | 1 in 1000 | Fever, ↓ hematocrit, hyperbilirubinemia, spherocytosis within 2–10 days of transfusion. | Supportive care. Evaluate for new alloantibody and avoid in the future. | An anamnestic response to undetected alloantibodies against minor antigens. | Occurs with reexposure to an antigen encountered during prior transfusion, transplantation, or pregnancy. |
| Transfusion-related acute lung injury (TRALI) | 1 in 5000 | Noncardiogenic pulmonary edema, ARDS, hypotension, and fever, usually within six hours of transfusion. | Supportive care as in ARDS. | Donor antibodies to recipient WBCs in pulmonary capillaries. | Recovery is usually complete within 96 hours. |
| Acute hemolytic transfusion areaction | 1 in 250,000 | Fever, chills, flank pain, red or brown urine, hypotension, and tachycardia within 24 hours of transfusion. DIC if severe. | Vigorous hydration to prevent ATN. Maintain urine output with diuretics, mannitol, or dopamine. | Preformed antibodies against donor RBCs usually 2/2 ABO incompatibility. | Usually due to an error. |

## Polycythemia Vera

A clonal proliferation of myeloid cells distinguished by ↑ RBC mass.

### SYMPTOMS/EXAM

- Presents with headache, dizziness, tinnitus, blurred vision, excessive sweating, **pruritus,** and GI complaints.
- The following are also seen:

- **Erythromelalgia:** Burning pain in the feet or hands accompanied by erythema, pallor, or cyanosis.
- **Acute gouty arthritis.**
- **Splenomegaly, plethora,** hypertension, and **engorged retinal veins.**

### DIFFERENTIAL

Must be distinguished from reactive erythrocytosis, which can be caused by COPD, high altitude, sleep apnea, and renal and liver lesions.

### DIAGNOSIS

- Diagnostic criteria from the **Polycythemia Vera Study Group** are as follows:
    - ↑ red cell mass **AND** arterial oxygen saturation > 92% **PLUS**
    - Splenomegaly **OR** any two of the following: platelets > 400,000, WBC count > 12,000, leukocyte alkaline phosphatase score > 100, serum vitamin $B_{12}$ > 900 pg/mL.
- **Low EPO** is > 92% specific for polycythemia vera, while ↑ EPO is 98% specific for 2° erythrocytosis.
- **Bone marrow biopsy** shows an ↑ number of megakaryocytes in a hypercellular marrow.
- **Endogenous erythroid colony formation** may be demonstrated using in vitro culture.

Polycythemia vera can be distinguished from 2° causes of erythrocytosis by ↑ RBC mass in the setting of normal oxygen saturation and low EPO.

### TREATMENT

- **Serial phlebotomy** to maintain hematocrit < 45% in men and < 42% in women.
- **Hydroxyurea** in patients at high risk for thrombosis—i.e., those > 60 years of age as well as those with a prior thrombosis, cardiovascular risk factors, or a platelet count > 1,500,000.
- **Anagrelide** for patients with a platelet count > 1,500,000 who are refractory to hydroxyurea.
- **Low-dose daily ASA** in all patients to prevent thrombotic complications.
- **Allopurinol** in patients with symptomatic hyperuricemia or ↑ risk of uric acid calculi based on levels of uric acid excretion.

### COMPLICATIONS

- Venous or arterial **thrombosis,** including Budd-Chiari syndrome and portal, splenic, and mesenteric vein thrombosis.
- Hemorrhage.
- Transformation to **acute myelogenous leukemia/myelodysplastic syndrome** occurs in 2–5% of cases
- Transformation to **myelofibrosis/myeloid metaplasia** occurs in 15% of cases. Risk ↑ with disease duration and most commonly occurs after 10 years.

### PROGNOSIS

The disease course is indolent. Median survival is 10–15 years. The most common cause of death is arterial thrombosis.

## Myelofibrosis

A clonal proliferative disorder of myeloid cells that → reactive bone marrow fibrosis and subsequent extramedullary hematopoiesis.

- **Ineffective erythropoiesis** → cytopenias → **fatigue and bleeding.**
- **Extramedullary hematopoiesis** (may occur in almost any organ) → **massive splenomegaly**/hepatomegaly → abdominal fullness.
- Tumor bulk and ↑ cell turnover → **constitutional "B" symptoms** (fever, night sweats, and weight loss).

### DIAGNOSIS

- CBC shows **severe anemia** with variable numbers of WBCs and platelets.
- Peripheral smear reveals **teardrop cells,** nucleated RBCs, immature WBCs, and giant degranulated platelets.
- Bone marrow aspirate yields a **dry tap.**
- Bone marrow biopsy shows significant fibrosis.

### TREATMENT

- Treat anemia with androgens and periodic transfusions.
- Splenectomy for symptomatic splenomegaly and anemia requiring frequent transfusions.
- Allogenic hematopoietic stem cell transplantation (HSCT) provides the only potential for cure and may be considered for young patients with an appropriate donor available.

### PROGNOSIS

Associated with a three-year survival rate of about 50%. Fewer than 5% transform into AML with a much worse prognosis. Bleeding and liver failure (caused by liver hematopoiesis and subsequent portal hypertension) are common causes of death.

## Essential Thrombocytosis

A chronic state of nonreactive thrombocytosis.

### SYMPTOMS/EXAM

- Often asymptomatic at presentation and diagnosed incidentally.
- May present with thrombosis and hemorrhage.
- Vasomotor symptoms may include headache, lightheadedness, atypical chest pain, acral paresthesia, and erythromelalgia (erythema, warmth, and burning of the hands and feet).
- Palpable splenomegaly may be present on exam.

### DIFFERENTIAL

Reactive thrombocytosis and other myelodysplastic or myeloproliferative disorders must be excluded. Causes of reactive thrombocytosis include iron deficiency anemia, rheumatoid arthritis, IBD, infection, inflammation, malignancy, and postsplenectomy status.

### DIAGNOSIS

- A **diagnosis of exclusion** that is made when the platelet count is chronically > 600,000 and there is no evidence of other myelodysplastic or myeloproliferative disorders, no causes for reactive thrombocytosis, and no Philadelphia chromosome identified.
- Bone marrow aspirate and biopsy show megakaryocytic hyperplasia.

- Patients < 60 years of age with no history of thrombosis or hemorrhage and a platelet count < 1,500,000 can be followed or treated with low-dose **aspirin.**
- Patients > 60 years of age or those with a history of thrombosis should be treated with **hydroxyurea** (preferred) or **anagrelide.**

*Patients with essential thrombocytosis have a normal survival rate.*

**PROGNOSIS**

Survival does not differ greatly from that of the control population, and there is a low rate of transformation.

## MISCELLANEOUS HEMATOLOGIC DISORDERS

### Multiple Myeloma

A neoplastic clonal proliferation of plasma cells producing a monoclonal immunoglobulin.

**SYMPTOMS/EXAM**

- The most common complaints are bone pain (especially back), weakness, fatigue, and weight loss.
- Symptoms are due to 2° organ or tissue impairment stemming from **anemia, hypercalcemia, renal insufficiency,** and **lytic bone lesions.**
- Neurologic disease may → radiculopathy, peripheral neuropathy, cord compression, and CNS involvement.
- An ↑ **incidence of infection** is seen.

**DIAGNOSIS**

- Diagnosed when the following are identified:
  - An **monoclonal (M) protein** in serum or urine on protein electrophoresis.
  - Clonal bone marrow **plasma cells (usually > 10%) on bone marrow exam** or plasmacytoma.
  - 2° organ or tissue impairment.
- **Skeletal survey will identify lytic lesions in the majority of patients** (they will not be seen on bone scan).
- $\beta_2$-microglobulin is usually ↑; higher values are a poor prognosticator.

*Lytic lesions 2° to multiple myeloma will not light up on bone scan (vs. those 2° to osteoblastic bony metastases).*

**TREATMENT**

- No treatment for smoldering multiple myeloma or asymptomatic stage I disease.
- **Autologous HSCT** offers the best opportunity for ↑ survival.
- **Chemotherapy:**
  - Initial treatment is with oral **melphalan** (an alkylating agent) and **prednisone.**
  - **Thalidomide** and bortezomib for relapsed or resistant disease.
- Prevention and treatment of complications include the following:
  - **Hypercalcemia:** Hydration, prednisone, or a bisphosphonate.
  - **Skeletal lesions: Bisphosphonates,** chemotherapy, local radiation, or surgical fixation.
  - **Infection:** Immunization with pneumococcal and influenza vaccines and aggressive treatment of bacterial infections. Consider prophylactic antibiotics and IVIG for recurrent infections.

- **Renal failure:** Hydration, avoidance of NSAIDs and IV contrast, and plasmapheresis for acute failure.
- **Hyperviscosity syndrome:** Plasmapheresis.

### PROGNOSIS

Median survival ranges from one to six years depending on the level of tumor burden and the availability of stem cell transplantation.

## Aplastic Anemia

Characterized by hypoplastic or aplastic bone marrow (with no dysplasia) → pancytopenia. There is a biphasic age distribution with a peak in adolescent and elderly years. May be congenital or acquired. Etiologies of acquired disease are as follows:

- **Idiopathic (most common).**
- Cytotoxic drugs and radiation.
- Toxic chemicals such as benzene.
- Idiosyncratic drug reactions to chloramphenicol, NSAIDs, and sulfa drugs.
- **Viral infections:** Parvovirus B19, EBV, HIV.
- **Immune disorders:** SLE, GVHD, thymoma.
- Paroxysmal nocturnal hemoglobinuria.
- Pregnancy.

### SYMPTOMS/EXAM

- Presents with fatigue, hemorrhage, and recurrent infections.
- Pallor and petechiae are seen in the absence of splenomegaly.

### DIAGNOSIS

- **Labs: Pancytopenia and absolute reticulocytopenia.**
- **Bone marrow:** Hypocellular with morphologically normal residual hematopoietic precursor cells.

### TREATMENT

- Hematopoietic cell transplantation is the only definitive therapy.
- Immunosuppression with antithymocyte globulin, cyclosporine, or prednisone for patients in whom hematopoietic cell transplantation is not an option.

### PROGNOSIS

Prognosis depends on the severity of the pancytopenia and the patient's age. Five-year survival rate varies from 20% to 80% depending on these factors.

## ACUTE LEUKEMIA

Neoplastic disorders characterized by proliferation of immature hematopoietic precursor cells in the bone marrow, and later in the peripheral blood and other organs and tissues. If untreated, death usually occurs within six months of diagnosis. ↑ **risk** is associated with the following:

- **Congenital disorders:** Down syndrome, Bloom's syndrome, Fanconi's anemia, ataxia-telangiectasia.
- **Acquired disorders:** Myeloproliferative disorders, myelodysplastic syndromes, aplastic anemia.

- **Environmental exposures:** Alkylating agents, radiation, cigarette smoke, benzene, organic solvents.

### SYMPTOMS/EXAM

Common presenting symptoms are usually 2° to anemia, thrombocytopenia, and neutropenia and include fatigue, fever, easy bruising and bleeding, purpura/petechiae, and infections.

### DIAGNOSIS

- **Peripheral smear:** ↑ circulating blasts as well as anemia and thrombocytopenia.
- **Bone marrow:** ↑ blasts.
- Immunohistochemistry, cytogenetics, and flow cytometry should also be done to aid in diagnosis, classification, and decision making.
- An **LP** should be performed on all patients with ALL and any AML patients who have **CNS symptoms.**

## Acute Lymphocytic Leukemia (ALL)

**Seen predominantly in children** (the most common cancer in children). Has a bimodal distribution with peaks at 10 years and 65 years. Classified as follows:

- Clonal cells may be B cells (75%) or T cells.
- Patients with T-cell ALL should be tested for **HTLV-1.**
- **Burkitt's leukemia** is a subtype of ALL with a proliferation of B cells. The **t(8;14) translocation** is universally seen in this subtype and → the aberrant expression of the **c-myc oncogene.**

### SYMPTOMS/EXAM

Findings that are more common in ALL than AML include the following:

- **Bone pain.**
- **Lymphadenopathy:** Occurs in > 50% of patients with ALL.
- **Hepatosplenomegaly:** Occurs in 66% of ALL patients.
- CNS involvement.

### TREATMENT

- Remission induction with combination chemotherapy to prevent resistance.
- **CNS prophylaxis** with **intrathecal chemotherapy** for all patients to prevent CNS relapse.
- Prolonged **postremission therapy** (1–3 years) to eliminate residual disease.

### COMPLICATIONS

The **long-term** disease-free survival rate is **30% for adults** and **66–85% for children.** Common sites of **solitary relapse (sanctuary sites)** are the **CNS and testes** because these sites are poorly penetrated by chemotherapy.

## Acute Myelogenous Leukemia (AML)

Represents 80% of all acute leukemia cases in adults. Most patients are > 65 years of age, and the incidence ↑ with age.

### SYMPTOMS/EXAM

Findings that are more common in AML than in ALL include the following:

- **Leukostasis:** Sludging of blasts in the microvasculature occurs when the blast count in the peripheral blood gets above 100,000/mm³. It commonly → CNS symptoms (**somnolence, seizure, stroke**) and pulmonary symptoms (**dyspnea**).
- **DIC:** Commonly associated with the promyelocytic subtype.
- **Leukemia cutis:** Violaceous raised lesions of the skin 2° to infiltration of leukemic cells; associated with monocytic subtypes.

### DIAGNOSIS

**Auer rods are pathognomonic for AML** (see Figure 7.4).

### TREATMENT

- **Induction chemotherapy** with **daunorubicin** and **cytarabine.**
- **Postremission therapy** options include the following:
    - **Consolidation chemotherapy.**
    - **Allogenic or autologous HSCT** may be considered, especially for patients who fail to achieve a complete remission or who relapse.

### PROGNOSIS

Although roughly 60–80% of patients achieve complete remission, the overall five-year survival rate is 10–35%.

## Acute Promyelocytic Leukemia (AML-M3 or APL)

- Associated with t(15;17) translocation, which juxtaposes the promyelocytic leukemia gene with the retinoic acid receptor alpha gene → a fusion protein.
- Commonly associated with DIC.
- **All-*trans*-retinoic acid** induces complete remission in 90% of patients with APL.

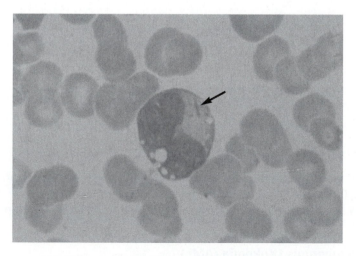

**FIGURE 7.4.** **Auer rod in acute myelocytic leukemia.**

The red rod-shaped structure (arrow) in the cytoplasm of the myeloblast is pathognomonic. (Courtesy of Dr. Peter McPhedran, Yale Department of Hematology.) (Also see Color Insert.)

## Chronic Lymphocytic Leukemia (CLL)

A monoclonal proliferation of immunologically **incompetent mature B cells.** CLL is the **most common adult leukemia** in the Western world, representing 30% of all cases of leukemia. The median age of onset is 65.

### SYMPTOMS/EXAM

- An **indolent** disease.
- Many patients are **asymptomatic at diagnosis.**
- Presenting symptoms include fever, night sweats, weight loss, fatigue, and weakness.
- **Generalized lymphadenopathy** and **hepatosplenomegaly** are common.
- Patients have an ↑ incidence of autoimmune diseases, including **AIHA,** autoimmune thrombocytopenia, and pure red cell aplasia.

### DIAGNOSIS

- **Peripheral smear shows isolated lymphocytosis.** Lymphocytes appear small and mature and are **monoclonal on flow cytometry.**
- **Smudge cells** are common on peripheral smear and occur when fragile malignant lymphocytes are disrupted during preparation of the smear (see Figure 7.5).

### TREATMENT

- **Treatment is palliative.**
- Asymptomatic patients may be followed without treatment.
- **Oral alkylating agents** (chlorambucil or fludarabine) are the mainstay of therapy for patients who are symptomatic, have rapidly progressive disease, or develop complications.

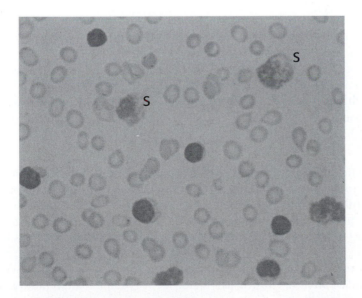

**FIGURE 7.5.** **Chronic lymphocytic leukemia.**

The numerous small, mature lymphocytes and smudge cells (S; fragile malignant lymphocytes are disrupted during blood smear preparation) are characteristic. (Courtesy of Dr. Peter McPhedran, Yale Department of Hematology.) (Also see Color Insert.)

- **Monoclonal antibodies** such as rituximab and alemtuzumab are options.
- **Corticosteroids** are used for treatment of AIHA or autoimmune thrombocytopenia.
- **Radiation therapy** is appropriate for large, bulky lymphoid masses.
- **Allogeneic bone marrow transplant** is being studied as an option for patients < 55 years of age.

### PROGNOSIS

The disease is associated with good short-term and poor long-term survival. Median survival is 8–10 years.

## Chronic Myelogenous Leukemia (CML)

A myeloproliferative disorder characterized by proliferation of myeloid cells that are capable of differentiation. It is associated with the **Philadelphia chromosome t(9;22)**. The clinical course may be divided into three phases defined by the number of blasts:

- **Chronic phase:** Blasts < 10%.
- **Accelerated phase:** Blasts 10–20%.
- **Blast phase:** Blasts > 20%.

### SYMPTOMS/EXAM

- Roughly **85% of patients present in the chronic phase and are typically asymptomatic.**
- Patients become increasingly symptomatic as they progress through the accelerated and blast phases.
- Common symptoms include fatigue, weight loss, night sweats, LUQ pain, and early satiety.
- Hepatosplenomegaly is common.
- Symptoms of leukostasis may be seen in the blast phase.

### DIAGNOSIS

- Peripheral smear shows leukocytosis and may show anemia, thrombocytopenia, basophilia, and eosinophilia.
- As noted above, **the number of blasts seen determines the phase.**
- **Leukocyte alkaline phosphatase is low.**
- The **Philadelphia chromosome** is present in **95% of patients** and may be diagnosed via cytogenetics or PCR for the bcr-abl gene product.

### TREATMENT

- **Allogenic HSCT** is the only curative treatment and should be considered in the **chronic phase** for younger patients who have a suitable donor available.
- **Imatinib mesylate (Gleevec)** is an oral tyrosine kinase inhibitor targeted to the fusion gene product. It may be used for patients in the accelerated or blast phase or for chronic-phase patients who are not candidates for HSCT. It is associated with a 95% rate of complete hematologic remission.
- Interferon-$\alpha$ (IFN-$\alpha$) plus cytarabine may be tried in patients who do not respond to imatinib but is associated with greater toxicity and fewer treatment responses.

### COMPLICATIONS

Has a poor prognosis, with a median survival of 4–6 years.

## Hodgkin's Lymphoma

A clonal **B-cell** malignancy in which **Reed-Sternberg cells** are the malignant cells. Has a bimodal age distribution with peaks in the 20s–30s and in those > 50 years of age.

### SYMPTOMS/EXAM

- Common presentations include the following:
  - A painless, enlarged, rubbery lymph node (70% of patients).
  - A mediastinal mass on CXR with possible retrosternal chest pain, cough, or shortness of breath.
  - **B symptoms:** Fever, night sweats, and weight loss.
- Hepatosplenomegaly and pruritus are common.
- Pain after alcohol consumption is uncommon but suggestive.

### DIAGNOSIS

- **Excisional lymph node biopsy** provides definitive diagnosis.
- Staging studies include CXR and CT of the chest, abdomen, and pelvis.
- Labs that may affect choice of therapy or staging include CBC with differential, ESR, LFTs, albumin, LDH, and calcium.
- Bone marrow biopsy should be done in patients with B symptoms, anemia, thrombocytopenia, or leukopenia or in those with clinical stages IIb–IV.

### TREATMENT

- Treat with irradiation and/or ABVD (Adriamycin, bleomycin, vinblastine, dacarbazine) depending on the stage and on whether bulky mediastinal disease is present.
- Treat relapsed disease with conventional chemotherapy or high-dose chemotherapy plus autologous HSCT.

## Non-Hodgkin's Lymphoma

Heterogeneous cancers of B and T cells. **Clinical classification** (with representative examples) is as follows:

- **Indolent:** Typically not curable, but even if left untreated, survival is measured in years. Patients may have prolonged survival even with partial treatment response.
  - **Follicular lymphoma:** Patients are typically middle-aged or older and present with painless peripheral lymphadenopathy.
  - **Mucosa-associated lymphoid tissue (MALT) lymphoma:** A form of marginal zone lymphoma. Gastric tumors have been linked to *H. pylori* infection, and the majority regress with antimicrobial therapy. Patients with gastric tumors may present with PUD or abdominal pain.
- **Aggressive:** Typically curable, but survival is measured in months if untreated.
  - **Diffuse large B-cell lymphoma:** Patients are typically middle-aged or older and often present with a rapidly enlarging neck or abdominal mass.
- **Highly aggressive:** Typically curable, but survival is measured in weeks if untreated. There is a high risk of tumor lysis syndrome.

- **Burkitt's lymphoma:** Exists in endemic, sporadic, and immunodeficiency-related forms. It is endemic in Africa, with up to 90% of cases related to EBV infection; presents as a tumor of the jaw or facial bone. Of sporadic cases, only about 20% are related to EBV infection. Typically presents as bulky abdominal disease.

### SYMPTOMS/EXAM

- B symptoms including fever, weight loss, and sweats.
- Systemic lymphadenopathy is seen with or without hepatosplenomegaly.

### DIAGNOSIS

- **Excisional lymph node biopsy** is preferable for definitive diagnosis, but FNA is acceptable.
- Staging studies include CXR, CT of the chest/abdomen/pelvis, and bone marrow biopsy.
- Labs that may affect choice of therapy or staging include CBC with differential, peripheral smear, LFTs, chem 10, LDH, and serum protein electrophoresis.

### TREATMENT

- **Indolent:** Treatment is aimed at alleviation of symptoms.
  - Early disease may be treated with locoregional or extended-field radiation therapy.
  - Options for advanced disease include single-agent chemotherapy with chlorambucil, cyclophosphamide, or fludarabine; combination chemotherapy with CVP (cyclophosphamide, vincristine, and prednisone); or monoclonal antibody therapy with rituximab.
- **Aggressive:** Treatment is aimed at cure.
  - Early disease may be treated with CHOP (cyclophosphamide, doxorubicin, vincristine, and prednisone) possibly followed by involved-field radiation.
  - Advanced disease is treated with **CHOP** or a CHOP-like regimen, often with **rituximab.**
- **Highly aggressive:** Enroll the patient in a clinical trial. CHOP is insufficient.

## BRAIN TUMORS

### 1° Brain Tumors

Classified by predominant cell type:

- **Gliomas:** Tumors derived from glial cells represent the most common 1° brain tumor. They are classified according to grade, with glioblastomas representing the highest grade. Various genetic syndromes may → a predisposition for these tumors, including tuberous sclerosis, neurofibromatosis 1, and Li-Fraumeni syndrome.
- **Medulloblastomas:** Embryonal tumors that are most often seen in children.
- **Meningiomas:** Arise from cells in the arachnoid membrane. The vast majority of these tumors are benign but are associated with morbidity due to their mass effect.

### SYMPTOMS/EXAM

- Present with headaches, seizures, nausea and vomiting, syncope, disturbance in memory or mood, personality changes, muscle weakness, sensory deficits, and aphasia.
- Headache features that suggest a possible brain tumor include a change in a prior headache pattern, an abnormal neurologic exam, positional changes, and associated nausea and vomiting.

### DIAGNOSIS

- **MRI** is the imaging of choice. CT or PET scans may be used adjunctively.
- Tissue biopsy for histologic confirmation is often obtained at the time of resection or may be done via stereotactic biopsy in cases where resection will not improve survival.

### TREATMENT

- High-grade gliomas should be treated with maximal surgical resection and adjuvant radiation therapy and chemotherapy. Chemotherapeutic agents include temozolomide and the PCV regimen (procarbazine, CCNU, and vincristine.)
- Asymptomatic meningiomas may be monitored with serial neuroimaging every 3–6 months. If they are symptomatic, expanding, infiltrative, or associated with significant surrounding edema, they should be surgically resected. Adjuvant radiation therapy may be offered for patients with high-grade lesions or incomplete resection.
- **Stereotactic radiosurgery** may be used instead of surgical excision for small tumors in sites where complete excision is difficult.

## Brain Metastases

Represent > 50% **of intracranial tumors** in adults. Some 10–15% of patients with solid tumors develop brain metastases.

### SYMPTOMS/EXAM

As with 1° brain tumors.

### DIAGNOSIS

- **Contrast-enhanced MRI** with characteristic findings suggesting metastasis, including multiple lesions, circumscribed margins, vasogenic edema out of proportion to the size of the lesion, and location at the gray–white matter junction.
- Brain biopsy if the diagnosis is in doubt.
- **CXR** to look for pulmonary metastasis or to establish a 1° site if it is unknown. Some 60% of patients with brain metastases have either a lung 1° or pulmonary metastases from their 1° tumor.

### TREATMENT

- Patients with a **favorable prognosis** include those < 65 years of age with a high performance status, a controlled 1° tumor, and no extracranial metastases. Median survival is about seven months. Aggressive treatment with **surgical resection or stereotactic radiosurgery** followed by **whole brain radiation therapy** is typically recommended.

> *Tumors that commonly metastasize to the brain—*
>
> *"Lots of Bad Stuff Kills Glia"*
>
> **L**ung
> **B**reast
> **S**kin (melanoma)
> **K**idney
> **G**I (colorectal)

227

- Patients with a **poor prognosis** have a poor performance status and a median survival of about two months. The following treatments are recommended:
  - **Whole brain radiation therapy** to improve neurologic deficits and prevent further neurologic deterioration.
  - **Corticosteroids** to control symptoms related to edema.

## SQUAMOUS CELL CARCINOMA (SCC) OF THE HEAD AND NECK

Most commonly associated with tobacco and alcohol use. Other risk factors include radiation, occupational exposures, and chronic viral infection with EBV, HPV, HSV, or HIV.

### SYMPTOMS/EXAM

- Neck mass.
- Ulcers or exophytic lesions in the nose, lips, mouth, or throat.
- Nasal obstruction, hoarseness, dysphagia, odynophagia, cervical lymphadenopathy, globus sensation, otalgia.

### DIAGNOSIS

- Physical exam should include bimanual examination of the tongue and the floor of the mouth.
- Panendoscopy should include laryngoscopy, bronchoscopy, and esophagoscopy to visualize the extent of tumor involvement.
- CT or MRI to better determine the size and location of lesions and nodes.
- Fine-needle biopsy of suspicious neck nodes should be performed.

### TREATMENT

Treatment is determined by the resectability of the lesion and the extent of advancement. Early lesions may be treated with radiotherapy or surgery alone, while more advanced lesions are usually treated with concomitant chemotherapy.

### Nasopharyngeal Carcinoma

- SCC of the nasopharynx.
- Rare in the West and associated with tobacco and alcohol, as with other SCCs of the head and neck. Endemic in southern China and associated with EBV, genetic predisposition, and dietary factors such as nitrates, salted fish, and Chinese herbs. There are endemic areas in southeast Asia and the Mediterranean as well.
- **Sx/Exam:** Neck mass, nasal obstruction, epistaxis, and otitis media.
- **Dx:** As with the diagnosis of other SCCs of the head and neck.
- **Tx:** Typically nonsurgical. Concomitant chemoradiation with cisplatin is commonly used.

## GENITOURINARY CANCERS

### Bladder Cancer

Risk factors for bladder cancer include exposure to chemicals, cigarette smoking, arsenic exposure, chronic cystitis, schistosomiasis, radiation, and cyclophosphamide use.

- **Hematuria** is the most common presenting symptom.
- Flank pain, suprapubic pain, hypogastric pain, and perineal pain may all result from invasive or metastatic disease.
- Irritative or obstructive voiding symptoms may be seen.

### DIAGNOSIS

- Hematuria in a patient > 40 years of age is urothelial cancer until proven otherwise and should be investigated with **cystourethroscopy, urine cytology,** and **CT with urography** or **IVP with renal ultrasound.**
- A CXR and bone scan may be used for screening patients with documented bladder cancer who are at high risk for metastasis.

### TREATMENT

- **Superficial bladder cancer** (superficial to the muscularis propria):
  - Cystoscopic resection of visible tumor (**transurethral resection of the bladder tumor, or TURBT**).
  - If the superficial cancer is high risk based on histology, number of lesions or recurrences, or failure to completely resect, then intravesical therapy with BCG (live attenuated *Mycobacterium bovis*) or other chemotherapeutic agents is recommended.
  - Aggressive post-treatment surveillance with urine cytology and cystoscopy is recommended.
- **Invasive bladder cancer:**
  - **Radical cystectomy** with bilateral pelvic lymph node dissection.
  - **Neoadjuvant or adjuvant chemotherapy:**
    - Gemcitabine plus cisplatin.
    - MVAC (methotrexate, vinblastine, doxorubicin, and cisplatin).

Risk factors for bladder cancer:

- *Chemicals*
- *Cigarette smoking*
- *Arsenic*
- *Chronic cystitis*
- *Schistosomiasis*
- *Radiation*
- *Cyclophosphamide*

Workers in these industries are at ↑ risk:

- *Aluminum*
- *Dye*
- *Paint*
- *Petroleum*
- *Rubber*
- *Textiles*

## Renal Cell Carcinoma (RCC)

Risk factors include smoking, obesity, hypertension, and end-stage renal disease. Associated with the von Hippel–Lindau gene mutation on chromosome 3, which is present in > 50% of sporadic cases and is the cause of hereditary clear cell renal carcinoma.

### SYMPTOMS/EXAM

- Although patients do not usually present with all three symptoms, the classic triad of symptoms includes flank pain, hematuria, and a palpable abdominal mass.
- Increasingly diagnosed in asymptomatic patients during incidental abdominal imaging.

### DIAGNOSIS

- Abdominal ultrasound is useful for distinguishing a benign cyst from a complex cyst or tumor.
- CT of the abdomen will show a multilocular mass with thickened, irregular walls and septae. It will enhance with contrast injection.
- Percutaneous biopsy is occasionally used.

### TREATMENT

- Patients with disease limited to the kidney (stages I and II) should undergo partial or radical nephrectomy.

- Patients with limited invasion (stage III) should undergo radical nephrectomy; those with extensive invasion or metastasis (stage IV) may have palliative nephrectomy.
- No chemotherapeutic regimen has been consistently shown to be effective in metastatic RCC.
- **Immunotherapy with IFN-α** or **interleukin-2** has been shown to induce an immune response against tumor cells and can be considered for metastatic RCC.

### COMPLICATIONS

Erythrocytosis, hypercalcemia, anemia, hepatopathy, and amyloidosis are all paraneoplastic syndromes associated with RCC.

## CARCINOMA OF UNKNOWN PRIMARY

A term used when patients present with a metastatic site and initial evaluation fails to identify a 1° tumor. Represents 2–5% of all cancer diagnoses. Classified in one of five histologic categories based on light microscopy of biopsied tissue:

- Adenocarcinoma
- SCC
- Neuroendocrine carcinoma
- Poorly differentiated carcinoma
- Poorly differentiated neoplasm (the pathologist cannot differentiate between carcinoma and other cancers)

### EXAM/DIAGNOSIS

- Begin with a complete history and physical (including genital and rectal exams).
- Initial labs should include a CBC and UA.
- Initial imaging should include a **CXR** and **CT of the chest, abdomen, and pelvis.**
- Biopsy with pathologic evaluation guides further studies. Examples:
  - **Poorly differentiated carcinoma:** HCG, AFP.
  - **Adenocarcinoma:** PSA, mammography, endoscopy.
  - **SCC of cervical nodes:** CT of the head and neck, laryngoscopy, nasopharyngoscopy, PET scan.

### TREATMENT

Table 7.10 outlines the treatment options for carcinoma of unknown primary.

## CHEMOTHERAPEUTIC AGENTS

Chemotherapeutic agents interfere with the cell cycle. There are two categories based on the kinetics:

- **Cell-cycle-specific (CCS) drugs:** Act specifically on cells that are cycling and are usually most active in one specific phase of the cycle.
- **Cell-cycle-nonspecific (CCNS) drugs:** Act on cells whether they are cycling or resting.

TABLE 7.10. Empiric Treatment for Carcinoma of Unknown Primary

| PATIENTS WITH: | TREAT AS: |
| --- | --- |
| SCC in cervical lymph nodes | Advanced head and neck cancer. |
| SCC in inguinal nodes | Do a careful exam of the anal canal and genitalia and consider lymphadenectomy and postoperative radiation +/– chemotherapy. |
| Women with peritoneal carcinomatosis | Advanced ovarian cancer. |
| Women with adenocarcinoma in axillary lymph nodes | Stage II breast cancer. |
| Men with bone metastases or an ↑ PSA | Advanced prostate cancer. |
| Young men with poorly differentiated carcinoma and a midline tumor | Extragonadal germ cell tumor. |
| Poorly differentiated carcinoma | Treat with empiric platinum/paclitaxel. |
| Poorly differentiated neuroendocrine carcinoma | Treat with empiric platinum/etoposide +/– paclitaxel. |

## Classes of Chemotherapeutic Agents

**Drug classes** are as follows:

- **Alkylating agents:** CCNS agents that alkylate nucleic acid bases → cross-linking, abnormal pairing, and breakage of DNA/RNA strands. Busulfan, chlorambucil, cyclophosphamide, ifosfamide, cisplatin, carboplatin.
- **Antimetabolites:** CCS agents that act primarily in the S phase of the cell cycle. They antagonize folate or nucleic acid bases, thus interfering with DNA/RNA synthesis. Methotrexate, mercaptopurine, thioguanine, cytarabine, fluorouracil, fludarabine, cytarabine, cladribine, gemcitabine, hydroxyurea.
- **Plant alkaloids:** CCS agents that are naturally occurring nitrogenous bases. Many act by inhibiting the mitotic spindle. Vinblastine, vincristine, etoposide, paclitaxel.
- **Antibiotics:** CCNS agents that intercalate adjacent nucleotides, thus causing DNA strand breaks. Doxorubicin, daunorubicin, bleomycin, mitomycin.
- **Hormonal agents:** Not directly cytotoxic, but down-regulate hormonally stimulated growth. Tamoxifen, leuprolide, goserelin.
- **Immunotherapeutic agents:** Rituximab, IFN-α.

## Toxicities

**Selected toxicities** include the following:

- **Cardiomyopathy:** Doxorubicin, daunorubicin.
- **Pulmonary fibrosis:** Bleomycin.
- **Hemorrhagic cystitis:** Alkylating agents, especially cyclophosphamide and ifosfamide.
- **Peripheral neuropathy:** Paclitaxel, vincristine, vinblastine.

HEMATOLOGY/ONCOLOGY

## Tumor Lysis Syndrome

A syndrome of metabolic disarray that results from rapid lysis of cancer cells. It is typically induced by chemotherapy or radiation but may rarely be caused by spontaneous necrosis. Most commonly associated with poorly differentiated lymphomas (e.g., Burkitt's lymphoma) and with leukemias, especially ALL. Rare in solid tumors.

*Risk factors for tumor lysis syndrome:*

- *Hyperuricemia*
- *Renal insufficiency*
- *Hypovolemia*
- *Chemosensitivity*
- *High tumor cell turnover*
- *Elevated LDH*

### DIAGNOSIS

- The diagnosis should be suspected in at-risk patients who develop ARF in the presence of hyperuricemia and/or hyperphosphatemia.
- Laboratory diagnosis may be based on two of the following: uric acid, potassium, or phosphate ↑ 25% from baseline, or calcium ↓ 25% from baseline.

### TREATMENT

- Patients at high risk for tumor lysis syndrome should be pretreated for at least two days prior to chemotherapy or radiation with allopurinol and fluids to maintain urine output > 2.5 L/day.
- Treatment includes management of electrolyte abnormalities, aggressive hydration, and diuretics to ↑ urine output.
- Hemodialysis may be needed for hyperkalemia, hyperphosphatemia, ARF, or fluid overload.

## Neutropenic Fever

Defined as a temperature > 38.3°C, or a temperature > 38°C sustained for one hour, in a patient with an absolute neutrophil count < 500. Etiologies are as follows:

- **Gram-⊖ rods** (especially *Pseudomonas*) have historically been the most common pathogens; however, **gram-⊕ cocci** have recently become more common.
- Fungal infections, especially *Candida* and *Aspergillus,* are commonly found with prolonged and severe neutropenia and prolonged antibiotic use.
- Viral infections also occur, especially with **human herpesviruses.**

### SYMPTOMS/EXAM

A thorough review of systems and exam should be done to localize a source of fever. Exam should include the skin, mucous membranes, oropharynx, sinuses, and perirectal area.

### DIAGNOSIS

- **Labs:** Should include CBC with differential, chem 7, a hepatic panel, and UA.
- **Microbiology workup:** Blood cultures through each line and one peripheral culture; sputum and urine Gram stain and culture. LP if indicated.
- **Imaging:** CXR; further imaging as indicated.

### TREATMENT

- **Empiric antibiotic therapy:**

- **Monotherapy:** Ceftazidime, cefepime, meropenem, or imipenem-cilastatin.
- **Combination therapy:** An antipseudomonal β-lactam plus an aminoglycoside (or a fluoroquinolone).
- Vancomycin should be added only in certain situations—e.g., in patients with a history of MRSA colonization, or with hypotension, mucositis, evidence of skin or catheter site infection, or recent quinolone prophylaxis. Discontinue if cultures are $\ominus$ at 72 hours.
- In patients with neutropenia and unexplained fever persisting for 5–7 days, an antifungal agent should be started.
- **Duration:**
  - If the source is known, complete a standard course of treatment.
  - For an unknown source:
    - If the ANC $\uparrow$ to > 500 and the patient becomes afebrile, then either continue antibiotics for 48 more hours or complete a minimum of a seven-day course.
    - If the patient becomes afebrile but remains neutropenic, consider completing a 14-day course.

## Graft-Versus-Host Disease (GVHD)

A syndrome that results when immunocompetent cells from a graft target the receiving patient's cell antigens. Occurs most often following an allogeneic bone marrow transplant. There are two categories of disease:

- **Acute GVHD:** Presents within the first 100 days after transplant and usually manifests in the skin, GI system, liver, and hematopoietic system.
- **Chronic GVHD:** Onset is > 100 days from the transplant and usually manifests in the skin, GI system, liver, and lungs.

### SYMPTOMS/EXAM

- **Acute:**
  - The most common presenting symptom is a **maculopapular rash** that may become confluent or form bullous lesions with diffuse desquamation.
  - Profuse watery or bloody **diarrhea, crampy abdominal pain,** nausea, vomiting, anorexia, and dyspepsia are also seen.
- **Chronic:**
  - Skin changes resemble those in scleroderma or SLE.
  - Also presents with dry oral mucosa with ulceration and pain, dysphagia, diarrhea, and weight loss.
  - Dyspnea and nonproductive cough are also seen.

### DIAGNOSIS

- Labs show **hyperbilirubinemia** and $\uparrow$ alkaline phosphatase if the liver is involved.
- Clinical diagnosis can be made in patients with a characteristic presentation.
- Biopsies of affected organ systems can be done to confirm.

### TREATMENT

- **Prophylaxis with methotrexate and cyclosporine** with or without T-cell depletion of the graft.
- **Corticosteroids are used for treatment.** For chronic disease, cyclosporine or tacrolimus may be used as well.

> A 63-year-old male patient presents with thoracic back pain six months after completion of treatment for renal cell carcinoma. He believes the pain started about four weeks ago, but he cannot recall precisely. He notices the pain more when he lies down in bed at night. He is afebrile, and his UA is unremarkable. Thoracic spine films show mild disc degeneration but are otherwise unremarkable. What is the next step? An MRI of the spine should be immediately obtained. Plain films cannot rule out spinal cord compression.

### Spinal Cord Compression

Usually caused by metastasis to the vertebral bodies. The prostate, breast, and lung are the most common 1° sites.

#### SYMPTOMS/EXAM

- The diagnosis should be considered in any patient with cancer who complains of **back pain.** It is usually the earliest symptom and may ↑ with recumbency, movement of the spine, or Valsalva.
- Functional deficits typically occur later and are progressive. They include weakness, sensory loss, and bowel and bladder dysfunction.
- There may be tenderness to palpation over the spine at the level of the lesion.
- Patients may be hyper- or hypotonic and hyper- or hyporeflexic depending on the acuity of the lesion.

#### DIAGNOSIS

- **MRI** of the entire spine should be done. Plain films cannot rule out compression.
- CT myelogram may be done as an alternative to MRI.
- Neurologic status at the time treatment is initiated is the most important prognostic factor, and therefore evaluation in symptomatic patients should be prompt.

#### TREATMENT

- Urgent **dexamethasone** 10 mg IV followed by 4 mg q 6 h. (Patients with paraparesis or paraplegia may be given 100 mg followed by 24 mg q 6 h.) Treatment should be started prior to the MRI if neurologic deficits are present.
- Emergent neurosurgical evaluation for possible surgical decompression followed by radiation therapy or radiation therapy alone if the patient is not a surgical candidate.
- Chemotherapy is occasionally used for sensitive tumors.

> A 32-year-old male smoker presents to your office with a complaint of a red face. On exam, you note distended neck veins in addition to his facial plethora. He denies dyspnea, and his oxygen saturation is 98% on room air. His CXR shows a widened mediastinum, and a contrast chest CT shows a mediastinal mass compressing the SVC as well as suspicious mediastinal nodes.

---

**Tumors that commonly metastasize to bone—**

**"BLT with Mayo, Mustard, and Kosher Pickle"**

**B**reast
**L**ung
**T**hyroid
**M**ultiple **M**yeloma
**K**idney (renal cell)
**P**rostate

---

> What is the next step? If there is no evidence of airway obstruction, treatment can be delayed until a definitive tissue diagnosis is established.

## Superior Vena Cava (SVC) Syndrome

Defined as compression of the SVC that is usually caused by mediastinal cancers such as lung cancer or lymphoma. It may also be caused by thrombosis.

### SYMPTOMS/EXAM

- Presents with dyspnea, facial swelling or plethora, cough, and arm swelling.
- Venous distention of the neck and chest wall is also seen.

### DIAGNOSIS

- CXR may show mediastinal widening and a pleural effusion.
- **Contrast chest CT** is the study of choice.

### TREATMENT

- SVC syndrome is a true emergency only if central airway obstruction is present. Otherwise, treatment may be delayed while an oncologic diagnosis is established, as chemoradiation may make subsequent diagnosis more difficult.
- Chemotherapy with or without radiation therapy is used for treatment-responsive tumors.
- An endovascular stent may be used for palliation in patients who are not good candidates for chemoradiation.
- Corticosteroids are frequently used for symptomatic relief but have not been shown to be effective.

## PARANEOPLASTIC SYNDROMES

Table 7.11 outlines common paraneoplastic syndromes and their causes.

**TABLE 7.11. Paraneoplastic Syndromes**

| SYNDROME | ASSOCIATED NEOPLASM | CAUSES |
|---|---|---|
| Lambert-Eaton syndrome | Small cell lung cancer, thymoma. | Autoantibodies against presynaptic calcium channels at the neuromuscular junction. |
| Erythrocytosis | RCC. | EPO. |
| Cushing's syndrome | Small cell lung cancer. | ACTH precursors. |
| SIADH | Small cell lung cancer, intracranial neoplasms, pancreatic cancer. | ADH or atrial natriuretic factor. |
| Hypercalcemia | Breast cancer; non–small cell lung cancer and other solid tumors metastatic to bone. | Local osteolysis by tumor cells. |
| | Multiple myeloma, lymphoma. | Osteoclast activating factors. |
| | Lymphoma, squamous cell lung cancer. | PTH-related protein. |

HEMATOLOGY/ONCOLOGY

# CHAPTER 8

# Pulmonary

Michael P. Grace, MD

**TABLE 8.1.** **Physical Findings Associated with Common Lung Conditions**

| | COPD | PNEUMONIA | ATELECTASIS | PNEUMOTHORAX | PLEURAL EFFUSION | TUMOR |
|---|---|---|---|---|---|---|
| Barrel chest (AP diameter > transverse) | + | – | – | – | – | If associated COPD |
| Retractions | + | + | – | | | – |
| Tracheal deviations | – | Ipsilateral | Ipsilateral | Contralateral | Contralateral (if large) | – |
| Fremitus | ↓ | ↓↑ | ↓ | ↓ | ↓ | ↑ |
| Percussion | Hyperresonant | Dull | Dull | Resonant to hyperresonant | Dull | Dull |
| Breath sounds | Distant | Bronchial | ↓ | ↓ or absent | ↓ or absent (based on size) | ↓ |
| Egophony | – | Ipsilateral | – | – | + or – | – |

### Lung Physical Findings

Table 8.1 depicts physical findings commonly associated with various lung conditions.

**Fremitus:** *Palpable vibration on chest while talking.*

### Lung Volumes

Common definitions pertinent to the measurement of lung volume are as follows (see also Figure 8.1):

**Egophony:** *Sounds that have a high-pitched, "bleating" quality on auscultation due to the presence of consolidation.*

- **Residual volume (RV):** Air in the lung at maximal expiration.
- **Expiratory reserve volume (ERV):** Air that can be exhaled after normal expiration.
- **Tidal volume (TV):** Air entering and exiting the lungs during normal respirations.
- **Inspiratory reserve volume (IRV):** Air in excess of TV that enters the lungs at full inspiration.
- **Functional reserve capacity (FRC):** RV + ERV.
- **Inspiratory capacity (IC):** TV + IRV.
- **Total lung capacity (TLC):** RV + ERV + TV + IRV.

### Cough

Cough is one of the most common reasons patients are prompted to visit their physicians. Healthy individuals rarely cough because mucociliary mecha-

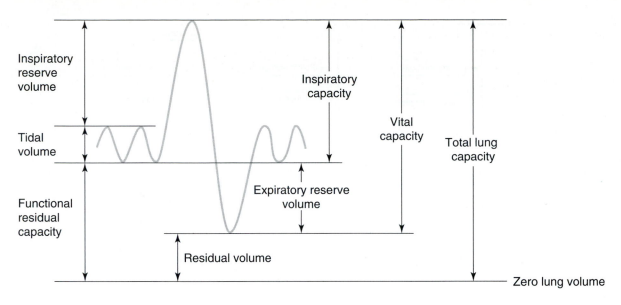

**FIGURE 8.1   Lung volumes.**

Lung volumes shown above as represented by spirogram tracing. (Reproduced, with permission, from Morgan GE Jr et al. *Clinical Anesthesiology*, 4th ed. New York: McGraw-Hill, 2006, Fig. 22-5.)

nisms are sufficient to clear normal bronchial secretions. Cough is important for clearing foreign bodies and secretions from the respiratory tract; however, it has the disadvantage of spreading illness through droplets and contamination of objects.

### SYMPTOMS

The following are some of the hallmarks of cough that may aid in determining its etiology (see also Figure 8.2):

- **Duration:**
  - **Acute cough:** < 3 weeks' duration.
    - Most commonly caused by viruses.
    - Other common causes include allergic rhinitis, acute bacterial sinusitis, COPD exacerbation, and infection with *Bordetella pertussis*.
    - Consider asthma, aspiration, and left heart failure, as cough may be the initial symptom of each.
  - **Subacute cough:** 3–8 weeks' duration.
    - Postinfectious cough is the most common cause.
    - Asthma, pertussis infection, and subacute bacterial sinusitis can also be causes of persistent cough in this time frame.
  - **Chronic cough:** > 8 weeks' duration.
    - Postnasal drip is the most common cause of chronic cough, followed by asthma and GERD.
    - Chronic bronchitis, bronchiectasis, and ACEI use are other common etiologies.
- **Productive vs. nonproductive:**
  - **Productive cough:** Points to an underlying inflammatory process (e.g., postnasal drip, acute or chronic bronchitis, or bacterial pneumonia).
  - **Nonproductive cough:** Points to a mechanical or irritative stimulus (e.g., ACEI cough).
- **Character:** A "brassy" cough may indicate major airway involvement, whereas a "barking/croupy" cough may signify laryngeal disease.

*Tactile fremitus is increased in pneumonia if it is alveolar; it is decreased in bronchoalveolar pneumonia, as bronchial mucous plugs dampen the tactile fremitus to make it softer.*

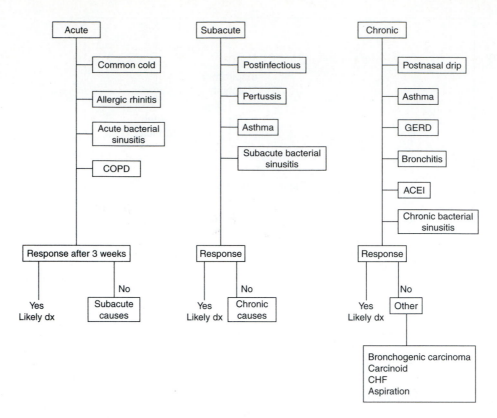

**FIGURE 8.2.** **Algorithm for the differential diagnosis of cough.**

(Reproduced, with permission, from Le T et al. *First Aid for the Internal Medicine Boards,* 1st ed. New York: McGraw-Hill, 2006: 555.)

- **Timing:**
  - **Nocturnal cough:** Associated with CHF or asthma.
  - **Mealtime cough:** Associated with esophagogastric disease.
  - **Cough upon awakening:** If cough results from the pooling of secretions from postnasal drip during sleep, it points to severe bronchitis or bronchiectasis.
- **Other:** Ask about postnasal drip symptoms, GERD, asthma, and smoking history.

### EXAM

- Focus on the nasal mucosa, lungs, and heart.
- Examine the fingers for clubbing.
- Boggy nasal mucosa and cobblestoning of the posterior oropharynx may suggest postnasal drip. Wheeze or cough on forced exhalation may be present in asthma.
- Listen for crackles or rhonchi.
- Examine for signs of CHF (e.g., elevated JVP, peripheral edema).

### DIAGNOSIS/TREATMENT

Diagnosis is largely based on symptoms/duration and on the patient's response to treatment of the presumed cause.

## COMPLICATIONS

Persistent and recurrent cough can → tussive syncope, retinal vessel rupture, persistent headache, chest wall and abdominal muscle strain (→ development of abdominal wall hernias), and rib fractures. Severe chronic cough can have a profound impact on activities of daily living, potentially → restriction of social activities, disruption of family life, and, in rare cases, attempted suicide.

*The most common causes of chronic cough are postnasal drip, asthma, and GERD.*

## Dyspnea

Defined as a feeling of difficulty breathing that is disproportionate to the stimulus and thus abnormally uncomfortable. It is often described by patients as feeling "breathless" or "short of breath."

### SYMPTOMS/EXAM

- Dyspnea can be caused by a multitude of conditions, necessitating a thorough history. Its onset can provide diagnostic clues:
  - **Sudden dyspnea** without provocation can represent pulmonary embolism, pneumothorax, or myocardial ischemia. Asthma can also present rapidly.
  - **Progressive dyspnea,** cough, and purulent sputum may represent a COPD exacerbation or pneumonia.
- To narrow the differential, attempt to identify the origin of the sensation, and try to document its impact on daily activities, its presence at rest, its time course, and the exertional distance traveled before symptoms force the patient to stop.
  - **Orthopnea:** Onset or worsening of dyspnea on becoming supine. Typically seen in heart disease and chronic lung disease.
  - **Paroxysmal nocturnal dyspnea:** Episodes of breathlessness that awaken patients from sleep. Usually points to chronic LV failure, but may also be seen in chronic pulmonary disease 2° to pooling of secretions.

### DIAGNOSIS/TREATMENT

- Order a CXR.
- Consider plasma brain natriuretic peptide (BNP) to determine if CHF is a possibility.
- PFTs should be among the initial studies considered.
- Consider ECG and echocardiography +/− stress testing.
- Testing for GERD may be necessary.
- Treat the underlying condition; whatever relieves dyspnea may also help diagnose the cause.

*The most common causes of chronic dyspnea are asthma, COPD, interstitial lung disease, and cardiomyopathy.*

## Hemoptysis

Defined as the coughing up of blood that **originates below the vocal cords.** Hemoptysis can range from trivial to massive in scope, with **massive hemoptysis** defined as any amount that is hemodynamically significant or threatens ventilation. Volume may range from 100 cc to > 600 cc in a 24-hour period.

### SYMPTOMS/EXAM

- Table 8.2 outlines a differential for hemoptysis based on anatomic location, with bolded causes the most common. Other common causes in-

**PULMONARY**

TABLE 8.2. Differential Diagnosis of Hemoptysis by Anatomic Location

| AIRWAYS | PULMONARY VASCULATURE | PULMONARY PARENCHYMA | IATROGENIC |
|---|---|---|---|
| **Bronchitis** | LV failure | Pneumonia | Transbronchial lung biopsies |
| **Bronchogenic carcinoma** | Mitral stenosis | Inhalation of crack cocaine | Anticoagulation |
| **Bronchiectasis** | Pulmonary emboli | Autoimmune disease: | Pulmonary artery rupture |
| | **AVMs** | Goodpasture's syndrome; | from balloon-tipped |
| | | Wegener's granulomatosis | catheter placement |

*Mitral stenosis is an often overlooked cause of hemoptysis, as it is associated with elevated pulmonary capillary pressure.*

clude aspergilloma, cystic fibrosis (CF), lung abscess, sarcoidosis, and TB.

- Hemoptysis can also be differentiated on the basis of **patient age:**
  - In patients < **40 years of age,** think bronchiectasis (if there is a prior history of recurrent pneumonia) or **mitral stenosis** (if a diastolic murmur is present).
  - In patients > **40 years of age,** consider **malignancy,** especially with a history of tobacco use, cachexia, and weight loss.
  - A URI prodrome and a benign exam in a young person may suggest bronchitis.

### DIAGNOSIS

- Lab work should include CBC with differential, UA, renal function tests, and coagulation studies.
- Obtain a CXR.
- Flexible bronchoscopy finds endobronchial carcinoma in 3–6% of patients with hemoptysis and a normal CXR (see Figure 8.3).
- If directed by the H&P, obtain sputum for cytology and acid-fast staining along with a chest CT (good for bronchiectasis, AVMs, central endobronchial lesions, and small peripheral malignancies).
- Additional tests include ABG analysis on room air as well as ANA, ANCA, and anti–glomerular basement membrane (anti-GBM) antibody assays to assess for autoimmune disease.

### TREATMENT

Treatment for hemoptysis is twofold: supportive if needed and then definitive.

- **Supportive care:** Consists of bed rest, supplemental oxygen, and blood products if needed. Ensure ventilation with airway protection, and intubate if necessary to achieve this objective. Avoid antitussives to allow blood clearance from airways.
- **Definitive treatment:**
  - **Nonmassive hemoptysis:** Identify and treat the specific cause.
  - **Massive hemoptysis:** A life-threatening condition whose treatment goal is to bring a rapid end to the bleeding.
    - If the bleeding site is known, place the patient in the decubitus position with the involved lung dependent. If bleeding is uncontrolled, urgent rigid bronchoscopy under general anesthesia allows for direct cautery or packing of bronchial lesions. A surgery consult may be necessary, but surgery is associated with high morbidity and mortality in this setting.
    - In stable patients, flexible bronchoscopy can identify the bleeding site, and angiography can embolize the involved bronchial arteries.

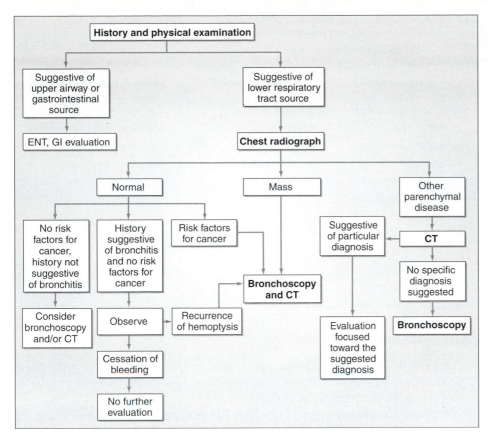

**FIGURE 8.3.** **Guidelines for the diagnosis of nonmassive hemoptysis.**

(Reproduced, with permission, from Kasper DL et al. *Harrison's Principles of Internal Medicine*, 16th ed. New York: McGraw-Hill, 2005: 208.)

- Angiography of the bronchial arteries can localize the bleeding site in > 90% of patients (< 10% of bleeds come from pulmonary arteries) and can then proceed to embolization, which is successful in > 90% of patients.

## Wheeze

A wheeze is an adventitious, "musical" lung sound produced by airflow through central and distal airways. Wheezes can be single toned or polyphonic and can occur on inspiration or expiration.

### SYMPTOMS/EXAM

- Wheezing is not always pathognomonic of an airway obstruction, and patients who have airway obstruction may not wheeze (e.g., with severe obstruction, there may not be enough air movement to generate a sound).
- A polyphonic wheeze (i.e., one with multiple notes) is often indicative of dynamic compression of larger, more central airways. Monophonic wheezes usually point to small airway disease. With upper airway obstruction, dyspnea on exertion usually occurs when the airway diameter is < 8 mm, and stridor is present with diameters < 5 mm.
- Table 8.3 outlines a differential for wheezing based on the location of the obstruction.

TABLE 8.3. **Differential Diagnosis of Wheezing**

| UPPER AIRWAY OBSTRUCTION | | LOWER AIRWAY OBSTRUCTION |
| --- | --- | --- |
| **EXTRATHORACIC** | **INTRATHORACIC** | |
| Vocal cord dysfunction | Tracheal stenosis | Asthma |
| Postnasal drip | Foreign body | Allergic bronchopulmonary |
| Laryngeal edema | Benign tumors | aspergillosis (ABPA) |
| Malignancy | Tracheomalacia | Aspiration |
| Relapsing polychondritis | Malignancy | Bronchiolitis |
| Wegener's granulomatosis | | Bronchiectasis |
| | | CF |
| | | COPD |
| | | CHF |
| | | Parasitic infections |
| | | Pulmonary embolus |

*"All that wheezes is not*

*asthma."*

### DIAGNOSIS/TREATMENT

■ PFTs with flow volume loops (see Figure 8.4) can be used to distinguish intrathoracic from extrathoracic obstruction. Treatment choices should be based on the specific cause of the wheeze.

■ Response to treatment helps confirm the diagnosis. Conversely, a lack of response should prompt the alteration of therapy (vs. looking for other potential causes).

## Hypoxemia

Hypoxia is defined as insufficient delivery of oxygen to the tissues. Hypoxemia is an **abnormally low arterial oxygen tension.** Under most situations, cardiac output is within a normal range, and **hypoxemia** is the most common cause of hypoxia. Generally, a $PaO_2$ of < 80 is considered hypoxemic (normal 80–100). With age, this number ↓ according to the formula 80 − [(age − 20)/4]. Hypoxemia is the result of any of a combination of five separate mechanisms:

1. **Hypoventilation:** Has multiple causes and essentially consists of a ↓ in **minute ventilation** (TV × breaths/minute) → an ↑ $PaCO_2$ and a **normal** alveolar-arterial (A-a) oxygen gradient.

2. **Right-to-left shunt:**
   ■ Occurs when blood bypasses the ventilated lung (e.g., vascular malformations or intracardiac shunts) or perfuses a nonventilated lung (e.g., pulmonary consolidation or pulmonary atelectasis) before returning to systemic circulation.
   ■ Always involves an ↑ in the A-a oxygen gradient. $PaCO_2$ may be low because of hyperventilation.
   ■ Failure of levels to improve with supplemental oxygen is characteristic of this condition (as blood is flowing past the nonventilated lung).

3. **Ventilation-perfusion (V/Q) mismatch:**
   ■ Failure to perfuse a ventilated lung (e.g., in pulmonary embolism).
   ■ Associated with an ↑ A-a oxygen gradient. Hypoxemia usually **improves** with supplemental oxygen (↑ $FiO_2$ [the fraction of inspired oxygen] in the ventilated lung will ↑ oxygen diffusion in the blood).

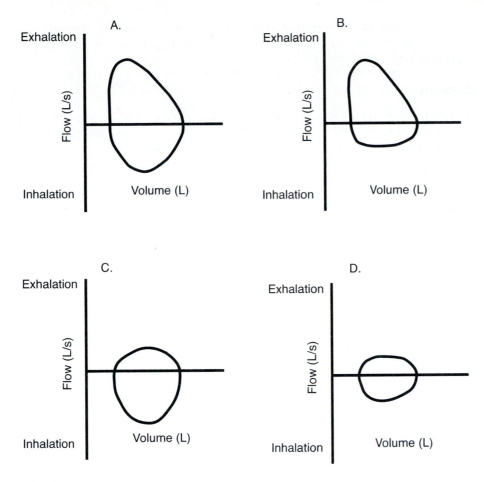

FIGURE 8.4. **Flow volume loops.**

A. normal pattern; B. variable extrathoracic obstruction; C. variable intrathoracic obstruction; D. Fixed obstruction. (Reproduced, with permission, from Le T et al. *First Aid for the Internal Medicine Boards,* 1st ed. New York: McGraw-Hill, 2006: 557.)

4. **Diffusion impairment:**
    - A situation in which there is a ↓ in the diffusion of gas across the alveolar-blood barrier.
    - Associated with an ↑ A-a oxygen gradient; hypoxemia improves with supplemental oxygen.
    - **Rarely** occurs in a clinically significant way.
5. **Low inspired oxygen:**
    - ↓ ambient oxygen pressure can → hypoxemia.
    - Seen at high altitudes—i.e., with lowered atmospheric pressure but preserved $FiO_2$ (21%). Also seen in closed-space rescues or structural fires.

### SYMPTOMS/EXAM

- The signs and symptoms of hypoxemia are nonspecific. Neurologic findings include agitation, headache, somnolence, coma, and seizures. Motor dysfunction may also be seen.
- Tachypnea and hyperventilation are frequent signs, but cyanosis is not a reliable predictor of hypoxemia.
- With chronic hypoxemia, polycythemia and pulmonary cachexia (weight loss as a result of ↑ energy requirements unbalanced by dietary intake)

may be present. At very low values of $PaO_2$ (< 20 mmHg), depression of the central respiratory drive is seen, and death usually results from respiratory failure.

### DIAGNOSIS

- Obtain an ABG if there is a suspicion of hypoxemia. Pulse oximetry, while noninvasive, is limited in that it does not assess ventilation and may lead to a delay in identifying clinically significant hypoxemia.
- Narrow the differential by calculating the A-a oxygen gradient, given by the formula $PiO_2 - (PaO_2 - PaCO_2/8)$.

### TREATMENT

- If possible, treat the underlying condition.
- Patients are eligible for and should be treated with long-term oxygen therapy when their arterial **$PaO_2$ is ≤ 55 mmHg** or their arterial oxygen saturation ($SaO_2$) is **≤ 88%.**
- If there is evidence of cor pulmonale, right heart failure, or erythrocytosis (hematocrit > 55%), patients who have a $PaO_2$ between 56 and 59 mmHg or an $SaO_2$ of 89% should also receive long-term oxygen.
- If sleep or exercise causes oxygen desaturations as above, oxygen therapy is warranted.

### DIAGNOSTICS IN PULMONARY MEDICINE

## Pulmonary Function Testing (PFTs)

Assessing lung function is important in pulmonary disease, and PFTs may significantly aid in diagnosis. The major types of PFTs include spirometry, measurement of lung volume, and quantitation of diffusing capacity. Indications for testing include the following (see also Table 8.4):

- Evaluation of various forms of pulmonary disease or for the presence of disease in patients with one or more risk factors (e.g., smoking).
- Evaluation of chronic persistent cough, wheezing, dyspnea, or exertional cough/chest pain.
- Objective assessment of bronchodilator therapy.
- Evaluation of work exposures.
- Assessing risk prior to major surgery.
- Objective assessment of impairment/disability.

**TABLE 8.4.** **Diagnostic Applications of PFTs**

| MODALITY | MEASURES | PATIENT SELECTION |
| --- | --- | --- |
| Spirometry | $FEV_1$, FVC, SVC | All smokers > 45 years of age to screen for COPD. |
| Forced inspiratory maneuvers | FIVC | Stridor heard over the neck or unexplained dyspnea. |
| Postbronchodilator spirometry | $FEV_1$, FVC | Obstruction on spirometry or suspicion of asthma. |
| Lung volumes | TLC | COPD. |
| Diffusing capacity | $DL_{co}$ | Restrictive/obstructive disease. |

## SPIROMETRY

Spirometry is the most useful and readily available of the PFTs. It includes measurement of forced expiratory volume in one second ($FEV_1$) and forced vital capacity (FVC). It may also include slow vital capacity (SVC), a measure that is useful when FVC is ↓, as slow exhalation → less airway narrowing, and lung volumes may prove to be normal (which can rule out restrictive disease).

- **Forced inspiratory maneuvers** (i.e., forced inspiratory vital capacity, or FIVC) can help detect variable airway obstruction, as is seen with vocal cord paralysis or dysfunction (see Figure 8.4).
- **Postbronchodilator spirometry** refers to the use of albuterol by measured-dose inhaler (MDI) during initial workup if baseline spirometry indicates obstruction or asthma is suspected. Spirometry should be repeated 10 minutes after treatment, and patients should be advised that proper MDI use is essential. An ↑ in $FVC_1 > 12\%$ or $> 0.2$ L indicates acute bronchodilator responsiveness.

## LUNG VOLUMES

Used to assess for restrictive lung disease, to show evidence of hyperinflation in obstructive lung disease, and to interpret the diffusing capacity for carbon monoxide ($DL_{CO}$). Can be done with helium dilution, nitrogen washout, **body plethysmography** (the gold standard), or CXR.

## DIFFUSING CAPACITY

Measurement of single-breath $DL_{CO}$. Can be used in restrictive disease to distinguish intrinsic lung disease (in which $DL_{CO}$ is ↓) from other causes of restriction in which $DL_{CO}$ is typically normal. In obstructive disease, diffusing capacity helps differentiate emphysema (characterized by a low $DL_{CO}$) from other causes of chronic airway obstruction. Obstruction from bronchitis typically has a normal $DL_{CO}$, whereas that associated with asthma has a normal to high $DL_{CO}$.

## Pulmonary Imaging Modalities

### CHEST X-RAY (CXR)

- CXR imaging has high clinical utility for infectious diseases as well as for screening patients at high risk for lung cancer.
- Can show infiltrates, nodules, masses, effusion, and, to a lesser extent, mediastinal and hilar abnormalities (see Tables 8.5 and 8.6).
- Generally includes both PA and lateral views.
- Lateral decubitus views are used to look for free-flowing pleural fluid, and apical lordotic views visualize the lung apices more effectively than the standard PA view.
- Portable views for acutely ill or otherwise bed-bound patients yield an AP view.

### COMPUTERIZED TOMOGRAPHY (CT)

- **Advantages of CT** over standard CXRs include the following:
  - Cross-sectional images show fluid collections, distinguish soft tissue structures, eliminate overlap, and define mediastinal structures.

TABLE 8.5.    Infiltrates Found on CXR

| UPPER LOBE | LOWER LOBE |
|---|---|
| Ankylosing spondylitis | Bronchiectasis |
| Sarcoidosis | Aspiration |
| TB | Dermatomyositis/polymyositis |
| Eosinophilic granulomatosis | Asbestosis |
| CF | Scleroderma |
| Silicosis | SLE, Sjögren's syndrome |
| Pneumonia | Rheumatoid arthritis (RA) |
| | Pneumonia |

Reproduced, with permission, from Le T et al. *First Aid for the Internal Medicine Boards,* 1st ed. New York: McGraw-Hill, 2006: 567.

- Scans can be obtained rapidly with detailed imaging of airways, vasculature, and parenchyma.
- Helical scans with IV contrast can rapidly detect pulmonary emboli or aortic dissection and, with reconstruction, detailed bronchial views
- High-resolution scans with thin slicing (1–2 mm) demonstrate bronchiectasis, emphysema, and interstitial lung disease.
- **Disadvantages** include cost, radiation exposure, and adverse reactions to IV radiocontrast media.

## VENTILATION/PERFUSION (V/Q) SCAN

- An imaging modality that aids in the diagnosis of pulmonary embolism using radioactive isotopes and a gamma camera.
- Albumin labeled with technetium-99m is injected and lodges in the pulmonary capillaries, showing the distribution of blood flow in the lung.
- Radiolabeled xenon gas can be inhaled to demonstrate the distribution of ventilation.
- In pulmonary embolism, defects in perfusion are not accompanied by a corresponding defect in ventilation and are thus called **mismatched defects.**

TABLE 8.6.    Masses found on CXR

| ANTERIOR MEDIASTINAL | POSTERIOR MEDIASTINAL |
|---|---|
| Teratoma | Bronchial cysts |
| Thymoma | Enterogenic cysts |
| Thymolipoma | Abscess |
| Thymic carcinoma/carcinoid | Non-Hodgkin's lymphoma |
| Thymic cyst | Neurogenic tumors |
| Thoracic thyroid | Pericardial cysts/plasmacytoma |
| Terrible lymphoma | Hodgkin's lymphoma |

Reproduced, with permission, from Le T et al. *First Aid for the Internal Medicine Boards,* 1st ed. New York: McGraw-Hill, 2006: 568.

PULMONARY

- Considered the **gold standard** for diagnosis of pulmonary embolism.
- Radiopaque contrast medium is injected into the pulmonary artery, allowing visualization of **filling defects** (defects in the lumen of a vessel) or an abrupt termination (**"cutoff"**) of the vessel.
- Can be used for suspected pulmonary AVMs.
- The **disadvantage** is that it is invasive. Used less and less frequently, since CT angiography delivers rapid imaging in a safer way.

- Provides a method to evaluate the airway/bronchial tree through direct visualization.
  - **Flexible bronchoscopy:** Performed on awake but sedated patients; can identify endobronchial pathology (e.g., tumors, granulomas, bronchitis, foreign bodies, bleeding sites) up to the level of subsegmental bronchi.
    - Samples can be obtained via washing, brushing, biopsy, and needle aspiration.
    - **Bronchial alveolar lavage** can reach the more distal pulmonary parenchyma and can recover organisms or cancer cells from the alveolar spaces.
  - **Rigid bronchoscopy:** Requires general anesthesia and is performed for massive bleeding and for the removal of large foreign bodies, blood clots, and tumors that may be obstructing airways.
- Complications stemming from bronchoscopy include hemorrhage, fever, transient hypoxemia, and pneumothorax.

## UPPER RESPIRATORY TRACT DISORDERS

A 44-year-old obese man comes to your office complaining of snoring and ↑ daytime sleepiness. His wife has reportedly witnessed apneic events while the patient sleeps. You suspect obstructive sleep apnea. What vital sign is most likely to be abnormal? The answer is blood pressure. Patients with this disorder have a 50% chance of being hypertensive.

## Obstructive Sleep Apnea (OSA)

Defined as complete or partial airway obstruction → apnea during sleep. Increasing respiratory efforts against the collapsed airway essentially suffocate the patient → repetitive arousals. Ultimately, clinical sequelae result from chronic sleep deprivation and recurrent oxyhemoglobin desaturation. Apnea is distinguished from hypopnea, or shallow breathing, as follows:

- **Apnea:** A temporary absence or cessation of breathing (airflow) during sleep, traditionally defined as **10 seconds** for adults.
- **Hypopnea:** Essentially "underbreathing"; breathing is present, unlike apnea, but is slower or more shallow than normal.

### SYMPTOMS/EXAM

- Patients' bed partners often complain of **loud snoring** and may witness actual apneic events. Patients often complain of **excessive sleepiness,** physically restless sleep, morning dry mouth and sore throat, personality changes, intellectual impairment, impotence, and **morning headache.**

- On exam, patients appear fatigued and often have ↑ BMI; collar size is frequently > 17 inches for men and > 16 inches for women.
- Systemic arterial **hypertension** is present in **50% of cases.**
- Airway crowding may be present as a result of adenotonsillar hypertrophy or redundant soft tissue of the soft palate together with an elongated uvula.

### DIFFERENTIAL

Excessive daytime sleepiness may also be caused by chronic sleep deprivation, narcolepsy, alcohol use, severe restrictive lung disease, medication and drug use, periodic restless leg syndrome, schedule disorders/shift work, and chronic pain and discomfort.

### DIAGNOSIS

- Although costly and labor-intensive, in-laboratory **nocturnal polysomnography** is the diagnostic gold standard for OSA.
- Results are reported in terms of the **apnea-hypopnea index** (AHI, or the number of episodes of apnea/hypopnea in an hour), also known as the respiratory disturbance index (RDI). Table 8.7 outlines the interpretation of AHI scores.

### TREATMENT

- **Conservative measures** (for patients with an AHI < 20): Avoid EtOH, weight loss, avoid sleeping on the back, intranasal steroids.
- **Continuous positive airway pressure (CPAP):** The **gold standard** for treatment; delivers constant air pressure through the nostrils to maintain a patent airway. Significantly improves quality of life and ↓ complications.
- **Aggressive treatment** (for patients with severe sleep apnea who cannot tolerate CPAP):
  - **Uvulopalatopharyngoplasty:** The most commonly performed procedure. Designed to ↑ the pharyngeal lumen by resecting redundant soft tissue.
  - **Nasal surgery:** Septal deviation repair, turbinectomy, polypectomy +/− surgical correction of craniofacial abnormalities.

### COMPLICATIONS

- Patients have a two- to threefold ↑ risk of motor vehicle accidents.
- **Cardiovascular complications:**
  - Contributes to difficult-to-treat systemic hypertension.

TABLE 8.7.    **Interpretation of AHI Results**

| AHI SCORE | INTERPRETATION |
| --- | --- |
| < 5 | Normal |
| 5–15 | Mild OSA |
| 16–30 | Moderate OSA |
| > 30 | Severe disease |

- Significantly ↑ the risk of stroke or death from any cause, with this ↑ independent of other risk factors, including hypertension.

## Nasal Polyps

Pale, edematous masses that are covered by mucosa and are frequently encountered in patients with allergic rhinitis. Nasal polyps arise from the sinuses (e.g., the **ethmoid sinuses**) and obstruct airflow by extending into the nasal cavity.

### Symptoms/Exam

- Patients may present with nasal obstruction, a diminished sense of smell, and rhinorrhea.
- Ask about a history of asthma, as up to 20–30% of asthmatics with nasal polyps have a sensitivity to aspirin (and the use of aspirin in these subjects may precipitate bronchospasm).
- Polyps appear as pale, gelatinous, rounded masses in the nasal cavity and are insensitive to pain.

### Differential

Chronic allergic rhinitis, sinusitis, Samter's triad, CF, Churg-Strauss syndrome, allergic fungal sinusitis.

### Treatment

- Intranasal steroids can block growth and may bring about regression. Systemic corticosteroids may → regression that can then be maintained with nasal steroids.
- Surgical removal may be necessary to relieve symptoms in patients in severe cases (e.g., those with intolerable nasal obstruction or recurrent sinusitis requiring multiple courses of antibiotics).

*Samter's triad consists of nasal polyps, asthma, and aspirin sensitivity.*

### Complications

The recurrence rate can be high, and thus preventive measures (e.g., controlling allergen exposure and maximizing medical therapy) are key.

## Epistaxis

Defined as bleeding from the nose, typically as a result of rupture of small vessels (Kiesselbach's plexus) in the mucosa overlying the anterior aspect of the cartilaginous nasal septum.

### Symptoms

Bleeding can occur from the anterior nasal cavity as above (95% of the time) or from the posterior cavity, either in the posterior half of the inferior turbinate or at the top of the nasal cavity. With posterior bleeds, there may be associated hemoptysis or hematemesis.

### Exam

- If possible, conduct the exam with the patient sitting upright to prevent ingestion or aspiration of blood. Wear protective eyewear and clothing.
- With a nasal speculum, examine both sides of the nose to assess the in-

251

tegrity of the septum and to identify bleeding sites. Examine the posterior oropharynx for 15 seconds to look for fresh blood flowing down the back wall, which may suggest a posterior source.

### DIFFERENTIAL

Nasal trauma (e.g., nose picking, foreign body, forceful nose blowing), rhinitis, dry nasal mucosa, deviated septum, chronic sinusitis, inhaled steroids, cocaine use, alcohol use, antiplatelet medications, thrombocytopenia, hemophilia, leukemia, Wegener's granulomatosis, nasal tumor.

### DIAGNOSIS

- Diagnose by exam as above. Obtain baseline vitals and monitor accordingly.
- Consider checking a platelet count and coagulation studies.
- The diagnosis may be difficult with large amounts of continued bleeding. The use of topical 4% cocaine or a topical decongestant plus a topical anesthetic (e.g., oxymetazoline and tetracaine, respectively), applied as a spray or on a cotton strip, can halt bleeding and aid in localization.

### TREATMENT

- **Anterior epistaxis:** Typically responds to continuous pressure to the nasal alae for 10 minutes.
  - Have the patient sit upright and lean forward.
  - Topical nasal decongestants such as a phenylephrine solution may be beneficial.
  - Silver nitrate or electrocautery can cauterize the bleeding site.
  - Anterior packing should be sufficient if bleeding persists.
- **Posterior epistaxis:** Likely calls for a referral. Treatment options include posterior pack placement to occlude choanae followed by anterior packing. Endovascular embolization vs. surgical ligation of the nasal arterial supply may be necessary.

## LOWER RESPIRATORY TRACT DISORDERS

A 23-year-old woman with a history of asthma previously managed by albuterol alone comes to your office complaining of an ↑ need for her inhaler over the past several months. She is coughing three days a week and has nighttime cough roughly once per week. What would be the next step in her asthma management? This patient meets the criteria for mild persistent asthma and thus requires a controller medication. The current preferred long-term controller treatment in mild persistent asthma is a low-dose inhaled corticosteroid.

### Asthma

Defined as inflammation of airways that may be idiopathic or caused by allergies or environmental factors that → an ↑ in airway secretions and subsequent contraction of the bronchial musculature. Acute inflammation produces asthma "attacks," but chronic inflammation can → narrowing and remodeling of the airways in the long term. Asthma is more common in nonwhite ethnic groups even after correcting for socioeconomic status. Five percent of Americans are affected, with asthma leading to > 450,000 hospitalizations and 5000 deaths per year.

### SYMPTOMS/EXAM

- Presents with episodic or chronic dyspnea, cough, wheezing, and chest tightness that worsen at night or in the early morning (see Table 8.8). Precipitants may be allergens such as dust mites, cockroaches, cat dander, or pollen. Nonallergic precipitants include exercise, cold air, URIs, stress, GERD, and secondhand smoke.
- Inquire about a history of atopy (the association is more common in younger patients).
- Exam may reveal prolonged expiration and diffuse wheezes.

### DIFFERENTIAL

CHF (cardiac asthma), GERD, pulmonary embolism, Churg-Strauss syndrome, conversion disorder.

### DIAGNOSIS

- Conduct spirometry ($FEV_1$, FVC, $FEV_1$/FVC) before and after the administration of a short-acting bronchodilator (see above).
  - Significant reversibility of obstruction is demonstrated by an ↑ of > 12% and 200 mL in $FEV_1$ or an ↑ of > 15% and 200 mL in FVC after bronchodilator use.
  - ABGs may show a respiratory alkalosis and an ↑ in the A-a oxygen gradient; in severe exacerbations, hypoxemia develops and the $PaCO_2$ normalizes.
  - If nondiagnostic, consider methacholine challenge.
  - An ↑ $PaCO_2$ and respiratory acidosis may portend respiratory failure.

**TABLE 8.8. Classification of Asthma Severity**

| STEP | GENERAL SYMPTOMS | NIGHTTIME SYMPTOMS | LUNG FUNCTION |
|---|---|---|---|
| Step 1: mild intermittent | Symptoms < 2 times per week. | ≤ 2 times per month. | $FEV_1$ or peak expiratory flow (PEF) ≥ 80% predicted. PEF variability < 20%. |
| Step 2: mild persistent | Symptoms > 2 times per week but < 1 time per day. Exacerbations may affect activity. | > 2 times per month. | $FEV_1$ or PEF ≥ 80% predicted. PEF variability 20–30%. |
| Step 3: moderate persistent | Daily symptoms. Daily use of an inhaled short-acting $\beta_2$-agonist. Exacerbations affect activity. Exacerbations ≥ 2 times per week; may last days. | > 1 time per week. | $FEV_1$ or PEF > 60% to < 80% predicted. PEF variability > 30%. |
| Step 4: severe persistent | Continual symptoms. Limited physical activity; frequent exacerbations. | Frequent. | $FEV_1$ or PEF < 60% predicted. PEF variability > 30%. |

Adapted, with permission, from South-Paul JE et al. *Current Diagnosis & Treatment in Family Medicine*, 1st ed. New York: McGraw-Hill, 2004, Table 26-7.

- Imaging may be obtained via CXR, but typically only hyperinflation can be seen.

### TREATMENT

Options include a combination of quick-relief therapy and long-term treatment based on asthma severity.

- **Quick-relief therapy:** Includes short-acting inhaled $\beta_2$-agonists (e.g., albuterol), anticholinergics (e.g., ipratropium), and glucocorticoids (e.g., oral prednisone). Intubation/ventilation may be necessary in cases of impending respiratory failure.
- **Long-term control therapy:** Involves use of inhaled and systemic (if necessary) corticosteroids, long-acting $\beta_2$-agonists (e.g., salmeterol), leukotriene modifiers (e.g., montelukast), mast cell stabilizers (e.g., cromolyn), and phosphodiesterase inhibitors (e.g., theophylline).

A 69-year-old white woman presents to the hospital with severe COPD along with a history of multiple hospital admissions, 30-step dyspnea on exertion, weight loss, weakness, and a resting $Pao_2$ of 59 mmHg. Which intervention will most likely affect her survival? Oxygen supplementation is the only treatment for severe COPD that has been shown to positively affect survival, ↓ dyspnea scores, and ↓ pulmonary artery pressure.

## Chronic Obstructive Pulmonary Disease (COPD)

A disease state characterized by **airflow limitation** that is no longer fully reversible. COPD includes **emphysema** (destruction and enlargement of lung alveoli) and **chronic bronchitis** (chronic cough and phlegm for three months or more over two consecutive years). Chronic airflow obstruction must be present in order for the diagnosis to be made. COPD is the **fourth leading cause of death in the United States,** and smoking is the most important risk factor. $\alpha_1$-antitrypsin deficiency is a rare genetic abnormality that → early-onset emphysema (1% of cases of COPD). Chronic bronchitis is frequently seen in patients in their 40s or 50s, whereas emphysema is more likely to appear in patients ≥ 60 years of age.

*Patients with emphysema are often called "pink puffers" because of a lack of cyanosis, their use of accessory muscles, and their pursed-lip breathing.*

*Patients with chronic bronchitis are called "blue bloaters" because of their more marked cyanosis and fluid retention.*

### SYMPTOMS/EXAM

- Symptoms typically arise in patients who have smoked > 1 pack of cigarettes per day for 20 years. On exam, patients may have distant breath and heart sounds, a barrel chest, prolonged expiration, and wheezing.
- Disease-specific symptoms are as follows:
  - **Chronic bronchitis:** Presents with a productive **cough** with sputum production for at least three months for two consecutive years. Patients with chronic bronchitis have more trouble getting air in and clearing their mucus.
  - **Emphysema:** Presents primarily with **exertional dyspnea** related to difficulty with exhaling, resulting in accessory muscle use → fatigue.

### DIFFERENTIAL

Acute bronchitis, asthma, bronchiectasis, CF, CHF.

Useful diagnostic tools include CXR, spirometry, and ABG analysis.

- **CXR:** Shows flattening of the diaphragm, ↓ lung markings, an enlarged retrosternal space, and blunting of the costophrenic angle.
- **Spirometry:** Can detect small changes in lung function relatively easily. Symptoms of COPD usually develop when $FEV_1$ ↓ to < 80% predicted. A PEF rate of < 350 L/min is a sign that COPD is likely present.
- **ABGs:** Acute exacerbations reveal hypoxemia and hypercarbia with acute respiratory acidosis.

*Oxygen therapy is the only therapy shown to ↓ mortality in hypoxemic patients with COPD.*

### TREATMENT

- **Nonpharmacologic:** The most important intervention is **smoking cessation,** as it improves lung function initially and slows annual loss of $FEV_1$. Hypoxemic patients should receive **supplemental oxygen.** Exercise and pulmonary rehabilitation can ↓ pulmonary symptoms and improve exercise tolerance.
- **Pharmacologic:**
  - **Inhaled anticholinergics** (e.g., ipratropium) have fewer side effects and yield better response than inhaled β-agonists. However, intermittent use of a **β-agonist inhaler** can be beneficial as an additional agent. Long-acting β-agonists may be useful as well, as they last through the night. **Tiotropium** is a long-acting anticholinergic that should serve as the bronchodilator of choice.
  - **Antibiotic therapy** may play a role in patients with chronic bronchitis who have ↑ volume or a purulent appearance to their sputum.
  - Inhaled **corticosteroids** can provide symptomatic relief as symptoms worsen, and oral steroid bursts during exacerbations can also ↓ symptoms.
- **Immunizations** for influenza and pneumococcus are recommended.

## Bronchiectasis

An abnormal and permanent **dilatation of bronchi** that is either focal or diffuse and is the result of repeated cycles of infection → pooling of secretions in the dilated airways. It is **caused by CF in 50% of cases.**

### SYMPTOMS/EXAM

- Presents with persistent or recurrent cough and purulent sputum production. **Hemoptysis is found in 50–70% of cases.**
- Patients may report a history of an initial severe pneumonia episode followed by chronic cough and sputum production. However, it may also have a more insidious onset.
- Nonproductive cough may represent "dry bronchiectasis" in an upper lobe. Dyspnea and wheeze may be a sign of extensive disease or underlying COPD. Infection may → ↑ sputum production and fever.
- Auscultation may reveal a combination of crackles, rhonchi, and wheeze. Clubbing of the fingernails may be present as well.

### DIFFERENTIAL

COPD, asthma, bronchiolitis, ABPA.

### DIAGNOSIS

The following studies can aid in making the diagnosis and/or clarify the underlying cause of bronchiectasis:

**PULMONARY**

- **CXR:** Findings are fairly nonspecific, but CXR may reveal **"tram tracks,"** which are dilated airways crowded in parallel due to atelectasis. In cross section, these produce **"ring shadows."**
- **High-resolution CT:** Offers good sensitivity for detecting bronchiectatic airways (ring shadows or tram tracks, depending on the CT plane of section).
- Obtain a sputum sample for bacterial and mycobacterial culture.
- CBC with differential.
- PFTs may show airflow **obstruction** from diffuse bronchiectasis.
- Sweat chloride levels for CF in cases of extensive lung involvement.
- Conduct skin testing/serology/sputum culture for *Aspergillus* if ABPA is suggested by the history (e.g., in an asthmatic person with proximal bronchiectasis).

### TREATMENT

- Treatment has four goals: to treat/eliminate the underlying condition causing bronchiectasis, to improve clearance of secretions, to control infection, and to reverse airway obstruction.
- Administer appropriate treatment when a treatable cause is found.
- **Airway clearance techniques:** Include chest physical therapy, flutter devices (which produce oscillatory positive pressure to assist the clearance of sputum), and percussive vests. Mucolytic agents to thin secretions are controversial (e.g., **DNase,** a medication that reduces mucus viscosity from DNA from degenerating neutrophils, is appropriate for CF but not for idiopathic bronchiectasis).
- **Antibiotics:** Commonly used in infrequent exacerbations when there is an ↑ in sputum quantity and purulence. Empiric coverage may include amoxicillin, TMP-SMX, or quinolone with an aminoglycoside if *Pseudomonas aeruginosa* is present. Chronic cases may warrant more prolonged courses or may benefit from intermittent but regular courses of single or rotating antibiotics.
- **Bronchodilators:** Agents such as β-agonists and anticholinergics improve obstruction and aid in the clearance of secretions.
- **Surgical resection:** Currently less common with the advent of improvements in medical therapy, but may be indicated with severe focal disease.

## Cystic Fibrosis (CF)

The most common lethal autosomal-recessive disorder in Caucasians, affecting 1 in every 3200 births; 1 in 25 is a carrier. It is caused by mutations affecting a membrane chloride channel (the cystic fibrosis transmembrane conductance regulator, or CFTR) and → multisystem dysfunction. Although CF is usually found in childhood, 7% of cases are diagnosed in adulthood, and with improvements in therapy, > 38% of patients are now adults.

### SYMPTOMS/EXAM

- Look for a history of failure to thrive, especially with recurrent infections of the airways (e.g., with *Pseudomonas*).
- Patients may have a history of pancreatic insufficiency, recurrent pancreatitis, sinusitis, intestinal obstruction, chronic hepatic disease, vitamin (fat-soluble) deficiencies, and male urogenital/infertility problems. Patients often have bronchiectasis. Symptoms include chronic or recurrent cough, sputum production, dyspnea, and wheezing.
- Exam may reveal digital clubbing, ↑ AP chest diameter, and apical crackles.

COPD, asthma, $\alpha_1$-antitrypsin deficiency, celiac disease, chronic sinusitis.

### DIAGNOSIS

Because of the large number of CF mutations, 1° diagnosis is typically made on the basis of clinical criteria and laboratory analysis of sweat Cl⁻ values.

- **PFTs** may show a mixed obstructive and restrictive pattern.
- **ABGs** reveal hypoxemia with compensated respiratory acidosis in advanced disease.
- Sweat chloride concentrations > 70 mEq/L help distinguish CF patients from those with other lung diseases.
- Genotyping, measurement of nasal membrane potential difference, semen analysis, and assessment of pancreatic function aid in diagnosis.
- Sputum cultures frequently show *S. aureus* or *P. aeruginosa* infections.
- CXR may show hyperinflation early; other findings include peribronchial cuffing, mucous plugging, bronchiectasis (seen effectively on high-resolution CT), and ↑ interstitial markings.

### TREATMENT

- **Acute exacerbations:** Treat with bronchodilators, DNase to thin sputum, antibiotics (at least two with antipseudomonal coverage), and chest physical therapy.
- **Longer-term therapy:**
  - Includes aerobic exercise, flutter devices, and external percussive vests to help with airway clearance.
  - Give pancreatic enzymes and the fat-soluble (A, D, E, and K) vitamins for malabsorption.
  - Nebulized DNase.
  - In severe cases, double-lung transplantation may extend survival (the donor lungs will not develop the CF phenotype).

## Interstitial Lung Disease (ILD)

A wide range of conditions (> 200) that are characterized by diffuse parenchymal lung involvement, often with significant morbidity and mortality. Conditions can be separated into those with predominant inflammation and fibrosis (e.g., idiopathic pulmonary fibrosis) and those that are predominately granulomatous (e.g., sarcoidosis).

### SYMPTOMS

- Patients may complain of onset of progressive **exertional dyspnea** or a persistent, nonproductive **cough.**
- Fatigue and weight loss are often seen. Chest pain, wheeze, and hemoptysis may be present but are less common.
- Acute presentation (days to weeks) is rare; subacute and **chronic presentations** are more common.
- Ask about smoking, occupational/environmental exposures, travel history, and a family history of lung conditions.

### EXAM

- Exam may reveal tachypnea and **bibasilar end-inspiratory dry crackles** (seen in inflammatory ILD but less often in granulomatous states).

- **"Inspiratory squeaks"** are late inspiratory high-pitched rhonchi heard in bronchiolitis. Look at the digits for cyanosis with clubbing, which develops in late disease.

### DIFFERENTIAL

- **Inflammation/fibrosis:** Asbestosis, drug reaction (e.g., amiodarone or chemotherapy), radiation exposure, idiopathic interstitial pneumonias, connective tissue diseases (e.g., RA, SLE), ulcerative colitis/Crohn's disease, heritable diseases (e.g., neurofibromatosis, tuberous sclerosis).
- **Granulomatous disease:** Hypersensitivity pneumonitis, sarcoidosis, eosinophilic granulomatosis, Wegener's granulomatosis, Churg-Strauss syndrome.

### DIAGNOSIS

- **Labs:** Can help confirm suspected connective tissue disorders.
- **Imaging:**
  - **CXR:** Most often nonspecific. May show a bibasilar reticular pattern, but often correlates poorly with the clinical or histopathologic stage of the disease. However, **honeycombing** may represent the pathologic findings of small cystic spaces and progressive fibrosis, signaling a poor prognosis.
  - **High-resolution CT:** Allows for early detection and confirmation of suspected ILD. Also serves to gauge the extent and distribution of the disease, and in some cases may effectively characterize the condition and prevent the need for biopsy.
- **PFTs:** Typically show a restrictive pattern, with a $\downarrow$ TLC, FRC, and RV. The $FEV_1/FVC$ ratio is usually normal or $\uparrow$. A $\downarrow$ in $DL_{CO}$ is common.
- **ABGs:** May be normal or reveal hypoxemia and respiratory alkalosis.
- **Lung biopsy:** The most effective way of confirming the diagnosis and assessing disease activity; can be transbronchial with fiberoptic bronchoscopy or open.

### TREATMENT

- Treatment is disease specific. The goals of treatment include permanent removal of the offending agent when known and suppression of the inflammatory process to limit further lung damage.
- Therapeutic measures include the following:
  - **Oxygen** for hypoxemia ($PaO_2 < 55$ mmHg) at rest and/or with exercise.
  - **Glucocorticoids** are often used despite a lack of evidence documenting their survival benefit.
  - **Immunosuppressive** agents such as cyclophosphamide and azathioprine have had variable success in some conditions.
- Lung transplantation may be considered in severe cases that do not respond to treatment as above.

## Pleural Effusion

Defined as an excess quantity of fluid in the pleural space caused either by $\uparrow$ pleural fluid formation or by $\downarrow$ removal by the lymphatic system. The fluid may be **transudative** or **exudative**.

- **Transudative effusion:** $\uparrow$ production of pleural fluid due to $\uparrow$ hydrostatic or $\downarrow$ oncotic pressures. Found in CHF, pulmonary embolism, cirrhosis, and nephrotic syndrome.

- **Exudative effusion:** ↑ production due to abnormal capillary permeability or ↓ lymphatic clearance of fluid. Found in malignancy, pneumonia, TB, pulmonary embolism, pancreatitis, esophageal rupture, collagen vascular disease, and chylothorax.

### SYMPTOMS/EXAM

- Patients may experience dyspnea with large effusions. They may also complain of pleuritic pain and may have symptoms of pneumonia such as productive cough, fever, and signs of consolidation.
- On exam, dullness to percussion and ↓ breath sounds may be found on the affected side. Look for signs of CHF such as JVD and edema. Ascites may point to cirrhosis as a cause.

### DIAGNOSIS

- **CXR:** On upright PA and lateral films, blunting of costophrenic angles may be present with effusions > 250 mL. Decubitus films can differentiate pleural fluid from pleural scarring and can aid in determining if the fluid is loculated.
- Via thoracentesis, pleural fluid should be sent for protein, glucose, LDH, cell count, Gram stain, and culture. Also obtain pH, fungal and mycobacterial cultures, and cytology. In appropriate settings, look for pleural fluid amylase, triglycerides, cholesterol, and hematocrit. Grossly purulent fluid represents empyema.
- **Exudates:**
  - Pleural fluid protein/serum protein > 0.5.
  - Pleural fluid LDH/serum LDH > 0.6.
  - Pleural fluid LDH more than two-thirds the upper limit of normal serum LDH.
- **Others:**
  - **Hemothorax:** A pleural hematocrit/peripheral hematocrit ratio > 0.5.
  - **Pancreatitis, pancreatic pseudocyst, adenocarcinoma of lung, or esophageal rupture:** ↑ pleural fluid amylase.
  - **Malignancy:** Cytology is only 50–60% sensitive for detection.
- Pleural biopsy can assist in the diagnosis of TB or cancer.

### TREATMENT

- **Transudative effusion:** Treat the underlying cause, and consider therapeutic thoracentesis if symptomatic.
- **Exudative effusion:**
  - **Parapneumonic:** Give appropriate antibiotics for infections; insert a chest tube for drainage if complicated (e.g., if pH < 7.2 **or** glucose < 60) or if empyema is present.
  - **Malignant:** Treat the underlying malignancy; repeat thoracentesis or chest tube insertion for symptom relief. Pleurodesis can ↓ reaccumulation of fluid.
  - **Hemothorax:** Rapid drainage via a large-bore chest tube to prevent fibrothorax.
  - **Tuberculous:** Usually resolves with treatment of TB.

## Pneumothorax

Defined as the presence of gas in the pleural space. Can be **spontaneous** (occurring without prior trauma to the thorax), **traumatic** (caused by penetrating or nonpenetrating chest injuries or iatrogenically following certain procedures), or **tension** (pressure in the pleural space is ⊕ throughout the respiratory cycle, as in mechanical ventilation or resuscitative efforts). In tension pneumothorax, ventilation is severely compromised and venous return can be ↓, reducing cardiac output and → a medical emergency. There are two types of spontaneous pneumothorax:

- 1°: Occur in individuals without clinically apparent lung disease (typically in tall, thin males 10–30 years of age, with smoking frequently a factor).
- 2°: Found in patients with underlying lung disease such as COPD, asthma, CF, TB, PCP, and ILD.

### SYMPTOMS/EXAM

- Patients may complain of acute onset of unilateral chest pain and dyspnea. Exam may be normal in mild cases.
- Findings include tachycardia, unilateral chest expansion, ↓ tactile fremitus, hyperresonance, and diminished breath sounds. Suspect tension pneumothorax if cyanosis, hypotension, and mediastinal or tracheal shift are present.

### DIFFERENTIAL

Costochondritis, rib fracture, pulmonary embolism, infectious pneumonia, viral pleuritis, empyema, MI.

### DIAGNOSIS

- On upright PA CXR, look for a thin visceral pleural line on expiration. In difficult or equivocal cases with a high degree of clinical suspicion, CT may be necessary.
- ABGs, if obtained, may show hypoxemia and acute respiratory alkalosis.

*If there is clinical suspicion of tension pneumothorax, initiate immediate needle thoracostomy with a 14- to 16-gauge needle in the second intercostal space at the midclavicular line. In an unstable patient, do not wait for x-ray confirmation.*

### TREATMENT

- Depends on the severity and nature of underlying disease.
  - Small (< 15% of a hemithorax), stable pneumothoraces may resolve spontaneously. Supplemental oxygen may hasten resolution.
  - Larger, spontaneous 1° pneumothoraces respond to simple aspiration drainage of pleural air with a small-bore catheter or a larger small-bore chest tube with a one-way valve. Follow patients with a daily CXR.
- 2° **spontaneous pneumothorax**, large pneumothorax, tension pneumothorax, or those with severe symptoms should have a chest tube placed under water-seal drainage. Suction should be applied until the lung expands, and the chest tube should then be removed after cessation of the air leak.
- Thoracoscopy or open thoracotomy may be necessary in recurrences of spontaneous pneumothorax, bilateral pneumothorax, and failure of tube thoracostomy. Surgery allows for the resection of blebs as well as for pleurodesis by mechanical abrasion and insufflation of talc.

> A 66-year-old man presents with increasing shortness of breath over the last 24 hours. He has no cough, fever, or hemoptysis and no prior history of lung disease. He denies any calf pain or swelling. There is no past history of cancer or thromboembolic disease. The man just returned from a long flight to Europe. His physical exam is remarkable for a heart rate of 107. You suspect pul-

monary embolism. What would be the next step to take to confirm your suspicion? Obtain a D-dimer and imaging (a helical CT if the kidneys are normal) given his history of immobilization, lack of an alternative diagnosis, and heart rate.

## Pulmonary Embolism

An obstruction of the pulmonary vasculature that most commonly results from a deep venous thrombosis (DVT) that has embolized. Rarely, other substances can cause an obstruction, such as air, fat, and amniotic fluid. Symptoms can range from mild to complete circulatory collapse and death. Risk factors include **hypercoagulable states,** as in certain cancers; recent trauma; immobility (e.g., postsurgery or long flights); pregnancy; and coagulation disorders such as factor V Leiden mutation and protein C, protein S, or antithrombin III deficiencies. **Venous stasis** and **endothelial damage** also predispose to DVT formation.

*The risk factors for DVT/pulmonary embolism are contained in Virchow's triad of venous stasis, endothelial damage, and hypercoagulable states.*

### SYMPTOMS/EXAM

- Patients most often complain of acute dyspnea. With peripheral pulmonary embolism, pleuritic pain, cough, or hemoptysis may be present. Tachycardia is the most common sign on exam. Patients may often appear anxious but are otherwise well.
- Patients may also exhibit low-grade fever, JVD, or a loud P2. With a massive pulmonary embolism, syncope, hypotension, or cyanosis may be seen.

### DIFFERENTIAL

MI/acute coronary syndrome, pneumonia, pericarditis, CHF, pleuritis, pneumothorax, pericardial tamponade, rib fracture, anxiety.

### DIAGNOSIS

Accurate diagnosis remains difficult, so pulmonary embolism should be on the differential for any patient presenting with sudden chest pain, dyspnea, and tachycardia in the setting of a normal CXR. Diagnostic modalities are as follows (see also Figure 8.5):

- **D-dimer:** Elevated in > 90% of patients, but not specific, and elevations are also seen in patients with MI, sepsis, and most systemic illnesses. Its high $\ominus$ predictive value can aid in excluding pulmonary embolism. The test should not be used alone.
- **ABGs:** In pulmonary embolism, both $P_{O_2}$ and $P_{CO_2}$ will often ↓. Respiratory alkalosis and an ↑ A-a oxygen gradient may also be seen.
- **ECG:** Frequently reveals sinus tachycardia; less often shows a new-onset atrial fibrillation/flutter or an **S1Q3T3** pattern (an S wave in lead I, a Q wave in lead III, and an inverted T in III). T-wave inversion in leads $V_1$–$V_4$ reflects RV strain.
- **CXR:** A normal CXR in a dyspneic patient may suggest pulmonary embolism. **Westermark's sign** (an area of lucency related to the abrupt tapering of the pulmonary vessel from the embolus), **Hampton's hump** (a peripheral wedged-shaped density from the pulmonary infarct), pleural effusion, or atelectasis may be present.
- **Lower extremity ultrasound:** In suspected cases of pulmonary embolism, a finding of DVT establishes the need for treatment and may thus make invasive pulmonary angiography unnecessary (see Figure 8.5). Of all pa-

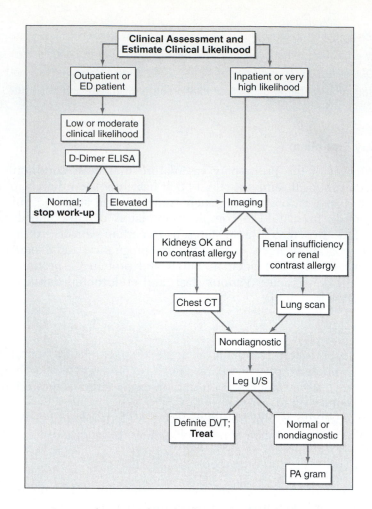

**FIGURE 8.5.** Systematic approach to the diagnosis of pulmonary embolism.

(Reproduced, with permission, from Kasper DL et al. *Harrison's Principles of Internal Medicine,* 16th ed. New York: McGraw-Hill, 2005: 1563.)

tients with pulmonary embolism, > 50% will not have evidence of DVT with imaging, and workup for pulmonary embolism should continue if there is a high clinical suspicion with a ⊖ ultrasound.

- **V/Q scan:** May show segmental regions of V/Q mismatch; results are expressed as normal-low, intermediate, and high probability for pulmonary embolism.

- **Spiral CT with contrast:** Effective for the diagnosis of large, central pulmonary embolisms. Can detect peripheral thrombi up to fifth-order branches. In patients without pulmonary embolism, lung parenchymal images may reveal other diagnoses that may explain the presenting symptoms.

- **Pulmonary angiography:** The **gold standard.** Largely being replaced by newer CT technology given its invasive nature and risk.

### TREATMENT

Options for management include anticoagulation to prevent further embolism, clot lysis with thrombolytic agents, or surgical removal of the clot.

- **Unfractionated heparin:** Administered intravenously. A weight-based nomogram for loading and maintenance improves the time needed to achieve adequate anticoagulation and ↓ bleeding risk. Drawbacks include the need for hospitalization and the risk of thrombocytopenia from heparin.

- **Low-molecular-weight heparin:** Suitable for lower-risk patients in place of unfractionated heparin. Can be used at home without the need for monitoring.
- **Warfarin:** Started promptly to achieve long-term anticoagulation; INR should be 2–3 before stopping heparin. Treatment duration is typically six months for a first episode when there is a reversible risk factor; 12 months after a first-episode idiopathic thrombus; and 6–12 months to indefinitely in those with recurrent disease or nonreversible risk factors.
- **Thrombolytic agents:** Reserved for patients with extensive embolism and/or hemodynamic instability.
- **Embolectomy:** Rarely performed, and usually a "last-ditch" effort to save a patient.

## Pulmonary Artery Hypertension (PAH)

An abnormal elevation in pulmonary artery pressure; defined as a resting pulmonary artery mean pressure of > 25 or > 30 with exercise. It can occur in isolation (idiopathic or 1° pulmonary hypertension) or may be 2° to a range of disorders, including connective tissue disease, advanced parenchymal lung disease, sleep-disordered breathing, congenital heart disease, advanced liver disease, HIV, chronic thromboembolic disease, and drugs. It is generally seen as a marker of advanced disease. 1° pulmonary hypertension is rare and occurs mostly in young to middle-aged women.

### Symptoms/Exam

- Difficult to recognize in the early stages because symptoms and signs may be attributed to underlying disease. Patients may complain of dyspnea initially on exertion and then at rest. Dull, substernal chest pain may be present. Fatigue and syncope on exertion may occur.
- Exam findings include narrow splitting of S2 with a loud P2 best heard at the apex. In advanced cases, tricuspid and pulmonary valve insufficiency and signs of right heart failure and cor pulmonale can be seen.

### Differential

LV systolic failure, LV diastolic dysfunction, causes of 2° pulmonary hypertension (see above).

### Diagnosis

- **Echocardiography:** May be the first test suggesting the presence of PAH. Most commonly reveals enlargement of the right ventricle and atrium with tricuspid regurgitation. Allows for the estimation of pulmonary artery pressure as well as the evaluation of LV function, valvular disorders, and congenital heart disease.
- **Blood chemistries:** In cases of suspected pulmonary hypertension, a CBC, a comprehensive metabolic panel, and coagulation studies may be obtained. Polycythemia may point to chronic, severe hypoxemia. Abnormal LFTs may suggest underlying hepatic disease. Look for connective tissue diseases with targeted testing such as ANA, ESR, and RF. HIV testing should be considered for all patients.
- **ABGs:** May show hypoxemia with respiratory alkalosis.

- **ECG:** Look for RVH, rightward axis, RV strain, and right atrial enlargement.
- **CXR:** Reveals cardiomegaly with enlarged central pulmonary arteries. May show evidence of parenchymal lung disease such as COPD.
- **V/Q scan vs. CT:** To look for possible occult thromboembolic disease.
- **Overnight oximetry:** Conduct in all patients to determine if hypoxemia worsens with sleep and requires treatment with supplemental oxygen.
- **Sleep study:** Conduct in patients with symptoms consistent with sleep-disordered breathing, as this may potentially reverse PAH.
- **Right heart catheterization:** Can definitively measure pulmonary artery pressure, cardiac output, and pulmonary vascular resistance as well as left-to-right shunts and evidence of left heart dysfunction.

### TREATMENT

Treatment is disease specific in 2° causes of PAH. Early detection is vital to disrupting the self-perpetuating cycle that can → rapid clinic progression.

- **Hypoxemic COPD:** Supplemental oxygen can slow progression.
- **High risk for thromboembolism:** Permanent anticoagulation in patients with chronic thomboembolic disease as a cause of their PAH.
- Vasodilatory agents (e.g., calcium channel blockers, hydralazine, nitroglycerin) have yielded disappointing results in the treatment of PAH.
- **1° PAH:** Continuous long-term IV infusion of prostacyclin (via a portable pump) has improved survival.
- Bilateral lung transplantation may be necessary after failure of medical therapy.

---

You are evaluating a 48-year-old man who requires a CXR for a physical exam through his work. He is otherwise healthy and denies a history of smoking. His CXR is clear with the exception of a 1-cm lesion with some central calcification in the left upper lobe. His PPD is negative. He has no prior chest films for comparison. What is your next step? The patient has a solitary pulmonary nodule. Given its size and appearance, it is more likely to be benign, but because of his age and smoking history, you decide to obtain a CT scan. On CT the lesion has a benign appearance, so you decide on close observation of the lesion with serial CT scan every 3–6 months for the next two years.

---

## Solitary Pulmonary Nodule

Defined as a solitary mass < 3 cm in size, surrounded by normal lung tissue and not associated with atelectasis or adenopathy. Historically referred to as **"coin lesions."** Often found incidentally when a CXR is obtained for a different purpose. Lesions > 3 cm are pulmonary masses and are much more likely to be malignant.

### SYMPTOMS/EXAM

- Patients are often asymptomatic but may have lung symptoms such as cough, hemoptysis, and dyspnea. Age, smoking history, environmental/infectious exposures, residence/travel, cancer history, and previous lung disease should be elicited.
- On exam, lungs may be entirely clear. A localized wheeze may indicate an endobronchial tumor. Look for clubbing and hypoxemia, and check for

lymphadenopathy (if localized to the supraclavicular/scalene nodes, it raises concern for cancer; generalized lymphadenopathy suggests lymphoma or an infectious etiology).

### DIFFERENTIAL

- **Benign:** Infectious granulomas, viral infections (measles, CMV), *Pneumocystis jiroveci* (formerly *P. carinii*), pneumonia, lung abscess, hamartoma, chondroma, pulmonary infarct, AVM, sarcoidosis, pulmonary amyloidosis.
- **Malignant:** Bronchogenic carcinoma, bronchial carcinoid tumors, metastatic tumors (colorectal, breast, renal cell, testicular, malignant melanoma, sarcoma).

### DIAGNOSIS

- Typically found incidentally on CXR. Figure 8.6 shows a diagnostic algorithm.
- Benign patterns on imaging include a **"bull's eye"** pattern of granulomas, a **"popcorn"** pattern of hamartomas, or a dense central core of calcifica-

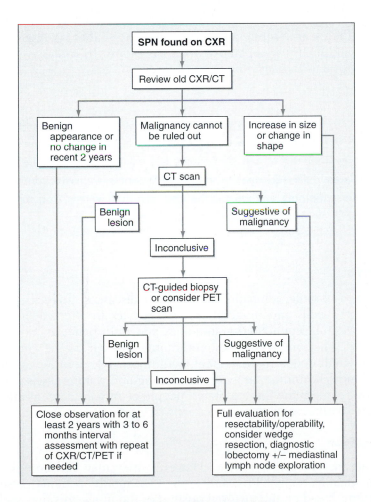

**FIGURE 8.6.** **Evaluation of the solitary pulmonary nodule.**

(Reproduced, with permission, from Kasper DL et al. *Harrison's Principles of Internal Medicine,* 16th ed. New York: McGraw-Hill, 2005: 513.)

PULMONARY

265

tion. Lesions lacking calcium or in a stippled or eccentric location raise more concern for malignancy.

- **Serial CXRs:** A **comparison** of serial CXRs can check for the stability of the lesion. No change in lesion size in two years indicates that the lesion is likely benign. The larger the lesion, the more likely it is to be malignant (although lesions < 1 cm have a 15% chance of malignancy).
- **Chest CT:** Best for further evaluating solitary pulmonary nodules, giving a better indication of size, calcification pattern, and nodule density. IV contrast can further aid diagnosis via enhancement of malignant lesions and can assess for mediastinal adenopathy.
- **PET scans:** Can be used to better evaluate indeterminate lesions; have sensitivities and specificities in the range of 85–95% and 75–85%, respectively.

### TREATMENT

- Patients with solitary pulmonary nodules who are felt to be low risk (e.g., nonsmoking patients, those < 35 years of age, and those with smaller lesions with a more benign appearance on radiography) can be followed with serial CTs every three months for one year and then yearly.
- Patients who are felt to be at higher risk for cancer (e.g., patients with a history of cigarette smoking; those ≥ 35 years of age; and those with larger lesions, lack of calcification, chest symptoms, interval growth of a lesion, or a ⊕ PET scan) require a histologic diagnosis either via resection or, for those with higher preoperative risk, via biopsy by video-assisted thoracoscopy or transthoracic fine-needle biopsy.

A 47-year-old African-American woman presents with a several-week history of fatigue and malaise. She complains of low-grade fevers, shortness of breath with exertion, and cough. Her exam is unremarkable. Her CXR shows bilateral hilar adenopathy, and her PPD is negative. What condition may explain her symptoms, and what is the next step in diagnosis? You suspect sarcoidosis and refer her for bronchoscopy for biopsy of her lesions.

## Sarcoidosis

Defined as a chronic, idiopathic multisystem disease distinguished by accumulation of T cells and mononuclear phagocytes in affected organs along with noncaseating epithelioid granulomas and disturbance in normal tissue architecture. The lung is the most commonly affected organ, with skin, eye, liver, and lymph node involvement also common. The disorder can be acute, subacute and self-limiting, or a chronic waxing and waning disease occurring over many years. In the United States, people of African descent are affected more than 10 times as often as Caucasians.

### SYMPTOMS/EXAM

- Patients may be asymptomatic. However, they may also complain of fatigue, malaise, weight loss, and fever. Commonly, patients present with symptoms based on the involved organ. For the lungs, this may include exertional dyspnea; dry, nonproductive cough; and vague chest pain.
- Exam findings include crackles +/– wheezing but may also be normal. Lymphadenopathy may be present.

TB, lymphoma, histoplasmosis, coccidioidomycosis, idiopathic pulmonary fibrosis, pneumoconiosis, syphilis.

## DIAGNOSIS

Diagnosed when clinical presentation and radiographic studies suggest the diagnosis and granulomatous inflammation is detected in an involved organ. Biopsy is necessary to exclude infection or malignancy.

- The H&P should focus on occupational and environmental exposures and on organs that are commonly affected, such as the lung, skin, eyes, and lymph nodes.
- CXR may show **bilateral hilar adenopathy**, but this is a nonspecific finding.
- **Fiberoptic bronchoscopy with transbronchial biopsy** most commonly makes the diagnosis, showing a "sarcoid granuloma," which is **a well-formed noncaseating epithelioid cell** granuloma surrounded by a rim of fibroblasts and lymphocytes.
- Other tests supportive of but not sufficient for diagnosis include angiotensin-converting enzyme (ACE) level and gallium scan.
- Baseline evaluation should include PFTs, ECG, ophthalmologic evaluation, CBC, a complete metabolic panel, and 24-hour urine calcium.
- On follow-up, periodic screening for other organ involvement is appropriate along with specialist referral as indicated.

## TREATMENT

Systemic corticosteroids as first-line therapy; methotrexate as a first alternative.

## Lung Cancer

The leading cause of cancer death in the United States, with a five-year survival rate of 15%. The various histologic types of bronchogenic carcinoma include **squamous cell carcinoma, adenocarcinoma, large cell carcinoma,** and **small cell carcinoma.** For purposes of staging and treatment, small cell lung cancer (SCLC) is separated from the three other subtypes (labeled together as non–small cell lung cancer, or NSCLC).

Squamous cell carcinoma and small cell carcinomas start centrally, whereas adenocarcinomas are more peripheral in origin. Large cell carcinomas can present centrally or peripherally.

### SYMPTOMS/EXAM

- Up to 15% of patients may be asymptomatic. Symptoms, when present, are a reflection of tumor location.
- With **central tumors,** patients may complain of cough, hemoptysis, wheeze and stridor, dyspnea, and fever/productive cough if postobstructive pneumonitis present.
- **Peripheral** tumor growth may cause pleuritic chest pain, cough, and dyspnea.
- **Regional** spread of tumor may cause tracheal obstructive symptoms, dysphagia (from esophageal compression), or hoarseness; hemidiaphragm elevation with dyspnea; or Horner's syndrome (ptosis, miosis, and anhidrosis on the unilateral side of face) from nerve compressions.
- Malignant effusions can → dyspnea.
- **Extrathoracic** metastatic disease is common and can affect nearly every organ system.
- **Paraneoplastic syndromes** can → anorexia, cachexia, weight loss, fever,

and suppressed immunity, while **endocrine syndromes** can → symptoms related to hypercalcemia, hypophosphatemia, and hyponatremia.

### DIAGNOSIS

- Screening of high-risk individuals with sputum cytology and CXR has not been shown to improve survival rate. Trials aimed at exploring screening with chest CT are currently under way. When the history/exam and screening tests are suggestive of lung cancer, tissue diagnosis is necessary.
- A biopsy can be performed with fiberoptic bronchoscopy, mediastinoscopy, surgical resection, percutaneous biopsy of an enlarged lymph node or pleural lesion, FNA under CT guidance, or cytology of a malignant pleural effusion.

### TREATMENT

Based on diagnosis and staging:

- SCLC shows early hematogenous spread and an aggressive course and is rarely amenable to resection. With limited disease, thoracic radiation may improve survival.
- NSCLC is slower to spread and more likely to be cured with early resection. Higher stages require multimodality therapy with chemotherapy and radiation.
- **Palliative therapy** can take many forms and may assist in relieving symptoms, whether it is photoresection with laser, external beam radiation, resection of brain metastases, or aggressive pain control in advanced disease. Referral to a palliative care specialist is recommended in advanced disease along with appropriate referral to hospice programs.

# Nephrology

Matthew Jaffy, MD

## Urinalysis

- Essential in patients with kidney disease as well as for many other indications. Plays no role in the screening of asymptomatic patients except in pregnancy. Consider screening in those with a family history of kidney disease.
- Involves midstream collection or bladder catheterization; analysis must be done within one hour of collection.
- Has two components:
    - **Dipstick testing**: Measures specific gravity, pH, protein, hemoglobin, glucose, ketones, bilirubin, nitrite, and leukocyte esterase.
    - **Microscopy**: Identifies crystals, cells, casts (see Table 9.1), infecting organisms, and oval fatty bodies in nephrotic syndrome.

## 24-Hour Urine Collection

- The **gold standard** for quantitative testing of proteinuria. Random urine may be more convenient if accuracy is not essential.
- Most commonly used to measure urine protein, creatinine, electrolytes, and urine volume.

## Renal Ultrasound

- Used to evaluate the thickness of the renal cortex (glomeruli) and echogenicity of renal as well as to assess any distention of the urinary collecting system. Can also determine kidney size and compare the two kidneys.
- Indications include the following:
    - The most appropriate initial test to exclude urinary tract obstruction.
    - Consider in patients presenting with renal failure of unknown etiology.

**T A B L E   9 . 1 .   Significance of Specific Urinary Casts**

| Type | Significance |
|---|---|
| Hyaline casts | Concentrated urine, febrile disease, after strenuous exercise, in the course of diuretic therapy (not indicative of renal disease). |
| RBC casts | Glomerulonephritis. |
| WBC casts | Pyelonephritis, interstitial nephritis (indicative of infection or inflammation). |
| Renal tubular cell casts | Acute tubular necrosis (ATN), interstitial nephritis. |
| Coarse granular casts | Nonspecific; can represent ATN. |
| Broad, waxy casts | Chronic renal failure (indicative of stasis in enlarged collecting tubules). |

Adapted, with permission, from Tierney LM et al. *Current Medical Diagnosis & Treatment,* 45th ed. New York: McGraw-Hill, 2006, Table 22-1.

- Rule out obstruction or abscess in pyelonephritis patients with incomplete response to appropriate antibiotics.
- Can help distinguish benign renal cysts from complex cysts or masses.
- Evaluation for malignancy in patients > 50 years of age with hematuria.
- Useful in screening for polycystic kidney disease, but less sensitive than CT scan.
- Used to localize the kidney for percutaneous procedures.

## Intravenous Pyelography (IVP)

- Requires administration of contrast; hence less popular than ultrasound or CT.
- Useful for the characterization of some structural disorders, such as medullary sponge kidney and papillary necrosis, or as part of the evaluation for malignancy in patients with hematuria.

## Computed Tomography (CT)

- **Noncontrast helical CT scan is the gold standard for detection of renal stones;** has 95% sensitivity and 98% specificity in patients presenting with acute flank pain.
- Allows for additional investigation of abnormalities identified on ultrasound, such as distinguishing a neoplasm from a simple cyst.
- Used for the evaluation and staging of renal cell carcinoma (RCC).
- Useful as part of evaluation for malignancy in patients > 50 years of age with hematuria.

## Magnetic Resonance Imaging (MRI)

- Nearly 100% sensitive and 96–98% specific for renal artery stenosis; has ↓ the role of renal artery angiography.
- Useful for the evaluation and staging of RCC in addition to CT.

## Voiding Cystourethrography (VCUG)

Used to detect vesicoureteral reflux, particularly in pediatric patients with UTI.

## Renal Biopsy

- Possible indications include the following:
  - Establishing an exact diagnosis in unexplained acute or chronic kidney disease.
  - Guiding future treatment in established diseases.
  - Acute nephritic syndrome.
  - Establishing renal involvement in systemic diseases such as SLE, Goodpasture's syndrome, and Wegener's granulomatosis.
- Relative **contraindications** are as follows:
  - Kidneys < 9 cm are generally indicative of irreversible changes.
  - Multiple bilateral cysts.
  - Renal neoplasm.
  - Uncorrectable bleeding disorders.
  - Severe, uncontrolled hypertension.

- Pyelonephritis or abscess.
- When the benefits of treatment options are outweighed by the risks.
- **Complications** include the following:
  - Bleeding into the collecting system, below the renal capsule, or into the perinephric space.
  - Pain due to obstruction of the ureter by a blood clot or renal capsular stretching due to hematoma.
  - Infection.
  - AV fistulas resulting from damage to an adjacent artery and vein.
  - "Page kidney," or chronic hypertension with persistent activation of the renin-angiotensin system from a large subcapsular hematoma.
  - Consider postprocedure observation for 24 hours, since 90% of complications occur within this time period.

## ACUTE RENAL FAILURE (ARF)

A 25-year-old woman presents to your clinic with fatigue, headache, ↓ appetite, swollen feet, and scant, bloody urine. The woman's son suffered a sore throat and fever about three weeks ago and was diagnosed with group A β-hemolytic streptococcal pharyngitis. A few days later, the woman developed similar symptoms but did not seek treatment. Her sore throat resolved, but two days ago she started developing the systemic symptoms above: Her BP is 165/102, and she has a mild fever and appears dehydrated. She also has 3+ lower extremity edema. A UA shows blood, and RBC casts are seen on microscopic exam. What is the most likely diagnosis, and which additional tests can confirm the diagnosis? This presentation is consistent with poststreptococcal glomerulonephritis (PSGN). Although most commonly found in children 2–6 years of age, PSGN can occur at any age. A UA showing blood and RBC casts on microscopy are pathognomonic for PSGN. Additional confirmatory tests include a rapid strep test and/or throat culture, which may be ⊖ by presentation, and an ASO titer. Further tests include CBC, ESR and/or CRP, BUN/creatinine, and complement levels. Penicillin, erythromycin, or cephalosporins can be used to treat strep pharyngitis, but this will not change the course of the glomerulonephritis, and it is not known whether treatment of the 1° infection can prevent PSGN. Treatment for PSGN is symptomatic, with > 95% of patients completely recovering within 3–4 weeks. The prognosis is worse in older patients and in those with a more severe initial presentation.

*Oliguria is defined as < 400 mL of urine in 24 hours and anuria as < 100 mL of urine in 24 hours in adults. A urine output < 300 mL/m² per 24 hours, < 0.5 mL/kg/hr in children, or < 1 mL/kg/hr in infants is consider oliguria.*

The accepted criteria for the diagnosis of ARF are as follows:

- A serum creatinine ↑ of 0.5 mg/dL above baseline.
- A 50% creatinine ↑ above baseline.
- A 50% GFR ↓ below baseline.
- A requirement for acute renal replacement therapy.

The mechanism underlying ARF may be prerenal, intrarenal, or postrenal. Tables 9.2 through 9.4 outline the etiologies and clinical presentation of each.

## EXAM/DIAGNOSIS

- Review the history and medications, and focus the physical exam on clinical volume status, including orthostatic changes, intake, and output.
- Obtain a UA with microscopy.
- Determine plasma and urine electrolytes: $Fe_{Na} = (U_{Na} \times P_{Cr}) / (P_{Na} \times U_{Cr}) \times 100$.
- $Fe_{Na}$ (fractional excretion of sodium) is the fraction of sodium filtered by the kidney that is ultimately excreted.
- Distinguish prerenal azotemia from ATN in the setting of oliguric renal failure (see Tables 9.2 through 9.4 for details).
- Renal ultrasound to rule out obstruction.

## TREATMENT

- Identify and treat the underlying cause or causes.
- Support renal function by maintaining adequate intravascular volume.
- Consider prompt referral for dialysis in accordance with the **AEIOU** mnemonic.
- Eliminate further exposure to nephrotoxic drugs and substances (see Table 9.5).
- Monitor and correct electrolyte abnormalities and urine output.
- Consider a nephrology consult and renal biopsy.
- Seek a urology consult for postrenal etiologies.

> **Indications for emergent dialysis—**
>
> **AEIOU**
>
> **A**cidosis
> **E**lectrolytes (hyperkalemia)
> **I**ngestions (severe acidemia)
> **O**verload (pulmonary edema)
> **U**remia

## CHRONIC KIDNEY DISEASE (CKD)

CKD is clinically defined in two ways:

- Kidney damage of three or more months' duration based on abnormal kidney structure seen on imaging studies or on abnormal kidney function as indicated by blood tests or UA.
- A GFR < 60 mL/min with or without evidence of kidney damage.

Kidney failure, or end-stage renal disease (ESRD), is defined as a GFR < 15 mL/min and/or a requirement for renal replacement therapy in the form of dialysis or transplantation.

**TABLE 9.2.** **Clinical Presentation and Diagnosis of Prerenal ARF**

| CAUSES AND SUGGESTIVE CLINICAL FEATURES | UA AND OTHER CONFIRMATORY TESTS |
|---|---|
| Volume depletion: | Hyaline casts |
| ▪ Thirst | $Fe_{Na} < 1\%$ |
| ▪ Vital sign changes: hypotension, tachycardia, weight loss | BUN/creatinine ratio > 20:1 |
| ▪ Overdiuresis | Urine specific gravity > 1.020 |
| ▪ Dry mucous membranes | Urine osmolality > 500 mOsm/kg |
| ▪ Decreased JVP | $U_{Na} < 10$ mmol/L |
| Low-output states: | Rapid resolution of ARF on restoration of renal perfusion |
| ▪ Heart or liver failure | |
| ▪ Nephrotic syndrome | |
| NSAIDs and ACEIs | |

**TABLE 9.3.** Clinical Presentation and Diagnosis of Intrarenal ARF

| CAUSES AND SUGGESTIVE CLINICAL FEATURES | UA AND OTHER CONFIRMATORY TESTS |
| --- | --- |

### Tubulointerstitial

| | |
| --- | --- |
| **Acute tubular necrosis (ATN):** | Muddy brown granular casts (see Figure 9.1) |
| ▪ Ischemic: | Tubular epithelial cell casts |
|   ▪ Prolonged prerenal azotemia | $Fe_{Na} > 1\%$ |
|   ▪ Hemorrhage or hypotension | BUN:Cr ratio 10–15:1 |
| ▪ Toxic: | Urine specific gravity < 1.015 |
|   ▪ Nephrotoxic drugs and substances (see Table 9.5) | Urine Osm < 350 mOsm/kg |
|   ▪ Rhabdomyolysis or tumor lysis | $U_{Na} > 30$ mmol/L |
|   ▪ Multiple myeloma | Elevated calcium, phosphate, uric acid, CPK |
|   ▪ Hypercalcemia | SPEP/UPEP for multiple myeloma |

| | |
| --- | --- |
| **Acute interstitial nephritis (AIN):** | WBC casts (see Figure 9.2), WBCs, RBCs, |
| ▪ Allergic: |   rarely RBC casts |
|   ▪ Recent drug ingestion (see Table 9.5) | Variable proteinuria |
|   ▪ Fever, rash, or arthralgias | Bacteria if infectious |
| ▪ Infection: | Consider a nephrology consult |
|   ▪ Pyelonephritis | Renal biopsy typically shows interstitial inflammation |
|   ▪ HIV, CMV, EBV, HCV | Treatment includes withdrawal or eradication of the |
| ▪ Autoimmune disorders: |   offending agent and corticosteroids |
|   ▪ Wegener's granulomatosis, sarcoidosis, SLE, Sjögren's syndrome | |

### Microvascular

| | |
| --- | --- |
| **Glomerulonephritis/vasculitis:** | RBC casts or granular casts |
| ▪ Symptoms: | RBCs and WBCs |
|   ▪ Hypertension | Proteinuria |
|   ▪ Hematuria | Blood cultures and echocardiogram for endocarditis |
|   ▪ Edema | Consider additional testing: |
|   ▪ Oliguria | ▪ ASO titers, complement levels (SLE, PIGN/PSGN) |
| ▪ Postinfectious (PIGN): | ▪ ANA, anti-dsDNA, anti-Smith antibodies (SLE) |
|   ▪ Classically seen 2–3 weeks after streptococcal pharyngitis or skin infection (PSGN) | ▪ Cryoglobulins, HCV, HBV, HIV (MPGN) |
| ▪ Endocarditis: | ▪ c-ANCA, anti-PR3 (Wegener's granulomatosis) |
|   ▪ Fevers | ▪ p-ANCA, anti-MPO (Churg-Strauss syndrome, PAN) |
|   ▪ New heart murmur | ▪ Anti-GBM (Goodpasture's syndrome) |
|   ▪ Predisposing factors: | Nephrology consult |
|     ▪ Abnormal heart valves, recent dental procedure, IV drug abuse | Renal biopsy is definitive |
| ▪ Other: | |
|   ▪ SLE | |
|   ▪ Membranoproliferative glomerulonephritis (MPGN) | |
|   ▪ IgA nephropathy | |
|   ▪ Wegener's granulomatosis | |
|   ▪ Polyarteritis nodosa (PAN) | |
|   ▪ Churg-Strauss syndrome | |
|   ▪ Goodpasture's syndrome | |

**TABLE 9.3.** Clinical Presentation and Diagnosis of Intrarenal ARF (continued)

| CAUSES AND SUGGESTIVE CLINICAL FEATURES | UA AND OTHER CONFIRMATORY TESTS |
|---|---|
| **Microvascular (continued)** | |
| **Hemolytic-uremic syndrome (HUS), thrombotic thrombocytopenic purpura (TTP), disseminated intravascular coagulation (DIC), preeclampsia:**<br>■ Fever, pallor, ecchymoses, neurologic abnormalities, edema, hypertension, bloody diarrhea<br>■ Recent medications or toxins (tacrolimus, cyclosporine, quinine) | May be normal, or may see RBCs, mild proteinuria, or, rarely, RBC casts or granular casts<br>Anemia, thrombocytopenia, schistocytes on blood smear, ↑ LDH, renal biopsy |
| **Macrovascular** | |
| **Renal artery thrombosis:**<br>■ Atrial fibrillation<br>■ Recent MI<br>■ Flank or abdominal pain | Mild proteinuria and occasional RBCs; ↑ LDH<br>Renal arteriogram |
| **Renal vein thrombosis:**<br>■ Nephrotic syndrome<br>■ Pulmonary embolism<br>■ Flank pain | Proteinuria and hematuria<br>IVC and renal vein imaging |
| **Atheroembolism:**<br>■ Age usually > 50 years<br>■ Recent surgery/procedure (angiography), administration of thrombolytics<br>■ Hypertension<br>■ Edema<br>■ Rash (livedo reticularis, subcutaneous nodules, palpable purpura) | Eosinophilia, low complement levels, skin biopsy, renal biopsy |

## EXAM/DIAGNOSIS

■ Screening:
- Screening for CKD is recommended for high-risk patients—e.g., those with diabetes, hypertension, recurrent UTIs, urinary obstruction, or systemic disease that can affect the kidneys.
- Consider screening all patients > 60 years of age.
- Screening methods include the following:
  - Serum creatinine to calculate GFR.
  - Random urine samples for proteinuria.
  - Consider renal imaging for patients with urinary obstruction, recurrent UTIs, vesicoureteral reflux, or a family history of polycystic kidney disease.

■ **Diagnosis:** Evaluation to establish the specific cause of CKD should include a thorough history, UA and microscopy, and renal imaging. Further testing should be guided by the patient's symptoms, past medical and family history, and physical exam.

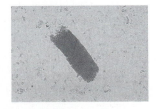

**FIGURE 9.1. Muddy brown cast.**

(Reproduced, with permission, from Le T et al. *First Aid for the Internal Medicine Boards*, 1st ed. New York: McGraw-Hill, 2006: 451.)

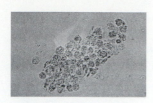

**FIGURE 9.2. White blood cell cast.**

(Reproduced, with permission, from Knoop KJ et al. *Atlas of Emergency Medicine,* 2nd ed. New York: McGraw-Hill, 2002: 676.)

**TABLE 9.4. Clinical Presentation and Diagnosis of Postrenal ARF**

| CAUSES AND SUGGESTIVE CLINICAL FEATURES | UA AND OTHER CONFIRMATORY TESTS |
| --- | --- |
| Urethral obstruction: | Frequently normal UA |
| ▪ Prostatic hypertrophy | Possibly hematuria |
| ▪ Urethral stricture | $Fe_{Na} < 1\%$ (acute) |
| Bladder, pelvic or retroperitoneal neoplasm | $Fe_{Na} > 1\%$ (few days) |
| Calculi | Plain films, renal ultrasound, IVP, |
| Neurogenic bladder | retrograde or anterograde |
| Anticholinergics, narcotics | pyelography, CT scan |
| All of the above: lower urinary tract symptoms, abdominal or flank pain, palpable bladder | |

▪ **Referral:**

- ▪ Consider referral to nephrology if the etiology remains unclear or there is an indication for renal biopsy; with rapid progression of renal disease or ARF on CKD; or when management is beyond the scope of primary care.
- ▪ Consider comanagement in stage 3 CKD (GFR 30–59 mL/min).
- ▪ A nephrology consult is essential in or beyond stage 4 CKD (GFR 15–29 mL/min) for dialysis access and possible transplant listing.

**TABLE 9.5. Nephrotoxic drugs and substances**

| DRUGS | SUBSTANCES |
| --- | --- |
| **Antimicrobials:** | Ethylene glycol (oxalic acid) |
| ▪ Aminoglycosides | Heavy metals (lead, arsenic) |
| ▪ Amphotericin B | Hemoglobin |
| ▪ Antivirals | Myeloma light chain deposition |
| ▪ Antiparasitics (pentamidine) | Myoglobin (rhabdomyolysis) |
| ▪ β-lactams | Radiocontrast agents |
| ▪ Cephalosporins | Uric acid |
| ▪ Fluoroquinolones | Cocaine |
| ▪ Rifampin | |
| ▪ Sulfonamides | |
| **ACEIs** | |
| **Anti-inflammatories:** | |
| ▪ NSAIDs | |
| ▪ COX-2 inhibitors | |
| **Other:** | |
| ▪ Phenytoin | |
| ▪ Allopurinol | |
| ▪ Cimetidine | |
| ▪ Furosemide | |
| ▪ Thiazide diuretics | |
| ▪ Lithium chemotherapeutics | |

## TREATMENT

- The following measures have been proven to **slow the progression of CKD:**
    - **Reduction of proteinuria with ACEIs/ARBs:** Beneficial for both diabetic and nondiabetic nephropathy.
    - **Treatment of hypertension:** Treat hypertension to < 130/80 with ACEIs (first-line therapy) or diuretics (second-line treatment).
    - Maintain glycemic control in diabetics.
- Treatment methods that **may prove beneficial** include lipid lowering with an LDL target < 100, treatment of anemia, protein restriction (controversial), and smoking cessation.
- Patients with stage 3 or 4 CKD should be periodically monitored with the following lab studies:
    - Hemoglobin/hematocrit
    - RBC indices
    - Reticulocyte count
    - Iron studies
    - Fecal occult blood test
    - Serum electrolytes
    - Calcium, phosphorus, and PTH
    - Serum albumin and total protein

## COMPLICATIONS

- Complications can be treated as follows:
    - **Anemia:** Erythropoietin (EPO) and repletion of iron stores.
    - **Hyperkalemia:** Dietary restrictions and diuretics.
    - **Acidosis:** Supplement $NaHCO_3$ to prevent $\ominus$ bone balance.
    - **Renal osteodystrophy:** Control phosphate and treat hyperparathyroidism.
    - **Dialysis-related problems:**
        - **Vascular catheter-related infections** (*S. aureus*, coagulase-$\ominus$ *Staphylococcus*): Treat empirically with an IV first-generation cephalosporin, and consider vancomycin coverage for MRSA. Tailor antibiotics to blood culture results from the catheter and a peripheral site. Consider removal of the catheter for fungal infections, sepsis, endocarditis, or persistent bacteremia.
        - **Peritoneal catheter-related infections** (*S. aureus*, *S. epidermidis*, enteric gram-$\ominus$ rods): Can often be treated with infusion of antibiotics into the peritoneum. Add IV antibiotics in severe cases and consider catheter removal.
        - **AV fistula thrombosis:** Treatment options include intravascular clot removal or thrombolytics.

*Cardiovascular disease is still the most common cause of death in CKD, with risk and mortality increasing in proportion to the ↓ in GFR.*

## NEPHROTIC SYNDROME

A 72-year-old man with a long-standing history of poorly controlled type 2 DM returns to your clinic with a 12-pound weight gain and leg swelling of one month's duration. He stopped taking his medications a few months ago and has not been to your office for six months. His BP is 173/91, and his UA shows 3+ proteinuria with microscopy revealing oval fat bodies. A CXR shows mild pleural effusions, but his heart size is normal. What additional testing and treatment should be considered? In addition to a cardiac etiology, consideration must be given to a renal source of this patient's presentation. Diabetes is the 1° cause of ESRD in the United States, and this could be consistent with nephrotic syndrome. Further evaluation should include quantitative analysis of proteinuria, assessment of renal function, and measurement of serum protein levels, glucose, HbA$_{1c}$, and lipids. An ACEI or an ARB, as well as a loop diuretic for peripheral edema, should be used for treatment. A renal biopsy may be needed if the diagnosis remains unclear.

A condition characterized primarily by significant proteinuria resulting from **noninflammatory** injury to the glomeruli. May be 1°/idiopathic or 2° to a variety of disorders.

- **1° or idiopathic causes:**
  - **Minimal change disease:** More common in children; characterized by sudden onset with heavy proteinuria. Responds to steroids, but often relapses. Renal failure is uncommon.
  - **Focal segmental glomerulosclerosis (FSGS):** More common in African-Americans; associated with a higher frequency of renal failure than the above. Treated with steroids, cyclosporin A, and cyclophosphamide.
  - **Membranous nephropathy:** More common in Caucasians; presents with proteinuria with occasional microhematuria and hypercoagulability (renal vein thrombosis). Has a 25% spontaneous remission rate with slow progression to renal failure. Treated with steroids, cyclosporin, cyclophosphamide, and chlorambucil.
  - **Membranoproliferative glomerulonephritis (MPGN):** Can present with nephritic or nephrotic features; HCV and cryoglobulin related. Treated with observation (non-nephrotic with stable renal function) or steroids. Associated with a 50% mortality rate or progression to ESRD within five years of renal biopsy.
- **2° causes:**
  - **Diabetic nephropathy:** The leading cause of ESRD in the United States. Onset is 5–10 years after diagnosis for type 1 DM but is more variable in type 2 DM. Treated with tight glycemic control, BP control (i.e., < 130/80), and lipid control (i.e., LDL < 100). ACEIs are first-line agents in type 1 DM; ACEIs or ARBs are used in type 2.
  - **Other etiologies:** Include malignancy (classically lymphoma or myeloma), infections (HIV, HBV/HCV, syphilis, leprosy, malaria), amyloidosis, and NSAID induced.

### SYMPTOMS/EXAM

Loss of appetite, fatigue and malaise, edema, dyspnea from pleural effusions, ascites, weight gain, muscle wasting, frothy urine, opportunistic infections, clotting disorders.

### DIFFERENTIAL/DIAGNOSIS

See Table 9.6 for a comparison of nephrotic and nephritic syndromes. Labs to order include the following:

- **UA and microscopy:** Reveals proteinuria. Oval fat bodies or "Maltese crosses" may be seen under polarized light.

- **24-hour urine collection:** To **quantify proteinuria.** Spot urine sampling for protein-creatinine ratio can approximate 24-hour protein excretion.
- Obtain additional labs (HbA$_{1c}$, SPEP/UPEP, complement levels, ASO titers, ANA, anti-dsDNA, and serologies for HBV, HCV, HIV, and syphilis) to determine 2° causes.
- Consider a nephrology consult and a renal biopsy.

### TREATMENT

- Control peripheral edema with loop diuretics.
- Maintain good nutrition.
- Administer ACEIs/ARBs to slow proteinuria.
- Institute lipid-lowering therapy with a target LDL generally < 100.
- Treat the underlying disease (see above).

## NEPHRITIC DISEASE

Typically consists of hematuria, hypertension, renal insufficiency, and edema due to **inflammatory** changes in the glomeruli. May be 1°/idiopathic or 2° to a variety of disorders.

- **1° or idiopathic causes:**
  - **Poststreptococcal glomerulonephritis (PSGN):** The leading cause of acute nephritic syndrome. Classically seen 2–3 weeks after pharyngitis or skin infection, and can present with nephritic or nephrotic features. Diagnosed via elevated ASO titers and anti-DNase B antibodies along with low complement levels. Treatment is supportive, and renal failure typically resolves within four weeks, with only 5% of cases requiring acute renal replacement therapy.
  - **IgA nephropathy:** More common among Asians and Hispanics. Presents with episodic hematuria +/− proteinuria, usually within 24 hours of a URI. Treated with ACEIs. Consider fish oil if proteinuria is < 3 g/day or steroids if > 3 g/day. Roughly 20% of cases progress to renal failure within 20 years.
  - **Anti-GBM disease:** A rare but rapidly progressive condition. Exposure to pulmonary toxins such as hydrocarbons ↑ risk. Presents with elevated serum anti-GBM antibody titers. Urgent treatments include plasmapheresis, steroids, and cyclophosphamide.
- **2° causes:**
  - **SLE:** Lupus nephritis can be the presenting feature. Diagnosed by anti-dsDNA and anti-Smith antibodies along with low complement levels. Some 8–15% of SLE patients progress to ESRD.
  - **Goodpasture's syndrome:** A constellation of glomerulonephritis, pulmonary hemorrhage, and anti-GBM antibodies that can present with rapidly progressive glomerulonephritis (RPGN). Diagnosed via anti-GBM antibodies as above. Urgent treatments include plasmapheresis, steroids, and cyclophosphamide.
  - **ANCA-related vasculitis:** Includes Wegener's granulomatosis, microscopic polyarteritis nodosa, and Churg-Strauss syndrome. Can present with RPGN. Diagnosed via c-ANCA, p-ANCA, antimyeloperoxidase (MPO) antibodies, anti-proteinase 3 (anti-PR3), and renal biopsy. Urgent treatments include plasmapheresis, steroids, and cyclophosphamide.

### SYMPTOMS/EXAM

About 50% are asymptomatic. Look for loss of appetite, fatigue and malaise, edema, headaches, vision changes, neurologic findings, nausea, vomiting, abdominal pain, hypertension, and dark urine (hematuria).

### DIFFERENTIAL

Table 9.6 distinguishes nephritic from nephrotic syndrome.

### DIAGNOSIS

- Diagnostic criteria are as follows:
    - Proteinuria < 3.5 g/day.
    - ARF over days to weeks.
    - Oliguria, edema, hypertension, and hematuria.
- Labs include the following:
    - **UA and microscopy:** Reveal RBC casts, dysmorphic RBCs, and WBCs.
    - **24-hour or spot urine sampling:** To determine the protein-creatinine ratio.
    - Obtain additional labs as indicated (complement levels, ASO titer, anti-GBM antibodies, c-ANCA, p-ANCA).
- Obtain a nephrology consult and consider a renal biopsy.

### TREATMENT

- Treatment should adhere to the same general principles as those associated with nephrotic syndrome.
- Treat the underlying disease as outlined above.

## HEMATURIA

Blood in the urine may be gross or microscopic and may stem from a number of conditions.

---

**TABLE 9.6.** Comparison of Nephrotic and Nephritic Syndromes

| | NEPHROTIC SYNDROMES | NEPHRITIC SYNDROMES |
|---|---|---|
| Findings | Proteinuria > 3.5 g/day | Proteinuria < 3.5 g/day |
| | Hypoalbuminemia (serum albumin < 3 g/dL) | ARF over days to weeks |
| | Edema | Oliguria |
| | Hyperlipidemia and lipiduria | Edema |
| | Hypercoagulability | Hypertension |
| | Oval fat bodies and "Maltese crosses" | Hematuria |
| 1° or idiopathic | Minimal change disease | PSGN (can present as nephrotic syndrome) |
| | FSGS | IgA nephropathy |
| | Membranous nephropathy | Anti–glomerular basement membrane (GBM) disease |
| | MPGN (can present as nephritic syndrome) | |
| 2° | Diabetic nephropathy | SLE (can present as nephrotic syndrome) |
| | Malignancy (lymphoma or myeloma) | Goodpasture's syndrome |
| | Infectious (e.g., HIV, HBV/HCV, syphilis) | ANCA-related vasculitis (Wegener's granulomatosis, microscopic polyarteritis nodosa, Churg-Strauss syndrome) |
| | Amyloidosis | |

- **Gross hematuria:** Can be 2° to a range of conditions other than bleeding in the urinary tract, including the following:
    - Medications (phenazopyridine, nitrofurantoin, NSAIDs).
    - Ingestion of beets or certain food dyes.
    - Myoglobinuria or hemoglobinuria.
    - Porphyria.
- **Microscopic hematuria:** Has glomerular as well as nonglomerular causes.
    - **Glomerular:**
        - 1° and 2° glomerulonephritis (see the discussion of ARF and nephritic disease).
        - Hereditary diseases.
        - Alport's syndrome (hereditary nephritis).
        - Thin basement membrane nephropathy (benign familial hematuria).
        - Vigorous exercise.
    - **Nonglomerular:**
        - **Renal:** Malignancy, vascular disease (malignant hypertension, AVM, nutcracker syndrome [left renal vein compression between the abdominal aorta and superior mesenteric artery], renal vein thrombosis, sickle cell trait/disease, papillary necrosis), infection (pyelonephritis, TB, CMV, EBV), hypercalciuria or hyperuricuria, hereditary disease (polycystic kidney disease, medullary sponge kidney).
        - **Nonrenal:** Malignancy (prostatic, ureteral, bladder), BPH, nephrolithiasis, coagulopathy (bleeding disorders or medication-induced disease), trauma (Foley catheter).

### SYMPTOMS/EXAM

- **Gross hematuria:** Generally associated with a red or brown color change of urine.
- **Microscopic hematuria:** Three or more RBCs/hpf in centrifuged urine. Often asymptomatic and discovered on urine dipstick or on a UA obtained for other purposes.
- A focused history can help guide further evaluation and should include the following:
    - **Recent symptoms:** URIs may point toward PSGN or IgA nephropathy. Look for urinary tract symptoms such as signs of infectious or obstructive processes as well as flank pain radiating to the groin.
    - **Other:** Ask about recent vigorous exercise or traumas; determine if there is a family history of renal diseases or sickle cell trait/disease. Review medications, including use of NSAIDs and anticoagulants.

### DIAGNOSIS

- **Gross hematuria:** Centrifuge urine.
    - **Red sediment:** Indicates hematuria.
    - **Red supernatant:**
        - **Heme-⊕ dipstick:** Indicates myoglobinuria or hemoglobinuria.
        - **Heme-⊖ dipstick:** Phenazopyridine, beets, porphyria, etc.
- **Microscopic hematuria:**
    - UA and microscopy to determine the number and morphology of RBCs, crystals, and casts.
    - Consider a urine culture.
    - Obtain screening blood work for electrolytes, kidney function, blood counts, and coagulation.

- Consider a repeat UA in a few days to determine if hematuria is transient or persistent.
- Further evaluation is indicated for single specimens with > 100 RBCs/hpf.
- Differentiate between **glomerular and nonglomerular causes:**
  - **Glomerular causes:** See the sections on ARF and nephritic diseases. Consider a referral to nephrology for further evaluation and possible renal biopsy.
  - **Nonglomerular causes:**
    - Radiographic evaluation with CT, renal ultrasound, and/or IVP.
    - Obtain urine cytology and consider a referral to urology for cystoscopy, especially for patients at risk for malignancies.
    - Look for the following risk factors:
      - Cigarette smoking
      - Occupational and environmental exposures (aluminum, certain paints and dyes, petroleum, rubber and textile industries)
      - Analgesic abuse (phenacetin)
      - High dietary consumption of fried meats and fats
      - Chronic cystitis
      - Schistosomiasis
      - Pelvic radiation and chemotherapy (cyclophosphamide)

### TREATMENT

- Consider a nephrology or urology referral as outlined above for glomerular vs. nonglomerular etiologies.
- Treat the underlying cause.
- Persistent unexplained hematuria is most likely due to a mild glomerulopathy or nephrolithiasis.
- Continued periodic UA and urine cytology are warranted, especially for those at risk for malignancy. Consider repeat renal ultrasound and/or cytoscopy at one year for those at high risk.

## SODIUM AND WATER DISORDERS

A 58-year-old man is admitted to the hospital with a CHF exacerbation. He recently stopped taking his diuretics because he was tired of going to the bathroom all the time. Exam reveals an elevated JVP and peripheral edema of 3+. Initial labs are as follows: Na+ 122, BUN 14, creatinine 1.4, and glucose 144. What type of hyponatremia is this, and how is it best treated? A plasma osmolality ($P_{osm}$) of 257 places this in the category of hypotonic hyponatremia. Clinical assessment of volume status further suggests that this patient is hypervolemic, which is congruent with his CHF exacerbation. The patient can be treated with both fluid restriction and diuretics; however, overly aggressive use of diuretics may induce a hypovolemic, diuretic-induced hyponatremia.

## Hyponatremia

Defined as a plasma sodium (Na+) level < 135 mEq/L. Figure 9.3 outlines an algorithm for the differential diagnosis of hyponatremia.

### SYMPTOMS/EXAM

- Symptoms and signs relate to the rate and severity of the decline in $Na^+$.
- Clinical presentation ranges from asymptomatic to nausea, vomiting, confusion, lethargy, seizures, or coma.

### DIAGNOSIS

- Obtain a thorough history to determine symptoms and identify potential causes of hyponatremia.
- See Figure 9.3.
- **Determine tonicity:** Plasma osmolality $(P_{osm}) = (2 \times Na^+) + (BUN/2.8) + (glucose/18)$.
- For hypotonic hyponatremias, **determine volume status:**
  - Perform a clinical exam looking for volume overload (elevated JVP, S3 gallop, ascites, edema) or volume depletion (dry mucous membranes, flat JVP).
  - Look for a urine $Na^+ < 10$ or a $Fe_{Na} < 1$ % (reliable only when the patient is oliguric and not taking diuretics).
  - $U_{osm} > P_{osm}$ or $U_{osm} > 1200$ mOsm/kg suggests a high ADH state due to hypovolemia or SIADH.

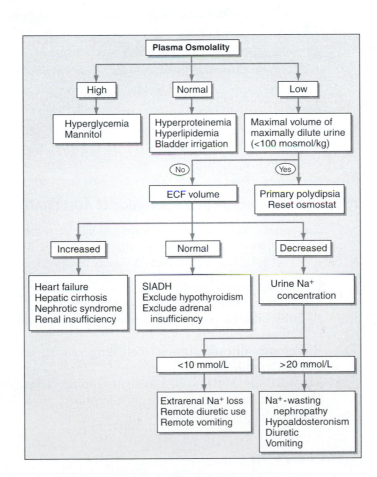

**FIGURE 9.3.**  **Evaluation and differential diagnosis of hyponatremia.**

Algorithm depicting clinical approach to hyponatremia. ECF, extracellular fluid; SIADH, syndrome of inappropriate antidiuretic hormone secretion. (Reproduced, with permission, from Kasper DL et al. *Harrison's Principles of Internal Medicine*, 16th ed. New York: McGraw-Hill, 2005: 256.)

To prevent central pontine myelinolysis, do not ↑ Na⁺ > 12 mEq/L over a 24-hour period.

***TREATMENT***

- Initiate fluid management according to patient's volume status.
  - **Hypervolemia:** Fluid restriction and/or diuretics.
  - **Euvolemia:** Fluid restriction or consider hypertonic (3%) saline.
  - **Hypovolemia:** Isotonic or, rarely, hypertonic saline.
- Correct Na⁺ according to the patient's symptoms and rapidity of onset of the abnormality.
  - **Acute symptomatic hyponatremia:**
    - Raise Na⁺ roughly 2 mEq/L per hour until symptoms resolve.
    - Consider careful use of hypertonic saline with a loop diuretic if volume overloaded.
  - **Chronic symptomatic hyponatremia:**
    - Raise Na⁺ more slowly (approximately 1 mEq/L per 1–2 hours).
    - Again, consider careful use of hypertonic saline.
  - **Chronic asymptomatic hyponatremia:**
    - Immediate correction is unnecessary.
    - Manage fluid according to volume status as above.
- Treat the underlying cause for long-term correction.

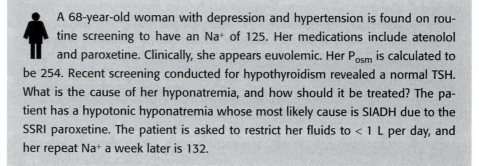

A 68-year-old woman with depression and hypertension is found on routine screening to have an Na⁺ of 125. Her medications include atenolol and paroxetine. Clinically, she appears euvolemic. Her $P_{osm}$ is calculated to be 254. Recent screening conducted for hypothyroidism revealed a normal TSH. What is the cause of her hyponatremia, and how should it be treated? The patient has a hypotonic hyponatremia whose most likely cause is SIADH due to the SSRI paroxetine. The patient is asked to restrict her fluids to < 1 L per day, and her repeat Na⁺ a week later is 132.

## Syndrome of Inappropriate Secretion of ADH (SIADH)

Small cell lung cancer is the malignancy most commonly associated with SIADH.

Occurs when antidiuretic hormone (ADH) is secreted independent of the body's need to conserve water → inappropriate water retention in the presence of Na⁺ loss. May result from a variety of disorders.

- **CNS disorders:**
  - **Head trauma:** SAH, subdural hematoma.
  - **Infection:** Meningitis, encephalitis, brain abscess.
  - **Other:** Neoplasm, CVA, MS.
- **Pulmonary disorders:** Small cell lung cancer, pneumonia, lung abscess, TB, pneumothorax.
- **Medications:** SSRIs, TCAs, carbamazepine, haloperidol, chlorpromazine, chlorpropamide, theophylline, amiodarone.
- **Other:** Malignant neoplasia.

***SYMPTOMS/EXAM***

The symptoms of SIADH are the result of hyponatremia and are the underlying cause of the disorder.

### DIAGNOSIS

- Low $P_{osm}$.
- Low uric acid and BUN due to serum dilution and ↑ renal losses.
- Euvolemic hyponatremia.
- $U_{osm} > P_{osm}$.
- SIADH is a diagnosis of exclusion.

### TREATMENT

- Water restriction.
- Consider hypertonic saline and a loop diuretic as second-line agents.
- Give demeclocycline for chronic SIADH.

## Hypernatremia

Defined as a plasma $Na^+$ level > 145 mEq/L. Grouped into four broad categories according to the underlying mechanism:

- **Inadequate intake and ↑ water loss** ($U_{osm} > 600$ mOsm/kg):
  - ↑ insensible or GI losses (↑ sweating, burns, diarrhea).
  - Barriers to accessible fluids or inadequate replacement.
- **↑ renal loss (polyuria):**
  - **Diabetes insipidus** ($U_{osm} < 600$ mOsm/kg): A defect in the secretion or action of ADH. Presents with hypernatremia with copious dilute urine (see the Endocrinology chapter).
  - **Postobstructive or post-ATN diuresis.**
  - **DM.**
- **1° hypodipsia:** Destruction of the hypothalamic thirst center due to neoplasm, vascular disease, granulomatous disease, or trauma.
- **Excess $Na^+$ retention** (rare): Due to accidental or intentional ingestion/infusion of hypertonic solution.

*Hypernatremia is almost always due to free-water deficits.*

### SYMPTOMS/EXAM

- Volume depletion is seen in the form of dry mucous membranes, hypotension, and low urine output.
- CNS symptoms include lethargy, weakness, irritability, confusion, seizures, and coma.
- Generally a defect in water intake.
- Hypernatremia → hyperosmolality, which in turn → cellular dehydration.

### DIAGNOSIS

- The diagnosis is usually apparent from the clinical situation.
- Review the patient's weight, intake and output, and types of IV fluid.
- $U_{osm}$ should be high in the hypovolemic patient as noted above (urine concentrates as kidney retains water).

### TREATMENT

- **Calculate the free-water deficit:** Normal body water (NBW) − current body water (CBW) = 0.5 × body weight in kilograms [(plasma $Na^+$ − 140)/140].
- **Replace the calculated free-water deficit:** Lower $Na^+$ approximately 1 mEq/L per hour, not to exceed 12 mEq/L in a 24-hour period. A general guideline is to correct 50% of the calculated free-water deficit in the first 12–24 hours, with the remainder corrected in the next 24–48 hours.

*In patients who are hypotensive and volume depleted, isotonic saline should initially be used and should be switched to hypotonic saline once tissue perfusion is adequate.*

## Hyperkalemia

↑ serum potassium ($K^+$) may result from a range of conditions:

- **High $K^+$ intake:** Supplements or dietary (rarely occurs without baseline renal dysfunction).
- **Extracellular $K^+$ shift** (↓ cellular entry or ↑ release):
  - Metabolic acidosis.
  - Insulin deficiency and hyperglycemia in uncontrolled diabetes.
  - Tissue damage from rhabdomyolysis, trauma, or burns or release during tumor lysis syndrome.
  - β-adrenergic blockade.
- **Impaired renal excretion:**
  - Renal failure.
  - ↓ effective circulating volume, as with severe CHF.
  - Hypoaldosteronism (hyporeninemic hypoaldosteronism, ACEIs/ARBs, NSAIDs, $K^+$-sparing diuretics, heparin, 1° adrenal insufficiency such as Addison's disease).

### SYMPTOMS/EXAM

May be asymptomatic or present with symptoms ranging from muscle weakness to ventricular fibrillation (VF).

### DIAGNOSIS

- Review the history, medications, and exam, focusing on muscle weakness, flaccid paralysis, and ileus.
- Obtain basic labs, including electrolytes, BUN, and creatinine.
- Consider additional labs as indicated by the history—e.g., CK for rhabdomyolysis; LDH, uric acid, phosphorus, and calcium for tumor lysis syndrome; $U_{osm}$ and $U_{K+}$ to calculate the transtubular $K^+$ gradient in hypoaldosteronism.
- ECG findings may be used as an indicator of severity. Figure 9.4 shows characteristically progressive changes with increasing serum potassium levels.
  - **Mild:** Normal or peaked T waves.
  - **Moderate:** QRS prolongation or flattened P waves.
  - **Severe:** VF.

### TREATMENT

- IV calcium gluconate to reduce cardiac excitability.
- ↑ $K^+$ entry into cells with insulin and glucose, $β_2$-adrenergic agonists (inhaled albuterol), and $NaHCO_3$.
- Give diuretics, cation-exchange resin (Kayexalate), or dialysis to remove excess $K^+$.

## Hypokalemia

↓ serum $K^+$ may result from the following:

- Low $K^+$ intake.
- Intracellular $K^+$ shift:
  - Metabolic alkalosis.
  - ↑ β-adrenergic activity in stress response.

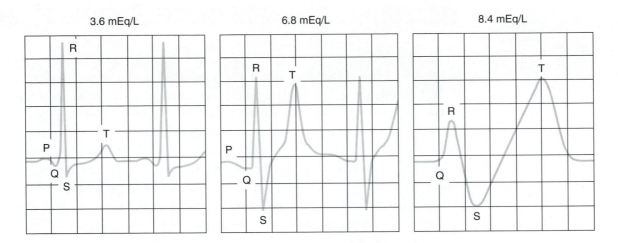

**FIGURE 9.4.** **Electrocardiographic effects of hyperkalemia.**

(Reproduced, with permission, from Morgan GE Jr et al. *Clinical Anesthesiology*, 4th ed. New York: McGraw-Hill, 2006, Fig. 28-6.)

- ↑ GI loss (diarrhea).
- ↑ renal excretion:
  - Loop and thiazide diuretics.
  - Vomiting.
  - Hyperaldosteronism (1° or 2° mineralocorticoid excess) from aldosterone-producing adrenal adenoma, pituitary adenoma (Cushing's disease), renal artery stenosis, or European black licorice ingestion.
  - Renal tubular acidosis (RTA).

### SYMPTOMS/EXAM

- Symptoms generally occur when $P_{K+} < 2.5–3.0$ mEq/L.
- May present with weakness, rhabdomyolysis, and cardiac arrhythmias.

### DIAGNOSIS

- 24-hour urine collection for $K^+$:
  - **Extrarenal:** < 25 mEq/day.
  - **Renal:** > 25 mEq/day.
- Spot urine for $K^+$ (more easily obtained, but less accurate):
  - **Extrarenal:** < 15 mEq/day.
  - **Renal:** > 15 mEq/day.
- See the Endocrinology chapter for evaluation of adrenal abnormalities.

### TREATMENT

- Replete $K^+$, usually as KCl.
  - The average $K^+$ deficit is 200–400 mEq when $P_{K+} = 3.0$ mEq/L.
  - Peripheral line replacement should not exceed 10 mEq/L per hour, or 20 mEq/L per hour for a central line.
- Consider $K^+$-sparing diuretics in patients with chronic urinary $K^+$ loss.

> A 17-year-old girl with type 1 DM is admitted to the ER with persistent vomiting. She has not been taking her insulin regularly for the past few days. She is tachycardic and tachypneic, but her BP is stable. Labs reveal $Na^+$ 136, $Cl^-$ 107, $HCO_3^-$ 14, and glucose 262. An ABG pH is 7.21. UA shows 3+ glucose and is ⊕ for ketones. What is the underlying acid-base disorder? This is an example of an anion-gap metabolic acidosis (AG = 15) due to diabetic ketoacidosis (DKA). Further evaluation would likely show that the patient's tachypnea is a compensatory respiratory alkalosis. Managing the underlying DKA with fluids, insulin, and close attention to other electrolytes, especially potassium, is the key to treatment.

## Metabolic Acidosis

**Anion-gap (AG) metabolic acidosis** is defined as the accumulation of unmeasured anions. It is quantified as follows:

- $AG = (Na^+) - [(Cl^-) + (HCO_3^-)]$.
- Normal AG is approximately 6–10.
- ↑ AG implies an AG metabolic acidosis even if plasma $HCO_3$ is normal.

**Non-AG (hyperchloremic) metabolic acidosis** is defined as loss of bicarbonate balanced by the accumulation of chloride.

### SYMPTOMS/EXAM

- Causes of AG metabolic acidosis are outlined in the mnemonic **MUDPILES**.
- Non-AG metabolic acidosis is associated with RTA and diarrhea.

### DIAGNOSIS

- A thorough history can often pinpoint the etiology of the metabolic acidosis.
- Calculate AG as above.
- Conduct further evaluation as indicated, including renal function, serum lactate, serum or urine ketones, calculation of osmolar gap to rule out ingestion of alcohol (ethanol, methanol, ethylene glycol), salicylate level, and calculation of urine AG to evaluate for RTA in non-AG metabolic acidosis.

### TREATMENT

- Treat the underlying cause.
- Bicarbonate therapy is controversial and, if used, is generally reserved for severe acidosis (arterial pH < 7.10–7.15).

## Metabolic Alkalosis

Has four main causes: hypovolemia, hypochloremia, hypokalemia, and hyperaldosteronism.

---

*Causes of AG metabolic acidosis—*

*MUDPILES*

**M**ethanol ingestion
**U**remia
**D**iabetic ketoacidosis
**P**araldehyde ingestion
**I**NH overdose
**L**actic acidosis
**E**thylene glycol ingestion
**S**alicylate ingestion

---

- Calculate the urine chloride ($U_{Cl^-}$) concentration:
    - **$U_{Cl^-}$ < 10 mEq/L:** Hypovolemia (the kidney tries to retain $Na^+$ and $Cl^-$, so $U_{Cl^-}$ is low).
    - Caused by GI loss, diuretics, or administration of $NaHCO_3$ or antacids.
    - Treat with NaCl infusion.
    - **$U_{Cl^-}$ > 10 mEq/L:** Chloride-resistant metabolic acidosis.
    - Hypertension implies mineralocorticoid excess (retain $Na^+$; lose $H^+$ and $K^+$).
    - Associated with 1° hyperaldosteronism or hyperreninemia, Liddle's syndrome (a rare autosomal-dominant disorder characterized by $Na^+$ and $H_2O$ reabsorption and $K^+$ excretion due to enhanced $Na^+$ channel activity in the collecting tubule), European black licorice ingestion, and 11- or 17-hydroxylase deficiency.
- **Normal BP:** Profound hypokalemia ($\rightarrow \uparrow$ ammonium production), Bartter's syndrome (a recessive disorder involving a defect in $Na^+Cl^-$ reabsorption in the ascending limb of the loop of Henle), refeeding alkalosis.
- Treat the underlying cause.

## Respiratory Acidosis

An $\uparrow$ in $P_{CO_2}$ (hypercapnia) due to $\downarrow$ alveolar ventilation. Etiologies are as follows:

- **Central:** Drugs (opiates, anesthetics, sedatives), stroke, infection.
- **Airway:** Obstruction (obstructive sleep apnea), asthma.
- **Parenchyma:** COPD, pneumonia or bronchitis, ARDS, barotrauma.
- **Neuromuscular:** Spinal cord injury, kyphoscoliosis, poliomyelitis, Guillain-Barré syndrome, myasthenia gravis, MS, severe hypokalemia or hypophosphatemia.

- **CNS symptoms:** Headache, blurred vision, restlessness, anxiety.
- **$CO_2$ narcosis:** Tremors, asterixis, delirium, somnolence.

- The diagnosis is often apparent from the history.
- Arterial pH < 7.40 and $P_{CO_2}$ > 40 mmHg.
- Distinguish intrinsic pulmonary from extrapulmonary disease using the alveolar-arterial (A-a) oxygen gradient.
    - At sea level, alveolar $P_{O_2}$ ($P_{AO_2}$) = 150 − ($P_{CO_2}$/0.8).
    - Arterial $P_{O_2}$ ($P_{AO_2}$) as measured by ABG.
    - A normal A-a gradient is 10–20 mmHg.
    - An A-a gradient > 20 implies intrinsic pulmonary disease causing impaired gas exchange.
- Initiate mechanical ventilation if necessary while correcting the underlying disorder.

## Respiratory Alkalosis

Defined as $\uparrow$ alveolar ventilation $\rightarrow$ a fall in $P_{CO_2}$ (hypocapnia). Etiologies include the following:

- CNS lesions (stroke or neoplastic)
- Pregnancy (progesterone)

- Endotoxins (gram-$\ominus$ sepsis)
- Salicylates
- Hepatic failure
- Hypoxemia
- Anxiety
- Pain

### SYMPTOMS/EXAM

- **Tachypnea.**
- **CNS symptoms:** Lightheadedness, altered mental status.
- **Hypocalcemia symptoms:** Paresthesias, circumoral numbness, carpopedal spasms.

### DIAGNOSIS/TREATMENT

- The diagnosis is often apparent from the history.
- Arterial pH > 7.40 and $P_{CO_2}$ < 40 mmHg.
- Use the A-a oxygen gradient as above.
- Correct the underlying disorder.

## Mixed Acid-Base Disorders

Independently coexisting disorders that are **not compensatory.** Can → dangerous extremes of pH. Consider the differential diagnosis associated with each of the disorders:

- A patient with DKA (metabolic acidosis) who develops pneumonia (respiratory acidosis).
- The "triple ripple": A patient overdoses on salicylates and has profuse vomiting caused by AG metabolic acidosis (salicylates) and metabolic alkalosis (vomiting) with respiratory alkalosis (salicylates directly stimulate the respiratory center).

## OTHER URINARY TRACT DISORDERS

A 27-year-old man presents to the ER with acute onset of dysuria and severe left flank pain radiating to the groin. UA shows 3+ blood, and specific gravity is > 1.030 but is $\ominus$ for nitrite and leukocyte esterase. Blood work for kidney function is normal. A helical CT scan for kidney stones reveals a 2-mm left ureteral–pelvic junction stone. The patient is treated with pain medications and IV fluids and is discharged to follow-up with his family medicine physician. What further evaluation and treatment should you recommend? The patient should ↑ his fluid intake to 2.5–3.0 L/day and should be given a urine strainer to try to collect the stone for analysis. Additional blood work for calcium, phosphorus, and uric acid can be obtained for a first stone, but further evaluation is not indicated at this time.

## Nephrolithiasis

### SYMPTOMS/EXAM

- Presents with flank pain +/− radiation to the groin.
- Urinary frequency, urgency, and dysuria are also seen.
- Microscopic or gross hematuria.

### DIAGNOSIS

- **Collect and analyze the stone!**
- **Labs:**
  - UA (blood and pH; rule out UTI).
  - Obtain electrolytes, BUN, creatinine, calcium, phosphorus, and uric acid. Consider PTH for hyperparathyroidism if calcium is high normal or elevated (more likely in women or older adults).
  - Consider 24-hour urine collection (to assess volume, pH, Na$^+$, calcium, oxalate, phosphorus, citrate, uric acid, cysteine, and creatinine) for recurrent nephrolithiasis, a large single stone, or patients in whom significant morbidity occurred or may occur with a recurrence.
- **Imaging:** Helical CT scan is the gold standard for nephrolithiasis.
  - Can consider plain film radiography for radiopaque stones (calcium oxalate and calcium phosphate), although less radiopaque stones (uric acid, cysteine, and magnesium ammonium phosphate [struvite]) may go undetected.
  - Even a helical CT scan may miss radiolucent stones due to HIV protease inhibitors, particularly indinavir. Occasionally, phleboliths overlying a ureter may be difficult to distinguish from ureteral stones.

*The majority of kidney stones are calcium oxalate.*

### TREATMENT

- ↑ urine volume through daily ingestion of 2.5–3.0 L of fluid.
- Additional treatment depends on the type of stone:
  - **Calcium:** Moderate protein intake; consider thiazides and potassium citrate. Calcium restriction has not been shown to reduce recurrences and may worsen osteoporosis.
  - **Uric acid:** Moderate protein intake; consider potassium citrate. Allopurinol is usually reserved for patients with elevated urinary uric acid levels.
  - **Cysteine:** Diagnostic of cysteinuria (a rare heritable disorder of cysteine transport in the proximal tubule). Urine alkalinization with potassium citrate or potassium bicarbonate. Na$^+$ restriction.
  - **Magnesium ammonium phosphate (struvite):** Results from a UTI with urea-producing bacteria such as *Proteus* or *Klebsiella*. Can develop into a staghorn calculus involving the entire renal pelvis and calyces. Initiation of appropriate antimicrobial therapy can slow progress, but generally requires surgical intervention.

# CHAPTER 10

# Dermatology

Graham Dresden, MD

Stephen Stukovsky, MD

## Terminology

Skin lesions may be characterized as 1° changes (i.e., caused by a 1° disease process; see Table 10.1) or as 2° changes resulting from a variety of factors (see Table 10.2). They may also be distinguished by their configuration (see Table 10.3) as well as by their distribution—e.g., whether the eruption is generalized, acral (affecting the hands, feet, buttocks, or face), or localized to a specific skin region. In general, skin lesions are described in reverse order from the presentation given above, beginning with distribution and followed by configuration, color, 2° changes, and 1° changes. For example, guttate psoriasis could be described as generalized discrete, red, scaly papules.

## Diagnostic Techniques

Key diagnostic techniques include the following:

- **KOH prep:** Used to diagnose fungal infection. Scrape with a blade or a glass slide, and add KOH (must be heated if not preserved with DMSO). KOH dissolves keratin but not hyphae walls. Look for branching structures.
- **Tzanck smear:** Used to test for HSV or VZV. Rupture the vesicle and take a sample (do not use a cotton swab).
- **Wood's lamp:** Emits UV light (the so-called "black light"). Can be used to diagnose tinea capitis, tinea versicolor, erythrasma, vitiligo, melasma, and porphyria.

**TABLE 10.1.  Differential of 1° Dermatologic Lesions**

| LESION | DESCRIPTION | EXAMPLE |
|--------|-------------|---------|
| Macule | Any circumscribed color change in the skin that is flat. | White (vitiligo), brown (café au lait spot), purple (petechiae). |
| Papule | A solid, elevated area < 1 cm in diameter whose top may be pointed, rounded, or flat. | Acne, warts, small lesions of psoriasis. |
| Plaque | A solid, circumscribed area > 1 cm in diameter, usually flat-topped. | Psoriasis. |
| Vesicle | A circumscribed, elevated lesion < 1 cm in diameter and containing clear serous fluid. | Blisters of HSV. |
| Bulla | A circumscribed, elevated lesion > 1 cm in diameter and containing clear serous fluid. | Bullous erythema multiforme. |
| Pustule | A vesicle containing a purulent exudate. | Acne, folliculitis. |
| Nodule | A deep-seated mass with indistinct borders that elevates the overlying epidermis. | Tumors, granuloma annulare. |
| Wheal | A circumscribed, flat-topped, firm elevation of skin resulting from tense edema of the papillary dermis. | Urticaria. |

**TABLE 10.2.**   **Differential of 2° Dermatologic Lesions**

| 2° Change | Description | Example |
|-----------|-------------|---------|
| Scales | Dry, thin plates of keratinized epidermal cells (stratum corneum). | Psoriasis, ichthyosis. |
| Lichenification | Induration of skin with exaggerated skin lines and a shiny surface resulting from chronic rubbing of the skin. | Atopic dermatitis. |
| Erosion and oozing | A moist, circumscribed, slightly depressed area representing a blister base with the roof of the blister removed. | Burns; bullous erythema multiforme. Most oral blisters present as erosions. |
| Crusts | Dried exudate of plasma on the surface of the skin following acute dermatitis. | Impetigo, contact dermatitis. |
| Fissures | A linear split in the skin extending through the epidermis into the dermis. | Angular cheilitis. |
| Scars | A flat, raised, or depressed area of fibrotic replacement of dermis or subcutaneous tissue. | Acne scars, burn scars. |
| Atrophy | Depression of the skin surface caused by thinning of one or more layers of skin. | Lichen sclerosus et atrophicus. |
| Color | The lesion should be described as red, yellow, brown, tan, or blue. Particular attention should be paid to blanching; failure to blanch suggests bleeding into the dermis (petechiae). | |

## Biopsy Procedures

- **Shave biopsy:** Performed by shaving tangentially to the skin with a blade. Indicated for elevated (exophytic) neoplasms.
- **Punch biopsy:** Done by exerting rotational torque. No closure is required for lesions ≤ 3 mm in diameter. Indicated for obtaining full-thickness skin specimens.

**TABLE 10.3.**   **Differential of Dermatologic Lesions by Configuration**

| CONFIGURATION | EXAMPLES |
|---------------|----------|
| Annular (circular) | Annular nodules represent granuloma annulare; annular scaly papules are more apt to be caused by dermatophyte infections. |
| Linear (straight lines) | Linear papules represent lichen striatus; linear vesicles, incontinentia pigmenti; and linear papules with burrows, scabies. |
| Grouped | Grouped vesicles occur in herpes simplex or zoster. |
| Discrete | Discrete lesions are independent of each other. |

- **Excisional biopsy:** Best performed with an elliptical incision to prevent "dog ears." Indicated for the diagnosis of suspected malignancy, melanoma therapy, complete excision of lesions, or cosmetic purposes.

## COMMON SKIN DISORDERS

A 15-year-old girl comes to your office asking for advice about the treatment of her acne. She has a few inflamed papules on her face but no nodules. She has been using daily cleansing soaps but no OTC acne treatments. How would you counsel or treat her? First-line therapy for mild inflammatory acne is benzoyl peroxide, an OTC medication. The girl should also be counseled not to squeeze lesions, as this can worsen inflammation and cause scarring. If this treatment does not succeed, then a topical antibiotic should be added. An oral antibiotic can be the next step, and in recalcitrant cases, isotretinoin (a topical retinoid) is often employed.

### Acne

Defined as chronic inflammation and blockage of the pilosebaceous units with ↑ production of sebum and colonization of *Propionibacterium acnes.* Exacerbated by medications such as glucocorticoids, anabolic steroids, lithium, some OCPs, and iodides. **Diet has not been proven to affect acne.**

#### SYMPTOMS/EXAM

Presents with noninflammatory comedones ("blackheads" and "whiteheads") as well as with inflammatory papules, pustules, and cysts (see Figure 10.1).

#### TREATMENT

- **First line:** Benzoyl peroxide; topical antibiotics (e.g., clindamycin).
- **Second line:** Oral antibiotics—e.g., tetracycline 500 mg BID × 4 months (also minocycline and doxycycline).

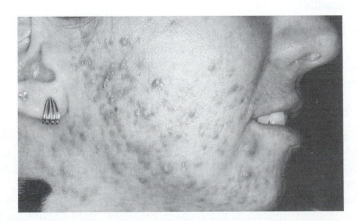

**FIGURE 10.1.** **Severe inflammatory acne with pustules and comedones.**

(Reproduced, with permission, from Kasper DL et al. *Harrison's Principles of Internal Medicine,* 16th ed. New York: McGraw-Hill, 2005: 295.) (Also see Color Insert.)

*Isotretinoin is teratogenic, so women must use two forms of birth control. Side effects include dry skin, cheilitis, hypertriglyceridemia, and transaminitis (therefore LFTs must be followed). Depression has also been associated with its use.*

*With recalcitrant acne in female patients, look for hirsutism and irregular menses, which may point to congenital adrenal hyperplasia, polycystic ovarian syndrome, or Cushing's disease.*

*Facial steroid creams can cause dermatitis resembling rosacea.*

- **Third line:** Isotretinoin (Accutane), a retinoid that is anti-inflammatory. OCPs can also be switched to a less androgenic variety.

## Rosacea

Chronic inflammatory facial dermatitis of middle-aged adults characterized by erythema and pustules.

### SYMPTOMS/EXAM

- The earliest symptom is **flushing**, followed by erythema, telangiectasia, papules, pustules, and occasionally lymphedema. Distribution is on the cheeks, nose, forehead, and chin.
- Triggered by **hot liquids, spicy food, alcohol, sun,** and **heat.**
- No comedones are seen (compared with acne).

### DIFFERENTIAL

- Acne, contact dermatitis, photosensitive eruptions, seborrheic dermatitis, SLE.
- Facial steroid creams can mimic rosacea.

### TREATMENT

- Avoid exacerbating factors.
- **Topical treatment: Metronidazole** gel or cream; sodium sulfacetamide lotion.
- **Oral treatment:** Tetracycline × 2–3 months. Appropriate in the presence of ocular involvement or if topical therapy is not effective. Erythromycin is second-line therapy.
- **Severe disease:** Isotretinoin (surgery is last line).

### COMPLICATIONS

**Rhinophyma** occurs primarily in middle-aged men with long-standing disease (see Figure 10.2). Blepharitis and conjunctivitis are also potential complications.

## Atopic Dermatitis

A chronic inflammatory skin disease that is considered familial with allergic features. It often occurs in patients with other atopic disorders, such as **asthma** and **allergic rhinitis.** Onset is usually before age 7. Thought to be immune related, with roughly 85% of patients having ↑ IgE.

### SYMPTOMS/EXAM

- Acute lesions can include vesicles (see Figure 10.3), and serous exudate may be seen in severe cases. Skin lesions in older individuals with more chronic disease are characterized by **lichenification** as well as by excoriated and fibrotic papules.
- The **flexural** areas (the neck, antecubital fossae, and popliteal fossae) are most commonly involved, with other common sites including the face, wrists, and forearms.
- Other physical findings that support the diagnosis include xerosis (dry skin), infraorbital skin folds (Dennie-Morgan lines), periorbital darkening, hyperlinear palms (accentuation of fine palmar skin lines), and keratosis

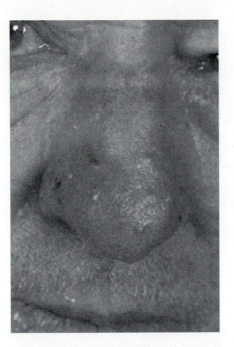

**FIGURE 10.2.** Rhinophyma and pustules on a male with rosacea.

(Reproduced, with permission, from Wolff K, Johnson RA, Suurmond D. *Fitzpatrick's Color Atlas & Synopsis of Clinical Dermatology*, 5th edition, Online Picture Gallery. New York: McGraw-Hill, 2007: Figure 1e-R5.) (Also see Color Insert.)

pilaris (follicular accentuation that is usually present on the extensor surfaces of the upper arms).

### DIFFERENTIAL

Contact dermatitis, seborrheic dermatitis, drug reactions, psoriasis (axillary, gluteal, or groin lesions are more characteristic of psoriasis).

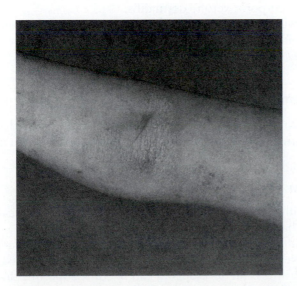

**FIGURE 10.3.** Atopic dermatitis in the antecubital region of a child.

(Reproduced, with permission, from Wolff K et al. *Fitzpatrick's Color Atlas & Synopsis of Clinical Dermatology*, 5th ed. New York: McGraw-Hill, 2005: Figure 2e-AD12.) (Also see Color Insert.)

### DIAGNOSIS

Diagnosed visually. Pruritus, a chronic recurring course, a ⊕ family history of atopy, and early age of onset are all suggestive of the diagnosis.

### TREATMENT

- **Skin hydration with lotions and emollients.**
- Eliminate exacerbating factors, including excessive bathing, low-humidity environments, emotional stress, xerosis (dry skin), rapid temperature changes, and exposure to solvents and detergents.
- Topical corticosteroids or topical calcineurin inhibitors (tacrolimus/pimecrolimus) are appropriate for patients with inflamed skin; antihistamines can be given for pruritus.
- Treat bacterial superinfection.

## Dyshidrotic Eczema (Pompholyx)

- An intensely pruritic, chronic recurrent dermatitis typically involving the palms and soles.
- **Sx/Exam:** Starts as an episode of intense itching followed by the formation of small vesicles. Desquamation occurs over 1–2 weeks, leaving fissures and erosions. Recurrences may be seen.
- **DDx:** Tinea; contact dermatitis.
- **Tx:** Treated with medium- to high-potency topical corticosteroids in mild cases and with a short course of systemic steroids in severe cases. Recalcitrant cases may respond to PUVA or UVA.

## Discoid (Nummular) Eczema

- Intensely pruritic dermatitis of unknown etiology.
- **Sx/Exam:** Presents with papules, scaling, crusting, and serous oozing. Lesions can be singular or multiple (up to 50) and are generally 2–10 cm in diameter and circular in shape. Distribution is over the trunk and lower extremities (the head is spared).
- **DDx:** Tinea corporis; xerotic dermatitis.
- **Tx:** Treat with a short course of high-potency topical steroids. Systemic corticosteroids may be needed for more severe cases. Avoid irritants (if identifiable).

## Seborrheic Dermatitis

A chronic inflammatory eruption hypothesized to be caused by *Malassezia furfur* yeast (formerly *Pityrosporum ovale*) colonization. Known as "cradle cap" in infants.

### SYMPTOMS/EXAM

- Presents with dry or **greasy,** yellow, sharply demarcated scales on an erythematous base.
- Primarily affects the scalp, **postauricular region,** central facial area (especially the **eyebrows** and **nasolabial folds**), and flexural areas.
- Crust and fissures can develop and can become superinfected.

### DIFFERENTIAL

Atopic or contact dermatitis, psoriasis (seborrheic dermatitis is usually more "pinkish-red" compared to the deep red of psoriasis), impetigo, rosacea.

*Parkinson's, stroke, and acutely ill patients can present with seborrheic dermatitis. If severe and recalcitrant, seborrheic dermatitis can also be a presenting symptom in patients with HIV.*

### TREATMENT

- **Scalp:** Treat with shampoos containing coal tar, zinc pyrithione, selenium sulfide, or 2% ketoconazole (Nizoral).
- **Face:** Topical steroids +/– 2% ketoconazole cream.
- **Intertriginous areas:** Low-potency steroids +/– ketoconazole cream.
- Treat infants with emollients and 1% hydrocortisone ointment or a miconazole-hydrocortisone combination.

## Psoriasis

A chronic, noninfectious, immune-mediated inflammatory dermatosis. Roughly 2% of the population is affected, with a bimodal distribution (peaks at 22 and 55 years of age). Triggered by environmental factors such as infection, stress, trauma, and drugs (β-blockers, lithium).

### SYMPTOMS/EXAM

- Presents with well-demarcated erythematous plaques covered by **waxy silvery-white scales** (see Figure 10.4). Characterized by bilateral involvement of the extensor surfaces, scalp, palms, and soles. Sometimes pruritic.
- **Nail pitting** is seen in half of cases.
- A severe form is seen in **HIV** infection.
- **Koebner's phenomenon** is a form of the disease that occurs at sites of trauma.
- **Guttate psoriasis** generally follows a **streptococcal** infection (e.g., strep throat) and presents with an acute symmetrical eruption of "droplike" lesions on the trunk and limbs.

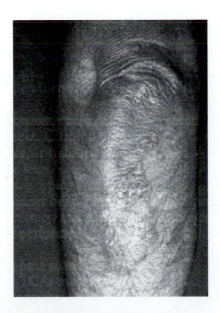

**FIGURE 10.4.** **Erythematous plaque of psoriasis.**

(Reproduced, with permission, from Bondi EE et al. *Dermatology: Diagnosis & Therapy*, 1st ed. Stamford, CT: Appleton & Lange, 1991.) (Also see Color Insert.)

DERMATOLOGY

### TREATMENT

- **Topical treatment:** Potent topical corticosteroids, a vitamin D analog (calcipotriene), topical retinoids.
- **Systemic treatment:** Phototherapy (UVB), photochemotherapy (PUVA), oral retinoids, methotrexate, cyclosporine, biologicals (efalizumab, infliximab).
- Penicillin VK or erythromycin is used to treat strep throat in guttate psoriasis.

### COMPLICATIONS

**Psoriatic arthritis** (affects 5% of patients, primarily affecting the DIP joints of hands); sacroiliitis.

## Pityriasis Rosea

An acute, self-limited disorder characterized by scaly oval papules and plaques. Generally found in adolescents and young adults in response to a viral infection (**HHV-7** has been implicated). **Affects females more often than males.**

### SYMPTOMS/EXAM

- Presents as a generalized rash preceded by the appearance of a 2- to 5-cm **herald patch.** Days later, many smaller plaques appear on the trunk, arms, and thighs (see Figure 10.5).
- Plaques are oval and pink with a delicate peripheral **"collarette of scale"** and are often distributed parallel to the lines of the ribs, creating the characteristic **"Christmas tree"** distribution.
- Accompanied by mild to moderate pruritus.

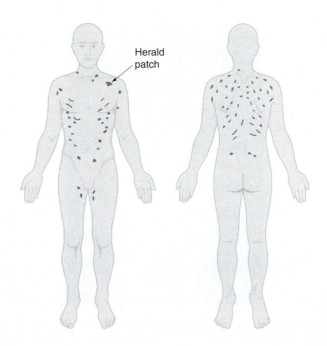

Herald patch

**FIGURE 10.5.** **Distribution of pityriasis rosea.**

(Reproduced, with permission, from Wolff K et al. *Fitzpatrick's Color Atlas & Synopsis of Clinical Dermatology,* 5th ed. New York: McGraw-Hill, 2005: 119.)

### DIFFERENTIAL

Guttate psoriasis, pityriasis versicolor, scabies, 2° syphilis.

### TREATMENT

Spontaneous resolution usually occurs in 1–2 months. Moderate-potency steroids may be given for itching.

## Lichen Planus

An eruption characterized by **purple, polygonal, pruritic papules** affecting the flexor surfaces, mucous membranes, and genitalia. Its cause is unknown but is thought to be immune related. Some two-thirds of cases occur in patients 30–60 years of age.

### SYMPTOMS/EXAM

- The rash starts symmetrically on the limbs, especially the wrists, and may spread to become generalized within four weeks but may also progress more slowly.
- Typical lesions are itchy, flat-topped polygonal papules a few millimeters in diameter (see Figure 10.6). They classically show a surface network of delicate white lines (Wickham's striae).
- Papules are initially red but become violaceous. Papules can flatten or become hypertrophic. Although 50% of cases clear within nine months, the condition often recurs.
- Associated with chronic **HBV and HCV.**

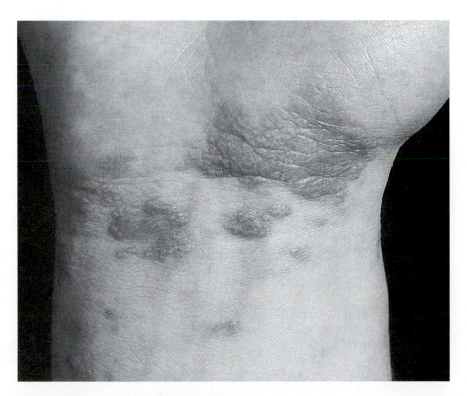

**FIGURE 10.6.**  **Lesions of lichen planus.**

(Reproduced, with permission, from Wolff K et al. *Fitzpatrick's Color Atlas & Synopsis of Clinical Dermatology*, 5th ed. New York: McGraw-Hill, 2005: 125.) (Also see Color Insert.)

### DIFFERENTIAL

Psoriasis, guttate psoriasis, pityriasis rosea, scabies.

### TREATMENT

- The disease is usually self-limited.
- Moderate- to high-potency topical steroids are indicated for symptomatic treatment.
- Oral lesions are treated with steroid-containing paste.

## Contact Dermatitis

Any dermatitis that results from direct contact between skin and a substance. The two variants are allergen and irritant. Irritants are responsible for 80% of cases.

### IRRITANT CONTACT DERMATITIS

- In irritant dermatitis, the trigger substance affects the skin by → breakdown of the normal epidermal barrier. Can → physical, chemical, or mechanical irritation.
- A reaction can be initiated by common irritants such as daily-use products (e.g., soap) or may result from one-time exposure to an allergen (e.g., bleach, alkali). Patients with compromised skin barriers (e.g., those with atopic dermatitis) are at higher risk.
- Sx/Exam:
  - Presents with erythema, fissures, and pruritus. In severe cases, bullae can develop.
  - Often affects the hands, especially the web spaces, but may also involve the face and eyelids
- Dx: Patch testing can distinguish the condition from allergic contact dermatitis.
- Tx:
  - Avoid triggers; restore the normal epidermal barrier; use emollients. More severe cases can be treated with topical corticosteroids.
  - Systemic steroids are generally not helpful without irritant removal.

### ALLERGIC CONTACT DERMATITIS

- In allergic dermatitis, a trigger substance induces a delayed type IV immune response in affected individuals. The first step takes 12–14 days to complete, and upon reexposure to an allergen, a dermatitis occurs in 12–48 hours.
- The most common allergen is plant oleoresin urushiol (found in poison ivy, poison oak, poison sumac, and mango skin). Other agents include nickel, formaldehyde, perfume, latex, and medications.
- Sx/Exam: Presents with an intensely pruritic rash that is papular and erythematous with indistinct margins. The rash can be linear (as in poison ivy) or can reflect the pattern of exposure to the allergen (e.g., rings, clothing, footwear; see Figure 10.7).
- Tx:
  - Avoid allergens.
  - Mild cases may be treated with medium- to high-potency topical steroids.

*Laundry detergent is only infrequently a cause of allergic contact dermatitis.*

*Patients with venous stasis dermatitis can often have contact dermatitis superimposed without clinical signs or symptoms. These patients typically fail to respond to conservative treatment of their stasis ulcers and may develop an allergic reaction to the treatment regimens.*

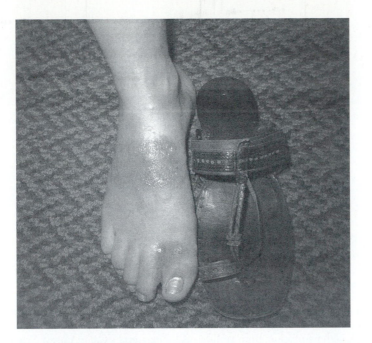

**FIGURE 10.7.**  **Contact dermatitis.**

(Reproduced, with permission, from Hurwitz RM. *Pathology of the Skin: Atlas of Clinical-Pathological Correlation.* Stamford, CT: Appleton & Lange, 1991: 3.)

- With more severe oozing, wet-dry compresses may facilitate application of topical steroids by drying skin out.
- Severe cases can also be treated with a short course of oral corticosteroids.

## Keratosis Pilaris

- Caused by plugging of the follicle by keratin that has failed to exfoliate → a red papule.
- **Sx/Exam:** Usually asymptomatic, but can → pruritus. Typically found on the lateral face, trunk, upper and lower extremities, thighs, and buttocks.
- **Tx:** Conservative treatment; exfoliation. Topical tretinoin may be tried for recalcitrant cases.

BACTERIAL INFECTIONS

## Folliculitis

- An acute pustular infection of hair follicles, usually due to S. *aureus*.
- **Sx/Exam:** Lesions are generally found in the hair-bearing areas. Men can get sycosis barbae in the beard area (see Figure 10.8).
- **DDx:** Furuncles, carbuncles.
- **Dx:** If possible, obtain a swab to identify the causative organism.
- **Tx:**
    - **Acute infections:** Systemic and topical antibiotics (usually empiric for *Staphylococcus*).

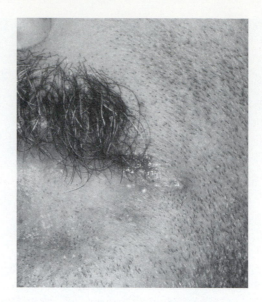

**FIGURE 10.8.** **Folliculitis in the beard area with impetigo at the corner of the mouth.**

(Reproduced, with permission, from Wolff K et al. *Fitzpatrick's Color Atlas & Synopsis of Clinical Dermatology*, 5th ed. New York: McGraw-Hill, 2005: 980.) (Also see Color Insert.)

- **Chronic infections:** Carrier sites (e.g., the nose) must be treated with topical mupirocin (Bactroban). Successive courses of systemic antibiotics may also be needed.
- **Hygiene** is key to treatment, along with weight loss and control of diabetes.
- **Cx:** Patients can get a gram-⊖ folliculitis (*Pseudomonas*) following prolonged treatment with antibiotics (e.g., for acne).

## Cellulitis

A bacterial infection of the skin with some extension into the subcutaneous tissues. Seventy percent of patients are men. Additional risk factors include leg ulcers, trauma, intertrigo, tinea pedis, venous insufficiency, obesity, and a history of cellulitis.

### SYMPTOMS/EXAM

- Presents with systemic symptoms such as fever, chills, and myalgias as well as rubor, calor, tumor, and dolor. Most commonly affects the extremities (73% of cases affect the lower extremities), but can involve any area of the body.
- Margins are generally not well demarcated (compared with erysipelas, which has distinct margins).
- Regional lymphadenopathy is common, and lymphangitis can be present.
- Abscess may be seen, as may macular erythema that is largely confluent.

### DIFFERENTIAL

DVT, contact dermatitis, drug and foreign body reactions, insect stings.

### DIAGNOSIS

- Pathogens associated with cellulitis include the following:
  - Cellulitis associated with furuncles, carbuncles, or abscesses is usually caused by *S. aureus*. Methicillin-resistant *S. aureus* (MRSA) can be seen.

- Cellulitis that is diffuse or unassociated with a defined portal is most commonly caused by streptococcal species. β-hemolytic streptococci, including groups A, B, and, less often, C and G, are common causative agents.
  - Facial cellulitis is associated with *H. influenzae* in children.
  - Cellulitis following puncture wounds is most often caused by *Pseudomonas aeruginosa*.
  - Exposure to fresh water or seawater is associated with *Aeromonas hydrophila* and *Vibrio* spp.
  - Animal bites point to *Pasteurella multocida* and *Erysipelothrix*.
- Cultures are usually not helpful, establishing the diagnosis in only 50% of cases, and generally do not result in a change of management (antibiotics).

### TREATMENT

- The guidelines set forth in 2005 by the Infectious Diseases Society of America suggest a penicillinase-resistant semisynthetic penicillin or a first-generation cephalosporin (A–I) unless streptococci or staphylococci resistant to these agents are common in the community.
- For penicillin-allergic patients, options include clindamycin or vancomycin.

### COMPLICATIONS

Necrotizing fasciitis, gas gangrene (see Figure 10.9).

## Impetigo

A superficial skin infection due to **staphylococci** and/or **streptococci (group A)**. Affects men and women in all age groups. Lesions are classically found on the face.

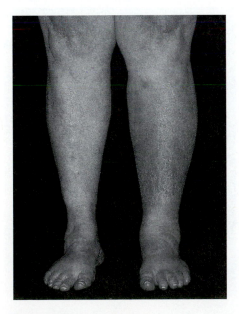

**FIGURE 10.9.   Cellulitis of the lower extremity.**

(Reproduced, with permission, from Knoop KJ et al. *Atlas of Emergency Medicine*, 2nd ed. New York: McGraw-Hill, 2002: 348.) (Also see Color Insert.)

*Bullous impetigo is usually caused by S. aureus.*

*Recurrent impetigo suggests nasal carriage of S. aureus. Treat with intranasal mupirocin.*

### SYMPTOMS/EXAM

- 1° lesions are thin-walled vesicles/pustules that easily rupture (see Figure 10.10).
- Lesions spread rapidly and become crusted and are classically described as **"honey-crusted."**

### DIFFERENTIAL

HSV, fungal infection.

### TREATMENT

- Removal of crusts via saline soaks and topical mupirocin.
- Systemic antibiotics (empirically directed against staph or strep) are appropriate for more severe cases.

## Erysipelas

An acute inflammation of the dermis by *Streptococcus pyogenes.* Elderly and immunocompromised patients are at higher risk.

### SYMPTOMS/EXAM

- Presents with well-demarcated erythema, edema, and tenderness (a type of cellulitis), typically affecting the face and lower legs (see Figure 10.11).
- Patients are generally systemically ill, presenting with fever, chills, and malaise.
- Lesions can rapidly advance.

### DIFFERENTIAL

Angioedema; allergic contact dermatitis.

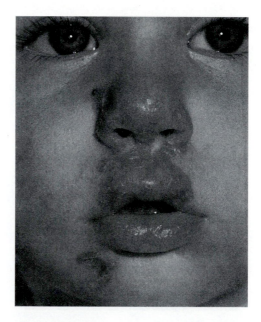

**FIGURE 10.10.  Lesions of impetigo.**

(Reproduced, with permission, from Wolff K et al. *Fitzpatrick's Color Atlas & Synopsis of Clinical Dermatology,* 5th ed. New York: McGraw-Hill, 2005: 589.) (Also see Color Insert.)

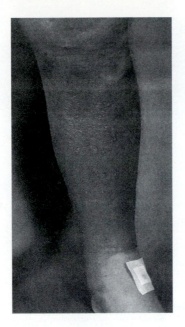

**FIGURE 10.11. Erysipelas.**

Note the well-demarcated borders of erysipelas as compared to general cellulitis. (Reproduced, with permission, from Wolff K et al. *Fitzpatrick's Color Atlas & Synopsis of Clinical Dermatology*, 5th ed. New York: McGraw-Hill, 2005: 607.) (Also see Color Insert.)

### TREATMENT

Treat with IV antibiotics directed against *Streptococcus*.

### COMPLICATIONS

Guttate psoriasis or acute glomerulonephritis can follow streptococcal infection.

## Anthrax

Caused by *Bacillus anthracis*, a gram-⊕, spore-forming aerobic rod; transmitted through the skin or mucous membranes, by inhalation of or contact with contaminated soil, by animals, or through biologic warfare.

### SYMPTOMS/EXAM

- Has three manifestations: cutaneous (95% of cases), GI, and pulmonary (woolsorters' disease).
- Presents as a nonspecific illness (fever, malaise, nausea and vomiting). Then, over 2–7 days, characteristic lesions develop.
- The 1° lesion is a small, erythematous macule that evolves into a papule with vesicles, significant erythema, and edema.
- One to three days later the papule ulcerates, leaving the characteristic **necrotic eschar.** No pain or tenderness is seen at this point.
- **Suppurative regional adenopathy** can develop.

### TREATMENT

- Treat with IV penicillin G. Oral tetracycline may be effective for mild disease.
- For penicillin-allergic patients, aminoglycosides, macrolides, or quinolones are second-line therapy.

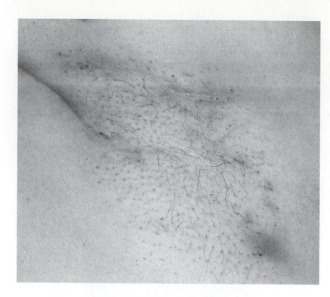

**FIGURE 10.12.** **Hidradenitis suppurativa.**

Note the bulging and depressed scars and draining sinus in the axillae. (Reproduced, with permission, from Wolff K et al. *Fitzpatrick's Color Atlas & Synopsis of Clinical Dermatology*, 5th ed. New York: McGraw-Hill, 2005: 15.) (Also see Color Insert.)

### COMPLICATIONS

Most cases resolve without sequelae, but 10–20% of untreated cases of cutaneous anthrax → death.

*Perianal hidradenitis suppurativa and Crohn's disease are similar and may be linked.*

## Hidradenitis Suppurativa

- A chronic, suppurative cutaneous process that results from occlusion of follicles and 2° inflammation of apocrine glands.
- Females are affected more often than males; more prevalent in hirsute women.
- Sx/Exam:
    - Presents with recurrent deep boils for > 6 months in flexural sites (see Figure 10.12).
    - Commonly affects the axillae, groin, vulva, and perineal or perianal areas, sparing the face (hence its proposed name, acne inversa). Lesions tend to recur.
- Tx:
    - Topical clindamycin is the treatment of choice. Antiandrogens and retinoids have been used but have yielded mixed results.
    - Severe disease requires surgical treatment.
    - Systemic antibiotics are usually not helpful.

### MYCOTIC INFECTIONS

## Tinea (Dermatophytes)

The most common type of fungal infection of skin and nails. Often called "ringworm." The appearance of tinea is variegated depending on location, but commonly it is seen as localized, erythematous, scaly lesions that form as pustules or vesicles with satellite lesions. Tinea is differentiated according to the site involved:

- **Tinea capitis ("cradle cap"):** Occurs primarily in children. Differentiate from seborrheic dermatitis in adults. Treated with griseofulvin; terbinafine and itraconazole may also be tried.
- **Tinea pedis ("athlete's foot"):** Chronic cases can usually be treated with a topical antifungal cream for four weeks. Interdigital tinea pedis, which is often macerated in appearance (see Figure 10.13), may require only one week of therapy. Resistant cases may require oral medication (beware of cost and side effects).
- **Tinea corporis ("ringworm"):** Lesions typically have sharply demarcated margins with scaling (see Figure 10.14). Treat with daily antifungal creams. Cases associated with contact sports (e.g., wrestling), called tinea corporis gladiatorum, generally respond better to oral antifungals (griseofulvin) and restriction from activity for 10–15 days.
- **Tinea cruris ("jock itch"):** Much more common in men. Obesity and sweaty physical activity are risk factors. Treat with topical antifungals. Use of talc or desiccant powders can help prevent recurrence.

*Tinea pedis is the most common cause of cellulitis in otherwise healthy patients.*

*Dermatophytid (id reaction) is a hypersensitivity reaction to a tinea infection on a distant body site (e.g., a patient with tinea pedis develops pruritic vesicles on the back).*

### TINEA VERSICOLOR

A chronic fungal infection characterized by pigmentary changes. Caused by overgrowth of *Pityrosporum orbiculare*. More common in humid or tropical locations. Typically affects young adults.

### SYMPTOMS/EXAM

- In fair-skinned people, presents with brown or pinkish, superficially scaly macules and patches that may be oval or round. Typically involves the trunk and the proximal parts of the limbs.
- In darker-skinned people, hypopigmentation is seen (see Figure 10.15).

### DIFFERENTIAL

Vitiligo, tinea corporis.

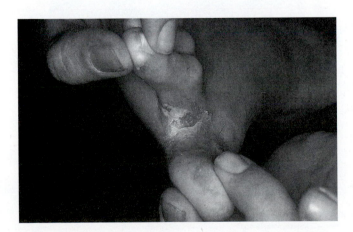

**FIGURE 10.13.   Interdigital tinea pedis.**

(Reproduced, with permission, from Knoop KJ et al. *Atlas of Emergency Medicine*, 2nd ed. New York: McGraw-Hill, 2002: 402.) (Also see Color Insert.)

DERMATOLOGY

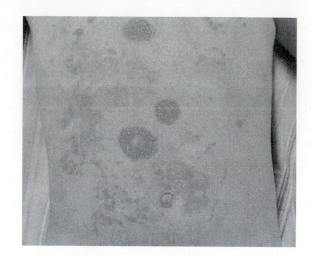

**FIGURE 10.14.** **Tinea corporis.**

Note the sharply demarcated margins with scale. (Reproduced, with permission, from Wolff K et al. *Fitzpatrick's Color Atlas & Synopsis of Clinical Dermatology*, 5th ed. New York: McGraw-Hill, 2005: 702.) (Also see Color Insert.)

### DIAGNOSIS

KOH scraping reveals hyphae and budding spores ("**spaghetti and meatballs**" appearance).

### TREATMENT

- Topical antifungal (clotrimazole or miconazole); selenium sulfide lotion; ketoconazole shampoo.
- A single dose of ketoconazole at a dosage of 400 mg → short-term cure in 90% of cases.

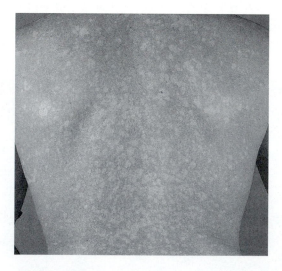

**FIGURE 10.15.** **Tinea versicolor.**

Note the hypopigmented macules on the back of a tanned individual. (Reproduced, with permission, from Wolff K et al. *Fitzpatrick's Color Atlas & Synopsis of Clinical Dermatology*, 5th ed. New York: McGraw-Hill, 2005: 731.) (Also see Color Insert.)

- Systemic antifungals (itraconazole) × 7 days can be used for resistant cases.

### COMPLICATIONS

Recurrence is common.

## Candidiasis/Intertrigo

A fungal infection that favors moist areas, with the intertriginous areas most commonly involved. Risk factors include DM, obesity, sweating, heat, maceration, and systemic and topical steroid use. Antibiotics and OCPs may also be contributory.

### SYMPTOMS/EXAM

- Initial vesiculopustules enlarge and rupture, becoming eroded and confluent.
- Brightly erythematous, sharply demarcated plaques are seen with scalloped borders (see Figure 10.16).
- Satellite lesions (pustular lesions at the periphery) may coalesce and become part of a larger lesion.

### DIAGNOSIS

KOH scraping shows pseudohyphae and yeast forms.

### TREATMENT

Keep affected areas dry; treat with topical antifungals (powders or creams).

*Diaper rash may be candidal diaper dermatitis. Look for satellite lesions.*

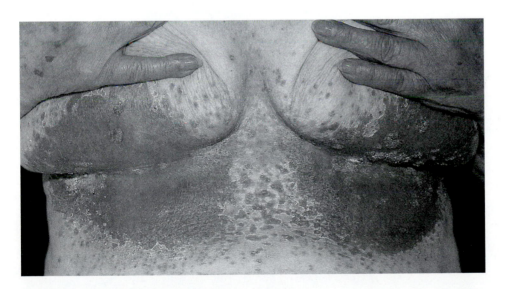

**FIGURE 10.16.    Cutaneous candidiasis—intertrigo.**

Small peripheral satellite papules and pustules coalesce to create a large eroded area in the submammary region. (Reproduced, with permission, from Wolff K et al. *Fitzpatrick's Color Atlas & Synopsis of Clinical Dermatology*, 5th ed. New York: McGraw-Hill, 2005: 719.) (Also see Color Insert.)

## Molluscum Contagiosum

Discrete, pearly-pink, umbilicated papules involving the trunk, face, and neck. Caused by a DNA poxvirus. Occurs mostly in children and young adults. Spread by direct contact (e.g., sexual contact, towels).

### SYMPTOMS/EXAM

- Presents with dome-shaped papules a few millimeters in size with central umbilication or puncta (see Figure 10.17).
- Lesions are usually multiple and occur in groups.
- If lesions are squeezed, a cheesy material can sometimes be expressed.

### DIFFERENTIAL

Viral warts, skin tags.

### TREATMENT

- The disease is self-limited.
- In adults or older children, lesions can be removed via expression with forceps, with curettage under local anesthesia, or with cryosurgery.
- Imiquimod may help (an off-label use).

### COMPLICATIONS

Infection can be especially severe in immunosuppressed patients.

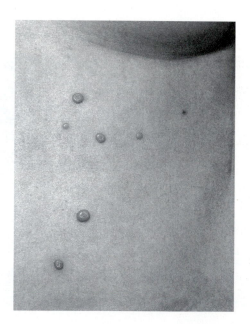

**FIGURE 10.17.** **Molluscum contagiosum on the chest of a female.**

Note the discrete, solid papules with central umbilication. (Reproduced, with permission, from Wolff K et al. *Fitzpatrick's Color Atlas & Synopsis of Clinical Dermatology*, 5th ed. New York: McGraw-Hill, 2005: 763.) (Also see Color Insert.)

## Viral Exanthem

- A rash associated with general features of a viral illness (myalgias, arthralgias, sore throat). Primarily seen in children and adolescents.
- **Sx/Exam:** The rash is erythematous and maculopapular with a blotchy appearance, generally affecting the trunk and limbs. The viral cause is generally not identified.
- **DDx:** Chickenpox, measles, rubella, fifth disease, coxsackievirus (hand, foot, and mouth disease).
- **Tx:** Treat with emollients or cooling agents (calamine).

*Infectious mononucleosis treated with amoxicillin → a rash similar to a viral exanthem.*

## PARASITIC INFECTIONS

A 14-year-old boy presents to your office with a pruritic, crusting rash on his feet of two weeks' duration. Topical corticosteroids have failed to improve his condition. How would you proceed? The skin should be scraped and examined under the microscope for characteristic mites. Treatment is usually begun with permethrin. Clothing and household contacts need to be treated as well.

## Scabies

Skin infection by the mite *Sarcoptes scabiei*. The female mite burrows into skin to lay eggs. The infection is highly contagious and spreads through prolonged contact with an infected host.

### SYMPTOMS/EXAM

- Presents with small pruritic papules, pustules, and burrows (see Figure 10.18). Lesions are intensely pruritic, especially at night.
- Infection usually spares the face and scalp and is classically located in the web spaces of the hands (see Figure 10.19). It is also common in the axil-

**FIGURE 10.18.** **Linear burrows of infection caused by scabies.**

(Reproduced, with permission, from Wolff K et al. *Fitzpatrick's Color Atlas & Synopsis of Clinical Dermatology*, 5th ed. New York: McGraw-Hill, 2005: 857.) (Also see Color Insert.)

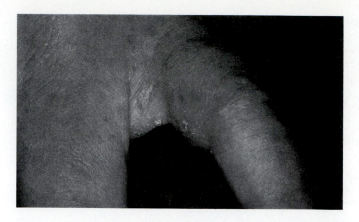

**FIGURE 10.19.** **Burrows of the scabies mite in the web spaces of the hands.**

(Reproduced, with permission, from Wolff K et al. *Fitzpatrick's Color Atlas & Synopsis of Clinical Dermatology*, 5th ed. New York: McGraw-Hill, 2005: 855.) (Also see Color Insert.)

*The symptoms of scabies may persist for weeks to months despite effectively treated scabies infection.*

lae, antecubital fossa, gluteal crease, feet, genitalia, nipples, and waistband (see Figure 10.20).
- Itching and rash are due to a type IV hypersensitivity reaction to the mite, eggs, and feces and → a two- to four-week delay between infection and onset of symptoms.
- Excoriations and crusts develop 2° to scratching.

### DIAGNOSIS

- Examine skin scrapings with microscopy to identify mites, ova, and fecal pellets (see Figure 10.21).
- The diagnosis should be confirmed with a skin scraping and viewed under a low-power microscope.

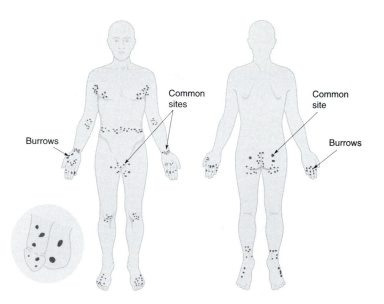

**FIGURE 10.20.** **Common sites of scabies infection.**

(Reproduced, with permission, from Wolff K et al. *Fitzpatrick's Color Atlas & Synopsis of Clinical Dermatology*, 5th ed. New York: McGraw-Hill, 2005: 856.)

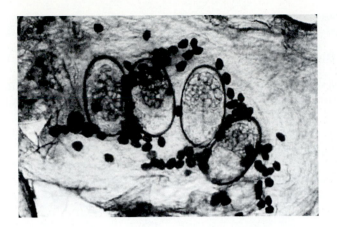

**FIGURE 10.21.** **Eggs and fecal pellets of the scabies mite found in skin scrapings under light microscopy.**

(Reproduced, with permission, from Tierney LM et al. *Current Medical Diagnosis & Treatment*, 45th ed. New York: McGraw-Hill, 2006.)

### TREATMENT

- Apply permethrin 5% below the neck. Leave on for eight hours and shower off. May be repeated in one week.
- Wash clothes and linens in hot water.
- STDs should be excluded.
- Consider treating family members who sleep in the same room.

## Pediculosis

Skin infection by lice. Lice do not transmit disease; their main effect is one of embarrassment. The female louse lays eggs (nits) at the base of the hair that adhere to the hair shaft as it grows. Lice do not jump or fly and are not passed by pets. Head and body lice are interchangeable; genital lice ("crabs") are another species.

### SYMPTOMS/EXAM

- Transmitted by direct contact or by fomites. May affect the head, body, or genital region.
- Patients may be asymptomatic or may present with pruritus resulting from allergy to lice saliva.
- Lice are visible to the naked eye and are 3–4 mm in size.

### DIAGNOSIS

Diagnosed by direct visualization on exam.

### TREATMENT

Permethrin 1% cream rinse is available OTC. Shampoo hair and towel dry. Apply permethrin cream rinse and rinse in 10 minutes. Treatment may be repeated in 7–10 days.

## Blistering Diseases

Pemphigus vulgaris and bullous pemphigoid are among the most common autoimmune blistering disorders. Table 10.4 outlines the presentation of both.

**TABLE 10.4.** Bullous Pemphigoid vs. Pemphigus Vulgaris

|  | BULLOUS PEMPHIGOID | PEMPHIGUS VULGARIS |
|---|---|---|
| Site of blistering | Subepidermal. | Intraepidermal. |
| Epidemiology | Affects patients > 60 years of age; the most common blistering disorder. | Affects patients 40–60 years of age. |
| Pruritus | Severe. | Not prominent. |
| Nikolsky's sign (superficial separation of skin with lateral pressure) | ⊖ | ⊕ |
| Frequency of oral mucosal lesions | Affect a minority of patients (< 30%). | Affect > 50% of patients. |
| Character of blisters and bullae | Intact, tense (see Figure 10.22). | Rupture easily; flaccid (see Figure 10.23) |
| Complications | Few complications. | Superinfection; high mortality from sepsis if untreated; ocular involvement dictates a referral. |
| Subtypes |  | Drug induced (penicillamine and ACEIs), paraneoplastic. |

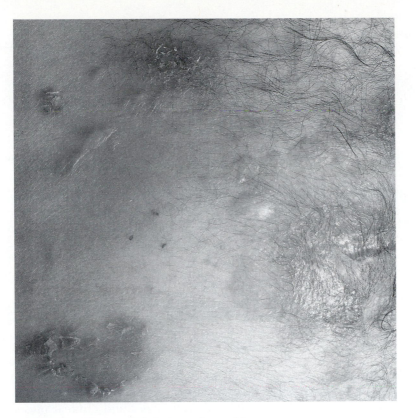

**FIGURE 10.22.** **Characteristic lesions of pemphigus.**

(Reproduced, with permission, from Wolff K et al. *Fitzpatrick's Color Atlas & Synopsis of Clinical Dermatology*, 5th ed. New York: McGraw-Hill, 2005: 104.) (Also see Color Insert.)

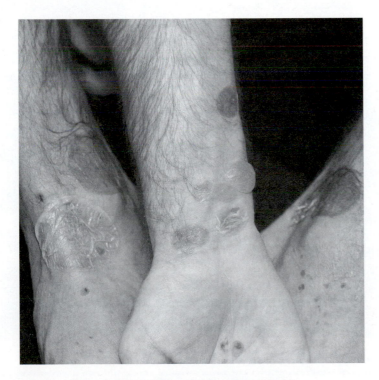

**FIGURE 10.23.** **Characteristic lesions of bullous pemphigoid.**

(Reproduced, with permission, from Wolff K et al. *Fitzpatrick's Color Atlas & Synopsis of Clinical Dermatology*, 5th ed. New York: McGraw-Hill, 2005: 108.) (Also see Color Insert.)

**TABLE 10.5.** Immunologic Mechanisms of Cutaneous Drug Reactions

| MECHANISM | EXAMPLES |
|---|---|
| Type I: classic immediate hypersensitivity | Urticaria, angioedema, anaphylaxis. |
| Type III: immune complex | Leukocytoclastic vasculitis, serum sickness, urticaria, angioedema. |
| Type IV: delayed hypersensitivity | Contact dermatitis, exanthematous reactions, photoallergic reactions. |
| Systemic infection impairing immune response | Mononucleosis, ampicillin-induced rash, HIV, sulfonamide-induced toxic epidermal necrolysis. |
| Unknown immunologic mechanisms | Lichenoid reactions, fixed drug eruptions. |

## CUTANEOUS DRUG REACTIONS

Mechanisms of dermatologic drug reactions may be immunologic (see Table 10.5) or nonimmunologic. Examples of nonimmunologic drug reactions include cutaneous phototoxicity with tetracycline use or the itching and erythema caused by mast cell mediator release in response to NSAIDs or radiographic contrast. Table 10.6 outlines the etiologies and clinical presentation of severe cutaneous drug reactions.

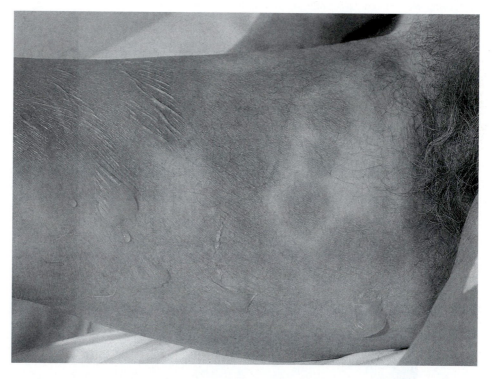

**FIGURE 10.24.** Lesions of Stevens-Johnson syndrome.

(Reproduced, with permission, from Wolff K et al. *Fitzpatrick's Color Atlas & Synopsis of Clinical Dermatology*, 5th ed. New York: McGraw-Hill, 2005: 145.) (Also see Color Insert.)

TABLE 10.6. Differential Diagnosis of Severe Drug Reactions

| DIAGNOSIS | MUCOSAL LESION | TYPICAL SKIN LESION | FREQUENT SYMPTOMS AND SIGNS | OTHER UNRELATED CAUSES | DRUGS MOST OFTEN IMPLICATED |
|---|---|---|---|---|---|
| Stevens-Johnson syndrome | Erosions are usually at two or more sites. | Small blisters on dusky purpuric macules or atypical targets (see Figure 10.24). Rare areas of confluence may be seen. Involves detachment of 10% or less of body surface area (BSA). | Some 10–30% present with fever. | Postinfectious erythema multiforme major (acute dermatitis characterized by distinctive, fixed target lesions, seen in Figure 10.25; caused by HSV or *Mycoplasma*). | Sulfa drugs, phenytoin, carbamazepine, lamotrigine, allopurinol. |
| Toxic epidermal necrolysis | Same as above. | Individual lesions like those of Stevens-Johnson syndrome (see Figure 10.26). ⊕ Nikolsky's sign; large sheet of necrotic epidermis. Involves > 30% of BSA. | Fever is nearly universal. "Acute skin failure" and leukopenia are also seen. | Viral infections, immunization, chemicals, *Mycoplasma* pneumonia. | Same as above. |
| Anticonvulsant hypersensitivity syndrome | Infrequent. | Severe exanthems (may become purpuric); exfoliative dermatitis. | Some 30–50% of cases present with fever, lymph-adenopathy, hepatitis, nephritis, carditis, eosinophilia, and atypical lymphocytes. | Cutaneous lymphoma. | Anticonvulsants. |
| Serum sickness | Absent. | Morbilliform lesions, sometimes with urticaria. | Fever, arthralgias. | Infection. | |
| Anticoagulant-induced necrosis | Infrequent. | Erythema; then purpura and necrosis, especially of fatty areas. | Pain in affected areas. | DIC. | Warfarin. |
| Angioedema | Often involved. | Urticaria or swelling of the face. | Respiratory distress or cardiovascular collapse. | Insect stings, foods. | NSAIDs, ACEIs, penicillin. |

DERMATOLOGY

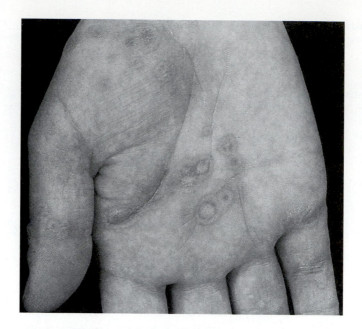

**FIGURE 10.25.** Lesions of erythema multiforme.

(Reproduced, with permission, from Wolff K et al. *Fitzpatrick's Color Atlas & Synopsis of Clinical Dermatology*, 5th ed. New York: McGraw-Hill, 2005: 141.) (Also see Color Insert.)

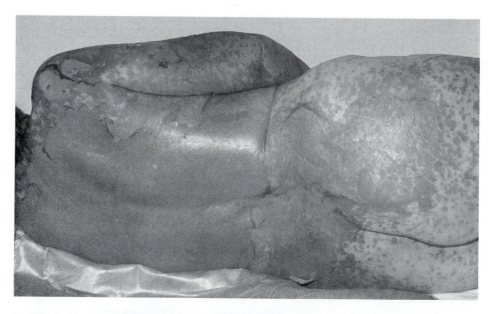

**FIGURE 10.26.** Lesions of toxic epidermal necrolysis.

(Reproduced, with permission, from Wolff K et al. *Fitzpatrick's Color Atlas & Synopsis of Clinical Dermatology*, 5th ed. New York: McGraw-Hill, 2005: 147.) (Also see Color Insert.)

## 1° Prevention of Skin Cancer

UVA and UVB both → photoaging, with UVB more commonly causing skin cancer. The following recommendations are for 1° prevention of skin damage and cancer:

- Minimize sun exposure during peak UVB midday hours (10–4 P.M.).
- Use sunscreen with at least SPF 15. Sunscreens should contain zinc oxide or titanium dioxide to block both UVA and UVB.
- Use wide-brimmed hats, sunglasses, and protective clothing.

## Atypical Nevi

- Benign growths sharing features of melanoma. Typically large (> 6 mm), hyperpigmented, and asymmetric, with irregular "fuzzy" borders ("fried egg" appearance).
- Sx/Exam:
  - Lesions may occur anywhere on the body but are more common in sun-exposed areas (e.g., the back).
  - Have variable appearance, but usually show the **ABCDE** appearance (see mnemonic).
- DDx: Melanoma.
- Tx: Excisional biopsy only if melanoma is suspected.
- Complications: The incidence of melanoma is ↑ in patients with atypical nevi.

> **The ABCDEs of skin cancer:**
>
> **A**symmetry
> **B**orders
> **C**olor
> **D**iameter
> **E**volution

## Melanoma

A malignancy of melanocytes that may occur on any skin or mucosal surface. It is the seventh most common cancer in the United States, with the incidence doubling every 10 years. Superficial spreading melanoma (which makes up 70% of cases) tends to stay "superficial" and has a better prognosis than nodular melanoma (15%), which tends to grow downward. Risk factors are expressed in the mnemonic **MMRISK**.

> **Malignant melanoma risk—**
>
> **MMRISK**
>
> **M**oles: atypical
> **M**oles: total number > 50
> **R**ed hair and freckling
> **I**nability to tan
> **S**evere sunburn, especially in childhood
> **K**indred: first-degree relative

### SYMPTOMS/EXAM

Presents with a changing mole (see Figure 10.27 and the mnemonic **ABCDE**) that may enlarge suddenly, begin to bleed, begin to itch, or become painful. May occur anywhere on the body, but more common in sun-exposed areas.

### DIFFERENTIAL

Atypical nevi; seborrheic keratosis.

### DIAGNOSIS

- Clinical exam and excisional biopsy.
- Tumor thickness (Breslow's classification) and lymph node spread are the most important prognostic factors.
- No staging workup is necessary if the lesion is < 1 mm in thickness, which is considered low risk.

### TREATMENT

- Excision with appropriate borders.
- Sentinel lymph node dissection for melanomas > 1 mm thick to determine if adjuvant therapy is needed.
- Close follow-up.

### COMPLICATIONS

Metastasis. Five-year survival rates with lymph node involvement and distant metastasis are 30% and 10%, respectively.

*The central face and ears are high-risk areas of ↑ recurrence and metastatic potential for basal cell carcinoma.*

## Basal Cell Carcinoma (BCC)

- The most common skin cancer (80%); occurs in sun-exposed areas, especially the central face and ears.
- **Sx/Exam:** Presents with a shiny "pearly" papule with an umbilicated center and telangiectasias (see Figure 10.28).
- **DDx:** Molluscum contagiosum.
- **Dx:** Shave biopsy.
- **Tx:** Excision or destruction (electrodesiccation and curettage) of the lesion. Patient education for sun avoidance is key to further prevention.
- **Complications:** Metastatic spread. Occurs in < 0.1% of patients.

## Actinic Keratosis

- A superficial keratotic lesion that is premalignant for squamous cell carcinoma. Prevention by avoidance of sun exposure is key.
- **Sx/Exam:** Presents as a discrete, reddish-pink keratotic lesion, usually with a white scale, that feels "rough" (see Figure 10.29). Found in sun-exposed areas, mostly on the face and dorsal hands.

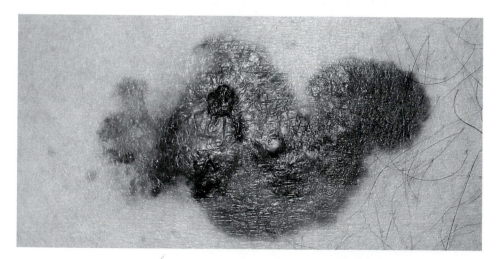

**FIGURE 10.27. Superficial spreading melanoma.**

A highly characteristic lesion with an irregular pigmented pattern and scalloped borders. (Reproduced, with permission, from Wolff K et al. *Fitzpatrick's Color Atlas & Synopsis of Clinical Dermatology,* 5th ed. New York: McGraw-Hill, 2005: 318.) (Also see Color Insert.)

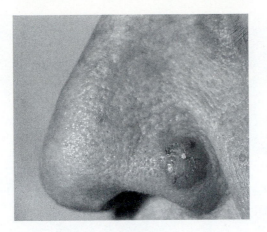

**FIGURE 10.28.** **Nodular basal cell carcinoma.**

A smooth, pearly nodule with telangiectasias. (Reproduced, with permission, from Wolff K et al. *Fitzpatrick's Color Atlas & Synopsis of Clinical Dermatology*, 5th ed. New York: McGraw-Hill, 2005: 283.) (Also see Color Insert.)

- **Dx:** Biopsy is not indicated. Diagnosed by clinical presentation on the basis of location and "rough" feel.
- **Tx:** Cryotherapy, topical 5-FU, or topical imiquimod.

### Squamous Cell Carcinoma (SCC)

- Represents 20% of all skin cancers. May arise within actinic keratoses, within HPV-induced lesions, and within burn and radiation scars. SCC is more common than BCC in immunocompromised individuals.

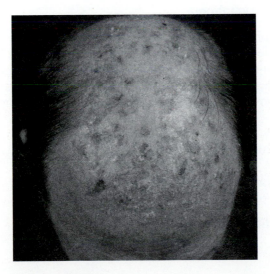

**FIGURE 10.29.** **Actinic keratosis.**

Multiple premalignant keratotic lesions on the bald scalp of this individual. (Reproduced, with permission, from Wolff K et al. *Fitzpatrick's Color Atlas & Synopsis of Clinical Dermatology*, 5th ed. New York: McGraw-Hill, 2005: 263.) (Also see Color Insert.)

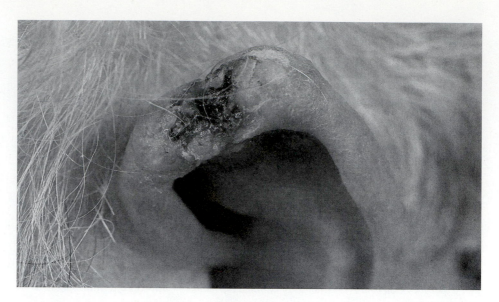

**FIGURE 10.30.** **Squamous cell carcinoma.**

A hyperkeratotic nodule with ulceration. (Reproduced, with permission, from Wolff K et al. *Fitzpatrick's Color Atlas & Synopsis of Clinical Dermatology*, 5th ed. New York: McGraw-Hill, 2005: 279.) (Also see Color Insert.)

*SCC is more common and more aggressive in the immunosuppressed.*

- **Sx/Exam:** Presents with a hyperkeratotic lesion with crusting and ulceration (see Figure 10.30). May occur anywhere, but most commonly seen in sun-exposed areas.
- **Tx:** Surgical excision with clear margins.
- **Cx:** Has a higher rate of metastasis than BCC. The five-year recurrence rate is 8% and the metastatic rate 5%.

## Cutaneous T-Cell Lymphoma

- **A T-cell lymphoma that begins in the skin;** the most common type is mycosis fungoides. Most often affects patients > 50 years of age. Twice as common in men and more common in African-Americans.
- **Sx/Exam:** Presents with pruritic, eczematous patches and plaques distributed over non-sun-exposed areas of skin. Tumors develop later in the disease course.
- **Cx:** Sézary syndrome is the leukemic form of T-cell lymphoma. Without treatment, patients succumb to opportunistic infections.

### MISCELLANEOUS DERMATOLOGIC DISORDERS

## Disorders Affecting the Hair

Table 10.7 outlines dermatologic disorders of the hair.

## Keloid

- A hypertrophic scar that is more common in those of African-American ethnicity.
- **Tx:** Intralesional corticosteroid injections. Surgical excision is **not** recommended, as lesions can recur larger than before.

TABLE 10.7.    Dermatologic Disorders Affecting the Hair

| DISORDER | HISTORY/EXAM | TREATMENT |
|---|---|---|
| Androgenic alopecia | Hereditary; affects those between 12 and 40, presenting with gradual progression of hair loss over the temple and crown area. | Topical minoxidil; finasteride. |
| Alopecia areata | Nonscarring autoimmune alopecia characterized by well-demarcated patches of hair loss. | Local steroid injection; topical steroids. |
| Telogen effluvium | Diffuse loss of scalp, axillary, and pubic hair occurring 2–4 months after an inciting event (psychological stressors, major surgery, postpartum, crash diets, endocrine disorders). | Treat the underlying cause. |
| Traction alopecia | Alopecia occurring in high-tension hair styles (tight braids, ponytails). May be permanent. | Change in hair style. |

## Melasma

- Splotchy hyperpigmented macules that affect sun-exposed areas of skin, most commonly on the face (see Figure 10.31). The cause is unknown.
- More common in women and darker-skinned persons (especially Hispanics).
- **Tx:** Topical therapy (hydroquinone cream) and strict sunscreen application. Can be chronic, but if associated with pregnancy it will usually regress within a year. If patients fail to respond, refer to a dermatologist for chemical peel or bleaching agents.

*Melasma occurs in 75% of pregnancies.*

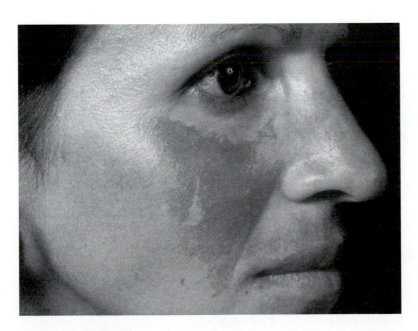

**FIGURE 10.31.    Melasma.**

Well-demarcated, hyperpigmented macules are seen on the cheek, nose, and upper lip. (Reproduced, with permission, from Wolff K et al. *Fitzpatrick's Color Atlas & Synopsis of Clinical Dermatology*, 5th ed. New York: McGraw-Hill, 2005: 349.) (Also see Color Insert.)

DERMATOLOGY

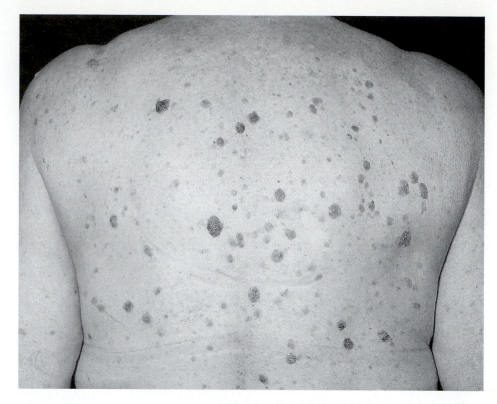

**FIGURE 10.32.** **Seborrheic keratosis.**

Multiple seborrheic keratoses with a "stuck-on" appearance are seen on the back. (Reproduced, with permission, from Wolff K et al. *Fitzpatrick's Color Atlas & Synopsis of Clinical Dermatology*, 5th ed. New York: McGraw-Hill, 2005: 207.) (Also see Color Insert.)

## Seborrheic Keratosis

- The most common benign epidermal growth.
- **Sx/Exam:** Usually asymptomatic; has a classic "stuck-on" appearance (see Figure 10.32).
- **Tx:** No treatment is necessary, but they can be frozen or excised if bothersome.

# CHAPTER 11

# Neurology

Tina Brueschke, MD, MHSA

NEUROLOGY

## Migraine Headache

Characterized as migraine without aura (formerly known as common migraine) and migraine with aura (also known as classic migraine). Onset is commonly between the ages of 10 and 30.

*Migraines are more common in women than in men.*

### SYMPTOMS/EXAM

- **Migraine without aura (common migraine):**
    - Recurrent headaches of 4–72 hours' duration with at least two of the following: **unilateral** distribution, **pulsatile** quality, severity limiting daily activities, and exacerbation by physical activity.
    - One of the following must also be present: **nausea** or **vomiting, photosensitivity,** and sensitivity to noise or smell.
- **Migraine with aura (classic migraine):**
    - Presents as described above, but with **headache preceded by an aura**—a reversible symptom indicative of focal cerebral dysfunction.
    - Aura symptoms include gradual onset and spread of scotomas, scintillations and/or hemianopic field defects, unilateral paresthesias or numbness, unilateral weakness, and speech disturbance. Symptoms may "march" from one area to another.
    - The elderly may have aura symptoms with gradual onset and spread without subsequent headache.
- Neurologic exam is generally normal.

### DIFFERENTIAL

Other forms of headache, intracranial mass, temporal (giant cell) arteritis, sinusitis, SAH, pseudotumor cerebri, TIA.

### DIAGNOSIS

Based on symptoms, a ⊕ family history, and lack of neurologic findings.

### TREATMENT

- **Acute attacks:** NSAIDs, triptans, ergotamines, narcotic analgesics, antinausea medications.
- **Prophylaxis:** β-blockers, calcium channel blockers, TCAs, anticonvulsants, methysergide. Avoidance or mitigation of triggers such as stress, missed meals, menses, and sleep deprivation.

### COMPLICATIONS

- Associated risk of rebound headaches with frequent analgesic use.
- Rarely may have lasting neurologic deficits.
- Migraine is a risk factor for stroke.

## Tension Headache

- The most common type of recurring headache.
- Sx/Exam:
    - Presents as a bilateral headache with pain in the frontal and occipital regions in a **bandlike distribution.** Exacerbated by stress, fatigue, glare, or noise.

- Often involves contraction of the scalp and posterior neck muscles.
- Neurologic exam is normal.
- **Dx:** Based on the history and lack of neurologic findings.
- **Tx:**
  - **Acute headache:** Aspirin, NSAIDs, ergotamines.
  - **Prophylaxis:** TCAs, SSRIs, β-blockers, relaxation techniques.
- **Cx:** Risk of rebound headaches with frequent analgesic use.

## Cluster Headache

- Occurs most often in middle-age men.
- **Sx/Exam:**
  - Recurrent, **unilateral, excruciating periorbital headaches** lasting from 15 minutes up to three hours. Headaches are nonpulsatile and constant.
  - Frequently occur at night.
  - Associated with **ipsilateral conjunctival injection** and **lacrimation**, nasal congestion, and Horner's syndrome (see Figure 11.1).
  - Recurrences take place in groups over days to weeks, occurring at the same time of day and in the same location.
  - Neurologic exam is usually normal.
- **DDx:** Migraine, glaucoma, sinusitis, uveitis, trigeminal neuralgia.
- **Dx:**
  - Based on the history and lack of neurologic findings. Often there is no family history of headache.
  - Consider a head CT or MRI for new headache onset after age 30.

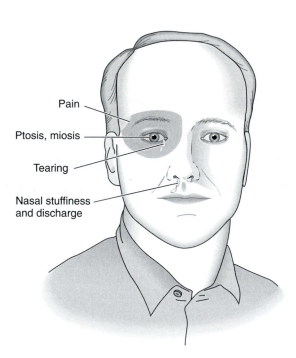

**FIGURE 11.1.  Symptoms of cluster headache.**

(Reproduced, with permission, from Aminoff M et al. *Clinical Neurology*, 6th ed. New York: McGraw-Hill, 2005: 91.)

- **Tx:**
    - **Acute attack:** 100% $O_2$, triptans, ergotamines, intranasal lidocaine, butorphanol.
    - **Prophylaxis:** Prednisone burst and taper following an episode to prevent acute recurrences. Other medications used are lithium, ergotamines, valproate, calcium channel blockers, and methysergide.
    - **Avoidance of triggers:** Alcohol, stress, vasodilating medications.
- **Cx:** Horner's syndrome. The severity of pain has driven some to suicide.


## Rebound Headache

- Chronic or nearly daily headache associated with **frequent use of medication for acute head pain.**
- **Sx/Exam:**
    - Presents with bilateral head pain in a bandlike distribution around the head, neck, and scalp.
    - Muscle contraction, tenderness, and photosensitivity are also seen. Neurologic exam is normal.
- **Dx:** Based on the history and lack of neurologic findings.
- **Tx:**
    - Discontinue the analgesics causing the rebound headaches.
    - **Acute attack:** Treat headaches during withdrawal with triptans or ergotamines.
    - **Prophylaxis:** TCAs, SSRIs, β-blockers, anticonvulsants.
    - Avoid headache triggers. Stretching, aerobic exercise, and relaxation techniques may be of benefit.
- **Cx:** One-third of patients relapse into analgesic overuse pattern.


## Post-traumatic Headache

- Commonly occurs following minor head injuries or hyperextension-flexion injuries ("whiplash"). Usually resolves in weeks to months.
- **Sx/Exam:**
    - Presents with a generalized constant headache associated with impaired attention, concentration, and memory. Onset is < 2 weeks from trauma.
    - Symptoms may become persistent within several weeks of injury. Acute cases last < 8 weeks. Chronic post-traumatic headache lasts > 8 weeks.
    - Dizziness, nausea, irritability, insomnia, and ↓ light and sound tolerance may also be seen.
    - Neurologic exam is typically normal.
- **DDx:** Migraine; tension headache; intracranial infection, mass, or bleed.
- **Dx:** Based on the history and a normal neurologic exam with a normal head CT and LP (if performed).
- **Tx:**
    - Supportive care; pain management.
    - Antiemetics and TCAs may be of benefit.
- **Cx:** ↓ patient functionality.

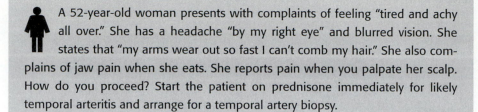

A 52-year-old woman presents with complaints of feeling "tired and achy all over." She has a headache "by my right eye" and blurred vision. She states that "my arms wear out so fast I can't comb my hair." She also complains of jaw pain when she eats. She reports pain when you palpate her scalp. How do you proceed? Start the patient on prednisone immediately for likely temporal arteritis and arrange for a temporal artery biopsy.

### Temporal Arteritis (Giant Cell Arteritis)

A treatable neurologic emergency characterized by subacute inflammation of the external carotid arterial system and vertebral arteries. **Most cases occur in women > 50 years of age.**

#### SYMPTOMS/EXAM

- Presents with temporal or diffuse headache unlike any the patient has had before, along with **transient visual loss, scalp tenderness, jaw claudication,** fever, myalgia, malaise, anorexia, weight loss, tenderness, and stiffness in the shoulders and hips.
- On exam, the temporal arteries may be dilated, tender, thickened, and nonpulsatile.
- Funduscopic exam may reveal a pale optic disk on the affected side. Cranial neuropathies are common.

#### DIFFERENTIAL

Glaucoma, uveitis, rheumatoid arthritis (RA), trigeminal neuralgia, retinal embolism, Takayasu's arteritis.

#### DIAGNOSIS

- Diagnosis is guided by the history and exam. History may reveal coexisting polymyalgia rheumatica.
- Biopsy of affected temporal arteries shows vasculitis with mononuclear cell infiltration or granulomatous inflammation.
- An ESR > 50 mm/hr is common (although rare cases may show a normal ESR). Normochromic, normocytic anemia with thrombocytosis is also common.

#### TREATMENT

Prednisone 60 mg daily for 1–2 months with slow taper and monitoring of symptoms and ESR. Aspirin ↓ the risk of stroke or visual loss.

#### COMPLICATIONS

Fifty percent of untreated patients suffer permanent visual loss, with half experiencing bilateral loss. Temporal arteritis is also associated with a risk of cranial neuropathy, TIA, stroke, and thoracic aortic aneurysm.

*"A sed rate over 50 in a patient over 50"–temporal arteritis.*

NEUROLOGY

An obese 37-year-old woman presents with headaches that worsen with lifting heavy objects and "ringing of the ears." She has also noted blurry vision. Exam shows limited abduction of her left eye, and funduscopy reveals optic disk swelling and hard exudates. How do you proceed, and what is the likely diagnosis? She is sent to the hospital for a head CT and an LP, which confirm the diagnosis of pseudotumor cerebri.

### Benign Intracranial Hypertension (Pseudotumor Cerebri)

A disorder consisting of **headache, ↑ ICP, and papilledema** unexplained by any other identifiable cause. The disorder is usually idiopathic and typically affects obese, hirsute-appearing young women.

#### SYMPTOMS/EXAM

- Presents with diffuse headaches that may worsen on straining.
- Visual loss or diplopia, transient visual obscurations, pulsatile tinnitus, limited abduction of one or both eyes, and ↓ level of consciousness are also seen.
- Funduscopic exam shows papilledema (see Figure 11.2). Visual function testing reveals an ↑ physiologic blind spot. Severe cases have constricted visual fields and ↓ acuity.

#### DIFFERENTIAL

Intracranial mass or bleed, hydrocephalus, dural venous thrombosis, migraine, glaucoma. Associated causative factors include hypervitaminosis A, hypoparathyroidism, Addison's disease, and medications (e.g., corticosteroids, tetracycline, OCPs).

#### DIAGNOSIS

- Findings include papilledema with possible abducens nerve palsy.
- Head CT or MRI may be normal or may show **slit-like ventricles.**
- LP shows elevated opening pressure with a normal CSF profile.

*Pseudotumor cerebri patients are typically **F**at, **F**emale, **F**ertile, and (under) **F**orty.*

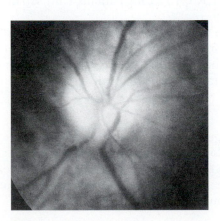

**FIGURE 11.2. Papilledema.**

(Reproduced, with permission, from Ropper A, Brown RH. *Adams and Victor's Principles of Neurology*, 8th ed. New York: McGraw-Hill, 2005: 212.)

NEUROLOGY

335

- Cerebral angiography or magnetic resonance venogram shows no dural sinus thrombosis.

### TREATMENT

- Start acetazolamide with or without a diuretic.
- Discontinue contributing medications or excessive vitamin A.
- Initiate corticosteroid treatment, especially if symptoms arose on withdrawal from corticosteroids.
- Repeated LPs or lumboperitoneal shunting for refractory cases. Weight reduction.

### COMPLICATIONS

Optic atrophy; permanent visual loss.

## Intracranial Arteriovenous Malformation (AVM)

Congenital abnormal connections between arterioles and venules without intervening capillaries. Usually **discovered on hemorrhage** of the malformation or related aneurysm. Most are supratentorial and are found by age 40.

### SYMPTOMS/EXAM

- Presents with persistent generalized or stereotyped unilateral headaches or seizure.
- Neurologic exam is usually normal without hemorrhage but may show progressive focal neurologic signs.
- Hemorrhage may be accompanied by an abnormal mental state, signs of meningeal irritation, seizure, signs of ↑ ICP, hemiparesis or paralysis, aphasia, and ↓ sensation.

### DIFFERENTIAL

Migraines, cluster headaches, intracranial mass, epilepsy, stroke, SAH, cerebral aneurysm, amyloid angiopathy.

### DIAGNOSIS

- Obtain an MRI/MRA. EEG for patients with seizure; head CT if hemorrhage is suspected.
- Perform an LP to examine CSF for blood if hemorrhage is suspected and CT is not diagnostic.
- Arteriography if hemorrhage, aneurysm, or AVM is detected (see Figure 11.3) or if the source remains unclear.

### TREATMENT

- Stop any anticoagulant or antiplatelet medications.
- Anticonvulsants for seizure activity.
- Neurosurgery for hemorrhage in patients with a reasonable life expectancy and an accessible lesion. Embolization or polymer occlusion of surgically inaccessible lesions.

### COMPLICATIONS

Headaches, hemorrhage, focal neurologic deficits, seizures, hydrocephalus.

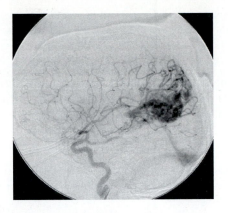

**FIGURE 11.3.** **Arteriovenous malformation.**

(Reproduced, with permission, from Ropper A, Brown RH. *Adams and Victor's Principles of Neurology*, 8th ed. New York: McGraw-Hill, 2005: 724.)

## Diagnosis of Dangerous Causes of Headache

Table 11.1 summarizes signs of underlying organic causes of headaches in the absence of other diagnostic features.

**TABLE 11.1.** **Presentation of Dangerous Causes of Headaches**

| SYMPTOM | POSSIBLE CAUSE |
|---|---|
| Sudden onset of "the worst headache of my life" | SAH. |
| Neck stiffness with severe headache | Bacterial meningitis. |
| Sudden ↓ level of consciousness | Intracranial bleed, intracranial mass. |
| Progressively worsening headache | Intracranial mass. |
| Daily headaches that awaken the patient from sleep or are severe on arising in the morning | Intracranial mass with ↑ ICP. (Migraine is the most common cause of morning headache.) |
| Onset of headaches after age 30 | Intracranial mass. |
| Progressive visual, motor, or balance disturbance | Intracranial mass, vascular lesion. |
| Onset of headache after age 50 | Temporal arteritis, intracranial mass. |

*Eighty-five percent of strokes are ischemic.*

*The risk of stroke doubles for each decade over age 55.*

*A head CT may not show ischemic lesions for the first 24–48 hours.*

NEUROLOGY

### Ischemic Stroke

Defined as a sudden brain dysfunction with **neurologic deficits lasting > 24 hours** resulting from occlusion of a vessel supplying the brain. Lacunar infarct is strongly associated with poorly controlled hypertension or diabetes.

#### SYMPTOMS/EXAM

- Presents with acute or abrupt onset of focal or multifocal neurologic symptoms that correlate with the area of the brain supplied by the affected arteries.
- Motor weakness, sensory deficits, ↓ reflexes, and mental status changes can occur.
- Cardiovascular exam may show a contributing arrhythmia or carotid or abdominal artery bruits.
- Common lacunar infarct syndromes include clumsy hand dysarthria, pure motor hemiparesis, pure hemisensory loss, and ataxic hemiparesis. The symptoms of some of these syndromes do not appear to follow classical neuroanatomy.
- Table 11.2 outlines the presentation of common stroke syndromes.

#### DIFFERENTIAL

Seizure, complicated migraine, subdural hematoma, dural sinus thrombosis, Bell's palsy, MS, intracranial mass, CNS infection, CNS inflammation, CNS arteritis.

#### DIAGNOSIS

- **Noncontrast CT:**
  - Ischemic lesions do not usually appear during the first 24–48 hours after stroke.
  - Lesions appear slightly hypodense (dark) when first seen and become more hypodense (darker) with evolution.
  - Lacunar infarcts may not be seen or may appear as small hypodense lesions.
- **MRI:** Shows ischemic changes within hours of the event as well as small infarcts missed by CT. Offers better visualization of the posterior fossa than CT.
- **Carotid and transcranial ultrasound or MRA plus ECG and echocardiogram with bubble study:** To assess for a cardioembolic source.

**TABLE 11.2. Key Stroke Syndromes**

| LEFT (DOMINANT) HEMISPHERE | RIGHT (NONDOMINANT) HEMISPHERE | BRAIN STEM | CEREBELLUM |
|---|---|---|---|
| Left gaze preference | Right gaze preference | Hemiparesis or quadriparesis | Gait ataxia |
| Aphasia | Neglect (of the left side) | Sensory loss in hemibody or all limbs | Truncal ataxia |
| Right visual field deficit | Left visual field deficit | Ipsilateral face and contralateral body | Ipsilateral limb ataxia |
| Right hemiparesis | Left hemiparesis | symptoms | Neck stiffness |
| Right hemisensory loss | Left hemisensory loss | Disconjugate gaze | |
| | | Dysphagia | |
| | | ↓ consciousness | |

- **Cerebral angiography:** The "gold standard" of cerebrovascular imaging. Shows the site and severity of occlusive disease. Also shows intracranial artery dissection if present.
- **Hypercoagulable workup:** Appropriate if the patient is < 55 years of age or has associated signs, symptoms, or risk factors.

### TREATMENT

- **Stabilize the patient:** Assess the airway. Avoid hypotonic IV fluids to prevent worsening cerebral edema.
- Bed rest to avoid orthostatic hypotension.
- **Antiplatelet therapy:** Give aspirin and/or clopidogrel.
- **Anticoagulation:**
  - Rule out coagulopathy.
  - Check a head CT for intracranial hemorrhage.
  - Heparin is relatively contraindicated in large infarcts with mass effect or hemorrhagic conversion. Warfarin may be given on an outpatient basis for cardioembolic events.
- **IV thrombolytic therapy:**
  - Potential tPA candidates can receive tPA within three hours of initiation of stroke symptoms. Most inclusion and exclusion criteria focus on the risk of bleeding. Head CT must show no hemorrhage, and bleeding disorders must be ruled out.
  - If the patient is not a tPA candidate and has no bleeding disorder, start antiplatelet therapy.
- Transient monocular blindness (amaurosis fugax) requires ophthalmologic evaluation.
- Elevated BP should be aggressively treated **only in a hypertensive emergency.**
- Discontinue any contributing hormone or oral contraceptive medications.
- **Carotid endarterectomy:** For 2° prevention if ipsilateral carotid artery stenosis is > 70%.
- **Speech and physical therapy;** swallow study before diet is started.

*Stroke is the third leading cause of death in the United States.*

### COMPLICATIONS

Cerebral edema with mass effect, hemorrhagic transformation, MI, aspiration pneumonia, disability, DVT, depression, death.

## Intracerebral Hemorrhage (ICH)

Defined as a rupture or aneurysm of an intracerebral artery that causes direct pressure on part of brain and ↑ ICP. **Hypertensive ICH is the most common subtype and evolves rapidly.** Can rupture into ventricles → potential for life-threatening transtentorial herniation. Risk factors include **male gender, age > 55, high alcohol intake,** anticoagulation, and uncontrolled DM.

*Hypertensive ICH evolves rapidly.*

### SYMPTOMS/EXAM

- Presents with sudden severe headache, nausea, vomiting, and a ↓ level of consciousness.
- Rapid onset of focal neurologic symptoms is seen.
- Meningeal irritation is possible and may → stiff neck (nuchal rigidity), leg pain, and low back pain. Papilledema may also be seen.

**NEUROLOGY**

### DIFFERENTIAL

Ischemic stroke, SAH, seizure, subdural or epidural hematoma, dural sinus thrombosis, intracranial mass, CNS infection, CNS inflammation.

### DIAGNOSIS

- CT shows **immediate high-density (bright) lesions in the brain parenchyma** (see Figure 11.4).
- In the presence of ventricle enlargement, consider neurosurgical ventriculostomy. Large cerebellar hemorrhages are rapidly fatal.
- Check bleeding times, platelet count, toxicology screen, and chem 12.

### TREATMENT

- **Neurosurgery:** Appropriate for any contributing treatable AVM, aneurysm, or excisable tumor or for decompression of superficial intracerebral hematomas. Can be lifesaving in the presence of a large cerebellar hemorrhage.
- Treat ↑ ICP with mannitol, hyperventilation, and cooling blankets.
- Supportive care; speech and physical therapy. Conduct a swallow study before diet is started.

### COMPLICATIONS

Permanent disability; mortality.

*Most nontraumatic SAHs are due to rupture of a saccular aneurysm.*

## Subarachnoid Hemorrhage (SAH)

Acute bleed into the subarachnoid space commonly resulting from trauma or rupture of an aneurysm, an AVM, or a neoplasm. The associated headache is often described as **"the worst headache of my life."**

### SYMPTOMS/EXAM

- Presents with sudden severe headache and nuchal rigidity.

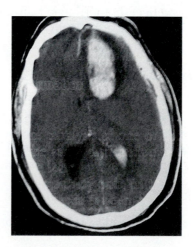

**FIGURE 11.4. Large frontal intracerebral hemorrhage.**

(Reproduced, with permission, from Stone C et al. *Current Emergency Diagnosis and Treatment*, 5th ed. New York: McGraw-Hill, 2004: 374.)

- Kernig's sign (passive extension of a flexed knee producing pain and resistance) and Brudzinski's sign (passive flexion of the neck causing flexion of the hips and knees) may be ⊕. Also associated with a ↓ level of consciousness.
- Nausea, vomiting, confusion, and irritability may be seen. Photophobia and visual disturbances are common.
- Focal neurologic deficits may be present, including cranial nerve palsies. Seizure is possible.
- Papilledema may be found on funduscopy.

### DIFFERENTIAL

Meningitis, ICH, ischemic stroke, migraine, hypertensive emergency, TIA, temporal arteritis.

### DIAGNOSIS

- **Head CT:** May show **hemorrhage into the subarachnoid space** (see Figure 11.5).
- **LP:** If the CT is normal but SAH is still suspected, obtain an LP to examine CSF for xanthochromia or blood.
- Cerebral arteriography can show the source when the patient is stable.
- Check for a history of Ehlers-Danlos syndrome, Marfan's syndrome, or polycystic kidney disease.

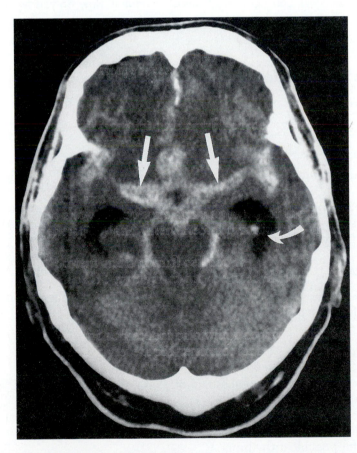

**FIGURE 11.5.    Subarachnoid hemorrhage.**

(Reproduced, with permission, from Tintinalli JE et al. *Emergency Medicine: A Comprehensive Study Guide,* 6th ed. New York: McGraw-Hill, 2004: 1445.)

### TREATMENT

- **Stabilize the patient:** Give IV osmotic agents or diuretics for suspected herniation.
- **Neurosurgery:** Appropriate for any contributing treatable AVM, aneurysm, or excisable tumor. Emergent decompression can be lifesaving for a large cerebellar infarct or hemorrhage.
- **Consider seizure prophylaxis:** Phenytoin is the usual choice.
- **Treat hypertension:** Gradually treat mean arterial BP > 130 mmHg but maintain SBP > 120 mmHg.
- Give analgesics and antiemetics. Advise patients to avoid exertion or straining.
- Recommend bedrest and smoking cessation.

### COMPLICATIONS

Rebleeding, stroke.

---

A 69-year-old man who takes "water pills" but "misses one here and there" presents to the ER with sudden right-sided arm and leg weakness and slurred speech. As his head CT is being arranged, he begins to regain function of his right arm and leg. When his CT is done, he clearly states, "I feel much better now. Can I go?" His head CT is normal. How do you proceed? Inform the patient that he has had a TIA and needs more tests.

---

## Transient Ischemic Attack (TIA)

Abrupt onset of focal neurologic symptoms **lasting < 24 hours** and often lasting only 5–20 minutes.

### SYMPTOMS/EXAM

- Multiple neurologic deficits related to a single "focus" of brain involvement.
- Transient monocular blindness (amaurosis fugax) and other visual disturbances can occur. Vertigo, diplopia, ataxia, and dysarthria are possible.
- Focal neurologic symptoms resolve within 24 hours.

### DIFFERENTIAL

Ischemic stroke, ICH, SAH, seizure, hypoglycemia, syncope, Bell's palsy, complicated migraine.

### DIAGNOSIS

- Head CT shows no acute changes.
- Check platelets, blood glucose, cholesterol, homocysteine level, and RPR for syphilis.
- Check a carotid duplex ultrasound and an echocardiogram for possible embolic sources or carotid stenosis.
- ECG for possible arrhythmia.

## TREATMENT

- **Antiplatelet therapy:** Aspirin and/or clopidogrel.
- **Anticoagulation:** For cases with a cardiac source of embolization. Rule out coagulopathy. Start IV heparin and switch to warfarin on an outpatient basis.
- **Carotid endarterectomy:** For carotid stenosis > 70% on the side of the source.
- **Treat contributing factors:** Arrhythmias, hyperlipidemia, hypertension, hyperviscosity, DM, arteritis. Recommend smoking cessation.

## COMPLICATIONS

Recurrent symptoms; risk for stroke.

## CEREBRAL LOBE DYSFUNCTIONS

## Aphasias

Acquired language disorders. Major aphasias are described as follows:

- **Broca's aphasia:** Speech that is **nonfluent, effortful,** sparse, and monotone. Also associated with impaired naming, repetition, and writing. **Comprehension is generally preserved.** The patient is often aware of the deficit. Right hemiparesis and depression are common.
- **Wernicke's aphasia:** **Fluent, possibly excessive** speech with frequent paraphasias and normal articulation. Also characterized by **impaired comprehension** of reading and speech as well as deficits in reading, writing, naming, and repetition. A right visual field cut may be present.
- **Global aphasia:** Involves impairment of all language functions, often accompanied by lethargy, right hemiparesis, hemisensory loss, apraxia, and visual field deficits.

> **W**ernicke's aphasia is **W**ord salad.
> **B**roca's aphasia speech is **B**roken and effortful.

## DIFFERENTIAL

Dementia, postconcussive syndrome, MS, partial status epilepticus.

## DIAGNOSIS

Diagnosis is based on neuropsychiatric evaluation and the clinical exam, including language functions such as repetition, spontaneous speech, comprehension, and naming.

## TREATMENT

Supportive care; speech therapy. Psychological support may be necessary.

## COMPLICATIONS

Those with deficits of comprehension (e.g., Wernicke's aphasia) have a poorer prognosis for functional improvement or recovery than do those with deficits of expression.

## Agnosia

Impaired recognition of familiar people or objects despite preservation of intelligence, attention, and perception. May involve visual, auditory, and/or tactile modalities. Subtypes are as follows:

- **Visual agnosia:** Inability to recognize familiar objects. May have an associated right visual deficit. Impairment may be limited to identification or discrimination of faces of known people (prosopagnosia), colors (color agnosia), known objects (object agnosia), or a whole item despite recognition of the parts (simultagnosia).
- **Auditory agnosia:** Inability to recognize familiar sounds despite the fact that hearing is intact. Impairment may be limited to words, environmental sounds, or music.
- **Astereognosia:** Inability to identify objects through tactile stimulation despite intact sensation of touch. Patients may be able to describe and draw an object and name it from its image in the drawing yet not recognize it through touch.

### DIFFERENTIAL

Dementia, mental retardation, postconcussive syndrome, Parkinson's disease.

### DIAGNOSIS

- Based on the exam, including language functions such as repetition, spontaneous speech, comprehension, and naming.
- MRI to examine for a possible underlying cause.

### TREATMENT

Supportive care. Treat any underlying condition.

## Dysarthria

- Poor articulation of appropriate words (slurred speech).
- **Sx/Exam:** Hoarseness and/or drooling may be seen. Reading comprehension and writing abilities remain intact.
- **DDx:** Developmental disability, postconcussive syndrome, dementia.
- **Dx:**
    - Based on the clinical exam, including normal language functions such as repetition, spontaneous speech, comprehension, and naming.
    - Head CT or MRI for any underlying cause.
- **Tx:** Speech and language therapy.

## Amnesias

Severe disturbance of retained memory with intact attention and language functions. Visuospatial functions are generally intact. These disturbances include the following:

- **Transient global amnesia:** Paroxysmal, **transient loss of recent memory** with preserved immediate recall and remote memory. Also involves impaired ability to retain new information. Confusion and anxiety are common, but **personal identity is retained.** Focal neurologic signs are absent. Typically lasts 30 minutes to 24 hours.
- **Korsakoff's syndrome:** Significant impairment of short-term memory with inability to form new memories and impaired remote memory. Patients have **apathy** and **lack of insight** into the disorder but are alert and responsive. Confabulation is common. Associated with peripheral neuropathy, hypothermia, nystagmus, and gait ataxia.

Seizure, TIA, conversion disorder, delirium, dementia, organic brain syndrome, malingering.

## DIAGNOSIS

- Based on the history and on the finding of anterograde amnesia with loss of recent memory. Otherwise neurologically normal in transient global amnesia. Peripheral neuropathy, nystagmus, and gait ataxia are present in Korsakoff's syndrome.
- Brain imaging to examine for an underlying condition.

## TREATMENT

- **Transient global amnesia:** Reassurance; neurology consult.
- **Korsakoff's syndrome:** Give thiamine prior to glucose to avoid precipitating Wernicke's encephalopathy → ataxia, ophthalmoplegia, nystagmus, and confusion. Recommend a recovery program for alcoholic patients.

## COMPLICATIONS

Korsakoff's syndrome → persistent vertical nystagmus, gait ataxia, and learning impairments.

*Transient global amnesia typically occurs in patients > 40 years of age.*

## SEIZURE

A mother brings her eight-year-old boy to the clinic because his teachers complain that he "daydreams too much" and has 20-second "staring spells" during which he stays still and does not react to anything said. He has good grades and many friends. His exam is unremarkable. How do you proceed? Suspecting absence seizures, you order an EEG.

Defined as a sudden change in neurologic function resulting from an abnormal, excessive, synchronous discharge of cortical neurons.

### Focal (Partial) Seizure

In **simple partial seizures,** patients preserve consciousness but may be aphasic. In **complex partial seizures,** consciousness is altered, there is amnesia for the event, and automatisms may be present. Focal seizures are further categorized according to location:

- **Temporal lobe seizure:**
  - The **most common seizure type in adults.**
  - Presents with unresponsive, quiet staring for 1–3 minutes.
  - Often **accompanied by an aura** (e.g., sensation of a particular smell, dizziness, nausea, or déjà vu).
  - Oral or ipsilateral manual automatisms may be present. Contralateral dystonic posturing of the arm and hand is common.
  - Postictal lethargy and confusion may last several minutes.
- **Frontal lobe seizure:**
  - Usually lasts 15–40 seconds without an aura or a postictal state.
  - Commonly occurs during sleep.

*Temporal lobe seizures are the most common seizures in adults.*

NEUROLOGY

- If the motor cortex is involved, rhythmic unilateral clonic activity may occur and spread across the body. Asymmetric tonic posturing is common with involvement of the supplemental motor area.
- **Occipital lobe seizure:**
    - Commonly begins with a visual aura that can range from spots or lights to formed visual hallucinations that are usually stereotyped from seizure to seizure.
    - May spread to the temporal lobe or to the motor cortex.

### DIFFERENTIAL

Syncope, orthostatic hypotension, hypoglycemia, hypoxia, migraine, TIA, panic attack, psychogenic seizure, narcolepsy, tics.

### DIAGNOSIS

- Obtain a detailed history of the event, prodromal symptoms, witnessed seizures, and postictal state. Evaluate for risk factors—e.g., head trauma, stroke, tumor, AVM, or a family history of seizures. Inquire if the event was preceded by sleep deprivation, stress, illness, medications, flickering lights, or stimuli.
- Check a CBC, a complete metabolic profile, and a toxicology screen as well as calcium, magnesium, alcohol, and ammonia levels.
- EEG and closed-circuit TV/EEG monitoring.
- MRI to elucidate the underlying cause.

### TREATMENT

- **Acute seizure:** Stabilize the patient. Administer lorazepam IV or IM; diazepam IV or per rectum in gel form; or midazolam IV or sublingually. Give glucose if the patient is hypoglycemic. Treat severe hypertension. Correct any metabolic causes.
- **Single, isolated seizure episode:** In the absence of risk factors, ongoing antiepileptic therapy is usually deferred. The recurrence rate is about 20%, and recurrences usually occur within one year.

### COMPLICATIONS

- May progress to a generalized tonic-clonic seizure.
- Falls and injuries. Patients are at risk for depression, anxiety, and psychosis.
- Side effects and drug interactions associated with antiepileptic medications.

## Generalized Seizure

Generalized seizures involve the whole brain and are categorized as follows:

- **Tonic-clonic (grand mal):**
    - No aura occurs. The tonic phase gradually progresses to a clonic phase, with each lasting about 30 seconds.
    - **Incontinence or tongue biting** may occur during the seizure.
    - The postictal state includes coarse breathing with gradual awakening over several minutes. Postictal acidosis with $\downarrow HCO_3$, $\uparrow CK$, and $\uparrow$ prolactin occurs within 30 minutes after a seizure.
- **Absence (petit mal):**
    - Sudden-onset **staring spells** usually **lasting about 10 seconds** with immediate recovery. Those lasting 20–30 seconds may also have simple automatisms.
    - **Eye fluttering** or altered postural tone is common and may occur many times per day.

- EEG shows **generalized spike-and-wave** discharges.
- Usually seen in neurologically normal **children 4–14 years of age.**
- **Myoclonic:**
  - Brief, **sharp muscle jerks** with no impairment of consciousness.
  - Movements may be symmetric, asymmetric, or multifocal.
  - EEG shows a **generalized polyspike-and-wave discharge.**
- **Tonic:**
  - Brief, sudden, bilateral, and symmetric tonic posturing with brief impairment of consciousness and rapid recovery.
  - EEG shows **sudden, diffuse low-voltage beta waves** or background attenuation.
  - Usually seen in neurologically abnormal patients.

*Absence seizures primarily affect patients 4–14 years of age.*

### DIFFERENTIAL

Syncope, psychogenic seizure, hypoglycemia, hypoxia, TIA, complex migraine, orthostatic hypotension, tics.

### DIAGNOSIS

- Obtain a detailed history of witnessed seizures that may be induced by sleep deprivation, stress, illness, medications, flickering lights, or stimuli. Look for a history of symptoms of prodrome, seizure, and/or postictal state. Evaluate for risk factors such as head trauma, stroke, tumor, AVM, or a family history of seizures.
- Check a CBC, a complete metabolic profile, and a toxicology screen as well as calcium, magnesium, alcohol, and ammonia levels.
- EEG and closed-circuit TV/EEG monitoring.
- MRI to determine the underlying cause.

### TREATMENT

- **Acute seizure:** Stabilize the patient. Administer lorazepam IV or IM; diazepam IV or per rectum in gel form; or midazolam IV or sublingually. Give glucose if the patient is hypoglycemic. Treat severe hypertension. Correct any metabolic causes.
- **Single, isolated seizure episode:** Ongoing antiepileptic therapy is usually deferred if there are no risk factors. The recurrence rate is about 20%. Recurrences usually occur in the first year.

### COMPLICATIONS

- Falls and injuries; accidental death due to impaired consciousness.
- ↑ risk of depression, anxiety, and psychosis.
- Side effects and drug interactions associated with antiepileptic medications.

*Most patients with > 3 seizure-free years on medication will not have recurrences.*

## Status Epilepticus

A neurologic emergency consisting of continuous seizure activity lasting > 10 minutes or repetitive seizures lasting > 30 minutes without a return to a baseline neurologic level between seizures.

### DIFFERENTIAL

Syncope, TIA, intracranial infection, migraine, hypoglycemia, Bell's palsy, psychogenic seizure.

### DIAGNOSIS

A clinical diagnosis in cases of sustained overt convulsions. An EEG may be needed for more subtle findings.

### TREATMENT

- Stabilize the patient and administer a loading dose and infusion of **fosphenytoin** with continuous ECG monitoring.
- If the patient is still seizing after 30 minutes, give a loading dose and infusion of phenobarbital. If seizing continues for 60 minutes, administer a pentobarbital loading dose and infusion.

### COMPLICATIONS

Respiratory failure, rhabdomyolysis, hyperthermia, neuronal cell damage.

## Epilepsy

- Epilepsy consists of a history of two or more unprovoked seizures due to underlying brain disease.
- **Sx/Exam:** History of recurrent seizures.
- **Dx:** Diagnosed by a history of recurrent, unprovoked seizures with documentation of seizure focus or an underlying brain lesion or disease.
- **Tx:**
  - Medication choice depends on seizure type. Generalized seizures should be treated with valproic acid; absence seizures with ethosuximide; and partial seizures with carbamazepine or phenytoin.
  - Antiepileptics are teratogenic. Perform a pregnancy test prior to starting any antiepileptic medication, and offer OCPs to young women.
  - Surgery to remove seizure foci is possible in many patients.
  - Ketogenic diets and vagal nerve stimulators are sometimes recommended.

*Most cases of epilepsy start before age 20.*

## CHRONIC DEGENERATIVE NEUROLOGIC DISORDERS

### Huntington's Disease

An **autosomal-dominant** disorder with gradual onset and progression of **chorea** and **dementia** usually starting between the ages of 35 and 50. Chromosome 4 shows excess **CAG trinucleotide repeats.**

### SYMPTOMS/EXAM

- Chorea, dystonia, tics, inhibitory pauses in voluntary movements, depression, and psychosis are common features.
- Also associated with irritability, moodiness, and antisocial behavior and later with dementia. Fidgetiness and restlessness may be seen early in the disease.

### DIFFERENTIAL

Wilson's disease, drug-induced tardive dyskinesia, Parkinson's disease, Sydenham's chorea, stroke, subdural hematoma, SLE.

### DIAGNOSIS

- Clinical suspicion is confirmed with genetic studies of the **HD (huntingtin) gene.** A family history usually elicits similar cases.
- A head CT shows cerebral and caudate nucleus atrophy (see Figure 11.6).

348

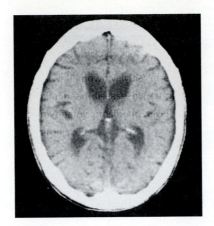

**FIGURE 11.6.** Cerebral and caudate nucleus atrophy in Huntington's disease.

(Reproduced, with permission, from Ropper A, Brown RH. *Adams and Victor's Principles of Neurology*, 8th ed. New York: McGraw-Hill, 2005: 912.)

### TREATMENT

- Supportive treatment. Dopamine receptor blockers for chorea symptoms; SSRIs to reduce aggression.
- Offer genetic counseling to family members.

### COMPLICATIONS

Usually fatal 10–20 years after clinical onset.

## Creutzfeldt-Jakob Disease

A **prion disease** characterized by **rapidly progressive dementia** in association with **diffuse myoclonic jerks.** Also known as subacute spongiform encephalopathy.

### SYMPTOMS/EXAM

- Presents with rapidly progressive dementia with late akinetic mutism and coma.
- Anxiety, **personality change,** depression, emotional lability, delusions, and hallucinations are also seen.
- Motor symptoms include myoclonus, cerebellar ataxia, rigidity, bradykinesia, tremor, chorea, and dystonia.

### DIFFERENTIAL

Alzheimer's disease, Parkinson's disease, progressive supranuclear palsy, intracerebral mass, hydrocephalus, multi-infarct dementia.

### DIAGNOSIS

- Definitive diagnosis is by immunodetection of the prion in brain tissue on biopsy.
- Brain MRI $T_2$-weighted images show hyperintense signals in the basal ganglia.
- EEG may show periodic sharp waves or spikes. CSF protein may be ↑.

*The dementia of Creutzfeldt-Jakob disease has rapid onset and progression.*

### TREATMENT

Treatment is supportive.

### COMPLICATIONS

Fatal within several months of diagnosis.

## SYNCOPE

Episodic loss of consciousness and postural tone with spontaneous recovery. Can occur with any global ↓ in cerebral perfusion. Incidence ↑ with age. **Vasovagal syncope is the most common subtype.** Cardiogenic syncope carries a worse prognosis.

*The most common form of syncope is vasovagal.*

### SYMPTOMS/EXAM

- Loss of consciousness with loss of postural tone and spontaneous recovery.
- Preceded by nausea, faintness, blurred vision, diaphoresis, vertigo, paresthesias, or pallor.
- **No post-event confusion.**
- Exam is likely unremarkable at the time of evaluation.

*Syncope has no post-event confusion.*

### DIFFERENTIAL

Stroke, TIA, seizure, hypoglycemia, benign paroxysmal positional vertigo (BPPV).

### DIAGNOSIS

- Check medications, activities, and position at the time of the event.
- Check for orthostatic BP changes.
- Tilt-table testing and the Valsalva maneuver are diagnostic for an orthostatic source.
- ECG for arrhythmia; echocardiogram for cardiac outlet obstruction.

### TREATMENT

Treat the underlying cause. Avoid precipitating factors and medications.

## PERIPHERAL POLYNEUROPATHIES

> A 41-year-old man comes to your office complaining of ↓ feeling and strength in both legs after he became acutely ill following dinner a few days ago. He also complains of "tingling" in his feet and some difficulty walking. Exam reveals ↓ lower extremity muscle strength with a lack of DTRs. The patient states that his arms now feel weaker as well. How do you proceed? You admit the patient to the hospital for monitoring of Guillain-Barré syndrome that progresses to require ventilation.

### Guillain-Barré Syndrome (Acute Idiopathic Polyneuropathy)

Symmetric, progressive ascending muscle weakness that usually starts in the legs and may be acute or subacute. The condition is life-threatening if

NEUROLOGY

respiratory or swallowing muscles are involved. Can follow minor infectious illness, inoculation, or surgical procedures. Carries a poorer prognosis when it follows *Campylobacter jejuni* infection.

### SYMPTOMS/EXAM

- The hallmark is **lack of DTRs.** Progressive weakness of two or more limbs typically begins with the proximal lower extremities.
- Shortness of breath, constipation, facial weakness, dysphagia, ophthalmoplegia, dysarthria, and sensory disturbances are commonly seen.
- Also associated with disturbances in BP, heart rate, and pulmonary function.
- Symptom progression halts in < 2–3 weeks.

### DIFFERENTIAL

Chronic inflammatory demyelinating polyneuropathy, HIV infection, transverse myelitis, intraspinal mass, porphyria, toxic neuropathy, poliomyelitis, botulism, tick paralysis, periodic paralysis syndrome.

### DIAGNOSIS

- CSF shows ↑ protein but a normal cell count, although sometimes this is not found in the first week.
- Electrophysiologic studies can show **marked slowing of motor and sensory conduction velocity** consistent with denervation and axonal loss.

### TREATMENT

- Plasmapheresis may improve recovery time and ↓ residual neurologic effects.
- IVIG is preferable in children and in cases involving cardiovascular instability.
- Symptomatic treatment. Severe cases should be monitored in the ICU.

### COMPLICATIONS

May have mild residual deficits. Relapse is possible years later. Fatal in 5% of cases.

## Chronic Inflammatory Demyelinating Polyneuropathy

- **Sx/Exam:** Presents with **relapsing or persistent ascending muscle weakness** beginning in the legs **without improvement after six months.** DTRs are absent. Paresthesias can develop, and fatigue is common.
- **Dx:** Diagnosed by electrophysiologic findings consistent with a demyelinating neuropathy with axonal degeneration. CSF protein is ↑ with a normal cell count.
- **Tx:** Treat with IVIG or plasma exchange. Often responds to long-term corticosteroids. Give azathioprine or cyclophosphamide if the patient is unresponsive to corticosteroids.

## BRACHIAL PLEXUS DISORDERS

Usually unilateral sensorimotor derangement attributable to one or more cords of the brachial plexus. Most cases have no apparent cause. May be due to trauma, radiation, infection, electrical injury, compression, or infiltration. Subtypes are as follows:

Guillain-Barré syndrome after a C. jejuni *infection is often severe.*

Corticosteroids can worsen Guillain-Barré symptoms.

NEUROLOGY

- **Whole plexus lesion:** The entire arm is paralyzed, with sensory loss complete past a line drawn from the shoulder to the middle third of the upper arm.
- **Upper brachial plexus paralysis:** Loss of shoulder abduction and elbow flexion. The affected arm is held internally rotated at the shoulder with the elbow extended and the forearm pronated. Sensory loss occurs over a small area of the deltoid muscle.
- **Lower brachial plexus paralysis:** Paralysis and wasting of the small muscles of the hand and of the long finger flexors and extensors → "claw hand" deformity. Sensory loss is found on the ulnar border of the hand and the inner forearm. Horner's syndrome is possible.
- **Lateral cord lesion:** Weakness of flexion and pronation of the forearm.
- **Medial cord lesion:** Combined median and ulnar nerve deficit. ↓ or absent hand sensation and finger flexor function are seen with atrophy of intrinsic hand muscles.
- **Posterior cord lesion:** Weakness of the deltoid muscle and extensors of the elbow, wrist, and fingers. Sensory loss is seen on the outer side of the arm.
- **Brachial neuritis:** Acute onset of excruciating and generally unilateral shoulder pain followed days later by weakness of shoulder and parascapular muscles. Numbness may also be seen.

### DIFFERENTIAL

Cervical radiculopathy, polymyalgia rheumatica, vertebral artery dissection.

### DIAGNOSIS

- Electrophysiologic testing of the affected muscles.
- AP and axillary lateral shoulder radiography for concerns of related fracture.
- MRI may reveal infiltrative processes.

### TREATMENT

- Physical/occupational therapy. Bracing prevents contractures.
- Possible surgery with nerve grafting and muscle or tendon transfers.
- Corticosteroids for brachial neuritis.

### COMPLICATIONS

Incomplete recovery. Chronic shoulder pain is possible in brachial neuritis.

## MONONEUROPATHIES

### Median Nerve Entrapment (Carpal Tunnel Syndrome)

Loss or impairment of superficial sensation in the palmar aspect of the thumb, the index finger, and often the radial half of the third finger.

*Nocturnal paresthesias in the median nerve distribution are classic for carpal tunnel syndrome.*

### SYMPTOMS/EXAM

- Presents with pain and paresthesias in the same distribution. **Symptoms ↑ at night.**
- Also characterized by thenar muscle weakness and atrophy. Abductor pollicis brevis and opponens pollicis muscle weakness is seen.
- Patients have a tendency to "flick" and wiggle the fingers in attempts to relieve **paresthesias.**
- **Tinel's** and **Phalen's signs** may be ⊕.

- Based on the history and exam. Check for a history of repetitive hand movements.
- Electrophysiologic studies can show slowing of sensory or motor conduction velocity at the wrist.
- Check for underlying conditions such as pregnancy, hyperparathyroidism, diabetes, amyloidosis, RA, sarcoidosis, acromegaly, or recent or poorly healed fractures.

*TREATMENT*

- Treat with NSAIDs, rest, vitamin $B_6$, nocturnal wrist splinting, and possible surgical decompression. Local corticosteroid injections can sometimes provide temporary relief.
- Treat any underlying conditions.

## Other Peripheral Mononeuropathies

- **Sx/Exam:** Findings are outlined in Table 11.3.
- **Dx:**
  - Diagnosed through clinical findings and EMG studies.
  - Spinal MRI imaging if spinal involvement is a concern; MRI of the affected area if symptoms are severe.

TABLE 11.3.    Selected Peripheral Mononeuropathy Symptoms

| NERVE | SYMPTOMS |
|-------|----------|
| Long thoracic nerve | Inability to raise the arm; **winging of the scapula** medial border with resistance against the outstretched arm. |
| Axillary nerve | **Paralysis of arm abduction;** atrophy of the deltoid muscle; ↓ sensation over the outer shoulder. |
| Radial nerve | **"Wrist drop":** Paralysis of elbow extension; supination of the forearm; extension of the wrist and fingers; extension and abduction of the thumb in the plane of the palm; flexion of the elbow with the forearm between pronation and supination. |
| Ulnar nerve | **"Claw hand" deformity:** Small hand muscle atrophy with finger hyperextension at the metacarpophalangeal joints and flexion at the interphalangeal joints. Sensory loss over the fifth finger and the ulnar aspect of the fourth finger and palm. |
| Lateral cutaneous nerve of the thigh | Paresthesias and ↓ sensation over the anterolateral aspect of the thigh from the inguinal ligament to above the knee. |
| Femoral nerve | Weakness of knee extension; atrophy of the quadriceps muscle; inability to fixate the knee. **No patellar reflex.** |
| Sciatic nerve | Lower leg pain and weakness. Weakness of knee flexion, foot eversion, and dorsiflexion. Absent ankle jerk; ↓ sensation over lateral shin, dorsal and distal foot, heel, sole, and toes. (In contrast, **sciatica** is associated with pain over the lumbosacral area and lateral leg; gluteal muscle weakness; and ↓ sensation over the posterior thigh, the posterior and lateral leg, and the sole.) |

NEUROLOGY

- **Tx:**
    - Treatment is symptomatic; supportive treatment for mild cases.
    - Treat the underlying cause.
    - Surgery for severe cases or threatened paralysis of affected musculature.

> A 58-year-old right-handed man notices left calf "stiffness" that causes him to trip frequently. Over several months, right arm muscle cramping and twitching have led to difficulty buttoning his shirt. He presents to your office with new difficulty swallowing and slurred speech. Exam reveals weakness and muscle atrophy in his extremities and hyperreflexia and fasciculations in the left lower extremity. An overactive gag reflex is present. What additional studies do you order? EMG and nerve conduction velocity studies confirm ALS.

### Amyotrophic Lateral Sclerosis (ALS)

A devastating neurodegenerative disease with **degeneration of lower and corticospinal motor neurons.** Most cases are sporadic.

#### SYMPTOMS/EXAM

- Presents with difficulty swallowing, chewing, coughing, breathing, and speaking (bulbar involvement).
- Vague sensory complaints and weight loss are common.
- **Upper and lower motor neuron (UMN/LMN) signs** in the bulbar region and upper and/or lower extremities include spasticity, hyperreflexia, atrophy, weakness or paralysis, fasciculations, hypotonia, and extensor plantar reflexes. Extraocular and sphincter muscles are generally spared. No sensory deficits.

#### DIFFERENTIAL

Progressive bulbar palsy (bulbar involvement), pseudobulbar palsy (UMN bulbar symptoms), progressive spinal muscular atrophy (primarily LMN deficit in the limbs), 1° lateral sclerosis (purely a UMN deficit in the limbs), poliomyelitis, MS, cervical myelopathy.

*ALS has progressive UMN and LMN signs.*

#### DIAGNOSIS

- Definitive diagnosis requires the presence of UMN and LMN signs in the bulbar region and in at least two other regions: cervical, thoracic or lumbosacral, or three spinal regions.
- EMG findings of diffuse degenerative signs with normal or near-normal nerve conduction (except in severe atrophy) are highly suggestive. Further workup is needed to eliminate other potential causes.

#### TREATMENT

- Riluzole ↓ presynaptic glutamate release and may slow symptom progression.
- Symptomatic and supportive care. Anticholinergics ↓ drooling and saliva pooling.
- Spasticity may be improved with baclofen or diazepam.
- Physical therapy to ↓ contractures; braces or walker to promote mobility.

Progressive and fatal, usually within 3–5 years of onset.

## DEMYELINATING DISEASES

A 29-year-old woman has fatigue and some right-sided "clumsiness." These symptoms wane over weeks. Months later, she notices blurry vision and decides to get new glasses. However, new-onset left-hand numbness and a "tingling" sensation around her trunk prompt her to visit your clinic first, where she is found to have focal areas of ↓ sensation. Which additional tests should be conducted, and what is the presumptive diagnosis? MRI finds three small periventricular white matter lesions. Further symptoms and subsequent tests over time confirm MS.

## Multiple Sclerosis (MS)

A chronic **multifocal demyelinating neurologic disorder** with involvement of different parts of the CNS at different points in time. Has a female-to-male ratio of 2:1. Prevalence ↑ with further distance from the equator. The disease takes **four forms**: relapsing and remitting, 1° progressive, 2° progressive, and progressive relapsing (see Table 11.4). Most cases are relapsing and remitting.

*The incidence of MS is highest among Caucasians.*

### SYMPTOMS

- Presents with focal limb weakness, numbness, paresthesias, a bandlike sensation around the trunk or a limb, and ataxia.
- Diplopia, dysarthria, intention tremor, and bladder dysfunction are also seen.
- **Optic neuritis** (sudden loss or blurring of vision in one eye) is the presenting symptom in 25% of cases.
- Symptoms are transient, lasting days to weeks. May present as spastic paraparesis and sensory deficit.

*MS is the most common acquired neurologic disability in young adults.*

### EXAM

Lhermitte's sign (an electric shock–like sensation down the spine with flexing of the neck) may be ⊕, with paresthesias in the trunk and limbs with neck flexion. An afferent pupillary defect may be seen. Focal areas of sensory deficit and weakness may be seen.

**TABLE 11.4.** **Types of Multiple Sclerosis**

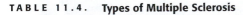

| TYPE | FEATURES |
|------|----------|
| Relapsing and remitting | Relapses followed by incomplete remissions. During relapses, symptoms can grow more severe. |
| 1° progressive | Gradual, steady progression of symptoms from initial presentation. |
| 2° progressive | Gradual progression of symptoms and disability over time following a period of relapsing-remitting disease. |
| Progressive relapsing | Gradual symptom progression over time accompanied by acute attacks of worse symptoms. |

NEUROLOGY

## DIFFERENTIAL

ALS, Bell's palsy, brain or spinal cord infection, HIV, trauma, sarcoidosis, stroke, syphilis, SLE, Lyme disease, TIA, trigeminal neuralgia.

## DIAGNOSIS

- Generally diagnosed on the basis of > 1 CNS lesion.
- MRI is the most sensitive study and shows white matter lesions (see Figure 11.7).
- Visual evoked potentials show prolonged responses, and CSF is ⊕ for **oligoclonal bands.**

## TREATMENT

- Disease-modifying therapy includes interferon-$\beta_{1b}$ or -$\beta_{1a}$, glatiramer acetate, mitoxantrone, and IVIG.
- Symptomatic therapy with corticosteroids.
- Canes, braces, walkers, wheelchairs, and assistance with daily functions.

## COMPLICATIONS

Relapsing and remitting courses may progress to a chronic progressive form. Residual impairment of color vision and depth perception is common. Chronic disability is frequent.

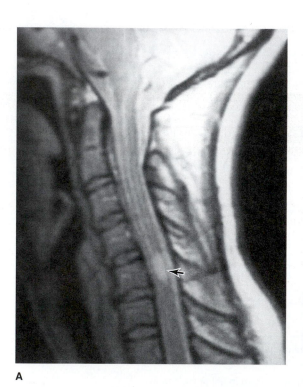 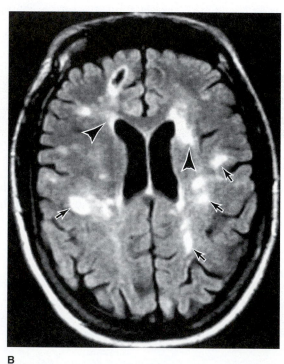

A          B

**FIGURE 11.7.** **MRI of the spine and brain in multiple sclerosis.**

(Reproduced, with permission, from Aminoff M et al. *Clinical Neurology,* 6th ed. New York: McGraw-Hill, 2005: 167.)

356

## Optic Neuritis

- Partial or total vision loss from optic nerve demyelination. Roughly half of all patients develop MS.
- **Sx/Exam:**
  - Presents with **eye pain** that may be preceded by loss of vision for 1–2 days.
  - An **afferent pupillary defect** is seen.
  - **Abnormal color vision.**
  - Funduscopic exam reveals papillitis and swelling or edema of the optic nerve head (may be normal in retrobulbar optic neuritis).
- **DDx:** Uveitis, retinal artery or vein occlusion, retinal detachment or hematoma.
- **Dx:** Findings as above. **Most cases are retrobulbar with a normal initial funduscopic exam.** CSF may show pleocytosis and ↑ IgG production.
- **Tx:** IV methylprednisolone for three days followed by oral prednisone. Treatment does not affect long-term vision outcomes.
- **Cx:** A high percentage (40–70%) of patients with isolated optic neuritis subsequently develop MS. There is also a risk of repeated attacks.

*Optic neuritis is a common presenting symptom of MS.*

*Retrobulbar optic neuritis initial exam: "The doctor sees nothing and the patient sees nothing."*

## Transverse Myelitis

- **Sx/Exam:** Presents with rapidly evolving symmetric or asymmetric paraparesis or paraplegia with ascending paresthesias, sensory loss, sphincter dysfunction, and loss of deep sensation in the feet. A sensory level on the trunk and bilateral extensor plantar signs are present.
- **Dx:** Diagnosed via CSF showing a moderate level of lymphocytes and an ↑ in total protein, although this may not be found early in the course of the disease. MRI shows focal demyelination in the expected level of the spinal cord. History may include infectious illness in the preceding weeks. Check for associated MS.
- **Tx:** Treat with IV glucocorticoids; switch to an oral form on discharge. Plasmapheresis is a second-line agent.

### NEUROMUSCULAR DISORDERS

A 32-year-old woman develops continuous "double vision." She attributes it to stress, but a vacation yields minimal improvement. Weeks later her problem worsens, and she becomes increasingly tired during the day, especially in the late afternoon to evening. She visits your office, where an exam reveals ptosis and voice hoarseness. What further evaluation should be conducted, and what is the diagnosis? A ⊕ Tensilon test and ↑ serum acetylcholine receptor antibodies confirm myasthenia gravis.

*The hallmark of myasthenia gravis is muscle weakness that worsens with activity and improves with rest.*

*Lambert-Eaton syndrome is associated with small cell lung cancer.*

### Myasthenia Gravis vs. Myasthenic Syndrome

Table 11.5 distinguishes the clinical presentation of myasthenia gravis from that of myasthenic syndrome.

TABLE 11.5. Myasthenia Gravis vs. Myasthenic Syndrome

| DISEASE | MYASTHENIA GRAVIS | MYASTHENIC SYNDROME (LAMBERT-EATON SYNDROME) |
|---|---|---|
| General | An **autoimmune disease.** Antibodies are usually against the postsynaptic muscle membrane acetylcholine receptors. Associated with **thymoma,** thyrotoxicosis, SLE, and RA. **Women are affected** more often than men. | Generally a **paraneoplastic syndrome.** Involves an immune-modulated defective release of acetylcholine in the neuromuscular junction. Associated with **small cell lung cancer** and **autoimmune diseases** such as pernicious anemia. |
| Symptoms/ exam | **Symptoms worsen with activity** and fluctuate during the day. Involves slow progression of **ptosis; diplopia; altered tone of speech;** limb weakness; and difficulty with chewing, swallowing, or respiration. Relapses and remissions for weeks. Myasthenic crisis consists of absent gag reflex, limpness of the body, and ↑ respiratory muscle weakness. | Presents with proximal limb **weakness that improves with activity.** Extraocular muscles are generally spared. May be associated with dry mouth, constipation, and impotence. ↑ environmental or body temperatures worsen symptoms. |
| Diagnosis | Electrophysiologic testing may show **decreasing response of muscle to repetitive motor nerve stimulation.** High serum acetylcholine receptor antibody levels are found in 80–90% of those with generalized disease. Edrophonium, the Tensilon test, or neostigmine improves symptoms. | Confirmed electrophysiologically by ↑ **response to repetitive nerve stimulation.** Serum **autoantibodies to the P/Q subtype of voltage-gated calcium channels** are highly sensitive and specific to this syndrome. |
| Treatment | Acetylcholinesterase inhibitors. Thymectomy for younger patients with weakness beyond the extraocular muscles. Corticosteroids initially worsen weakness. Azathioprine, plasmapheresis, IVIG, mycophenolate mofetil. | Plasmapheresis, corticosteroids, azathioprine, or IVIG. Guanidine hydrochloride may help severe cases but carries the risk of renal failure and bone marrow suppression. Treat the underlying condition. |
| Complications | Respiratory complications can be fatal. | Worsens over time. Respiratory compromise may result. |

## MUSCULAR DISORDERS

*The most common muscular dystrophy is Duchenne's.*

### Muscular Dystrophies

- **Sx/Exam:** Present with progressive muscle weakness and muscle wasting. Age at onset and distribution of symptoms depend on type (see Table 11.6).
- **Dx:** Diagnosed by muscle biopsy histology, which distinguishes different types of muscular dystrophy. EMG reveals myopathic findings and/or myotonia.

TABLE 11.6.    Presentation of Common Muscular Dystrophies

| Type | Age at Onset | Mode of Inheritance | Distribution and Symptoms | Prognosis | Serum CK |
|---|---|---|---|---|---|
| Duchenne's | 1–5 | X-linked recessive | Affects the pelvic and shoulder girdle muscles and then the extremities and respiratory muscles. Presents with muscular pseudohypertrophy. Also associated with mental retardation, deformities, and contractures. | Rapid progression. Fatal 15 years after onset. | Markedly ↑ |
| Becker's | 5–25 | X-linked recessive | Affects the pelvic and then the shoulder girdle muscles. | Slow progression. | ↑ |
| Limb-girdle | 10–30 | Autosomal recessive; dominant or sporadic | Affects the pelvic or shoulder girdle muscles; then progresses to other muscles. Presents with calf hypertrophy. | Variable. May be severe in midlife. | Mildly ↑ |
| Fascioscapulo-humeral | Any | Autosomal dominant | Affects the face and shoulder girdle muscles; then progresses to the pelvic muscles and lower extremities. | Slow progression; minor disability. | Can be normal |
| Myotonic | Any | Autosomal dominant | Weakness and myotonia (i.e., "spasming") of facial, sternocleidomastoid, and distal extremity muscles. Associated with baldness, cataracts, gonadal atrophy, cardiac abnormalities, mental retardation, and endocrinopathy. | Variable. | Normal or mildly ↑ |

- Tx: No specific treatment is available. Physical therapy can prevent or improve contractures or deformities. Surgical intervention may be necessary.

## Inflammatory Myopathies

Defined as muscle fiber destruction and inflammatory infiltration of muscles. Associated with some **autoimmune disorders,** including SLE, Sjögren's syndrome, scleroderma, and RA. Peak incidence is in the **fifth and sixth decades. More women are affected** than men. Subtypes are as follows:

- **Polymyositis:**
  - Presents with muscle pain, weakness, and atrophy, especially of the proximal limb muscles. Begins with leg weakness and progresses to arm weakness. Dysphagia and respiratory difficulties are also seen.
  - Raynaud's phenomenon, malaise, arthralgias, low-grade fever, and weight loss are common.

**NEUROLOGY**

359

*Dermatomyositis is associated with lung, breast, ovarian, and GI cancers.*

- **Dermatomyositis:**
  - Presents as above but with a **heliotrope rash,** an erythematous rash appearing over the eyelids, around the eyes, or on the extensor surfaces of the joints.
  - Erythema over the face, neck, shoulders, and upper chest → **"shawl sign."**
  - **Gottron's sign** consists of scaly patches over the dorsa of the proximal hand joints, periungual erythema, and nail bed capillary dilation.
  - Skin or muscle **calcinosis** is common.
- **Inclusion body myositis:** Painless proximal weakness of the lower extremities and then the upper extremities, especially the quadriceps and finger flexors. Has a progressive course with early loss of patellar reflexes.

### DIFFERENTIAL

Myasthenic syndrome, myasthenia gravis, MS, ALS, polymyalgia rheumatica, trichinosis, hypothyroidism, HIV myopathy.

### DIAGNOSIS

*Muscle biopsy is the gold standard for diagnosis of polymyositis and dermatomyositis.*

- Muscle biopsy shows necrosis of muscle fibers and inflammatory cell infiltration with distinctions made for polymyositis vs. dermatomyositis.
- Labs show ↑ serum CK and aldolase.
- EMG reveals short, low-amplitude, polyphasic motor unit potentials, possibly with abnormal spontaneous activity.
- Antinuclear antibodies are likely present.

### TREATMENT

- Anti-inflammatory drugs. Prednisone should be initiated and then lowered as serum muscle enzyme levels ↓. Second-line agents are methotrexate and azathioprine.
- Physical therapy to preserve function.
- For inclusion body myositis, immunosuppressive therapy is preferred.

### COMPLICATIONS

Up to 25% of patients with dermatomyositis have an occult malignancy. Patients with respiratory muscle involvement can have hypercapnia and respiratory failure. Severe muscle inflammation can precipitate rhabdomyolysis and subsequent renal failure.

## METABOLIC MYOPATHIES

### Congenital Metabolic Myopathies

Muscle pain and cramps due to insufficient energy production related to hereditary defects in glycogen (e.g., glycogen storage diseases), lipid, adenine nucleotide, or mitochondrial metabolism.

### SYMPTOMS/EXAM

- **Glycotic/glycogenolytic disorders:**
  - Presents with muscle pain, cramps, stiffness, and/or swelling with high-intensity exercise. Patients are easily fatigued with exertion.
  - Recurrent myoglobinuria (cola-colored urine that is heme ⊕ and ⊖ for RBCs) may occur.

- **Disorders of lipid metabolism:**
    - Muscle pain or tightness and/or myoglobinuria induced by prolonged exercise or prolonged fasting, infection, exposure to cold, general anesthesia, or a low-carbohydrate, high-fat diet.
    - Recurrent episodes of hypoketotic hypoglycemia may occur.
    - Hypertrophic or dilated cardiomyopathy and fatty liver may occur.
- **Mitochondrial myopathies:** Muscle weakness, poor endurance, and/or exertional myoglobinuria.

### DIFFERENTIAL

Muscular dystrophy, myasthenia gravis, MS, infection.

### DIAGNOSIS

- Check chem 12 and LFTs. Determine serum levels of lactate, CK, pyruvate, LDH, uric acid, carnitine, ketones, ammonia, and myoglobin.
- Check urine ketones, dicarboxylic acid, and myoglobin excretion at rest and with exercise.
- EMG for cases with fixed weakness (vs. intermittent for most cases).
- Obtain muscle biopsy after blood and urine testing.
- **Glycotic/glycogenolytic disorders:** CK may be elevated at rest.
- **Disorders of lipid metabolism:**
    - ↓ carnitine concentrations may be found in plasma and tissue, as may an ↑ ratio of serum free fatty acids to ketones. ↑ urine dicarboxylic acid level may be found.
    - Hypoketosis with hypoglycemia.
- **Mitochondrial myopathies:**
    - Elevated serum lactate and pyruvate levels.
    - Ragged red fibers on muscle biopsy.

### TREATMENT

- Reduction in intense or prolonged physical activity.
- Treatment of myoglobinuria as needed.
- Avoidance of skipped meals; dietary changes depending on the disorder.

### COMPLICATIONS

- Rhabdomyolysis can occur with severe myoglobinuria.
- Progressive symptoms may in some cases → respiratory failure.

## Endocrine Myopathies

- **Sx/Exam:** Present with proximal muscle pain and weakness.
- **Dx:** Diagnosed by the symptoms and exam outlined above in the setting of an **endocrinopathy** such as hypo- or hyperthyroidism, hypo- or hyperparathyroidism, hypo- or hyperadrenalism, hypopituitarism, or acromegaly with no other source.
- **Tx:** Treat the underlying endocrine disorder.

## Alcoholic Myopathies

- **Sx/Exam:** Muscle pain, swelling, proximal limb weakness, and possible dysphagia develop 1–2 days after heavy drinking. Weakness may be focal or asymmetric.

- **Dx:** ↑ serum CK; myoglobinuria. Associated with a heavy alcohol history.
- **Tx:** Potassium and phosphorus correction. Recommend nutrition counseling and alcohol cessation.

### Drug-Induced Myopathies

- **Sx/Exam:** Present with symmetric proximal muscle weakness, myalgia, and fatigue.
- **Dx:** ↑ serum CK; myopathic EMG findings. Look for a history of contributory medications such as potassium-depleting drugs, corticosteroids, chloroquine, clofibrate, bretylium, colchicine, HMG-CoA reductase inhibitors (e.g., statins), aminocaproic acid, cocaine, or zidovudine.
- **Tx:** Discontinuation of the implicated drug.
- **Cx:** Severe rhabdomyolysis → myoglobinuric renal failure.

## VERTIGO

The perception of movement of the body or the environment when no movement occurs. May be central or peripheral.

### Central Vertigo

#### SYMPTOMS/EXAM

*Central vertigo symptoms are not ↓ or abolished with provocative maneuvers.*

- The illusion of movement of the body or environment in conjunction with nausea, vomiting, or gait ataxia.
- Associated with vertical, unidirectional, or multidirectional nystagmus that may be different in the two eyes.
- **No extinguishing of symptoms or symptom latency occurs with provocative maneuvers** such as the Dix-Hallpike (or Nylen-Bárány) maneuver.
- Diplopia, dysarthria, facial motor or sensory asymmetry, ↓ gag reflex, and asymmetry of tongue protrusion are possible.
- Other motor or sensory deficits, hyperreflexia, extensor plantar responses, or limb ataxia may be present.

#### DIFFERENTIAL

Stroke, intracerebral hemorrhage, Ménière's disease, orthostatic hypotension, drug toxicity, TIA, postconcussion syndrome, MS.

#### DIAGNOSIS

Diagnosed by the exam results shown above. A plain head CT can reveal the source, with MRI showing smaller lesions and infarcts as well as a better view of the posterior fossa.

#### TREATMENT

Patients should be referred to a neurologist or a neurosurgeon.

#### COMPLICATIONS

Possible surgical complications; continued symptoms if the lesion is untreatable.

## Peripheral Vertigo

### SYMPTOMS/EXAM

- Presents in the same manner as central vertigo, but symptoms are generally intermittent and more distressing.
- **Hearing loss or tinnitus** is common.
- **Unidirectional or rotational nystagmus** (not vertical) may be present. Eyes drift toward the affected side.
- Provocative maneuvers such as the Dix-Hallpike (or Nylen-Bárány) maneuver elicit symptoms and nystagmus with symptom latency and extinguishment on repetition.

### DIFFERENTIAL

- BPPV, labyrinthitis, Ménière's disease (recurrent episodes of vertigo, nausea, vomiting, tinnitus, and hearing loss), drug toxicity.
- Side effects of anticonvulsants, antibiotics, hypnotics, analgesics, or alcohol.

### DIAGNOSIS

- Provocation of symptoms with the Dix-Hallpike (or Nylen-Bárány) maneuver.
- Obtain a fasting chem 12, ESR, TSH, RPR, and CBC to look for underlying contributing conditions.

### TREATMENT

- Meclizine for BPPV. Correct any underlying metabolic disorders.
- Discontinue or taper contributing medications.
- Offer education on desensitization exercises and canalith repositioning procedures.

## MOVEMENT DISORDERS

## Ataxias

Incoordination and irregularity of voluntary movement. Categorized as follows:

- **Vestibular ataxia:** Ataxia with unilateral nystagmus that ↑ with gaze away from the affected side. Romberg's sign is ⊕, and patients fall toward the affected side.
- **Cerebellar ataxia:**
    - Presents with hypotonia and irregularities in the rate, amplitude, and force of voluntary movements. Terminal dysmetria, "overshooting," and terminal intention tremor are seen.
    - Complex movements are performed as a series of individual movements.
    - Nystagmus, gaze pareses, and defective saccadic and pursuit movement are possible.
- **Proprioceptive ataxia:**
    - Symmetrically affects the legs and gait with limited or no arm involvement.
    - Involves impairment of vibratory sense, joint position sense, and proprioception.
    - Also associated with numbness or tingling in the legs.

- Improved balance is achieved with use of a cane or other support or by watching one's own feet while walking. Symptoms worsen when the patient's eyes are closed.
- Romberg's sign is ⊕, and patients exhibit a wide-based, high-stepping gait and poor heel-to-toe walking.

### DIFFERENTIAL

Vertigo, sensory deficit, toxins.

### DIAGNOSIS

Based on exam findings. Neuroimaging for suspected cerebellar causes.

### TREATMENT

Supportive treatment; treat any underlying conditions.

*Friedreich's ataxia is the most prevalent inherited ataxia.*

### FRIEDREICH'S ATAXIA

An idiopathic **progressive spinocerebellar disorder** beginning between the ages of 4 and 20. The most common hereditary ataxia. Typically **autosomal recessive** with an expanded GAA trinucleotide repeat on chromosome 9 in the frataxin gene. Associated progressive **kyphoscoliosis** can → **restrictive lung disease** and **cardiomyopathy**.

### SYMPTOMS/EXAM

- **Progressive mixed sensory and cerebellar gait ataxia** involves all limbs within two years of onset.
- Extensor plantar responses occur within five years.
- ↓ knee and ankle reflexes are seen along with cerebellar dysarthria and impaired leg and joint position and vibratory senses. Weakness of the legs and arms is found late in the course of the disease.
- **Pes cavus** and kyphoscoliosis are common, and nystagmus, paresthesias, tremors, vertigo, spasticity, and ↓ vision and hearing are also seen.

### DIFFERENTIAL

Vitamin E deficiency, ataxia-telangiectasia, Refsum disease, abetalipoproteinemia, spinocerebellar ataxia.

### DIAGNOSIS

- Diagnosis is guided by the clinical history and exam.
- Sensory nerve action potentials are absent or ↓.
- MRI reveals cervical spinal cord atrophy and minimal cerebellar atrophy; chest and spine x-rays show kyphoscoliosis.
- Echocardiography reveals associated ventricular hypertrophy.

### TREATMENT

Supportive care and treatment of associated cardiac and endocrine disorders. Orthopedic procedures can assist with foot deformities.

### COMPLICATIONS

Disability with inability to walk unassisted may occur within five years of onset. Patients are typically bedridden 10–20 years after onset. The average life span is 35 years.

## ATAXIA-TELANGIECTASIA

An inherited **autosomal-recessive** disorder characterized by **cerebellar ataxia,** progressive pancerebellar degeneration, variable **immunodeficiency,** impaired organ maturation, predisposition to malignancy, and **ocular and cutaneous telangiectasia.** Onset is in infancy, and the disease is usually fatal in adolescence.

### SYMPTOMS/EXAM

- Presents with nystagmus, cerebellar dysarthria and gait, and **limb and trunk ataxia.** Loss of vibration and position sense, **choreoathetosis,** areflexia, and disorders of eye movement are seen.
- **Oculocutaneous telangiectasia** appears during the teen years, first on the eyes and then on sun-exposed areas of the skin.
- Mental deficiency appears in the second decade.
- Recurrent sinopulmonary infections are seen, as are progeria-like skin and hair changes, hypogonadism, and insulin resistance.

### DIFFERENTIAL

Refsum disease, Niemann-Pick disease, Friedreich's ataxia, cerebral palsy, familial spinocerebellar atrophies, cerebellar tumor.

### DIAGNOSIS

- Guided by the history and exam.
- Look for ↑ levels of AFP and CEA and/or chromosomal abnormalities such as inversions and translocations in chromosomes 7 and 14.
- IgA is ↓ or absent; IgG is ↓ or normal; IgM is ↑ or normal; and IgE is ↓ or absent.
- Low lymphocyte count; poor skin test response to common antigens.

### TREATMENT

- Avoid all x-rays in light of patients' abnormal cellular sensitivity to ionizing radiation.
- Supportive care; antibiotics for any bacterial infections.

### COMPLICATIONS

Death usually occurs in adolescence. Associated with a risk of leukemia and lymphoma.

## Chorea and Athetosis

Clinically distinguished as follows:

- **Chorea:** Rapid, irregular, involuntary, and purposeless movement that goes from one body part to another. **Facial grimacing** and tongue movements are common. Ranges from a restless or clumsy appearance to forceful limb and head movements and an unsteady, **"dancing gait."** Full muscle strength is preserved, and attempted muscle contraction is intermittent. **"Explosive speech"** has irregular volume and tempo. No symptoms occur in sleep.
- **Athetosis:** Slow, **sinuous, writhing movements** that may be generalized or restricted to one area of the body. Symptoms are ↑ by emotional stress and voluntary activity and are not present during sleep. In some cases, symptoms occur only during specific activities, such as speaking or writing.

### DIFFERENTIAL

Huntington's disease, Wilson's disease, Parkinson's disease, cerebral palsy, Sydenham's chorea, drug toxicity, SLE, stroke.

### DIAGNOSIS

Diagnosis is guided by the history and exam. Check for underlying conditions or causes such as polycythemia vera or thyrotoxicosis in chorea.

### TREATMENT

Treat any underlying disease. Supportive care.

## Tremor

Rhythmic oscillatory movement characterized by the action taken during symptoms. Categorized as follows:

- **Postural tremor:** Tremor with sustained posture of an extremity. Symptoms ↑ with emotional stress or sleep deprivation and are not present during sleep. They also ↑ with use of TCAs, valproic acid, lithium, and bronchodilators.
- **Intention tremor:** Tremor during movement that ↑ as a target is approached. May be associated with cerebellar signs. No tremor at rest.
- **Resting tremor:** Tremor at rest. May affect the fingers, hands, forearms, or feet. Has a **frequency of 4–6 Hz.** Associated with hypokinesia or rigidity when due to parkinsonism.

### DIFFERENTIAL

- **Postural tremor:** Physiologic tremor, benign essential tremor, cerebellar disorders, Wilson's disease.
- **Intention tremor:** Cerebellar or brain stem disease, Wilson's disease, drug toxicity.
- **Resting tremor:** Basal ganglia lesions, parkinsonism, Wilson's disease, heavy metal poisoning, hyperthyroidism, anxiety, drug withdrawal/toxicity, benign hereditary tremor.

### DIAGNOSIS

Diagnosis is guided by the history and exam. In intention tremor, MRI may show a lesion of the superior cerebellar peduncle.

### TREATMENT

Treat any underlying condition. β-blockers or anticonvulsants may reduce benign essential tremor. Severe intention tremor may be treated with thalamus stereotactic surgery or high-frequency stimulation via an implanted device.

*Postural tremor is usually an exaggeration of normal physiologic tremor.*

## Tics

- Repetitive, stereotyped movements or vocalizations.
- **Sx/Exam:** May present as blinking, sniffing, stretching of the neck or mouth, or touching something repetitively. Voluntary suppression may produce anxiety, while performing the tic may relieve tension. Symptoms ↑ with emotional stress and ↓ with voluntary activity. No symptoms occur during sleep.

- **DDx:** Tourette's syndrome, encephalitis, chorea, Huntington's disease, Wilson's disease, seizure, tardive dyskinesia, tuberous sclerosis.
- **Dx:** Based on the history and exam.
- **Tx:** Benzodiazepines or clonidine may be helpful. Antipsychotic medications such as haloperidol may be used for severe cases. Injected botulinum toxin can also ↓ symptoms.

## Restless Legs Syndrome

- Leg "restlessness" along with crawling, itching, or stretching sensations in the calves relieved by movement.
- **Sx/Exam:** Symptoms worsen when the patient lies down at night or sits while at rest. Sleep may be disturbed.
- **DDx:** Akathisia, periodic movements of legs, peripheral neuropathy.
- **Dx:** Clinical diagnosis. Check for **pregnancy, iron deficiency anemia,** or peripheral neuropathy. Family history is often ⊕. Associated with periodic limb movement disorder → involuntary leg twitching or jerking every 10–60 seconds during sleep.
- **Tx:** Treat the underlying condition. Levodopa, ropinirole, pramipexole, clonazepam, propoxyphene, and clonidine are commonly used.
- **Cx:** Daytime somnolence; development of tolerance to treatment.

*Eighty percent of patients with restless legs syndrome have periodic limb movement disorder.*

- **Sx/Exam:**
    - High-pitched noise in the ear that may last for several minutes or persist. When symptoms are severe, they may interfere with concentration or sleep.
    - Otologic exam may be normal.
    - Cerumen impaction is common, and head or neck carotid bruit may be present.
- **DDx:** Conductive hearing loss, palatal myoclonus, otosclerosis, otitis media, head trauma, glomus tumor, jugular venous hum, Ménière's disease.
- **Dx:**
    - Guided by the history. Examine for hearing loss and obtain a complete audiographic evaluation.
    - In the presence of a pulsatile tinnitus suggestive of a vascular etiology, MRI angiography is warranted.
    - If tinnitus is asymmetric or unilateral, an MRI of the internal auditory canals is needed to check for possible acoustic tumor.
    - "Clicking" tinnitus may be due to palatal myoclonus.
- **Tx:**
    - Amplification of normal sounds or music; "white noise" to mask the symptoms.
    - Treat related sleep interference with nortriptyline 50 mg PO at night.
    - Surgical ablation of any contributing vascular anomaly or tumor.
    - Caution patients to avoid excessive noise and ototoxic medications. Recommend stress reduction.

*Tinnitus is strongly associated with some degree of hearing loss.*

NEUROLOGY

### Internuclear Ophthalmoplegia

- Disconjugate gaze with impaired adduction and nystagmus of the abducting eye due to a lesion of the **medial longitudinal fasciculus.** In young adults or in those with bilateral involvement, the most common cause is **MS.** Vascular disease is likely in older patients or in those with unilateral involvement.
- **Sx/Exam:** The ipsilateral eye fails to adduct when the patient looks toward the opposite side (see Figure 11.8). Instead of complete paralysis of adduction, there may be slow adducting saccades in the affected eye. Nystagmus is present in the unaffected eye.
- **DDx:** MS, vascular disease, brain stem encephalitis, intrinsic brain stem tumors, syringobulbia, drug toxicity, Wernicke's encephalopathy, myasthenia gravis, SLE.
- **Dx:** Guided by the exam. Neuroimaging is required to look for possible etiologies.
- **Tx:** Treat any underlying cause.

### Nystagmus

- Rhythmic involuntary eye movement. Subtypes include the following:
  - **Pendular nystagmus:** Involuntary rhythmic eye oscillation with equal velocity in both directions.
  - **Jerk nystagmus:** Slow phase of rhythmic, involuntary eye movement in one direction and fast phase in the opposite direction. May be horizontal, vertical, or rotatory.
- **Sx/Exam:** Symptoms can occur at the extremes of gaze under normal conditions. Vertigo, hearing loss, tinnitus, or cranial nerve abnormalities are possible depending on the cause.
- **DDx:** Associated causative factors include drug toxicity (anticonvulsants or sedatives), alcohol intoxication, brain stem disorders, lithium toxicity ($\rightarrow$ vertical jerk nystagmus), BPPV, and head trauma.

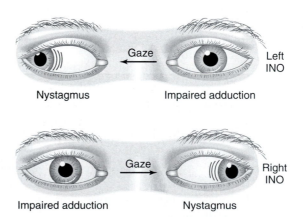

**FIGURE 11.8.** **Eye movements in internuclear ophthalmoplegia.**

(Reproduced, with permission, from Aminoff M et al. *Clinical Neurology*, 6th ed. New York: McGraw-Hill, 2005: 143.)

- **Dx:**
    - Guided by the history and exam. Neuroimaging is appropriate for those without an identifiable cause.
    - Vertigo may be present when the cause is a vestibular lesion.
    - Hearing loss or tinnitus is associated with peripheral lesions or those of the corticospinal tract. Cranial nerve abnormalities point to a central lesion.
- **Tx:** Discontinue contributory medications. Treat any identified cause, including surgery if necessary. Neurology referral for unidentifiable causes.

*The direction of jerk nystagmus is named for the direction of the fast phase.*

## Horner's Syndrome

- Unilateral **miotic pupil** with **ipsilateral mild ptosis** often associated with **ipsilateral anhidrosis** (see Figure 11.9).
- **Sx/Exam:** Response to light and accommodation is normal. The ipsilateral conjunctiva may be acutely injected, and the ipsilateral face may be warm and hyperemic. Slow pupillary dilation is seen on the affected side.
- **DDx:** Argyll Robertson pupil (associated with late syphilis; the pupil accommodates but does not react), neuroblastoma, history of ocular trauma. Associated causative factors include cervical cord lesion, pulmonary apical or mediastinal tumor, neck trauma or mass, cluster headache, carotid artery thrombosis, and brain stem infarct.
- **Dx:** Based on the history and exam. MRI for numbness of the ipsilateral face and contralateral extremities or ipsilateral abducens palsy; CXR for suspicion of chest tumor. Concomitant neck pain may be associated with carotid artery dissection and warrants an MRA.
- **Tx:** Treat the underlying cause.

## Bell's Palsy

- Abrupt onset of **LMN facial weakness** or paralysis that is usually **unilateral.**
- **Sx/Exam:**
    - Symptoms progress over hours to 1–2 days. An **impaired sense of taste, hyperacusis,** and **lacrimation** are common.
    - The ipsilateral eye may be difficult to close. Pain around the ipsilateral ear is possible.

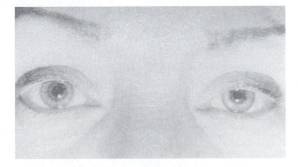

**FIGURE 11.9.** **Left-sided Horner's syndrome.**

(Reproduced, with permission, from Aminoff M et al. *Clinical Neurology,* 6th ed. New York: McGraw-Hill, 2005: 140.)

**NEUROLOGY**

- Patients have difficulty eating.
- No abnormalities are found beyond the facial nerve territory.
■ **DDx:** Intracranial tumor, stroke, Ramsay Hunt syndrome, Lyme disease, sarcoidosis, AIDS, acoustic neuroma, Guillain-Barré syndrome.
■ **Dx:**
  - Based on the history and exam. Nerve conduction studies can point to the prognosis.
  - Labs or studies are needed to exclude other causes if the history or exam is not conclusive. Although the cause is usually **idiopathic,** it may be associated with **pregnancy** or **diabetes,** Lyme disease, HIV, or herpesvirus infection.
■ **Tx:** Treatment with oral corticosteroids and acyclovir is controversial. Lubricating eye drops may be used along with an ipsilateral eye patch if the eye is difficult to close. Most patients have complete recovery within weeks to months without treatment.
■ **Cx:** Severe pain, older age, hyperacusis, and complete palsy at diagnosis are associated with a poorer prognosis, with disfigurement affecting about 10% of patients.

### Ramsay Hunt Syndrome

■ **Ipsilateral facial weakness with herpetic eruption** of the ear, palate, pharynx, or occipital scalp.
■ **Sx/Exam:** May involve deafness, tinnitus, or vertigo.
■ **DDx:** Bell's palsy, stroke, TIA, Guillain-Barré syndrome.
■ **Dx:** Based on clinical findings.
■ **Tx:** Treat acutely with **acyclovir** and **corticosteroids.**
■ **Cx:** Postherpetic neuralgia in the affected areas or persistent facial weakness. Fewer than half of patients achieve a complete recovery.

> A 62-year-old woman presents with an intermittent dull ache on the lower right side of her face that is worsened by chewing and is not relieved by OTC analgesics. Her symptoms have been occurring for a month and are now "stabbing" and ↑ even with talking. Exam elicits pain on touching the lower right side of the patient's face. Head CT is ⊖. What is the diagnosis? Trigeminal neuralgia.

### Trigeminal Neuralgia

An **idiopathic facial pain syndrome** that is more common in mid- to late life. The male-to-female incidence ratio is 2:3. Idiopathic cases usually occur in the sixth decade. Consider MS in cases that are bilateral or in those that occur in younger, female patients.

#### SYMPTOMS/EXAM

■ Presents as **stabbing, brief unilateral pain** in the areas of the **second and third branches of the trigeminal nerve** (see Figure 11.10). Touching the affected area, eating, or a draft of air over the face elicits the pain.
■ Symptoms radiate from the corner of the mouth to the ipsilateral eye, ear, or nostril. Symptoms during sleep are rare.
■ Otherwise neurologically normal.

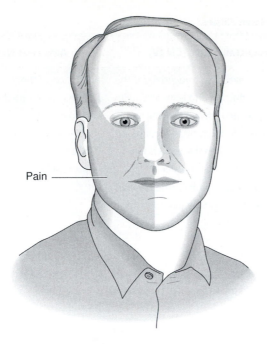

Pain

**FIGURE 11.10.** **Distribution of symptoms in trigeminal neuralgia.**

(Reproduced, with permission, from Aminoff M et al. *Clinical Neurology*, 6th ed. New York: McGraw-Hill, 2005: 83.)

### DIFFERENTIAL

Temporal arteritis, TMJ dysfunction, atypical facial pain, glaucoma, brain stem tumor, MS, dental abscess, postherpetic neuralgia.

### DIAGNOSIS

Guided by the history and exam. Head CT is ⊖. In a young patient, suspect MS and obtain evoked potential testing, an MRI, and CSF tests.

### TREATMENT

**Carbamazepine** and **oxcarbazepine** are first-line agents but require monitoring of cell counts and LFTs. Baclofen and gabapentin are second-line and adjunctive therapies.

### COMPLICATIONS

Spontaneous remissions can occur for months, but some patients have progression of the disorder with more frequent symptoms and possibly persistent low-grade pain.

### Selected Cranial Nerve Palsies

Table 11.7 compares the clinical presentations of selected cranial nerve palsies.

### DIFFERENTIAL

- Myasthenia gravis, trauma, thyroid ophthalmopathy.
- Associated causative factors if the pupil is dilated and nonreactive include aneurysm, hemorrhage, tumor, and uncal herniation. Other associated

*Treatment of trigeminal neuralgia with carbamazepine is diagnostic and therapeutic.*

NEUROLOGY

371

**TABLE 11.7.** **Presentation of Selected Cranial Nerve Palsies**

| OCULOMOTOR NERVE (CN III) | TROCHLEAR NERVE (CN IV) | ABDUCENS NERVE (CN VI) |
|---|---|---|
| The affected eye is **deviated down and out.**<br>**Ptosis** and paralysis of accommodation are seen.<br>Diplopia is seen except in lateral gaze toward the affected side. Pupillary function may be impaired. | The eye is elevated in forward gaze. This ↑ with adduction and is greatest with the head tilted toward the affected side. The effect ↓ with abduction and is abolished when the head is tilted away from the affected side. Downward gaze adducts the affected eye and worsens diplopia. Tilting of the head ↓ diplopia. | Adduction of the involved eye at rest.<br>Failure of attempted abduction.<br>Diplopia is seen on lateral gaze to the affected side.<br>Esotropia (a cross-eyed appearance) is present. |

causative factors include **hypertension, diabetes,** MS, sarcoidosis, atherosclerosis, tumor, ischemia, and aneurysm.

### DIAGNOSIS

*In oculomotor (CN III) palsy, the affected eye is "down and out."*

- Based on the clinical exam.
- CT or MRI may be needed if pupillary function is impaired, a structural lesion is suspected, the patient is > 40 years of age or has associated pain, other neurologic findings are present, or symptoms persist past several weeks.
- Conduct a Bielschowsky head-tilt test for CN IV palsy (⊕ if head tilt toward the side of the affected eye yields elevation of the affected eye and marked diplopia).

### TREATMENT

- Treat the underlying condition.
- Surgery for severe, persistent symptoms.
- Prisms can reduce diplopia.
- May resolve spontaneously in 6–12 months. Possible surgery if symptoms persist. Alternate eye patching in young children for CN VI palsy.

## SPINAL CORD DISORDERS

### Spinal Arteriovenous Malformation

#### SYMPTOMS/EXAM

- Presents with weakness or paralysis of one or both legs along with numbness or paresthesias in the same distribution. An upper, lower, or mixed motor deficit is seen in the legs.
- Associated with acute, **lancinating pain in the back or legs that worsens with recumbency.** Hyperreflexia is seen caudal to the lesion. Sphincter function is compromised.
- Symptoms are also present in the arms with cervical lesions.
- A bruit, cutaneous angioma, or dermatomal nevus may be present over the affected area of the spine.

#### DIFFERENTIAL

Guillain-Barré syndrome, spinal cord infarction, transverse myelitis, MS, stroke, cauda equina syndrome.

NEUROLOGY

### DIAGNOSIS

- Based on **selective angiography.**
- MRI of the spine or CT myelography shows one or more enlarged and tortuous draining vessels in the subarachnoid space, usually at the lower spinal cord. The spine may appear enlarged in the area of the lesion.
- CSF shows high protein but little or no cellular reaction.
- Associated with **SAH** or myelopathy.

### TREATMENT

Embolization of the lesion or ligation of its feeding vessels and excision of the anomalous AVM nidus.

### COMPLICATIONS

Increasing gait disability can progress to the point at which the patient is bedridden.

## Cervical Spondylosis

### SYMPTOMS/EXAM

- Presents with limited head and neck movement with neck pain or stiffness.
- Pain in the arms, muscle atrophy, and occipital headache are also seen. Lhermitte's sign is often ⊕.
- A segmental motor or sensory deficit may be present in the arms with UMN deficits in the legs.
- If the C5–C6 interspace is affected → hyperreflexic triceps reflex with absent biceps and supinator reflexes.

### DIFFERENTIAL

MS, motor neuron disease, subacute combined degeneration of the spinal cord, spinal mass, syringomyelia.

### DIAGNOSIS

- Supportive history and exam.
- Cervical x-rays show **osteophytes** and **narrowing of the disk space** (cervical disk degeneration) and intervertebral foramina (→ **impingement of nerve roots**).
- CSF shows ↑ protein and a normal cell count.
- MRI of the neck or CT myelogram may be needed for confirmation.

### TREATMENT

↓ cervical movement and subsequent pain with a cervical collar. Surgical intervention may be needed to prevent progression or for severe or refractory pain.

### COMPLICATIONS

Chronic pain or weakness.

## Subacute Combined Degeneration of the Spinal Cord

- Sx/Exam:
  - Presents with distal extremity weakness and paresthesias starting in the hands.

- Also associated with ↓ sensation with deficits in vibratory and joint position senses.
- Later symptoms include **spastic paraparesis** and **ataxia** due to ↓ postural sensation in the legs.
- Extensor plantar responses are present.
- Visual impairment with optic atrophy is seen. Psychosis is possible.
- **DDx:** MS, ALS, spinal mass, cervical spondylosis.
- **Dx:** By exam. Labs show macrocytic megaloblastic anemia and low serum vitamin $B_{12}$ if not treated. The Schilling test is abnormal if the source is pernicious anemia.
- **Tx:** IM vitamin $B_{12}$ injections.
- **Cx:** Progression without treatment → ataxia, visual impairment, and psychosis.

# CHAPTER 12

# Surgery

Sarah Lowenthal, MD

Family medicine physicians must be familiar with methods of risk-stratifying patients and for providing appropriate interventions prior to cardiac and non-cardiac procedures.

- One in six surgical patients will develop at least one perioperative or post-operative complication.
- Each year, 50,000 patients have perioperative MIs, and approximately 40% die as a result.
- The overall mortality rate for end-stage renal disease patients undergoing surgery is 4%.
- Venous thromboembolism, a highly preventable complication, can occur in up to 80% of patients undergoing total hip replacement and in as many as 60% of those undergoing total knee replacement.

*Nonselective imaging and lab screening tests have been shown to be of minimal value in assessing operative risk. Routine preoperative CXRs and CBCs are seldom useful except to evaluate patients for a specific preexisting condition.*

## Cardiac Risk Evaluation

A preoperative cardiac risk assessment should address **three major components:**

1. The patient's risk of a major cardiac complication (see Table 12.1).
2. The patient's current functional status (see Table 12.2).
3. The cardiac risk associated with the planned procedure (see Table 12.3).

Guidelines for further cardiac evaluation and for the mitigation of cardiac risk are outlined in Figure 12.1 and below.

*The indications for coronary revascularization in the preoperative patient are no different from those in patients not facing surgery. "Prophylactic" CABG and/or angioplasty/stenting should not be done unless it is likely to ↑ survival.*

## Perioperative β-Blockers

Growing evidence indicates that perioperative β-blockers ↓ cardiac-related mortality in patients with known or suspected CAD. All studies used $\beta_1$-selective agents. Recommendations for use include the following:

- β-blockers are most appropriate for intermediate-risk patients with good functional status; intermediate-risk patients with poor functional status but with a ⊖ noninvasive stress test (NST); and high-risk patients with a ⊖ NST.
- β-blockers are contraindicated in patients with high-grade conduction system disease.
- Optimal dosage is controversial.

**TABLE 12.1.** **Cardiac Risk Stratification**

| MAJOR | INTERMEDIATE | MINOR |
|---|---|---|
| MI within 6 months with persistent ischemic symptoms | MI > 6 months ago | Advanced age |
| Decompensated CHF | Stable/mild angina | Abnormal ECG |
| Significant arrhythmias | Compensated or prior CHF | Rhythm other than sinus (e.g., atrial fibrillation) |
| Severe valvular disease | DM | Poor functional capacity |
|  | Renal insufficiency | History of stroke |
|  |  | Uncontrolled hypertension |

**TABLE 12.2. Functional Status Assessment**

| Excellent (> 7 METs)[a] | Moderate (4–7 METs) | Poor (< 4 METs) |
|---|---|---|
| Squash | Cycling | Vacuuming |
| Jogging (10-minute mile) | Climbing a flight of stairs | Activities of daily living (e.g., |
| Scrubbing floors | Golf (without cart) | eating, dressing, bathing) |
| Singles tennis | Walking 4 mph | Walking 2 mph |
| | Yardwork (e.g., raking leaves, | Writing |
| | weeding, pushing a power | |
| | mower) | |

[a] MET = metabolic equivalent.

*Incentive spirometry ↓ the risk of complications and should be taught to pulmonary patients preoperatively.*

*PFTs and ABGs are not part of a routine pulmonary risk assessment and should be obtained only if you would do so even if the patient were not undergoing surgery.*

- β-blockers should be started before the induction of anesthesia and may be initiated up to one month before the procedure.
- Continue at least until discharge from the hospital and longer if possible.

## Management of Preoperative Anticoagulation

- **Warfarin** should generally be stopped four days before surgery and replaced with IV heparin.
- **Heparin** should be stopped 6–12 hours before surgery, and the PTT should be allowed to return to normal to ensure adequate intraoperative hemostasis.
- **Aspirin and NSAIDs** should be stopped approximately seven days before surgery.

## Pulmonary Risk Evaluation

The risk factors for perioperative pulmonary complications include the following:

**TABLE 12.3. Degree of Cardiac Risk Associated with Surgical Procedures[a]**

| Low: "ABCDE-TURP" | Intermediate: "CHOPIN" | High: "EVA" |
|---|---|---|
| **A**mbulatory procedures | **C**arotid endarterectomy | **E**mergency major procedures |
| **B**reast procedures | **H**ead procedures | **V**ascular procedures |
| **C**ataract procedures | **O**rthopedic procedures | **A**nticipated prolonged surgical |
| **D**ermatologic procedures | **P**rostatectomy | procedures associated with large |
| **E**ndoscopic procedures | **I**ntraperitoneal and intrathoracic procedures | fluid shifts or blood loss |
| **T**ransurethral resection of the prostate | **N**eck procedures | |

[a] Cardiac risk is stratified as follows: low risk = < 1%; intermediate risk = < 5%; high risk = > 5%.

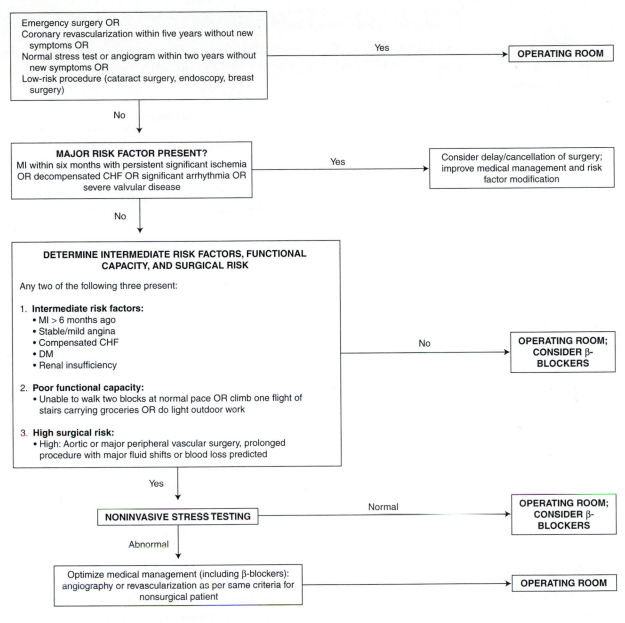

**FIGURE 12.1.** **Algorithm for further cardiac evaluation and intervention.**

(Reproduced, with permission, from Le T et al. *First Aid for the Internal Medicine Boards,* 1st ed. New York: McGraw-Hill, 2006: 359.)

- Surgery on the chest or abdomen
- Chronic lung disease
- Current tobacco use
- Morbid obesity
- Age > 60
- Prior stroke
- Altered mental status
- Neck or intracranial surgery

*Poor glycemic control is associated with a higher incidence of infection and delayed wound healing.*

*Average-risk patients (those without additional major risk factors) should be treated with unfractionated heparin (5000 U SQ BID) or TEDS if anticoagulation is contraindicated.*

*Sucralfate and $H_2$ receptor blockers both → at least a 50% reduction in the likelihood of GI bleeding but have known disadvantages such as ↓ absorption of medications and a possible ↑ risk of nosocomial pneumonia.*

Table 12.4 outlines the perioperative management of common chronic diseases. Table 12.5 discusses indications for perioperative prophylaxis.

**TABLE 12.4.** Perioperative Management of Chronic Diseases

| CONDITION | POTENTIAL COMPLICATIONS | PREOPERATIVE MANAGEMENT | POSTOPERATIVE MANAGEMENT |
|---|---|---|---|
| DM, on insulin as outpatient | Hypo- and hyperglycemia; DKA; infection. | Give 50% of usual long-acting insulin the morning of surgery (the exception being glargine, which should be given at the usual dose the evening before surgery) with glucose drip. | Strongly consider insulin drip titrating to normoglycemia; otherwise restart long-acting insulin with supplemental short-acting insulin (with rapid titration of long-acting insulin). |
| DM, not on insulin | Hypo- and hyperglycemia; nonketotic hyperosmolar state. | Omit oral hypoglycemic the day prior to surgery. | Consider insulin drip; use regularly scheduled short-acting insulin if needed and restart oral agent when possible. |
| Chronic steroid use (especially greater than the equivalent of prednisone 20 mg for three weeks) | Adrenal crisis (rare). | Continue usual dose. | Can usually just give chronic dose; consider "stress-dose" steroids for longer/major surgeries—hydrocortisone 100 mg q 8 h × 2–3 days. |
| Liver disease | Mortality, hemorrhage, infection. | Optimize treatment of underlying complications; high morbidity and mortality rates are seen in Child-Pugh Class C patients. | Optimize treatment of underlying complications. |

Reproduced, with permission, from Le T et al. *First Aid for the Internal Medicine Boards,* 1st ed. New York: McGraw-Hill, 2006: 360.

TABLE 12.5. Indications for Perioperative Prophylaxis

| CONDITION | AT-RISK GROUPS | RECOMMENDATIONS |
|---|---|---|
| Bacterial endocarditis | Patients with known valvular disease, most congenital heart disease, hypertrophic cardiomyopathy, prosthetic valves, and prior endocarditis. | **Procedures above the diaphragm:** PO amoxicillin, IV ampicillin, or IV/PO clindamycin 30–60 minutes before the procedure.<br>**Procedures below the diaphragm:** IV ampicillin plus gentamicin 30 minutes before the procedure followed by PO amoxicillin or IV amoxicillin six hours after the procedure; or IV vancomycin plus gentamicin 30 minutes before. |
| DVT | All surgical patients are at risk for DVT, especially those undergoing major surgery, those having orthopedic surgery, and those > 40 years of age or with additional DVT risk factors. | **"Minidose" heparin:** Usually 5000 U SQ BID.<br>**Low-molecular-weight heparin:** Enoxaparin 30 mg BID or 40 mg QD.<br>Thromboembolic disease stockings (TEDS).<br>Sequential compression devices.<br>**Warfarin:** Dose adjusted; for very high risk patients only. |
| GI bleeding (2° to stress-induced gastric mucosal disease) | At especially high risk for GI bleeding are patients with coagulopathy; those with respiratory failure requiring mechanical ventilation; and those with a history of trauma, burns, sepsis, or hepatic or renal dysfunction. | $H_2$ receptor blockers (can be given PO or IV), sucralfate, antacids.<br>PPIs are relatively unproven for the prophylaxis of GI bleeding and are therefore considered second-line therapy. |
| Constipation | All postoperative patients on narcotic pain medications. | Docusate sodium (e.g., Colace). |

## POSTOPERATIVE CARE

Recovery from surgery can be divided into three phases: (1) the immediate postoperative phase; (2) an intermediate postoperative phase encompassing the hospitalization period; and a (3) convalescent phase.

### The Immediate Postoperative Period

The principal causes of complications and death following major surgery are acute cardiac, pulmonary, and fluid derangements. For this reason, all patients who have undergone major surgery should be monitored until cardiopulmonary and neurologic function has returned to baseline. Patients who require ongoing ventilatory or circulatory support are transferred to an ICU.

### The Intermediate Postoperative Period

During the time from complete recovery from anesthesia until discharge from the hospital, the patient must recover basic bodily functions and become self-sufficient. Measures with which to achieve these goals are outlined below.

*Check an ECG immediately after surgery and daily for the next two days given that postoperative MI and angina often present atypically and have a peak incidence during the first three postoperative days.*

SURGERY

*Accurate intake/output records and daily weight measurements are extremely important in postoperative patients! Remember to account for intraoperative and/or PACU losses/gains in fluid balance.*

*It is not necessary to measure serum electrolytes in most postoperative patients receiving short-term IV fluid replacement.*

*Sepsis ↑ capillary permeability and can → pulmonary edema. In the absence of cardiac function derangement or fluid overload, the development of pulmonary edema should be regarded as evidence of sepsis.*

## FLUID AND ELECTROLYTE MANAGEMENT

The fluids of choice in postoperative patients are generally 5% dextrose in normal saline or lactated Ringer's. Additional guidelines for postoperative fluid replacement should be based on the following considerations:

- Maintenance requirements.
- Extra needs resulting from systemic factors (e.g., burns, fever).
- Losses from drains.
- Requirements resulting from **third-space** losses (e.g., tissue edema, ileus).

### ESTIMATING FLUID REQUIREMENTS

- Daily maintenance requirements in the adult are approximately 1500–2500 mL depending on the patient's age, gender, weight, and body surface area.
- A rough estimate of daily fluid requirements in adults can be obtained by multiplying the patient's weight in kilograms by 30 (e.g., 1800 mL/24 hr in a 60-kg patient).

### PULMONARY CARE

Pulmonary function in the postoperative period is compromised for many reasons, including changes in pulmonary physiology due to surgery and anesthesia as well as shallow breathing and immobilization. Vital capacity ↓ to about 40% of the preoperative level 1–4 hours after surgery and does not return to normal until the second postoperative week. Functional residual capacity ↓ to 70% of the preoperative level by 24 hours postoperatively and does not return to normal until the tenth postoperative day. The following measures should be addressed to ↓ the likelihood of postoperative pulmonary complications:

- Minimizing atelectasis by deep inspiration (can be facilitated through use of incentive spirometry).
- Early mobilization.
- Careful monitoring of fluid balance.
- Early treatment of cardiac failure.

### GASTROINTESTINAL CARE

Peristalsis returns in the small intestine within 24 hours postoperatively, in the right colon by 48 hours, and in the left colon by 72 hours, but gastric function returns more slowly. After operations involving the stomach and upper intestine, normal gastric function may not return for 3–4 days.

- **Overall guidelines:**
  - In general, patients should remain NPO until there is evidence of peristalsis (e.g., appetite, audible bowel sounds, passage of flatus).
  - Opioid pain medications contribute to postoperative ileus; thus, all patients receiving such medications need a stool softener and/or laxative medication.
- **Nasogastric (NG) tube intubation:**
  - An NG tube should be considered in patients with marked ileus; in those with a very low level of consciousness (to prevent aspiration);

and in those with postoperative emesis or marked abdominal distention.

- In patients with an NG tube, GI fluid loss is usually < 500 mL/day and can be replaced by an ↑ IV fluid rate to account for the loss. Add 20 mEq/L of KCl to every liter used to replace these GI losses.
- **NG tube management is as follows:**
    - Low intermittent suction.
    - Frequent irrigation (to ensure patency).
    - Leave in place for 2–3 days or until there is evidence of normal peristalsis.
    - Patients should fast for 24 hours after NG tube removal and should then advance to a clear liquid diet.

*"Clamping" an NG tube overnight to check residual volumes is not necessary and may ↑ the risk of aspiration.*

### PAIN MANAGEMENT

Postoperative pain serves no practical function and can give rise to a range of complications, including the following:

- Splinting of the diaphragm → reluctance to breathe → atelectasis.
- Limited motion → venous stasis → DVT.
- Release of catecholamines → vasospasm and hypertension → stroke, MI, and bleeding.

Factors that influence postoperative pain include:

- **Type of operation:** Some 60% of patients who have undergone intrathoracic, intra-abdominal, and major bone or joint procedures have what they describe as "severe" pain. In contrast, > 15% of patients who have undergone superficial operations on the head and neck, limbs, or abdominal wall describe their pain as severe.
- **Patient characteristics:** Physical, emotional, and cultural characteristics → differing perceptions of pain even in patients who undergo the same procedure.
- **Physician-patient communication:** Frequent reassurance, attention to patients' needs, and genuine concern do more to relieve pain than many physicians realize.
- Table 12.6 outlines options for postoperative pain management.

### ANTIBIOTICS

Patients receiving prophylactic antibiotics are usually given only one dose prior to an operative procedure. Only if the operation is particularly complex and/or long may a second dose of antimicrobials be warranted. There is no evidence that the ongoing administration of postoperative antimicrobial agents provides any additional benefit in patients who lack the signs and symptoms of active infection.

*Routine postoperative antimicrobial use should be discouraged, as it is costly and is associated with ↑ rates of microbial drug resistance.*

## The Convalescent Period

The final postoperative phase begins when a patient is discharged from the hospital. The following support services should be considered to ensure a smooth transition home, minimize postoperative complications, and hasten the patient's recovery from surgery:

- Visiting/home nursing agencies
- Physical/occupational therapy

TABLE 12.6. **Postoperative Pain Medications**

| ROUTE/ MEDICATION CLASS | EXAMPLES | ADVANTAGES | SIDE EFFECTS |
|---|---|---|---|
| IV opioids | Morphine, meperidine, hydromorphone, methadone | Potent analgesia. | Respiratory depression, nausea, vomiting, altered sensorium. |
| IV nonopioid analgesics | Ketorolac tromethamine (an NSAID) | Analgesic and anti-inflammatory. | Potential for gastric ulcer; impaired coagulation; ↓ renal function with long-term use. |
| PO analgesics | Acetaminophen with codeine (T#3); hydrocodone with acetaminophen (Vicodin) | Acetaminophen acts as an antipyretic and allows patients to be "transitioned" home with adequate pain relief. | Tolerance with long-term use. |
| Patient-controlled analgesia | Usually morphine | Controlled by the patient. The possibility of overdose is limited because the patient must be awake to self-administer. The maximum dose and timing are preset by the physician. | Respiratory depression, nausea, vomiting, altered sensorium, inadequate analgesia if the patient is unable to depress the button. |
| Continuous epidural analgesia | Morphine with or without bupivacaine (topical to the epidural space) | Intense and prolonged segmental analgesia, ↓ respiratory depression, longer pain relief, ↓ alteration of sensorium than IV opioids. | Pruritus, nausea, respiratory depression, hypotension, urinary retention (usually requires a bladder catheter). |
| Intercostal block | Bupivacaine | Useful for diminishing pain following thoracic and abdominal procedures. | Risk of pneumothorax. |

- Rehabilitation services
- Wound care specialists

Consider a short stay at a **skilled nursing facility** for patients with more intense nursing needs and/or poor support at home.

## SURGICAL WOUNDS

Wound healing can be thought of as a **stepwise process** proceeding from coagulation and inflammation through fibroplasia, matrix deposition, angiogenesis, epithelialization, collagen maturation, and wound contraction. The process is generally divided into **first-intention (1°)** and **second-intention (2°) healing**. These two forms may be combined in **delayed 1° closure.**

- **First-intention (1°) healing:** Occurs when tissue is cleanly incised and reapproximated and repair occurs without complication.
- **Second-intention (2°) healing:** Occurs in open wounds through the formation of granulation tissue and eventual coverage of the defect by spontaneous migration of epithelial cells.
- **Delayed 1° closure:** Combines 1° and 2° healing. A wound is allowed to

SURGERY

heal open (under an occlusive dressing) for about five days and is then reapproximated using suture or other ligature.

## Types of Skin Closures

The exact method of wound closure may be less important than how well the closure is performed. General guidelines are as follows:

- Sutures should be placed as far apart as possible consistent with approximation of tissue. Sutures placed too tightly and too close together obstruct blood supply to the wound.
- In healthy patients, the ideal closure for **small superficial wounds** (e.g., skin lacerations) consists of fine **interrupted sutures** placed loosely and conveniently close to the wound edge.
- **Mattress sutures** (horizontal and vertical) promote wound edge eversion and minimize tension on skin edges.
- **Running subcuticular sutures** are useful for long wounds in which the tension has been already minimized by deep sutures.
- **Deeper abdominal wounds** require closure of fascia layers (but not necessarily the peritoneum) with **continuous nonabsorbable** or slowly absorbable sutures.

*Gentle handling of tissue is of utmost importance; excellent hemostasis should always be the goal. Minimal and skillful use of electrocautery, ligatures, and sutures is desirable.*

## Suture Selection

The ideal suture is flexible, strong, easily tied, and securely knotted; excites little tissue reaction; and will not serve as a nidus for infection. Some general suture types and their relative advantages and disadvantages are listed in Table 12.7.

## Postoperative Wound Care

Recommendations for postoperative wound management include the following:

- **General guidelines:**
  - Sterile dressings applied in the OR should remain intact until the third or fourth day postoperatively unless they are soaked.
  - Any handling of a wound in the first 24 hours postoperatively should be done using aseptic technique.
  - Skin sutures or skin staples may be removed by the fifth postoperative day and replaced by tapes (Steristrips).
  - If the incision is healing normally, the patient may shower or bathe by the seventh postoperative day.
  - Skin sutures should be left in longer (e.g., two weeks) in incisions under tension, crossing creases (groin), or on the extremities as well as in debilitated patients.
  - Fever without another source and/or ↑ wound pain raise concern for postoperative wound infection.
  - Sutures should be removed if a suture tract shows signs of infection.
  - Any drainage from an infected wound should be sent for Gram stain and culture.
  - In patients with venous stasis, a lower extremity wound heals faster if it is elevated.
  - Wound healing is faster if there are no nutritional deficits (e.g., vitamin C, vitamin A, trace minerals).

*The quantity and quality of drainage should be recorded and contamination minimized.*

SURGERY

TABLE 12.7. Types of Sutures

| SUTURE | CHARACTERISTICS | ADVANTAGES | DISADVANTAGES | EXAMPLES OF CLINICAL USE |
|---|---|---|---|---|
| **Absorbable** | | | | |
| *Natural* | | | | |
| Catgut (plain or chromic) | Made from sheep intestine. | Quickly absorbed (good for fast-healing areas). | Poor tensile strength; high tissue reactivity (both drawbacks are minimized with chromic). | OB/Gyn (e.g., perineal lacerations). |
| *Synthetic* | | | | |
| (e,g., Dexon, Vicryl, PDS) | Made of chemical polymers; absorbed by hydrolysis; may be monofilament or multifilament. | Strong with predictable rates of loss in tensile strength; minimal tissue reaction. | Some have high tissue drag; coatings can reduce knot security. | Deep (dermal or buried) closures. |
| **Nonabsorbable** | | | | |
| *Natural* | | | | |
| Silk | Made of raw silk spun by silkworms; may be coated in wax. | Excellent handling. | High tissue reactivity; risk of infection. | Rarely used. Intraoral surgery. |
| Stainless steel wire | Made of a stainless steel alloy and comes in monofilament and multifilament. | High tensile strength. | May kink and break. | Cardiothoracic surgery; neurosurgery and orthopedics. |
| *Synthetic* | | | | |
| (e.g., Nylon, Dacron, Prolene) | Generally inert; may be monofilament or multifilament. | Low tissue reactivity; high tensile strength. | High memory (requires 3–4 knot throws to hold). | Superficial (subcuticular) skin closures. |

*When there has been little or no drainage, a drain may be withdrawn at once or progressively over a period of a few days.*

- Anticipate problems with wound healing in patients taking corticosteroids (e.g., consider delaying the removal of skin sutures).
- **Drains:** The purpose of drains is twofold: to prevent or treat unwanted accumulation of fluid (pus, blood, or serum) and to evacuate air from the pleural cavity. Types include the following:
    - **Closed drains (e.g., Jackson-Pratt or JP):** Connected to a suction device.
    - **Open drains (e.g., Penrose):** Not connected to a suction; collapses closed when fluid is not running through it.
    - **Sump drains (e.g., Davol):** Connected to a suction device; has an airflow system that keeps the drain open when fluid is not passing through it.

SURGERY

TABLE 12.8. Risk Factors for Wound Dehiscence

| HOST FACTORS | OPERATOR FACTORS |
|---|---|
| Smoking | Tissue injury |
| Starvation | Poor blood supply |
| Steroids | Poor apposition of tissues (unclosed dead |
| Infection | space, unreduced fracture) |
| Hypoxia and hypovolemia | |
| Radiation | |
| Trauma | |
| Uremia | |
| DM | |
| Drugs (especially chemotherapeutic agents) | |
| Advanced age | |

## Causes of Wound Dehiscence

- **Dehiscence** is defined as undesired spontaneous separation of wound edges.
- The most common causes are **infection** and **excessively tight sutures.**
- Wound dehiscence can be caused by **host factors** and/or operator **factors** (see Table 12.8).

## SURGICAL INFECTIONS

**Three elements** are common to surgical infections: an infectious agent, a susceptible host, and a closed space. These elements must be fully understood in order to optimize patient care.

## Infectious Agents

Any organism can cause a surgical infection, but some pathogens are more frequently implicated than others. Common examples are listed in Table 12.9.

## Susceptible Hosts

**Immunosuppression,** usually representing a combination of defects in the multifaceted human immune system, is the most common cause of a susceptible host. Both disease processes and iatrogenic causes (e.g., corticosteroids) can → immunosuppression. Types of immunity are as follows:

- Specific immunity:
  - Contributes little to the severity of ordinary surgical infections.
  - Depends on prior exposure to an antigen; involves mobilization of T and B lymphocytes and synthesis of specific antibodies.
  - Examples of impaired specific immunity include AIDS, transplant immunosuppression, and agammaglobulinemia.
- Nonspecific immunity:
  - The principal means by which hosts defend against abscess-forming and necrotizing infections.

387

TABLE 12.9. **Common Pathogens Causing Surgical Infections**

| ORGANISM | CHARACTERISTICS |
|---|---|
| Staphylococci (*S. aureus*) | The most common pathogen in wound infections; associated with foreign bodies. |
| Streptococci | Can invade minor skin breaks and spread through connective tissue. |
| *Klebsiella* | Often invades the inner ear, enteric tissues, and lung. |
| Enteric organisms (Enterobacteriaceae and enterococci) | Often found with anaerobes such as peptostreptococci, *Bacteroides,* and *Clostridium.* |
| *Clostridium* | Anaerobic; often found in ischemic tissue. |
| *Pseudomonas* | Opportunistic in critically ill or immunosuppressed patients. |
| Fungi, yeast, and parasites | Cause abscesses. |

- Limits damage during the first few hours after infection.
- Depends on phagocytic leukocyte migration, ingestion, and cidal activity for microorganisms.
- **Immunity in DM:**
  - Well-controlled diabetics resist infection normally except in tissues made ischemic by arterial disease; uncontrolled diabetics do not.
  - The mechanism is unknown but may be due to impaired leukocyte function in the face of ↑ blood glucose and low insulin.
  - Insulin is consumed in wounds and other poorly perfused spaces → low ambient insulin levels.

### The Closed Space

- A closed, poorly vascularized space is a form of local immunosuppression.
- Poor perfusion → local hypoxia, hypercapnia, and acidosis, all of which predispose to infections.

### Management of Infection

- An infected surgical site **must be opened** either partially or entirely, depending on the extent of infection.
- Perform Gram stain and culture of purulent drainage.
- Administer empiric antibiotics.
- Switch to narrow-spectrum antibiotics once Gram stain and culture reveal a likely organism.

## ACUTE ABDOMEN

Any sudden spontaneous nontraumatic disorder whose chief manifestation is in the abdominal area and for which urgent operation may be necessary.

## SYMPTOMS

- Abdominal pain, fever, anorexia, nausea, vomiting, diarrhea, or constipation.
- **Jaundice, hematemesis, hematochezia,** or **hematuria** may also be seen.

## EXAM

The following common exam findings may be absent in specific cases:

- **General:** Rigidly motionless, pale, tachycardic, hypotensive, and hypo- or hyperthermic.
- **Abdominal examination** (see also Table 12.10):
    - **Inspection:** Tensely distended; old surgical scars.
    - **Auscultation:** Silent bowel sounds.
    - **Percussion:** Tenderness and tympany.
    - **Palpation:** Guarding and/or rebound tenderness.
- **Rectal exam must be performed** in all patients with an acute abdomen.

## DIFFERENTIAL

- Acute appendicitis, acute cholecystitis, acute pancreatitis.
- **Other:** Bowel obstruction, incarcerated hernia, ruptured ectopic pregnancy, dissecting aortic aneurysm, perforated peptic ulcer (and others).

## DIAGNOSIS

- **Labs:** Leukocytosis and anemia may be seen on CBC; chem 7 may reveal ↑ BUN/creatinine and metabolic acidosis. Obtain LFTs to look for ↑

**TABLE 12.10.  Physical Exam Findings Associated with Acute Abdomen**

| CONDITION | APPEARANCE | PALPATION | AUSCULTATION |
|---|---|---|---|
| Perforated viscus | Scaphoid abdomen | Tense; guarding and rigidity. | Diminished bowel sounds; loss of liver dullness. |
| Peritonitis | Motionless patient | Guarding and rebound tenderness. | Absent bowel sounds (late). |
| Inflamed mass or abscess | Variable distention | Tender to palpation; special signs (Murphy's, psoas, obturator). | Variable bowel sounds. |
| Intestinal obstruction | Distention; visible peristalsis (late) | Diffusely tender to palpation; hernia or mass (some). | Hyperactive (early) or hypoactive (late) bowel sounds. |
| Paralytic ileus | Distention | No localized tenderness. | Hypoactive bowel sounds. |
| Ischemic or strangulated bowel | No distention (until late) | Severe pain but little tenderness to palpation; rectal bleeding (some). | Variable bowel sounds. |
| Bleeding | Pallor, shock; distention | Pulsatile (aneurysm) or tender (e.g., ectopic pregnancy) mass; rectal bleeding. | Variable bowel sounds. |

transaminases and/or hyperbilirubinemia. An ↑ lipase level may indicate acute pancreatitis. A urine pregnancy test must be performed on all females of reproductive age!

- **Imaging:**
  - Upright CXR may reveal subdiaphragmatic air (perforated viscous) or lower lung pathology that may mimic an acute abdomen.
  - AXR may show signs of bowel obstruction or free air.
  - Ultrasound is useful for evaluating the biliary tree.
  - A CT scan should routinely be obtained.
  - Consider MRI, GI contrast studies, and endoscopy.

### TREATMENT

In a patient with true acute abdomen, **urgent exploratory laparotomy** is often necessary before the precise diagnosis is known.

## APPENDICITIS

A bacterial infection in the wall of the appendix that is due to obstruction of the proximal lumen. Can eventually → gangrene and perforation.

> A 16-year-old boy presents to your office on a weekday afternoon with severe abdominal pain. On further history, his mother states that he vomited dinner last night and did not eat breakfast this morning. When she dropped him off at school, he was complaining of mild periumbilical pain. By 10 A.M. he was curled up on the classroom floor unable to move and was complaining of generalized abdominal pain. On presentation, he is febrile, tachycardic, and mildly hypotensive. Physical exam reveals abdominal guarding and tenderness at McBurney's point with ↓ bowel sounds. CBC shows leukocytosis with a left shift. CT scan reveals an inflamed mass in the RLQ consistent with appendicitis. The patient is taken to the operating room for emergent appendectomy.

### Acute Appendicitis

#### SYMPTOMS

- Often begins with vague midabdominal pain followed by **anorexia, nausea, vomiting,** and **low-grade fever.**
- Classically progresses to localized tenderness to palpation in the RLQ.

#### EXAM

- Temperature is only slightly ↑ (e.g., 37.8°C) in the absence of perforation.
- Patients with early (nonperforated) appendicitis often appear quite well.
- Abdominal tenderness with guarding and possible rebound can be seen in later stages.
- Tenderness is seen at **McBurney's point,** one-third the distance from the anterior superior iliac spine to the umbilicus.
- Patients may also have pain on flexion of the hip (**psoas sign**), pain on internal rotation of the hip (**obturator sign**), or pain on the right side when pressing on the left (**Rovsing's sign**).
- **Appendicitis in pregnancy** can present with **RUQ tenderness** due to the gravid uterus.

PID (especially in women 20–40 years of age), ectopic pregnancy, ovarian torsion, cholecystitis, diverticulitis, gastroenteritis, psoas abscess, right inguinal hernia, mesenteric adenitis.

### DIAGNOSIS

- **Labs: Leukocytosis** is seen (usually > 10,000/μL). May have WBCs and/or RBCs in urine (especially in retrocecal or pelvic appendicitis).
- **Imaging:**
    - **AXR:** May show localized air-fluid levels, localized ileus, or ↑ soft tissue density in the RLQ. Less common findings include a calculus, an altered right psoas shadow, or an abnormal right flank stripe.
    - **CT:** Most useful when the clinical presentation and/or lab findings are less than typical and a ⊕ CT scan would be an indication for surgery. Classic findings include an **enlarged appendix with wall thickening or enhancement or periappendiceal fat stranding.**
    - **RLQ ultrasound:** Much less reliable than CT.

### TREATMENT

- Open or laparoscopic appendectomy.
- Prophylactic preoperative antibiotics (usually a single-drug regimen using a cephalosporin).
- Antibiotics alone if surgery is contraindicated or unavailable.

### COMPLICATIONS

- **Perforation:** Usually due to delay in seeking medical care. Occurs late (> 12 hours after onset of symptoms) and associated with more severe pain and a higher fever. Affects patients < 10 or > 50 years of age.
- **Peritonitis:** Can be localized or generalized; results from microscopic perforation of a gangrenous appendix or gross perforation into the peritoneal cavity, respectively.
- **Appendiceal abscess:** Occurs when the infection is walled off by adjacent omentum or viscera.
- **Pylephlebitis:** A suppurative thrombophlebitis of the portal venous system.

## Chronic Appendicitis

- **Sx/Exam:**
    - Presents with pain of ≥ **3 weeks' duration.**
    - History reveals an **acute illness** at some time in the past that was managed nonoperatively and is **compatible with acute appendicitis.**
    - A chronically **inflamed or fibrotic appendix** can be seen.
- **Tx:** Symptoms **resolve with appendectomy.**

## SMALL BOWEL OBSTRUCTION (SBO)

There are numerous disorders of the small intestine, including acute enteritis, regional enteritis (Crohn's disease), mesenteric adenitis, blind loop syndrome, and intestinal fistulas. This section will focus on the **most common surgical disorder of the small intestine, small bowel obstruction.** Etiologies include **adhesions, neoplasms, hernias, intussusception, foreign bodies, and gall-**

**stones.** Obstruction can be mechanical or functional; proximal, middle, or distal; and complete or partial.

### SYMPTOMS

- **Proximal (high) obstruction:** Presents with abdominal pain and vomiting.
- **Mid- or distal obstruction:** Presents with periumbilical or poorly localized abdominal cramping along with distention and constipation/obstipation. Feculent vomitus may also be seen.
- **Dehydration** and mild fever are seen.

### EXAM

- Vital signs are normal in the early stages.
- Peristalsis may be visible beneath the abdominal wall in thin patients.
- Exam reveals mild abdominal tenderness.
- Peristaltic rushes, gurgles, and **high-pitched tinkles** are sometimes audible.

### DIFFERENTIAL

- **Postoperative ileus:** Gas in the colon on AXR rules out obstruction.
- **Large bowel obstruction:** Obstipation and colonic dilation on AXR.
- **Intestinal pseudo-obstruction:** Symptoms and signs of obstruction without evidence of obstruction. Associated with SLE, drugs and amyloidosis.
- **Other:** Acute gastroenteritis, acute appendicitis, acute pancreatitis.

### DIAGNOSIS

- **Labs:** Can be normal. Leukocytosis, evidence of dehydration, and/or electrolyte abnormalities may be seen.
- **Imaging:**
  - **AXR (abdominal radiographs):** Supine and upright AXRs reveal a ladderlike pattern of dilated small bowel loops with air-fluid levels (see Figure 12.2).

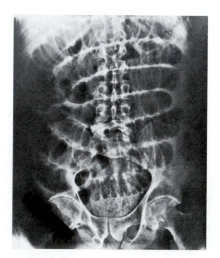

**FIGURE 12.2.    Small bowel obstruction.**

(Reproduced, with permission, from Doherty GM, Way LW. *Current Surgical Diagnosis & Treatment*, 12th ed. New York: McGraw-Hill, 2006: 666.)

- **CT:** Highly accurate in making the diagnosis and confirming the level of SBO.

### TREATMENT

- **Partial obstruction (gas seen in the colon on AXR):** Can be managed expectantly with **NPO and an NG tube** as long as the patient is passing flatus and stool.
- **Complete obstruction:**
    - Requires **operation,** in part to rule out **strangulation** (bowel dilation that impairs blood supply, which can eventually → necrosis, sepsis, perforation, and death).
    - Patients must be NPO, have an NG tube, and be fluid and electrolyte resuscitated prior to the procedure.
    - Antibiotics should be given if strangulation is suspected.
    - The timing and details of the operation vary according to the patient and the underlying cause of the obstruction.

### LARGE BOWEL OBSTRUCTION (LBO)

Approximately 15% of intestinal obstructions in adults occur in the large intestine, most commonly in the **sigmoid colon.** The most common cause of LBO is carcinoma; the remainder of cases are caused by diverticular disease, volvulus, inflammatory disorders, benign tumors, fecal impaction, and miscellaneous rare problems.

### SYMPTOMS/EXAM

- Presents with abdominal cramping, borborygmus, constipation and/or obstipation, and vomiting.
- Exam reveals abdominal distention, tympany, high-pitched "tinkles" on auscultation of bowel sounds, and tenderness to palpation +/– signs of peritonitis (rebound tenderness).

### DIFFERENTIAL

SBO, paralytic ileus, pseudo-obstruction (Ogilvie's syndrome).

### DIAGNOSIS

- **Labs:** May be normal. Leukocytosis and electrolyte abnormalities are seen with progression of disease.
- **Imaging:**
    - **AXR:** Demonstrates a dilated colon (distinguished from the small intestine by its haustral markings, which do not cross the entire lumen of the distended colon) with air-fluid levels.
    - **Barium enema:** Confirms the diagnosis and identifies the location of the obstruction.
    - **CT:** The best study for identifying the exact location and etiology of the bowel obstruction.

### TREATMENT

- Almost always **needs an operation.**
- The patient may require a **staged operation** consisting of an initial colonic resection and diverting colostomy followed by a later reanastomosis.

## Diverticular Disorders

Approximately 65% of adults in the Western world develop diverticula by age 80, most commonly in the colon. Colonic diverticula are classified as false because they consist of mucosa and submucosa that have herniated through the muscular coats. True diverticula (containing all layers of bowel) are rare in the colon.

### DIVERTICULOSIS

- Defined as the presence of multiple false diverticula.
- **Sx/Exam:** Usually asymptomatic. Exam reveals mild tenderness in the LLQ.
- **DDx:** Diverticulitis, colon cancer.
- **Dx:**
    - **Labs:** Fever and leukocytosis are absent in patients with diverticula (and no diverticulitis).
    - **Imaging: Barium enema** reveals segmental spasm and muscular thickening that narrows the lumen, giving it a **sawtoothed appearance.**
- **Tx:** High-fiber diet; bulking agents (psyllium); education and reassurance; surgical resection for massive hemorrhage or to rule out carcinoma.

### DIVERTICULITIS

A complication of diverticulosis that can range from mild inflammation to colonic perforation with peritonitis.

#### SYMPTOMS/EXAM

- Presents with acute onset of LLQ pain.
- Also associated with constipation and/or diarrhea.
- Nausea, vomiting, or dysuria may be seen depending on the location and extent of inflammation.
- Peritoneal signs are seen if the disease presents late (with perforation).
- Exam reveals low-grade fever, mild abdominal distention, LLQ tenderness, and an LLQ mass.

#### DIFFERENTIAL

Appendicitis, mesenteric ischemia, bowel obstruction, Crohn's disease.

#### DIAGNOSIS

- **Labs:** Leukocytosis; ⊖ fecal occult blood (if present, suggests malignancy).
- **Imaging:**
    - **AXR:** Reveals free air in the presence of a perforation. Shows ileus and partial obstruction +/− LLQ mass.
    - **CT: The best initial study (preferably with IV and oral contrast).** May reveal **pericolic fat stranding,** an abscess, or a fistula.
    - **Barium enema: Contraindicated** 2° to the possibility of barium leaking into peritoneal cavity.

#### TREATMENT

- **Expectant management:**
    - NPO, NG tube placement, IV fluids.
    - Broad-spectrum antibiotics with colonoscopy 4–6 weeks after the acute attack.

- Surgical management:
    - Indicated for **perforation or failure of expectant management;** may sometimes be managed with percutaneous drainage of paracolic abscesses.
    - Severe cases usually require laparotomy and **possible colectomy** (often done as a **staged operation**). Laparoscopic operations are difficult in the setting of inflammation.

## Sigmoid Volvulus

Rotation of a segment of the intestine on an axis formed by its mesentery can → obstruction of the lumen and circulatory impairment of the bowel. The sigmoid is the segment that is most commonly involved in colonic volvulus.

### SYMPTOMS/EXAM

Presents with intermittent cramplike pain and obstipation. Exam reveals abdominal distention.

### DIFFERENTIAL

Cecal volvulus and other causes of LBO (carcinoma, benign tumors, fecal impaction, diverticular disease).

### DIAGNOSIS

- **AXR:** A single, greatly distended loop of bowel that has lost its haustral markings is usually seen rising up out of the pelvis (sometimes termed **"megacolon"**).
- **Barium enema:** The pathognomonic finding is the **"bird's beak"** or **"ace of spades"** deformity, named for the way the barium column tapers toward the volvulus (see Figure 12.3).

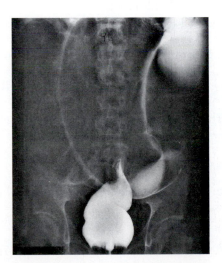

**FIGURE 12.3.** **Sigmoid volvulus showing "bird's beak" or "ace of spades" deformity.**

(Reproduced, with permission, from Doherty GM, Way LW. *Current Surgical Diagnosis & Treatment*, 12th ed. New York: McGraw-Hill, 2005: 721.)

## TREATMENT

- **Endoscopic decompression** with a flexible colonoscope or sigmoidoscope.
- **Emergent operation (partial or total colectomy):** Performed if strangulation or perforation is present or if attempts at decompression are unsuccessful.

### ANORECTAL DISORDERS

A 70-year-old African-American man with a history of CAD calls your answering service on Sunday night complaining of "bright red blood in my stool" for a few days. He had a normal colonoscopy six months ago and has no history of weight loss or anemia. When you see him in the office on Monday morning, he has stable vital signs and no abdominal pain, and anoscopy reveals a friable internal hemorrhoid. CBC reveals a stable hemoglobin/hematocrit. You prescribe a stool softener and advise your patient to increase fluid intake, get regular exercise, and limit time spent on the commode.

## Hemorrhoids

Hemorrhoidal tissues that cause bleeding, pain, or mucus are pathologic, usually occurring in the setting of ↑ intra-abdominal pressure such as that which occurs in pregnancy, in the presence of obesity, and with lifting or straining.

### SYMPTOMS

- **Internal hemorrhoids:** Painless; present with bright red blood per rectum, mucous discharge, and rectal fullness or discomfort. Classification is based on history:
    - **First degree:** Hemorrhoids bleed.
    - **Second degree:** Hemorrhoids bleed and prolapse but reduce spontaneously.
    - **Third degree:** Hemorrhoids bleed and prolapse and require manual reduction.
    - **Fourth degree:** Hemorrhoids bleed, cannot be reduced, and may strangulate.
- **External hemorrhoids:** Present with severe perianal pain and perianal mass.

### EXAM

Exam reveals vascular dilation, friable mucosa, and local perineal irritation.

### DIFFERENTIAL

Malignancy, diverticular disease, IBD, adenomatous polyps.

### DIAGNOSIS

- **Labs:** CBC to rule out anemia 2° to chronic bleeding.
- **Anoscopy:** Allows direct visual inspection of the anal canal.

### TREATMENT

- **Medical:** Best for first-degree and second-degree internal hemorrhoids. Consists of dietary changes (eliminating constipating foods and increasing fiber), exercise, and limiting toilet time.
- **Surgical:** Used when medical management fails. The three classic techniques are elastic band ligation, sclerosis, and excisional hemorrhoidectomy.

### COMPLICATIONS

Bleeding, pain, necrosis, and, rarely, perianal sepsis.

### THROMBOSED EXTERNAL HEMORRHOID

Acute intravascular thrombosis that develops within an external hemorrhoid → severe perianal pain.

### SYMPTOMS/EXAM

- Presents with sudden, severe perianal pain that peaks within 48–72 hours.
- Exam reveals a purplish-black, edematous, tense subcutaneous perianal mass.

### DIFFERENTIAL

Nonthrombosed external hemorrhoid, internal hemorrhoid, skin tag.

### DIAGNOSIS

Anoscopy allows direct visual inspection of the anal canal.

### TREATMENT

- **< 48 hours after onset of symptoms:** Excision or hemorrhoid/clot evacuation.
- **48–72 hours after onset of symptoms:** Warm sitz baths, high-fiber diet, stool softeners, reassurance.

## Anal Fissure

A split in the anoderm that results from forceful dilation of the anal canal, most commonly during defecation.

### SYMPTOMS/EXAM

- Presents with pain with defecation along with blood on the tissue and stool or dripping into the toilet water (but not mixed in the stool). Constipation is common.
- Exam reveals disruption of the anoderm in the anterior or posterior midline involving the epithelium immediately distal to the dentate line.

### DIFFERENTIAL

Crohn's disease, anal TB, anal malignancy, abscess or fistula disease, HSV.

### DIAGNOSIS

**Anoscopy** may reveal the classic triad of a proximal hypertrophied anal papilla above a fissure with the sentinel pile at the anal verge.

### TREATMENT

- **Medical:** Stool softeners, bulking agents, sitz baths.
- **Surgical:** Consider surgery for chronic (> 1-month) or chronic recurrent ulcers. Lateral internal anal sphincterectomy is the procedure of choice.

## Anorectal Abscess and Fistula

When glands in the anorectum become infected, they can develop into an abscess and an associated fistula tract.

### SYMPTOMS/EXAM

- Presents with severe, continuous throbbing anal pain.
- Anal swelling, fever, urinary retention, and sepsis may be seen.
- Exam reveals a tender perianal or rectal mass. A fistula tract may not be discovered until exam is performed under anesthesia.

### DIFFERENTIAL

Crohn's disease, pilonidal disease, hidradenitis suppurativa, diverticulitis, anal fissure.

### DIAGNOSIS

- No imaging is necessary in uncomplicated cases.
- Sinography, transrectal ultrasound, CT, and MRI can be useful in complex or recurrent cases.

### TREATMENT

Surgical drainage under general anesthesia.

## Pilonidal Disease

An acquired infection of natal cleft hair follicles, which, when obstructed, become distended and rupture into the subcutaneous tissue, forming an abscess. The highest incidence is in white males 15–40 years of age, with a peak incidence in those between 16 and 20.

### SYMPTOMS/EXAM

- Presents with pain, tenderness, purulent drainage, inspissated hair, and induration near the perianal region.
- Patients are typically overweight, hirsute males who perspire profusely.
- Exam of the coccyx or sacrum reveals small pits or abscesses on or close to midline.

### DIFFERENTIAL

Abscess-fistula disease, hidradenitis suppurativa, furuncle, actinomycosis.

Physical exam is adequate for diagnosis.

### TREATMENT

- Surgical incision, drainage, and curettage of the abscess cavity to remove hair nests and skin debris.
- Meticulous skin care, hygiene, and shaving of the surrounding area for at least three months after the surgical procedure.
- May require more definitive surgery (e.g., excision of pits, marsupialization).

## Fecal Impaction

May develop after excisional hemorrhoidectomy, in chronically debilitated patients, or from the use of constipating pain medications without stool softeners and fiber.

### SYMPTOMS

- Diarrhea (only liquid stool is able to pass the obstructing inspissated fecal bolus).
- Pelvic pain and fullness.

### EXAM

DRE (digital rectal exam) reveals hard, dry stool that obstructs the rectum. Abdominal exam may reveal a pelvic or abdominal mass.

### DIFFERENTIAL

Sigmoid malignancy or other obstructing lesion.

### TREATMENT

- Digital disimpaction at the bedside.
- Treatment in the operating room with local or regional anesthesia may be necessary to provide pelvic floor relaxation and pain control.

## ABDOMINAL WALL HERNIAS

An abnormal protrusion of intra-abdominal tissue through a fascial defect in the abdominal wall. Approximately 75% occur in the groin, most of these being inguinal hernias (see Table 12.11). Hernias can be completely reducible, incompletely reducible, or nonreducible, depending on the ability to manually push the herniated tissue back into the abdomen. Bowel strangulation is a dreaded complication that usually occurs in nonreducible hernias.

SURGERY

TABLE 12.11.   Types of Hernias

| Type | Pathophysiology | Location | Characteristics |
|------|-----------------|----------|-----------------|
| Indirect inguinal | A persistent processus vaginalis. | The groin **lateral** to the inferior epigastric vessels. | May present at birth. Can descend into the scrotum. |
| Direct inguinal | A defect of the transversalis fascia in Hesselbach's triangle.[a] | The groin **medial** to the inferior epigastric vessels. | Most occur in middle-aged or elderly patients. |
| Femoral | Occurs through the femoral canal. | The upper thigh medial to the femoral vein. | Less common; usually occurs in women. Can easily become incarcerated or strangulated. |
| Incisional/ventral | Breakdown of fascial closure from prior surgery. | At the site of a previous surgical incision. | Often asymptomatic. May become larger upon standing or with ↑ intra-abdominal pressure. |
| Umbilical | Occurs through the fibromuscular umbilical ring. | The umbilicus. | Repair only if it persists beyond age two. |
| Obturator | Occurs through the large obturator canal. | Deep structures of the pelvis/thigh (not visualized externally). | Has a female-to-male ratio of 6:1. Can present as bowel obstruction. |

[a] Hesselbach's triangle is defined inferiorly by the inguinal ligament, laterally by the inferior epigastric arteries, and medially by the conjoined tendon.

> A 30-year-old woman who is otherwise healthy presents to you for the first time because she wants to be tested for the "breast cancer gene." She is concerned because her 52-year-old mother was diagnosed with metastatic breast cancer at age 38. You advise her that she is likely a candidate for BRCA1/BRCA2 mutation testing given that she has a first-degree relative with premenopausal breast cancer. You refer her for genetic testing.

## BREAST CANCER

The second deadliest cancer in women. Risk factors include the following:

- A ⊕ family history, particularly of premenopausal breast cancer.
- Mutations of BRCA1 and BRCA2.
- Age > 40.
- Estrogen exposure; HRT.
- Age at menarche < 12; age at first birth > 30; age at menopause > 55.
- Alcohol use.
- A history of a benign breast biopsy.
- A history of atypical hyperplasia on breast biopsy.
- OCP use is probably **not** a risk factor in average-risk women but may be in those with a ⊕ family history.

Screening methods include the following:

- **Breast self-examination:** Not standardized, and **not shown to have benefit.**
- **Clinical breast exam:** Not standardized; has a sensitivity of approximately 50%. There is insufficient evidence to recommend for or against routine CBE alone or in combination with screening mammography.
- **Mammography:** Screening should start at age 40 and should continue until age 70 (controversial for those < 40 and > 70 years of age). Sensitivity is 90% and is higher in older women. Screen patients in their 40s every year (cancer is more aggressive even though it is less prevalent) and every 1–2 years for patients ≥ 50 years of age.
- **BRCA1/BRCA2 mutation testing:** Appropriate for patients with the following:
    - A ⊕ family history of **premenopausal** breast cancer.
    - A known breast cancer.
    - Coexisting breast and ovarian cancer.
    - A family history of male breast cancer.

### DIFFERENTIAL

Fibrocystic disease, fibroadenoma, abscess, adenosis, scars, mastitis.

### DIAGNOSIS

- Breast cysts can be evaluated with ultrasound and then aspirated.
- Breast masses require either FNA or core needle biopsy, possibly followed by excisional biopsy.
- Any mass that is felt on exam **must** be further evaluated with biopsy even if no abnormality is seen on mammography.
- **Algorithm:** Mass → bilateral mammogram → tissue sampling → possible further workup depending on tissue findings.

### TREATMENT

Treatment for **early-stage breast cancer** is as follows:

- **Ductal carcinoma in situ (DCIS):** A premalignant condition that is high risk for becoming breast cancer. Treatment consists of excision (lumpectomy) with ⊖ margins and radiation therapy to the breast.
- **Lobular carcinoma in situ (LCIS):** A condition associated with an ↑ risk of breast cancer arising elsewhere in the breast. Treatment with tamoxifen may be considered, but close follow-up and observation are usually indicated.
- **Invasive ductal or lobular carcinoma:** Lumpectomy followed by radiation therapy is equivalent to mastectomy. Mastectomy for large tumors or for patient preference.
- **Sentinel lymph node biopsy:** Indicated for invasive disease and may be indicated in certain cases of carcinoma in situ.
- **Adjuvant therapy:**
    - In general, any patient with an infiltrating ductal or lobular cancer > 1 cm or with ⊕ lymph nodes should receive adjuvant therapy.
    - Hormone therapy with tamoxifen (for five years) is effective only with estrogen- or progesterone-receptor-⊕ (ER- or PR-⊕) breast cancers. Where appropriate, tamoxifen ↓ the risk of recurrence by 40%.
    - Polychemotherapy reduces the risk of recurrence by 25%.

The treatment approach for **advanced (metastatic) breast cancer** includes the following:

- **ER/PR-⊕ masses:**
  - **First-line therapy:** For postmenopausal women, first-line treatment consists of an **aromatase inhibitor.** Aromatase inhibitors prevent conversion of adrenal androgens into estrogens by aromatase enzymes in muscle and fat.
  - **Second-line hormonal therapy:** Includes megestrol acetate or tamoxifen.
- **ER/PR-⊖ masses (or progression of disease despite first-line treatment in hormone receptor-⊕ patients):**
  - Initial chemotherapy can be multiagent, but once patients progress after first-line treatment, single-agent treatment is commonly used.
  - Active chemotherapy drugs include paclitaxel, docetaxel, doxorubicin, methotrexate, vinorelbine, capecitabine, and 5-FU.
- **Patients with HER2 receptor overexpression:**
  - Overexpression of the HER2 receptor is associated with a poorer prognosis in breast cancer.
  - Trastuzumab (Herceptin) is a humanized monoclonal antibody against the HER2 receptor found on breast cancer cells.
  - Patients with HER2 overexpression show responses to trastuzumab alone or in combination with chemotherapy.

# CHAPTER 13

# Pediatric and Adolescent Medicine

Eve Paretsky, MD

Reina Rodriguez, MD

# PEDIATRIC MEDICINE

## The Newborn Exam

An infant's first exam is an important time to identify neonatal distress and also helps practitioners become aware of congenital abnormalities and correctable defects. Pertinent information to obtain on H&P includes the following:

- **History:** Elicit information on family history, maternal labs, maternal health during pregnancy and labor, outcomes of previous pregnancies, and potential toxic exposures.
- **Apgar scores:** Performed at one and five minutes; may be repeated at ten minutes if indicated (see Table 13.1).
- **Exam:**
  - **Skin:**
    - **Acrocyanosis:** May be normal, but generalized cyanosis may be a sign of a congenital heart defect and warrants immediate evaluation.
    - **Birthmarks:** Benign birthmarks include capillary hemangiomas and Mongolian spots. Those that raise concern include café-au-lait spots (> 6 may point to neurofibromatosis type 1; see Figure 13.1) and ash leaf spots (a sign of tuberous sclerosis).
  - **Head:**
    - **Caput succedaneum:** Edema over the presenting part. Crosses suture lines.
    - **Cephalhematoma:** Swelling over one or both parietal bones contained within suture lines. Generally benign.
    - **Subgaleal hemorrhage:** Bleeding beneath the scalp; can → extensive blood loss.
  - **Eyes:** An abnormal light reflex may be a sign of glaucoma, cataracts, or a tumor such as retinoblastoma.
  - **Ears:** Low-set ears may be associated with congenital anomalies; preauricular pits may point to congenital hearing loss.
  - **Nose:** Congenital defects such as choanal atresia may → respiratory distress, as infants are obligate nose breathers.

*More than six café-au-lait spots may be indicative of neurofibromatosis type 1.*

TABLE 13.1.  **Apgar Scores**

| SIGNS | POINTS SCORED | | |
|---|---|---|---|
| | **0** | **1** | **2** |
| Heartbeats per minute | Absent | Slow (< 100) | > 100 |
| Respiratory effort | Absent | Slow, irregular | Good, crying |
| Muscle tone | Limp | Some flexion of extremities | Active motion |
| Reflex irritability | No response | Grimace | Cry or cough |
| Color | Blue or pale | Body pink; extremities blue | Completely pink |

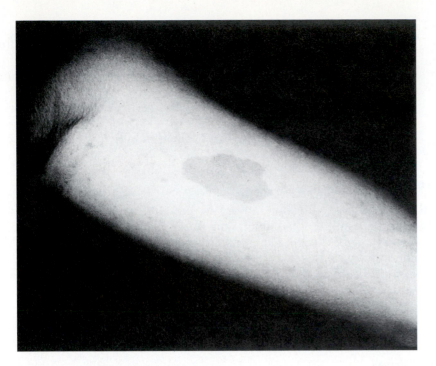

**FIGURE 13.1. Café-au-lait spot.**

(Reproduced, with permission, from Ropper A, Brown RH. *Adams and Victor's Principles of Neurology*, 8th ed. New York: McGraw-Hill, 2005: 869.)

- **Oropharynx:** Check for cleft lip or palate. Epstein pearls at the junction of the hard and soft palates are epithelial retention cysts and are considered normal.
- **Chest:** Fractured clavicles may result from delivery complicated by shoulder dystocia and are indicated by crepitus, bruising, and tenderness.
- **Heart:** Murmurs in the immediate newborn period are common and are usually benign (see the Cardiology section). Cyanosis, abnormal pulses, and signs of CHF are more frequent indicators of serious disease.
- **Abdomen:**
  - An abnormal mass is most often associated with kidney disease (tumor, hydronephrosis, multicystic kidney disease).
  - Consider diaphragmatic hernia in an infant with scaphoid abdomen and respiratory distress.
  - Prune belly (absence of abdominal musculature) is sometimes associated with congenital kidney abnormalities.
- **Genitalia:** Cryptorchidism may be present in up to 3% of term male infants but generally resolves by the first birthday.
- **Musculoskeletal:**
  - **Spine:** Pits or hair tufts at the base of the spine may be a clue to spina bifida occulta.
  - **Upper extremities:** ↓ movement may indicate a brachial plexus injury, especially following shoulder dystocia. Roughly 80% of cases resolve by 13 months of age.
  - **Lower extremities:** A clunk felt on Barlow's or Ortolani's maneuver indicates congenital hip dysplasia.
- **Neurologic:**
  - **Suck:** Observed by 14 weeks' gestation.

- **Rooting:** Develops by 28 weeks' gestation.
- **Grasp:** Develops by 28 weeks' gestation and disappears by three months of age.
- **DTRs:** Several beats of ankle clonus and presence of the Babinski reflex are normal.
- **Moro reflex:** Develops by 28 weeks' gestation and disappears by three months.
- **Tonic neck reflex:** Disappears by eight months.

## Circumcision

- **Risks:** Bleeding, infection, injury to the urethra or other surrounding structures, removal of too much skin, unsatisfactory cosmetic outcome.
- **Benefits:** Slightly ↓ the risk of penile cancer, UTIs, and possibly HIV infection.
- **Contraindications:** Genital abnormalities (e.g., hypospadias) or bleeding disorder.

## Problems in the Neonatal Period

### BIRTH TRAUMA

Complications associated with birth trauma include the following:

- **Intraventricular hemorrhage:** Most commonly occurs in preterm infants.
- **Hypoxia:** Related to chronic intrauterine conditions such as placental insufficiency or to acute events such as cord prolapse or maternal hypoxia. Low five-minute Apgar scores correlate with an ↑ risk of death in the first year as well as with cerebral palsy.
- **Fractures:** May occur with traumatic delivery. Clavicle fractures are most common.
- **Peripheral nerve injuries:** May occur with traumatic delivery or in the absence of any apparent cause. Most brachial plexus injuries resolve spontaneously in the first year. Physical therapy may be of benefit.

### NEONATAL JAUNDICE

- More than half of newborns will develop clinical jaundice in the first week of life. Risk factors include maternal diabetes, male gender, prematurity, and Asian ethnicity. Etiologies are outlined in Table 13.2.
- **Sx/Exam:** Early symptoms of bilirubin encephalopathy include lethargy, hypotonia, and poor suck.
- **Dx:** A nomogram correlating safe bilirubin levels with age should be used to determine the bilirubin concentration at which to consider intervention. A bilirubin concentration of 20 mg/dL is generally considered the level at which brain damage (kernicterus) is likely to occur, but treatment is generally initiated sooner.
- **Tx:** Hydration, ↑ feeding, phototherapy and exchange transfusion.
- **Cx:** Long-term complications of kernicterus include movement disorders and deafness.

*The rate of kernicterus fell sharply following the introduction of phototherapy and exchange transfusions, but recently it has risen again with the ↑ in early hospital discharges.*

*Any jaundice that arises in the first 24 hours of life should be considered pathologic and requires further evaluation.*

**Causes of neonatal jaundice—**

**CHIMPS**

**C**ephalohematoma
**H**emolysis
**I**nherited disorders
**M**ilk
**P**hysiologic
**S**epsis

**TABLE 13.2.** **Etiologies of Neonatal Jaundice**

| | CAUSE | DIAGNOSIS/COMMENTS |
|---|---|---|
| Hemolytic | Rh and ABO incompatibility | Check maternal Coombs' antibody for signs of isoimmunization. |
| | Hereditary spherocytosis | Spherocytes may be noted on peripheral smear. Confirm with a red cell osmotic fragility test. |
| | G6PD deficiency | An X-linked disorder seen most commonly in African, Mediterranean, and Asian families. |
| Nonhemolytic | Enclosed hemorrhage (cephalohematoma) | As blood is resorbed, bilirubin levels will ↑. |
| | Inherited disorders of conjugation | Examples include Crigler-Najjar and Gilbert syndrome. |
| | Physiologic (normal) | May be due to ↑ hematocrit (even in the absence of true polycythemia) and initial lack of gut flora. In order for jaundice to be physiologic, it must appear after the first 24 hours of life, may not rise by > 5 mg/dL per day, and should not exceed 15 mg/dL total. Bilirubin levels should peak on day 4 or 5 of life; jaundice typically resolves by the first week. |
| | Breast milk jaundice | Most likely related to free fatty acids in breast milk, which can → ↑ enterohepatic circulation of bilirubin. Typically appears after the first week and may persist for many weeks. |
| | Breast-feeding jaundice | Related to dehydration while the mother's milk supply is coming in; resolves when feeding is well established. |
| | Infection | Congenital and acquired infections may → jaundice. |

## NECROTIZING ENTEROCOLITIS

- More common among premature infants. The etiology may be related to ischemia and infection.
- **Sx/Exam:** Presentation may include abdominal distention, feeding intolerance, and blood in the stools.
- **Dx:** Radiographs may reveal pneumatosis intestinalis (intramural air).
- **Tx:** Initially treated with broad-spectrum antibiotics and parenteral nutrition, but surgery may be necessary.

## ESOPHAGEAL ATRESIA AND TRACHEOESOPHAGEAL FISTULA

- **Sx/Exam:** Pregnancy may be complicated by polyhydramnios 2° to the fetus being unable to swallow amniotic fluid. Infants present shortly after with copious secretions, choking, cyanosis, and respiratory distress. An NG tube cannot be passed to the stomach.
- **Dx:** Confirm with CXR after placement of an NG tube to the point of resistance. If a tracheoesophageal fistula is present in the distal esophagus, gas will be present in the bowel. In cases of esophageal atresia without tracheoesophageal fistula, there is no gas in the bowel.
- **Tx:** Surgical treatment is necessary. Keep the NG tube for suctioning while awaiting repair to prevent aspiration.

## NEONATAL SEPSIS

Risk factors for neonatal sepsis include prolonged rupture of membranes (>18 hours), maternal fever, and prematurity.

### SYMPTOMS/EXAM

*Screening and chemoprophylaxis for maternal GBS has ↓ the incidence of neonatal GBS sepsis. This benefit has been somewhat offset by a rise in non-GBS neonatal sepsis, especially in preterm and low-birth-weight infants.*

- **Early sepsis (first week of life):**
  - Usually presents in the first 24 hours.
  - Characterized by respiratory distress, hypotension, and poor perfusion.
  - Common pathogens include group B β-hemolytic streptococcus (GBS) and gram-⊖ bacteria such as *E. coli.*
  - Pneumonia is a common source.
- **Late-onset sepsis (after the first week):**
  - May present with poor feeding, temperature instability, lethargy, and apnea.
  - Causal organisms include S. *aureus*, GBS, *Enterococcus*, *Pseudomonas*, and other gram-⊖ organisms.
  - Meningitis is more common in this period.

### DIAGNOSIS

Laboratory abnormalities may include a low or high WBC count, thrombocytopenia, metabolic acidosis, hypoglycemia, and ↑ CRP.

### TREATMENT

Broad-spectrum antibiotics are appropriate while awaiting culture results (blood, urine, and CSF). Ampicillin with gentamicin is a common regimen.

---

Shortly after the delivery of a term baby boy by cesarean section, you are called to the nursery to evaluate the infant. His respiratory rate is 55, and he is noted to be a bit dusky when he tries to breast-feed. His $O_2$ saturation is good, but he has some mild retractions with respiratory effort. What is your management strategy? Start a sepsis workup with CBC, cultures, and CXR. If the sepsis workup appears ⊖, the most likely diagnosis is transient tachypnea of the newborn. The infant should be closely monitored and supported with $O_2$ as needed. In some cases, mechanical ventilation is necessary until the condition improves.

---

### TRANSIENT TACHYPNEA OF THE NEWBORN

- Transient tachypnea of the newborn is a consequence of retained fetal lung fluid. Risk factors include precipitous delivery, cesarean delivery, and maternal diabetes.
- **Sx/Exam:** Respiratory distress is generally present within several hours of birth. Respiratory rate typically exceeds 60 breaths/minute.
- **Dx:** CXR reveals streaky opacities in the hilar region.
- **Tx:** Management is supportive, and the syndrome typically resolves in 12–24 hours.

## MECONIUM ASPIRATION

- Can → chemical pneumonitis and pulmonary hypertension.
- Risk factors include low amniotic fluid volume, postdate pregnancies, and intrauterine growth retardation (IUGR).
- **Tx:** Resuscitation should include suction of the hypopharynx under direct visualization **if the infant is depressed.** Vigorous infants do not require suctioning. Routine suctioning at the perineum is no longer recommended.

## HYALINE MEMBRANE DISEASE

- A condition caused by absence of surfactant. Occurs almost exclusively in preterm infants.
- **Sx/Exam:** Poor lung compliance and atelectasis → ↑ work of breathing and eventual respiratory failure.
- **Tx:** Treated with exogenous surfactant and mechanical ventilation.

## Genetic and Congenital Disorders

### CHROMOSOMAL ABNORMALITIES

- Trisomies:
    - **Trisomy 21 (Down syndrome):** Incidence is 1 in 600 live births; risk is greatest among women > 35 years of age. Presents with moderate to severe mental retardation, short stature, characteristic facies (epicanthal folds, midface hypoplasia), heart defects, and GI tract disorders. Complications include an ↑ risk of leukemia and ↑ rates of Alzheimer's dementia.
    - **Trisomy 18 (Edwards' syndrome):** Affects 1 in 6000–8000 live births, with females three times more likely to be affected than males. Characterized by severe mental retardation, IUGR, hypertonicity, abnormal facies, overlapping fingers, and "rocker-bottom" feet. Most affected infants die within the first year of life.
    - **Trisomy 13 (Patau's syndrome):** Incidence is 1 in 6000 live births. Affects slightly more females than males. Presents with mental retardation, midline facial defects, polydactyly, syndactyly, blindness, deafness, and heart defects. Complications include seizures. Few infants survive.
- Abnormal sex chromosomes:
    - **Klinefelter's syndrome (XXY):** Incidence is 1 in 1000 live births. Affected individuals are phenotypically male until puberty, when they may be noted to have small testicles (micro-orchidism), gynecomastia, and ↓ facial hair. Mild mental retardation is common, but IQ may be normal. Treat with testosterone replacement.
    - **Turner's syndrome (XO):** Affects 1 in 10,000 live births. Most fetuses conceived with this disorder are spontaneously miscarried. Presents with short stature, absence of 2° sexual characteristics, the characteristic "shield chest," webbed neck, edema of the hands and feet, and coarctation of the aorta. Estrogen replacement is needed for sexual maturation, and growth hormone is used for the treatment of short stature. Complications include amenorrhea and learning disabilities.

### AUTOSOMAL-DOMINANT DISORDERS

- **Neurofibromatosis type 1 (von Recklinghausen's disease):** Neurofibromas are benign but have malignant potential and may compress nerves.

*Although women > 35 years of age have an ↑ risk of having an infant with Down syndrome, most infants with Down syndrome are born to women with no risk factors.*

---

***Diagnostic criteria for neurofibromatosis type 1—***

**CAFÉ SPOT**

Two or more of the following:

**C**afé-au-lait spots (six or more)

**A**xillary, inguinal freckling

**F**ibroma

**E**ye—Lisch nodules

**S**keletal (e.g., bowing leg)

**P**edigree/**P**ositive family history

**O**ptic **T**umor (glioma)

Affected individuals are also at risk for other CNS tumors as well as for optic tumors and pheochromocytomas.

- **Neurofibromatosis type 2:** Acoustic neuromas and other CNS neoplasms. Cutaneous manifestations are much less prevalent.
- **Tuberous sclerosis:** Presents with cutaneous lesions (ash leaf spots and shagreen patches). Associated with mental retardation, seizures, CNS tumors, and tumors in the pancreas, kidney, liver, and spleen.
- **Marfan's syndrome:** A triad of musculoskeletal changes (long limbs and ligamental laxity), lens dislocation, and aortic aneurysm. Penetrance is variable.

### AUTOSOMAL-RECESSIVE DISORDERS

- **Cystic fibrosis (CF):** Occurs most frequently in Caucasians in North America and northern Europe (1 in 3000). May be caused by mutations in the CFTR protein (a chloride channel). In the past, the disease was generally fatal in childhood, but with improved therapy, median survival is now > 30 years.
- **Inborn errors of metabolism:** Absence of certain enzymes. The best-known type is phenylketonuria (PKU), in which affected individuals are unable to convert phenylalanine to tyrosine → CNS damage and mental retardation. Treatment involves avoidance of phenylalanine in the diet.

### X-LINKED DISORDERS

- **Duchenne muscular dystrophy:** Occurs in about 1 in 3500 live births. Symptoms develop in the second or third year of life, presenting with proximal muscle wasting and distal muscle hypertrophy. The disease is progressive, with almost all affected individuals requiring the use of a wheelchair by age 12. Life expectancy is in the 20s, with respiratory failure and cardiomyopathy the leading causes of death.
- **Hemophilia A and B:** Occur in roughly 1 in 5000 live births. Hemophilia A (factor VIII deficiency) is much more common than hemophilia B (factor IX deficiency). Treatment involves prevention of injury along with factor replacement in the setting of active hemorrhage.
- **Fragile X syndrome:** An example of genetic anticipation. Caused by a trinucleotide repeat on the long arm of the X chromosome that expands with each generation. Female carriers may be mildly affected, but their male offspring represent the full phenotype of mental retardation, macroorchidism, and behavioral problems.

### OTHER CONGENITAL DISORDERS

- **Cleft lip/palate:** Isolated cleft palate is more likely than cleft lip+ palate to be part of a syndrome. Complications include feeding difficulties, speech delay, and recurrent otitis media.
- **Neural tube defects:** Encompasses a broad range of defects, including myelomeningocele, spina bifida, encephalocele, and anencephaly. Causes include genetic abnormalities, folate deficiency and exposures (alcohol, anticonvulsants). Often idiopathic.
- **Fetal alcohol syndrome:** Presents with short palpebral fissures, epicanthal folds, a flat midface, absent philtrum, a thin upper lip, mental retardation, behavioral problems, and poor coordination (see Figure 13.2). Heart defects and epilepsy are sometimes seen.

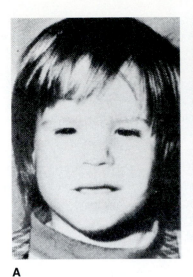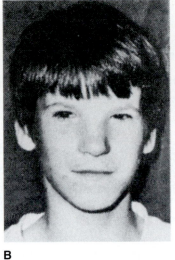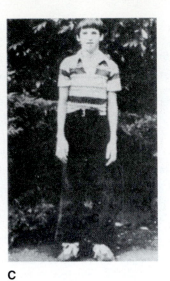

A  B  C

**FIGURE 13.2.  Fetal alcohol syndrome.**

(A) At 2 1/2 years. (B, C) At 12 years. Note the persistence of short palpebral fissures, epicanthal folds, flat midface, hypoplastic philtrum, and thin upper vermilion border. This child also has the short, lean prepubertal stature characteristic of young males with fetal alcohol syndrome. (Reproduced, with permission, from Cunningham FG et al. *Williams Obstetrics*, 22nd ed. New York: McGraw-Hill, 2005: 347.)

■ **Congenital hypothyroidism:** Roughly 80% of cases are caused by thyroid agenesis; less commonly related to inborn errors of metabolism or maternal antithyroid antibodies. Early diagnosis and treatment can prevent the severe mental retardation formerly known as cretinism.

### HEMOGLOBINOPATHIES

■ **Thalassemias:** Most common in individuals of Mediterranean, South Asian, and African descent. Severity depends on the number of damaged genes. Characterized by a four-locus code for α-hemoglobin and a two-locus code for β-hemoglobin. Severe disease presents with hemolysis, jaundice, and high-output cardiac failure.
■ **Sickle cell disease:** Most often affects individuals of African descent. Caused by a defect in β-hemoglobin. Heterozygotes are generally asymptomatic and have some protection against malaria. Homozygotes present with painful crises.

## THE FIRST YEAR OF LIFE

### Pyloric Stenosis

■ Most common in firstborn sons.
■ **Sx/Exam:** Usually presents after several weeks of life with projectile, non-bilious vomiting. An olive-sized mass may be felt in the epigastrium.
■ **Dx:** Ultrasound is diagnostic.
■ **Tx:** Pylorotomy is curative.

**TABLE 13.3.** Differential Diagnosis of Intestinal Obstruction in Infants

| SITE OF OBSTRUCTION | CLINICAL FINDINGS | PLAIN RADIOGRAPHS | CONTRAST STUDY |
|---|---|---|---|
| Duodenal atresia | Down syndrome (30%); early vomiting that is sometimes bilious. | "Double bubble" sign (dilated stomach and proximal duodenum; no air distal). | Not needed. |
| Malrotation and volvulus | Bilious vomiting with onset at any time in the first few weeks. | Dilated stomach and proximal duodenum; paucity of air distally (may be a normal gas pattern). | UGI shows a displaced duodenojejunal junction with a "corkscrew" deformity of twisted bowel. |
| Jejunoileal atresia, meconium ileus | Bilious gastric contents of > 25 mL at birth; progressive distention and bilious vomiting. | Multiple dilated loops of bowel; intra-abdominal calcifications if in utero perforation occurred (meconium peritonitis). | Barium or osmotic contrast enema shows microcolon; contrast refluxed into the distal ileum may demonstrate and relieve meconium obstruction (successful in about 50% of cases). |
| Meconium plug syndrome, Hirschsprung's disease | Distention; delayed stooling (> 24 hours). | Diffuse bowel distention. | Barium or osmotic contrast enema outlines and relieves plug; may show transition zone in Hirschsprung's disease. Delayed emptying (> 24 hours) suggests Hirschsprung's disease. |

Reproduced, with permission, from Hay WW et al. *Current Diagnosis & Treatment in Pediatrics,* 18th ed. New York: McGraw-Hill, 2007: 47.

## Intestinal Obstruction

Forms of intestinal obstruction in infants can be distinguished according to clinical and radiographic findings, as outlined below and in Table 13.3.

### BOWEL ATRESIA

- Most obstructions are bowel atresias, which are believed to be caused by an ischemic event during development. Approximately 30% of cases of duodenal atresia are associated with Down syndrome.
- **Sx/Exam:** Proximal atresias have earlier bilious vomiting and less distention; distal atresias present later and have more distention.
- **Dx:** AXR shows distended bowel loops and air-fluid levels (see Figure 13.3).
- **Tx:** Surgical resection of the affected area.

> You are preparing to discharge a two-day-old male infant delivered by the normal spontaneous vaginal route when the nurse tells you that he has not yet passed any stool. The baby is breast-feeding but seems to spit up most of what goes down, and his mother is becoming discouraged. You examine the infant and note that his belly is somewhat distended. You are not sure if you can feel a mass in the left side of the abdomen. What is the next step in

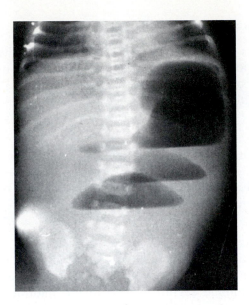

**FIGURE 13.3.** **Intestinal obstruction in the newborn.**

This child has jejunal atresia. Several loops of distended bowel can be seen with air-fluid levels. (Reproduced, with permission, from Brunicardi FC et al. *Schwartz's Principles of Surgery*, 8th ed. New York: McGraw-Hill, 2005: 1488.)

evaluation? This picture raises concern for Hirschsprung's disease or an atresia. An AXR would be a good starting point, although a contrast enema may also be needed to make a definitive diagnosis.

### HIRSCHSPRUNG'S DISEASE

Hirschsprung's disease results from an absence of ganglion cells in the mucosal and muscular layers of the colon when neural crest cells fail to migrate appropriately. The aganglionic segment is of normal caliber or slightly narrowed, with dilation of the normal colon proximal to the aganglionic segment. The disease is four times more common in boys than in girls, and 10–15% of patients have Down syndrome.

#### SYMPTOMS/EXAM

- Early signs include failure to pass meconium, vomiting, abdominal distention, and reluctance to feed.
- Later signs may include fever and explosive diarrhea. A dilated colon full of stool may be palpable through the abdomen, but no stool will be appreciated in the rectum on digital exam.

#### DIAGNOSIS

AXR may reveal a dilated proximal colon and absence of gas in the pelvic colon. Barium enema shows a narrowed segment distally with a sharp transition to a dilated proximal colon.

#### TREATMENT

Surgery to resect the aganglionic section of bowel.

### MALROTATION/VOLVULUS

Malrotation occurs early in development and may → volvulus. Volvulus occurs when a section of bowel rotates, occluding the superior mesenteric artery. Associated congenital anomalies (especially cardiac) occur in > 25% of symptomatic patients.

### SYMPTOMS/EXAM

- Early signs include recurrent bile-stained vomiting or acute small-bowel obstruction.
- Later signs include intermittent intestinal obstruction, malabsorption, protein-losing enteropathy, and diarrhea.

### DIAGNOSIS

- An upper GI series shows the duodenojejunal junction on the right side.
- The diagnosis can be further confirmed by barium enema, which may demonstrate a mobile cecum located in the midline, RUQ, or left abdomen.

### TREATMENT

Malrotation is treated surgically even when volvulus is not immediately present given the risk of developing volvulus. Midgut volvulus is a surgical emergency, as it may result in bowel necrosis.

## Colic

*The typical infant will cry for about two hours a day at two weeks and three hours a day at six weeks, and will return to one hour a day at three months.*

- **Sx/Exam:** Presents with the **rule of 3's:** crying for more than **three hours** a day **three days** a week for **more than three weeks.**
- **DDx:** If crying has developed suddenly, exogenous sources (e.g., hair tourniquets, corneal abrasion, infection) should be ruled out.
- **Tx:** Ranitidine may be tried if GERD appears to be implicated, or formulas may be changed. However, most cases are variations of normal behavior and resolve at about four months of age.

## Foot Problems

Most flexible deformities are 2° to intrauterine posture and usually resolve spontaneously.

### METATARSUS VARUS

- A common congenital foot deformity characterized by inward deviation of the forefoot.
- **Sx/Exam:** A vertical crease in the arch may be present when the deformity is rigid. The angulation is at the level of the base of the fifth metatarsal, and this bone will be prominent.
- **Tx:** If the deformity is rigid and cannot be manipulated past the midline, it is worthwhile to correct with a cast changed at two-week intervals.
- **Cx:** Roughly 10–15% of affected children also have hip dysplasia.

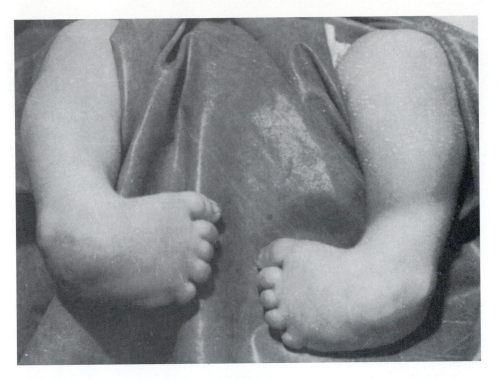

**FIGURE 13.4.** **Talipes equinovarus (clubfoot).**

(Reproduced, with permission, from Brunicardi FC et al. *Schwartz's Principles of Surgery*, 8th ed. New York: McGraw-Hill, 2005: 1718.)

### TALIPES EQUINOVARUS (CLUBFOOT)

- May be idiopathic, neurogenic, or syndromic (e.g., arthrogryposis, Larsen's syndrome). Idiopathic clubfeet may be hereditary.
- **Dx:** Presents with plantar flexion of the foot at the ankle joint (equinus), inversion deformity of the heel (varus), and medial deviation of the forefoot (varus) (see Figure 13.4). Infants should be carefully examined for associated anomalies, especially of the spine.
- **Tx:** Treat with manipulation of the foot to stretch the contracted tissues followed by splinting to hold the correction. Serial casting (the Ponseti technique) is generally effective, but if the deformity is rigid, surgical release may be necessary.

### Developmental Dysplasia of the Hip

- Inadequate pressure of the femoral head against the acetabulum that → a shallow socket with risk of future dislocation and gait abnormalities. Risk factors include a ⊕ family history, breech presentation, and female gender.
- **Sx/Exam:** Perform Barlow's and Ortolani's maneuvers to assess for a dislocatable hip. Asymmetric thigh or gluteal skin folds may be present, and in older children one knee may be lower than the other when patients are examined on their backs with the hips and knees flexed (Galeazzi test).
- **Dx:** Ultrasound is used for diagnosis until four months of age, as radiographs do not detect the uncalcified femoral head before this time.
- **Tx:** A Pavlik harness is used to hold the hips in abduction. Triple diapering is contraindicated, as it may maintain the hip in a dislocated position.

## Microcephaly

- Defined as a head circumference > 2 SDs below the mean or a declining rate of head growth over time. The fontanelle may close early, and sutures may be prominent.
- Etiologies include trisomies, fragile X syndrome, TORCHeS infections, fetal alcohol syndrome, metabolic disorders, perinatal infections (GBS meningitis, herpes encephalitis), anoxic brain injury, and neurodegenerative disorders (e.g., Tay-Sachs disease). **Treatable causes include hypopituitarism, hypothyroidism, and severe protein-calorie undernutrition.**
- **Dx:** TORCHeS titers, metabolic workup, head CT, karyotype. Screen for maternal PKU.
- **Tx:** Correct endocrine or metabolic disorders if present. Otherwise, treatment is largely supportive.

## Macrocephaly

- Defined as a head circumference > 2 SDs above the mean.
- Etiologies include progressive hydrocephalus, subdural effusion, arachnoid cyst, porencephalic cyst, brain tumor, external hydrocephalus, benign enlargement of the subarachnoid spaces, neurofibromatosis, and tuberous sclerosis.
- **Sx/Exam:** An excessive rate of growth is suggestive of ↑ ICP (hydrocephalus, extra-axial fluid collections, neoplasms). Macrocephaly with normal head growth rate suggests familial macrocephaly.
- **Dx:** Imaging is not necessary if the infant is normal neurologically and head growth is consistent with catch-up or familial macrocephaly. Ultrasound may be used if the fontanelle is still open. Otherwise, CT or MRI is appropriate.
- **Tx:** Surgical resection or drainage of lesions as appropriate.

## Cryptorchidism

- May be unilateral or bilateral. Approximately 3% of full-term male newborns have an undescended testis at birth. In > 50% of these cases, the testes descend by the third month, and by one year of age 80% of all undescended testes are in the scrotum.
- **Tx:** Surgical orchidopexy if descent has not occurred by one year of age.
- **Cx:** Infertility and testicular malignancy. The risk of malignancy (although lower) persists even following placement into scrotum.

## Ambiguous Genitalia

- The most common cause is congenital adrenal hyperplasia, which can → both XX virilization and XY feminization. Other causes include testicular regression syndrome, androgen insensitivity, testosterone biosynthesis disorders, and chromosomal abnormalities
- **Sx/Exam:** Initial evaluation should include a history, physical exam, and karyotype. Measure gonadotropins (LH, FSH), adrenal steroids (cortisol, 17-OHP, ACTH stimulation test), testosterone precursors (DHEA, androstenedione), testosterone, dihydrotestosterone, and hCG (hCG stimulation test).
- **Tx:**
  - Replace glucocorticoids, mineralocorticoids, and sodium as necessary in CAD.

- Provide hormone replacement as needed.
- Surgical reassignment is controversial. In the past, early surgery was recommended, but as children reached adolescence, some rejected their gender assignment. This has raised the issue of waiting and allowing the child to express a preference.
- Surgical resection of dysmorphic or abdominal testes is necessary to prevent malignancy.

## DEVELOPMENT

Table 13.4 outlines major developmental milestones in pediatric patients from one month to five years of age.

**TABLE 13.4.** **Developmental Milestones**

| AGE | MOTOR | LANGUAGE/COGNITIVE | SOCIAL |
|---|---|---|---|
| 1–2 months | Holds head up; rolls from side to back. | Vocalizes. | Spontaneous smile; recognizes parents. |
| 3–5 months | Reaches for objects; sits with support; rolls from back to side. | Orients to voice. | Laughs; responds to facial expressions. |
| 6–8 months | Sits alone briefly; rolls from back to stomach; passes objects between the hands. | Babbles. | Sleeps through the night; stranger anxiety begins. |
| 9–11 months | Stands alone; pulls to stand; plays "pat-a-cake" and "peek-a-boo"; starts using pincer grasp. | Follows one-word commands; uses "mama" and "dada" nonspecifically; develops the concept of object permanence. | Waves "bye-bye." |
| 1 year | Walks independently; stacks two cubes. | Uses "mama" and "dada" appropriately. | Points to desired objects. |
| 18 months | Stacks 3–4 blocks; throws ball; walks up/down stairs with help. | Uses 4–20 words; follows two-step commands. | Feeds self with hands; stranger anxiety peaks. |
| 2 years | Stacks 6–7 blocks; kicks ball; can stand on one foot. | Uses **two-word phrases;** uses pronouns; 50% of speech is comprehensible. | Helps dress self; mimics parents; stranger anxiety subsides. |
| 3 years | Builds tower of 9–10 blocks; rides a tricycle. | Uses **three-word phrases;** copies a circle; knows own name. | Dresses self; feeds self with utensils. |
| 5 years | Runs and turns without losing balance; can stand on one foot for ten seconds. | Counts to four; answers questions appropriately. | Magical thinking; plays with peers. |

**NUTRITION**

### Normal Weight Gain/Feeding in Childhood

- **Newborns to six months:**
  - Weight loss in the first days is normal, but the infant should be back to birth weight by the tenth day of life. Loss of > 8–10% of birth weight raises concern for dehydration.
  - "Breast is best"—breast-feeding ↓ the incidence of obesity and diabetes, improves immune defenses, ↓ allergies later in life, and facilitates mother-infant bonding.
  - Exclusive breast or formula feeding should continue until 5–6 months of age to meet the infant's nutritional needs and ↓ the risk of developing allergies.
  - The American Academy of Pediatrics recommends that all babies receive 200 IU of vitamin D per day starting in the first two months of life.
  - Weight typically doubles by 5–6 months.
- **Six to twelve months:**
  - Begin to add enriched cereals, fruits, vegetables, and meats to the diet. Add only one new item per week both to ↓ the incidence of food aversions and to allow allergic reactions to be readily correlated with a new food. To prevent infant botulism, honey should not be introduced until after one year of age.
  - Continue breast-feeding for at least one year or longer as desired. Formula should be continued until one year of age and should then be switched to cow's milk. Whole milk is best from age one year until age two years, at which time low-fat milk should be introduced.
  - Iron-rich foods should be introduced by six months of age.
  - Birth weight triples by one year.
- **Twelve months and beyond:** Growth decelerates dramatically. Use the growth curve to assess adequacy.

*Absolute contraindications to breast-feeding are TB or HIV in the mother and galactosemia in the infant.*

### Failure to Thrive (FTT)

- **Sx/Exam:** Presents with persistent weight loss or a weight curve that declines across two major percentile lines. Etiologies include the following:
  - **Familial short stature:** Normal readjustment of both weight and height on the growth curve to reflect genetic potential. Obtaining a family history is helpful.
  - **Constitutional growth delay:** May closely resemble FTT, but the family history reveals a tendency toward later growth spurts.
  - **Endocrine dysfunction:** In congenital hypothyroidism, height slows before weight.
  - **Genetic syndromes:** Examples include Turner's and Down syndromes.
- **Dx:**
  - **Organic:** Consider GERD, problems with chewing/swallowing, malabsorption, and protein-wasting nephropathy.
  - **Nonorganic:** Assess for inappropriate or inadequate feeding by caregivers. May be related to lack of knowledge about feeding, bonding issues, socioeconomic issues, or abuse. Can have a mixed picture, with frustration or anxiety over organic illness → inadequate feeding.
- **Tx:** Institute a high-calorie diet with particular attention paid to protein intake. Outpatient treatment is often sufficient, but hospitalization may be necessary.

## Obesity

- **Sx/Exam:** Defined as a body mass index (BMI) greater than the 95th percentile for age and gender. At-risk children are between the 85th and 95th percentiles. Diagnosis should not be made until after age two, although at-risk children may be identified earlier.
- **Tx:** Lifestyle modification must involve the entire family. Limit sedentary activities such as watching television. For most children, maintaining current weight while linear growth catches up is adequate.
- **Cx:** Dyslipidemia, insulin resistance, type 2 DM, orthopedic problems, sleep apnea.

## Vitamin and Nutrient Deficiencies

- **Scurvy:** Vitamin C deficiency. Presents with bleeding gums, osteoid deficiency, and poor healing. Anorexia, FTT, irritability, and apathy may also be seen.
- **Rickets:** Vitamin D deficiency. Presents with craniotabes (thinning of the skull), rachitic rosary (thickening of the costochondral junctions), bowed legs, and tooth defects.
- **Kwashiorkor:** An isolated protein deficiency presenting with edema and FTT.
- **Marasmus:** A protein and calorie deficiency that presents with generalized wasting and FTT.
- **Calcium deficiency:**
  - Results in bone loss and failure to achieve maximal bone density. May contribute to later development of osteoporosis.
  - Premature infants and adolescents with poor dairy intake are at ↑ risk.
  - Absorption of calcium from breast milk is greater than that from cow's milk.

> *Vitamin D deficiency—*
>
> **RICKETS**
>
> **R**eaction of the periosteum (may occur)
> **I**ndistinct cortex
> **C**oarse trabeculation
> **K**nees, wrists, and ankles are predominantly affected
> **E**piphyseal plates are widened and irregular
> **T**remendous metaphysis (cupping, fraying, splaying)
> **S**pur (metaphyseal)

## PREVENTIVE MEDICINE

## Immunizations

Vaccine schedules are updated annually. Current recommendations may be found at www.cdc.gov/nip/ACIP. Diseases targeted by immunizations include the following:

- **Diphtheria:** Toxin mediated. Infection → pseudomembranous pharyngitis and myocarditis.
- *Haemophilus influenzae* **type B (Hib):** Infection → meningitis, cellulitis, epiglottitis, bacteremia, osteomyelitis, and pneumonia. Before the introduction of the Hib vaccine, 1 in 200 U.S. children < 5 years of age developed invasive disease. Use of the vaccine has ↓ disease incidence by 97%.
- **HAV:** Vaccination is recommended for children in communities with a high incidence as well as for travelers.
- **HBV:** The three-injection series confers 95% immunity.
- **Influenza:** Annual vaccination is recommended for children 6–23 months of age as well as for older children with risk factors such as asthma. Children < 9 years of age need two shots one month apart if they are receiving the vaccine for the first time. Allergy to eggs is an absolute contraindication.
- **Measles:** The series of two vaccinations confers 99% immunity.

*With the exception of the introduction of clean drinking water and effective sewage systems, immunizations have ↓ morbidity and mortality more than any other public health intervention.*

*The MMR vaccine and its components do not cause of autism.*

*Smallpox was the first disease for which a vaccine was created and was eliminated globally in 1977.*

- **Meningococcus:** Vaccination is recommended for young people entering large group situations (e.g., college freshmen and military recruits) as well as for those with asplenism and complement deficiencies.
- **Mumps:** The vaccination series confers 99% immunity, but outbreaks still occur.
- **Pertussis:** Infection → whooping cough. It is highly contagious, and close contacts of infected individuals require antibiotic prophylaxis (erythromycin). The vaccine is acellular in order to ↓ adverse reactions.
- **Pneumococcus:** All children < 2 years of age should be immunized. Children > 2 years of age who have not been immunized should receive the vaccine based on risk stratification. Sickle cell disease, asplenism, diabetes, and HIV infection are among the indications.
- **Polio:** The inactivated poliovirus vaccine (IPV) is now used in the United States because the risk of vaccine-associated poliomyelitis 2° to use of the attenuated live oral poliovirus vaccine (OPV) is greater than the risk of inadequate immunity with IPV.
- **Rubella:** Vaccination is used primarily to prevent infection in pregnant women, as rubella → significant birth defects. The vaccine is contraindicated during pregnancy, and nonimmune women should receive the vaccine in the postpartum period.
- **Tetanus:** Occurs via exposure of open tissue to anaerobic spores in the soil. The toxin → painful muscle spasms and trismus ("lockjaw").
- **Varicella:** The vaccine is live and should not be given to pregnant women or immunocompromised individuals.

## Anticipatory Guidance

### GROWTH

Plotting a child's growth on a standardized graph at all well-child checks is helpful in diagnosing FTT and growth abnormalities at a point when interventions may still be effective.

### DENTAL CARE

- Teething may begin as early as five months.
- Encourage use of a cup by one year of age. Do not allow a bottle in bed (→ "baby bottle tooth decay").
- Fluoride supplementation should start at six months if the water supply is not fluoridated. Fluoride varnish may be applied at well-child checks by a trained medical provider.
- Infants should start brushing as soon as teeth appear. The first dental visit should occur by age three.

### ELIMINATION AND TOILET TRAINING

- Newborns typically have 6–8 wet diapers per day; older infants will usually have 4–6. Checking the number of diapers is a useful means of gauging hydration.
- Newborns often stool after every feed, but at 2–3 months this will become much less frequent. Breast-fed infants can go as long as a week without stooling.
- Toilet training is generally initiated around 2–3 years of age but varies depending on the child's readiness and parental expectations.

## SLEEP

- Roughly 70% of infants sleep eight hours at a time by three months, 80% by six months, and 90% by twelve months of age.
- Sleep disorders affecting children include the following:
    - **Night terrors:**
        - Occur during non-REM sleep in about 3% of children.
        - **Sx/Exam:** Children present with inconsolable screaming and thrashing. Episodes can last as long as 30 minutes and may be associated with sleepwalking. The next day, the child has no recollection of events.
        - **Tx:** Focused on reassurance of parents and prevention of injury to the child. Waking the child several minutes before the usual time of occurrence for several days may break the cycle.
    - **Nightmares:**
        - Occur during REM sleep in 25–50% of children. Most common in children 3–5 years of age.
        - **Sx/Exam:** The child can be awakened and consoled.
        - **Tx:** Generally, no intervention is required.

## BEHAVIOR

- **Temper tantrums:**
    - Common in children 1–4 years of age, as children learn to express desires and frustrations. Most episodes ↓ with age.
    - **Tx:** Focused on protecting the child and others from harm and helping the child develop better forms of expression.
- **Breath holding:**
    - An involuntary response to minor injury or anger in which the child stops breathing after expiration. Loss of consciousness may occur.
    - **Dx:** Occasionally associated with pica or iron deficiency anemia. Most children grow out of this behavior by age six. Frequent episodes require workup for a CNS tumor or seizure disorder.
    - **Tx:** Focused on preventing injury but not acceding to the child's demands.

## INJURY PREVENTION

- Injuries are the leading cause of death in children and adolescents after the first year of life.
- The well-child check is an opportunity to counsel on injury prevention strategies such as keeping poisons stored locked and out of reach, drowning prevention, and "baby-proofing" to prevent falls and aspirations.
- Specific strategies include the following:
    - **Car seats/seatbelts:**
        - Car seats and booster seats should be in the back seat of the car.
        - Rear-facing infant seats should be used for children weighing < 20 pounds and < 1 year of age; forward-facing car seats are appropriate for children 20–40 pounds or > 1 year of age.
        - Booster seats should be used for children who have outgrown car seats.
        - A combination lap/shoulder belt should be used when a child has grown enough to fit the seat belts (usually when they are four feet tall).

423

*Injuries are the leading cause of death in children and adolescents after the first year of life.*

- **Bicycle helmets:**
  - Head trauma is the greatest cause of bicycle fatalities.
  - Although > 85% of brain injuries can be prevented through the use of bicycle helmets, < 25% of children wear a bike helmet when riding.
  - Community interventions can greatly influence the rate of helmet use.

## Laboratory Tests

### IRON DEFICIENCY ANEMIA

- Risk factors include preterm or low-birth-weight births, multiple and/or closely spaced pregnancies, iron deficiency in the mother, use of nonfortified formula or cow's milk before 12 months of age, and an infant diet that is low in iron-containing foods. Infants and toddlers consuming > 24 ounces of cow's milk per day are also at risk, as are children with chronic illness or restricted diets.
- Screen at-risk children at 9–12 months of age and again at 15–18 months. Screening may be done annually if indicated until five years of age. Premature and low-birth-weight infants may need testing before six months of age.
- Universal anemia screening at 9 and 15 months of age is appropriate for children in communities or populations in which anemia is found in ≥ 5% of those tested.

### LEAD SCREENING

- The most common source of lead exposure is lead-based paint, which has been banned since 1977. Children may eat or inhale contaminated particles.
- High levels of lead are associated with seizures and coma. Moderate elevations are associated with behavioral problems and learning disabilities that persist into later life. Even low elevations are correlated with lower intelligence quotients.
- The CDC recommends universal screening in communities with a large number of old buildings or a high percentage of children with ↑ blood lead levels.

## COMMON CHRONIC PROBLEMS

## Atopic Conditions

### ALLERGIES

- An array of disorders related to heightened immune response, including rhinoconjunctivitis, atopic dermatitis, urticaria, angioedema, and anaphylaxis. Caused by exposure to an allergen → the production of IgE and eosinophils and subsequent release of allergic mediators from mast cells and basophils. Common allergens include dusts, pollens, animal dander, medications, foods, and insect bites.
- **Sx:** Sneezing, hives, wheezing, vomiting, anaphylaxis.
- **Tx:** Intranasal steroids or oral antihistamines. Immunotherapy is used when desensitization might be helpful. Anaphylaxis may be treated in the field using diphenhydramine (Benadryl) and an epinephrine pen, but re-

ferral to an emergency department is often required for the **ABCz**: Adrenaline (epinephrine), **B**enadryl, **C**orticosteroids, **Z**antac.

### ECZEMA (ATOPIC DERMATITIS)

- Genetic susceptibility and environmental factors combine to produce skin with ↓ ability to hold water. The stratum corneum shrinks, leaving cracks in the epidermal barrier. Affected skin is at risk for 2° infection.
- **Sx/Exam:** Patients present with areas of dry, cracked skin (see Figure 13.5), with distribution varying by age. In infants, the cheeks and trunk are most often affected; in children, the flexor surfaces are most frequently involved. In adolescents, the hands are the most common site.
- **Tx:** For flares, use topical steroids, moisturizers, and antibiotics as needed. For chronic treatment, prevent excessive drying with short, less frequent baths and showers, nonirritant soaps and lotions, and frequent moisturizing. Topical immunosuppressants (e.g., tacrolimus) may be used for a limited time in children > 2 years of age.

> *The ABCz of anaphylaxis treatment:*
>
> **A**drenaline (epinephrine)
> **B**enadryl
> **C**orticosteroids
> **Z**antac (an $H_2$ antagonist)

An eight-year-old girl is brought to your office by her father. She has been to the ER twice in the last month for wheezing and has missed three or four days of school. She has a nebulizer at home but lost her albuterol inhaler. Her father thinks she has a cold because she has woken up coughing during the night once or twice in the last week. On exam, she is comfortable and has some faint expiratory wheezes. What is your evaluation and management? This child has moderate persistent asthma. She needs to be placed on an inhaled steroid and probably a long-acting bronchodilator in addition to her rescue inhaler. Above all, she and her family need education and an action plan.

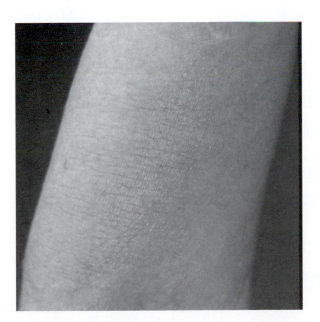

**FIGURE 13.5.   Atopic dermatitis.**

(Reproduced, with permission, from Wolff K et al. *Fitzpatrick's Color Atlas & Synopsis of Clinical Dermatology,* 5th ed. New York: McGraw-Hill, 2005: 39.) (Also see Color Insert.)

## ASTHMA

A chronic inflammatory disorder of the airways characterized by reversible bronchoconstriction, asthma is one of the most common diseases of childhood. Up to 25% of children will have one or more attacks, with 3–5% going on to have symptoms into adulthood. Risk factors include poverty and non-white ethnicity. Smooth muscle constriction, ↑ mucus production, inflammation, and basement membrane thickening → symptoms (see Figure 13.6).

### SYMPTOMS/EXAM

- Acute attacks present with dyspnea, expiratory wheezing, nasal flaring, retractions, hypoxia, and a prolonged expiratory phase. Some patients present only with cough, and some are symptomatic only during or after exercise.
- The disease is often associated with other forms of atopy (e.g., allergies, eczema).

### DIFFERENTIAL

Croup, foreign body aspiration, reflux disease, CF, tracheomalacia.

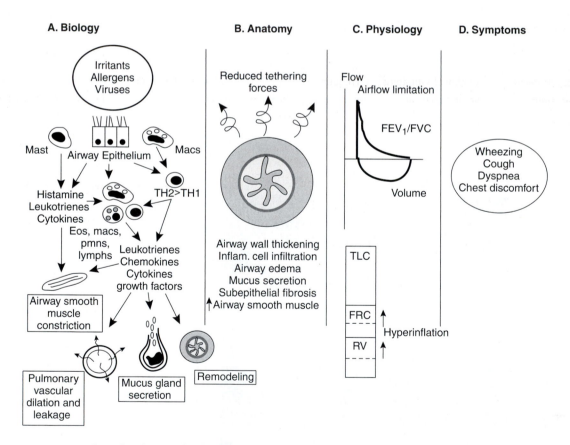

**FIGURE 13.6. Overview of asthma pathophysiology.**

(Reproduced, with permission, from Hanley ME, Welsh CH. *Current Diagnosis & Treatment in Pulmonary Medicine,* 1st ed. New York: McGraw-Hill, 2003: 68.)

## DIAGNOSIS

- ↓ $FEV_1/FVC$ ratio and > 10% improvement in $FEV_1$ following administration of a short-acting bronchodilator.
- In equivocal cases, a methacholine challenge may be diagnostic.

## TREATMENT

Use of a stepwise approach and action plan is most effective (see Table 13.5).

## COMPLICATIONS

In the long term, asthma results in airway remodeling and loss of lung function as measured by forced expiratory volume. Aggressive management may limit this progression.

> **Precipitating factors for asthma—**
>
> **ASTHMA**
>
> **A**llergies (dust mites, pollens, dander)
> **S**ports
> **T**emperature (cold, wet, windy weather)
> **H**eredity
> **M**icrobes (e.g., viruses, *Mycoplasma*)
> **A**nxiety

## Diabetes Mellitus (DM)

- Type 1 DM is more common among children; it is immune mediated and associated with an interaction between genetic susceptibility and environmental factors → the production of autoantibodies.

**TABLE 13.5.** **Evaluation and Treatment of Asthma**

| DISEASE SEVERITY | SYMPTOMS | NIGHTTIME SYMPTOMS | LUNG FUNCTION | MAINTENANCE THERAPY |
|---|---|---|---|---|
| Step 4: severe persistent | Continual symptoms; limited physical activity; frequent exacerbations. | Frequent. | $FEV_1$ or peak expiratory flow (PEF) < 60% predicted; PEF variability > 30%. | Choose all needed:<br>■ High-dose inhaled corticosteroid<br>■ Long acting bronchodilator<br>■ Leukotriene modifier<br>■ Oral steroid |
| Step 3: moderate persistent | Daily symptoms affecting function; daily use of short-acting β-agonists; exacerbations more than twice per week. | > 1 per week. | $FEV_1$ or PEF 60–80% predicted; PEF variability < 30%. | Low- to medium-dose inhaled corticosteroids plus a long-acting bronchodilator. |
| Step 2: mild persistent | Symptoms more than twice a week but not daily. May affect function. | > 2 per month. | $FEV_1$ or PEF > 80% predicted; PEF variability 20–30%. | Choose one:<br>■ Low-dose inhaled corticosteroid<br>■ Cromolyn<br>■ Leukotriene modifier |
| Step 1: mild intermittent | Symptoms less than twice a week; asymptomatic and normal PFTs between exacerbations. | < 2 per month. | $FEV_1$ or PEF > 80% predicted; PEF variability < 20%. | No daily medication needed. |

Adapted from the National Heart, Lung, and Blood Institute (NHLBI). *NAEPP Expert Panel Report: Guidelines for the Diagnosis and Management of Asthma—Update on Selected Topics 2002,* 1st ed. Bethesda, MD: NIH, 2002.

- Type 2 DM is seen more often in adults and teens; it is associated with insulin resistance and caused by genetic predisposition and obesity. Mature-onset diabetes of the young includes a number of inherited autosomal-dominant forms of type 2 DM that present early in life.
- **Sx/Exam:** Presents with polyuria, polydipsia, weight loss, hyperglycemia, and glucosuria +/− ketonuria and acidosis.
- **Dx:** Fasting glucose > 126 mg/dL or random glucose > 200 mg/dL with symptoms.
- **Tx:** Education, monitoring, medications (insulin for type 1; oral medication is first-line treatment for type 2).
- **Cx:** Long-term complications include vision loss, kidney failure, cardiovascular disease, peripheral neuropathy, and gastroparesis. Acute complications include DKA, hyperosmolar nonketotic state, and hypoglycemia.

## Hearing Loss

- Many states mandate universal screening for hearing loss at birth. Routine clinical screening at well-child checks is essential. A child should turn toward a sound at six months and locate the source of a sound by nine months. Attention to language acquisition landmarks is essential.
- **Sx/Exam:** Distinguish conductive from sensorineural hearing loss.
  - **Conductive hearing loss:**
    - Most often 2° to otitis media and its sequelae (middle ear effusion). May also be caused by canal stenosis, impaction (cerumen or foreign body), and middle ear abnormalities (stapes fixation, ossicular malformation).
    - Hearing loss 2° to middle ear infusion is typically mild and temporary but may affect language acquisition if it occurs during critical developmental periods.
  - **Sensorineural hearing loss:** Damage to the inner ear or the auditory nerve (CN VIII). May be congenital or acquired (more often congenital). Either may be genetic.
    - **Genetic congenital:** Most cases are autosomal recessive and nonsyndromic. Inner ear dysplasia is the most common defect.
    - **Nongenetic congenital:** Associated with prenatal infections, teratogenic drugs, and perinatal injury (e.g., hypoxia).
    - **Genetic postnatal:** More often syndromic (e.g., Alport's syndrome, Klippel-Feil syndrome).
    - **Nongenetic postnatal:** Associated with infections (e.g., syphilis), trauma, ototoxic drugs, metabolic disorders, and neoplastic disease.
- **Dx:** In children old enough to cooperate with this exam, the Weber and Rinne tests may be helpful.
  - **Weber test:** A tuning fork is applied to the forehead in the midline. In a normal exam, the sound is heard equally in both ears. In sensorineural hearing loss, the sound is heard best in the normal ear. In conductive hearing loss, the sound is heard best in the affected ear.
  - **Rinne test:** A tuning fork is applied to the mastoid process. When the sound is no longer appreciated, the fork is held next to the auditory meatus. In conductive hearing loss, the sound cannot be heard by air conduction after bone conduction has ceased. In sensorineural hearing loss, air conduction is significantly better than bone conduction.
- **Tx:** Language acquisition programs (verbal and sign), hearing aids, surgical implants.

## Gastroesophageal Reflux Disease (GERD)

- Reflux of stomach contents into the esophagus caused by inappropriate relaxation of the LES. Children with neurologic deficits have a higher incidence of this condition.
- **Sx/Exam:** Spitting up, vomiting, apnea, colic, FTT.
- **Dx:** A clinical diagnosis is generally sufficient. Twenty-four-hour pH testing may be useful if symptoms are atypical. EGD may lead to overdiagnosis of the condition but is helpful in identifying esophagitis.
- **Tx:**
  - Conservative treatment includes small feeds at shorter intervals. Medical options include $H_2$ receptor antagonists and PPIs.
  - Indications for surgery include persistent vomiting with FTT, esophagitis, and apnea or pulmonary symptoms that persist following several months of medical treatment.
- **Cx:** Prolonged symptoms may → esophagitis, occult blood loss, anemia, esophageal stricture, and inflammatory esophageal polyps. Aspiration pneumonia, coughing, and wheezing may result if gastric secretions reflux into the airways.

## Sickle Cell Disease

An autosomal-recessive disorder in which abnormal hemoglobin is produced. Deoxygenated HbS polymerizes → distorted RBC morphology, ↓ RBC deformability, and ↑ blood viscosity. Affects roughly 1 in 400 African-American children.

### SYMPTOMS/EXAM

The earliest symptom is often dactylitis (pain in the hands or feet). Pain crises, which are triggered by hemolysis and episodes of vaso-occlusion, may affect any part of the body.

### DIAGNOSIS

- Neonatal screening by hemoglobin electrophoresis detects the disease.
- Other lab abnormalities include mild to moderate anemia, hyperbilirubinemia, and ↑ reticulocyte count.

### TREATMENT

- **Acute:** Acute episodes may require $O_2$, hydration, hydroxyurea, blood transfusion, and pain management.
- **Chronic:** Chronic management includes penicillin prophylaxis from two months to five years of age.
- The pneumococcal conjugate vaccine should be given in addition to other routine childhood vaccines.

### COMPLICATIONS

- Splenic infarct occurs in almost all patients and → functional asplenia, which ↑ susceptibility to infection from encapsulated organisms.
- Other complications include sepsis, stroke, avascular necrosis of the hip, gallstones, MI, multiorgan failure, and acute chest syndrome (lung injury from vaso-occlusion, infarct, embolism, or infection).

*Reflux disease in children is usually self-limited. Roughly 85% of cases resolve by 6–12 months.*

---

**Common complications of sickle cell anemia—**

**HbS PAIN CRISIS**

**H**emolysis, **H**and-foot syndrome
**B**one marrow hyperplasia/infarction
**S**troke (thrombotic or hemorrhagic), **S**ubarachnoid bleeds, **S**kin ulcers (primarily leg)
**P**ain episodes, **P**riapism, **P**sychosocial problems
**A**nemia, **A**plastic crisis, **A**vascular necrosis
**I**nfections—CNS, pulmonary, GU, bone, joints
**N**octuria, urinary frequency from hyposthenuria
**C**holelithiasis, **C**ardiomegaly, **C**ongestive heart failure, **C**hest syndrome
**R**etinopathy, **R**enal failure, **R**enal concentrating defects
**I**nfarction—bone, spleen, CNS, muscle, bowel, renal
**S**equestration crisis involving the spleen or liver
**I**ncreased fetal loss during pregnancy
**S**epsis

## Juvenile Rheumatoid Arthritis (JRA)

The majority of cases of JRA improve with age, and many patients become asymptomatic after puberty. Unfortunately, joint damage acquired during active disease may contribute to later disability even in the absence of an ongoing disease process. Late-onset JRA (in the teen years) is more likely to persist into adulthood. Subtypes are as follows:

*Unlike adults, children with RA generally have a ⊖ RF.*

- **Systemic JRA:**
  - Also known as Still's disease.
  - **Sx/Exam:** Presents with fever, rash, arthritis, hepatosplenomegaly, and leukocytosis. Systemic symptoms generally regress within one year. Arthritis may regress but may also continue and become extremely destructive.
  - **DDx:** Reactive or postinfectious arthritis; other connective tissue disease (e.g., SLE); malignancy (e.g., leukemia).
  - **Dx:** Daily symptoms for > 6 weeks. ANA and RF are usually ⊖.
  - **Tx:** NSAIDs, corticosteroids, methotrexate, other immune-modifying agents.
- **Polyarticular JRA:**
  - **Sx/Exam:** Presents with symmetric chronic arthritis that may wax and wane. Systemic symptoms may be present but are generally mild. Iridocyclitis rarely occurs.
  - **Dx:** ↑ ESR; mildly ⊕ ANA.
  - **Tx:** NSAIDs; disease-modifying medications (e.g., methotrexate, TNF-α blockers).
- **Pauciarticular JRA:**
  - **Sx/Exam:** Chronic inflammation in a few joints (typically weight bearing). Iridocyclitis is a significant risk, and children require frequent ophthalmologic exams.
  - **Dx:** Arthritis in four or fewer joints for at least six weeks. ESR and WBC are normal; RF is ⊖ but ANA is ⊕. Other causes of arthritis (e.g., reactive) must be ruled out.
  - **Tx:** Treatment is the same as that for polyarticular JRA.

*Iridocyclitis or uveitis is one of the more serious complications of JRA. It is most often seen in pauciarticular disease but is occasionally seen in the other forms as well. If untreated, this complication can → blindness.*

## Constipation/Encopresis

- Encopresis is overflow incontinence of stool associated with chronic constipation and stool dilation. Initiating constipation is most often behavioral and is related to control issues or fear of using school or public toilets. Physiologic causes include dehydration, lack of bulk, and anal fissure.
- **DDx:** Newborns will often stool after every feed, but after a few months stools will become much less frequent. Breast-fed infants can go as long as a week without stooling. An appearance of straining with bowel movements in infants is normal and should not trigger treatment.
- **Tx:**
  - Constipation may be treated with stool softeners to make the passage of stool less painful.
  - Encopresis requires disimpaction followed by regular use of a stool softener +/– a stimulant laxative for several weeks to months to establish a regular routine of 1–2 soft bowel movements a day.
  - Referral to psychiatry may be necessary if significant behavioral problems persist.

## Enuresis

- Nocturnal enuresis (bedwetting) may persist in 15% of five-year-olds and 1–2% of 15-year-olds. May be 1° or 2°.
    - **1° enuresis:** Enuresis in which the child has never had an extended period of dryness. May be related to small bladder capacity, abnormal ADH secretion, sleep disorders, or, on rare occasions, psychological issues.
    - **2° enuresis:** Recurrence of bedwetting after a period of six months or more. 2° enuresis and daytime wetting are more often related to psychosocial issues.
- **DDx:** UTI, neurologic disorders, structural abnormalities.
- **Tx:**
    - **Behavioral:** Behavior modifications include reducing fluid intake in the evening and emptying the bladder before bedtime; bladder training to ↑ capacity; and bed alarms.
    - **Pharmacologic:** Medical therapies include intranasal desmopressin (DDAVP) and imipramine.
    - Enuresis often recurs after medication is stopped, but medical treatment may be helpful for sleepovers or camp. Some families use medications until the child "grows out" of bedwetting, but this can be expensive.

## Strabismus

- Misalignment of the visual axes of the eyes. **Esotropia** is a form of strabismus characterized by convergent axes; **exotropia** refers to strabismus with divergent axes.
- **Dx:** Intermittent esotropia may occur in normal infants up to 5–6 months of age. To confirm suspected strabismus, check the following:
    - **Light reflex:** The corneal light reflex from a penlight held along a toy that the child focuses on should appear symmetric.
    - **Cover test:** In an abnormal test, when the dominant eye is covered, the weaker eye will move to focus on an object.
- **Tx:** Esotropia is more serious and often requires surgery. Exotropia may initially be treated with patching and exercises but may also need surgical correction.
- **Cx:** Amblyopia (↓ visual acuity in the less dominant eye); diplopia (double vision); contracture of the extraocular muscles. Acquired strabismus (occurring after the first year of life) is of more concern and may be the result of a significant visual deficit or CNS disease.

## Limping

An 18-month-old child is brought to your office for fussiness and fever. He is demanding to be held and will not stand on his own. The child will not allow you to bend his leg at the knee or hip. What should you include in your workup? Workup should include CBC, radiographs, and ESR. In this child, suspicion must be high for osteomyelitis or septic joint. The infection may be in either joint (knee or hip), with pain in the other joint being an example of referred pain that can be misleading or confusing. Even if the x-ray is ⊖, it is often necessary to proceed with MRI (sensitive for osteomyelitis) and/or joint aspiration (for septic joint). Start broad-spectrum antibiotics while awaiting blood culture results. In this age, *S. aureus* or *H. influenzae* is the most likely culprit.

### SLIPPED CAPITAL FEMORAL EPIPHYSIS

- Disruption at the growth plate → displacement of the proximal femoral epiphysis. Most common in overweight adolescent boys.
- **Dx:** Generally presents with vague progressive pain and limp, but may occur suddenly with trauma. X-rays reveal the classic appearance of an ice-cream scoop slipping off its cone.
- **Tx:** Surgical pinning.
- **Cx:** Avascular necrosis (see Figure 13-7) may occur in up to one-third of cases.

### SEPTIC ARTHRITIS

- Causative organisms vary with age:
  - **Less than four months:** *S. aureus* and GBS.
  - **Four months to four years:** *H. influenzae* and *S. aureus.*
  - **Four years and older:** *S. aureus* and *S. pyogenes.*
  - **Adolescence:** Consider gonococcus.
- **Sx/Exam:** Presents with pain, fever, malaise, and ↓ range of motion (ROM). Early changes may not be seen on radiographs; late changes include destruction of the joint space.
- **Tx:** Drainage is key. The knee may be aspirated or washed arthroscopically, but the hip generally requires surgical drainage. Broad-spectrum IV antibiotics are used while awaiting culture results and may be switched to

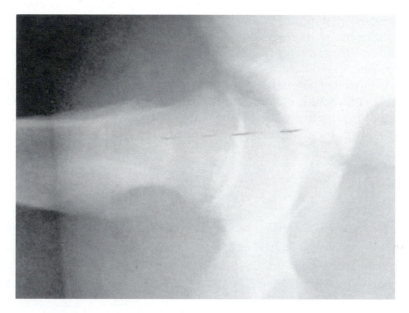

**FIGURE 13.7. Avascular necrosis.**

(Reproduced, with permission, from Brunicardi FC et al. *Schwartz's Principles of Surgery,* 8th ed. New York: McGraw-Hill, 2005: 1716.)

oral medications to complete a two- to three-week course when the patient is afebrile and clinically improved.

### LEGG-CALVÉ-PERTHES DISEASE

- Avascular necrosis of the proximal femur. Most frequently occurs between four and eight years of age; five times more common in boys.
- Sx/Exam: Presents with persistent pain, limp, and limited ROM.
- Dx: X-ray changes occur over several weeks. At several weeks, ↓ bone density, a necrotic center, and femoral head sclerosis are apparent.
- Tx: ↓ weight bearing and protection of the hip.

### OSGOOD-SCHLATTER SYNDROME

- Tendonitis of the patellar tendon from overuse; seen in girls 11–13 and boys 12–15 years of age.
- Sx/Exam: Presents with pain at the tibial tubercle, especially with eccentric exercises.
- Dx: Radiographs may reveal fragmentation at the tibial tubercle.
- Tx: Rest, ice, anti-inflammatories.

### OSTEOMYELITIS

- Infection occurring in the bone resulting from either direct or hematogenous spread of bacteria. *Staphylococcus* infection is most common, but *Streptococcus* and *Pseudomonas* are also seen. Infants are more susceptible to infection of the epiphysis, as blood supply is shared across the growth plate.
- Sx/Exam: Infants may present with fussiness and pseudoparalysis of a limb. Older children will generally have fever and acute tenderness and will refuse to bear weight on the affected limb.
- Dx: ↑ WBC, CRP, and ESR. X-ray findings lag behind clinical findings and should not delay treatment. Aspiration of the bone for culture is useful in identifying an organism and narrowing the antibiotic spectrum.
- Tx: Broad-spectrum IV antibiotics with surgical debridement as indicated.

## Rotational and Angular Disorders of the Lower Extremities

- **Genu varum and genu valgum:** Varum (bowlegs) is normal until age two, after which many children develop genu valgum (knock knees), which may persist until about age eight. Persistence of either condition beyond these ages requires referral and possible surgical repair or splinting.
- **Tibial torsion:** Internal rotation of the leg between the knee and the ankle is normal in the newborn but justifies referral for splinting if it persists beyond 18 months.
- **Femoral anteversion:** Internal rotation at the hip causes the appearance of intoeing. Treatment is generally not necessary unless passive external rotation is not possible.

> In genu val**GUM,** the knees are **GUM**med together.

## Scoliosis

- Lateral curvature of the spine associated with rotation of the vertebrae. Idiopathic disease is most common and usually presents around 8–10 years of age, but on rare occasions it may be seen in toddlers.

- There is an association with Marfan's syndrome, cerebral palsy, muscular dystrophy, and neurofibromatosis. The disease is seen four times more often in girls and frequently runs in families.
- **Dx:** First noted by the family or on exam. To assess severity, check x-rays to calculate the angle of defect. There is no evidence to support universal screening.
- **Tx:** Treatment should be based on symptoms, obviousness of the deformity, and the likelihood of progression. Mild disease may be followed with serial exams and bracing as required; more severe disease may require surgery to correct obvious deformity and preserve respiratory capacity.

## Autism

> *Signs of autism—*
>
> **AUTISM**
>
> **A**loneness
> **U**nderstanding (lack of)
> **T**ouch (hypersensitivity to)
> **I**rrelevant and metaphorical language
> **S**ameness (desire for)
> **M**emory (rote)

- A pervasive developmental disorder characterized by deficits in interpersonal relationships accompanied by speech and language delay. It is an uncommon condition (4 in 10,000) with a male-to-female ratio of 3:1. The cause is unknown, but its higher incidence within families suggests a genetic component. It is **not** linked to vaccinations.
- **Sx/Exam:** Presents between one and three years of age. Early signs are poor eye contact, lack of stranger anxiety, and poor attachment to parents. Later signs include peculiar interests, stereotypic behaviors, and low IQ (generally < 70). There has been a recent ↑ in the diagnosis of this condition, but this may be related to ↑ recognition rather than to ↑ incidence.
- **DDx:** In Asperger's syndrome, lack of awareness of others and poor social functioning are similar to that seen in autism, but mental retardation and language delay are generally absent.
- **Tx:** Early intervention with behavioral education focused on sensory clues and appropriate interactions.

## Attention-Deficit Hyperactivity Disorder (ADHD)

Characterized by a triad of symptoms consisting of inattention, impulsivity, and hyperactivity. The disorder may be classified as inattentive, impulsive, or combined. To make the diagnosis, symptoms must be present in two areas of social interaction (home plus school); must have been present since before the age of seven; must have persisted for > 6 months; and must be maladaptive or inappropriate for the child's developmental stage.

### DIAGNOSIS

- Six of the symptoms in one or both of these categories must be present:
  - **Impulsivity/hyperactivity:**
    - Fidgetiness
    - Difficulty remaining seated in the class
    - Excessive running or climbing
    - Difficulty engaging in quiet activities
    - Is always "on the go"
    - Excessive talking
    - Blurting out answers before questions have been completed
    - Difficulty awaiting turn
    - Interrupting and intruding on others
  - **Inattentiveness:**
    - Failure to pay close attention to detail
    - Difficulty sustaining attention in tasks
    - Failure to listen when spoken to directly

- Failure to follow instructions
- Difficulty organizing tasks and activities
- Reluctance to engage in tasks that require sustained attention
- Losing utensils (e.g. pencils, books) necessary for tasks or activities
- Easy distractibility
- Forgetfulness in daily activities

- Comorbid psychiatric problems are common and include mood and conduct disorders. All children should be evaluated for learning disabilities.

### TREATMENT

- Components include medication, behavior modification (often with a token economy that rewards good behavior), and environmental interventions such as preferential seating and ↓ stimuli.
- The most commonly used medications are stimulants such as methylphenidate (Ritalin), complications of which include loss of appetite and growth delay.
- Intensive behavioral therapy may be helpful but is generally less effective than medication. Counseling is generally ineffective for ADHD itself but may be an important part of managing comorbid conditions such as depression and anxiety.

*Stimulants used for the treatment of ADHD are associated with anorexia and may → inadequate growth. Some families opt not to use the medication on weekends or during holidays from school in order to let their children regain appetite and growth.*

## Developmental Delay

- Children who fail to meet developmental milestones must be evaluated early in order to initiate appropriate therapies.
- **DDx:** Environmental causes (abuse/neglect), sensory causes (vision/hearing loss), motor delay (coordination defect → speech delay), psychiatric conditions.
- **Dx:** Workup includes a careful physical exam to assess for the presence of features consistent with a syndrome (Down, fetal alcohol, Turner's syndromes), supplemented by chromosome analysis and fragile X testing. Cognitive tests include the Wechsler and Stanford-Binet scales. Loss of skills raises concern for a metabolic disorder or a neurodegenerative condition.
- **Tx:** Special education classes; appropriate occupational therapy.

## Growth Delay

Although height and weight percentiles may adjust during the first two years of life, a persistent ↑ or ↓ in height percentiles between two years of age and the onset of puberty warrants further evaluation. Workup includes hand x-rays for bone age, CBC and ESR to evaluate for infection, kidney function and UA to assess for occult renal disease, stool studies to examine for malabsorption, karyotype for girls to assess for Turner's syndrome, TSH to evaluate for hypothyroidism, and IGF-1 to look for growth hormone deficiency. Table 13.6 compares three common causes of growth delay.

*The anticipated height of a child can be determined by calculating the mean parental height and adding 6.5 cm for boys or subtracting 6.5 cm for girls.*

## Cerebral Palsy

- A spectrum of disorders that are nonprogressive and originate from some type of cerebral insult or injury. The injury may occur before birth, during delivery, or in the perinatal period.

**TABLE 13.6.** Common Causes of Growth Delay

| FAMILIAL SHORT STATURE | CONSTITUTIONAL GROWTH DELAY | GROWTH HORMONE DEFICIENCY |
|---|---|---|
| Parents are short. | Parents are not necessarily short, but there may be a family history of late growth ("late bloomers"). | Characterized by ↓ growth velocity and delay in skeletal maturation. Growth delay may begin in infancy or later in childhood. |
| Children are typically born with normal weight and length but adjust to a lower percentile in the first two years of life. They will then have normal growth along that growth curve. | Growth pattern is similar to that of familial short stature. | May be isolated or occur with other pituitary hormone deficiencies. |
| Skeletal maturation and the timing of puberty are consistent with chronologic age. | Skeletal maturation and puberty are delayed, and linear growth continues beyond the typical age for reaching full height. | Treatment is recombinant human growth hormone. |
| No treatment is necessary. | No treatment is necessary. | |

- **Sx/Exam:** The most common form involves spasticity of the limbs. The second most frequent presentation is ataxia. Associated neurologic deficits can include seizure, mental retardation, speech delay, and sensory loss.
- **Tx:** Physical, occupational, and speech therapy; orthopedic interventions as necessary.

## COMMON ACUTE CONDITIONS

### Respiratory Distress

In all cases of respiratory distress, look for nasal flaring, grunting, and suprasternal, intercostal, and subcostal retractions, and listen for wheezing, crackles, and ↓ air movement. Signs of significant hypoxia include cyanosis around the mucous membranes and nail beds.

#### APNEA

Defined as cessation of breathing for > 20 seconds or for 10–20 seconds with signs of hypoxia. Subtypes are as follows:

- **Central:** Frequently identified early in infancy. May be related to infection, metabolic abnormalities, anemia, hypoxia, or CNS dysfunction.
- **Obstructive:** Occurs in later infancy and childhood. Obstruction → cessation of airflow despite respiratory effort.

#### DIAGNOSIS

- In infants, check for metabolic imbalance with a basic metabolic panel and BUN/creatinine. Look for signs of infection (CBC, UA, and CXR; consider CT and LP); check for RSV and pertussis; consider an ECG.
- Consider an EEG if the patient has altered mental status or if a seizure focus is suspected. Admit for apnea monitoring.
- In older children, consider upper pharyngeal lesions such as tonsillitis and pharyngitis or laryngomalacia.

A panicked father presents to your office with his two-month-old daughter, who is coughing and wheezing. The child was entirely well and playing "tea party" with her older sister when the father started doing laundry, but she looked ill when he returned. She has no significant past medical history and no sick contacts. She is afebrile, is slightly pale, and has an inspiratory wheeze. Her $O_2$ saturation is normal, and her CXR is significant only for mild hyperinflation of the right lung. What is your diagnosis? This child almost certainly inhaled something nonradiopaque into her right bronchus while at her tea party. She needs urgent evaluation for removal of this object under direct visualization by ENT.

### UPPER AIRWAY OBSTRUCTION

May be caused by a foreign body or by epiglottitis or croup, distinguished as follows (see also Figure 13.8):

- **Foreign body:**
  - **Sx/Exam:** Abrupt onset with no fever; not positional; presents with inspiratory **and** expiratory stridor.
  - **Dx:** CXR shows possible object and hyperinflation.
  - **Tx:** Removal via laryngoscopy or bronchoscopy.
- **Epiglottitis:**
  - Most common in children 2–5 years of age. Most often caused by S. *pyogenes*, S. *pneumoniae*, and S. *aureus*; on rare occasions, H. *influenzae* may be implicated (a significant ↓ in incidence has been seen 2° to routine vaccination).
  - **Sx/Exam:** Rapid onset with high fever; presents with drooling and sore throat. Patients remain sitting or leaning forward. Primarily inspiratory stridor.
  - **Dx:** A lateral neck x-ray reveals the characteristic "thumbprint sign" (see Figure 13.9).
  - **Tx:** Secure the airway; send blood cultures and start broad-spectrum antibiotics.
- **Croup:**
  - Most common in children six months to three years of age, occurring during the fall and winter months. Caused by parainfluenza virus.
  - **Sx/Exam:** Gradual worsening; low-grade fever; normal WBC. Inspiratory and expiratory stridor are also seen.
  - **Dx:** CXR shows subglottic narrowing (the "steeple sign").
  - **Tx:** Treat mild disease with humidified $O_2$. Moderate to severe disease should be treated with steroids and nebulized racemic epinephrine.

*The key feature of upper airway obstruction is inspiratory stridor.*

### LOWER AIRWAY OBSTRUCTION

Causes in children include bronchiolitis, asthma, pneumonia, and foreign body obstruction. In infants, it can be associated with congenital anomalies of the airway (tracheal web, cysts, vascular rings, lobar emphysema).

- **Bronchiolitis:**
  - An acute lower airway respiratory disease that → small airway obstruction, typically occurring in the wintertime. It primarily affects children < 12 months of age and is caused by RSV.

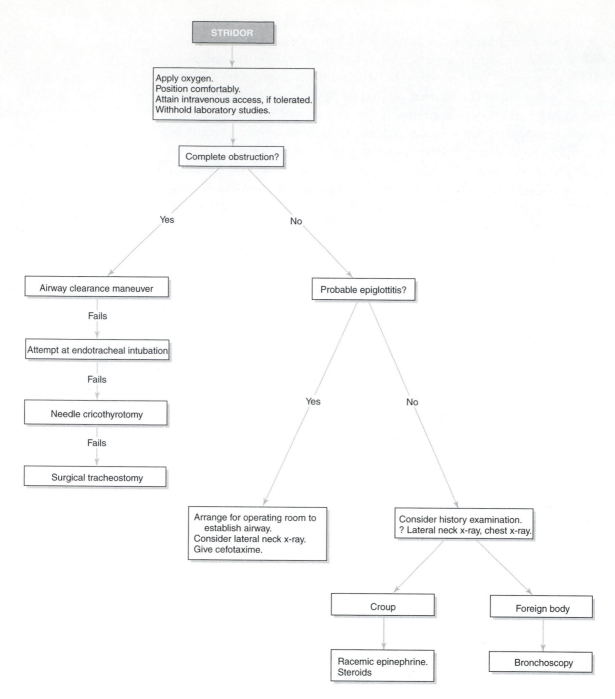

**FIGURE 13.8.** **Diagnosis and treatment of upper airway obstruction.**

(Reproduced, with permission, from Stone CK, Humphries RL. *Current Emergency Diagnosis & Treatment*, 5th ed. New York: McGraw-Hill, 2004: 1054.)

- **Sx/Exam:** Cough, coryza, and upper respiratory symptoms, usually with fever, precede wheezing and dyspnea.
- **Dx:** WBC count is normal, and CXR shows shifting patterns of hyper-aeration and atelectasis. Hypercapnia, hypoxemia, or both may be present. Obtain a nasal swab/wash for RSV.

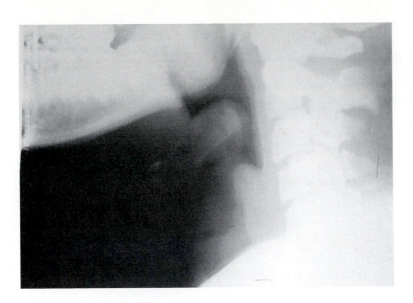

**FIGURE 13.9.** The "thumbprint sign" of epiglottitis.

(Reproduced, with permission, from Stone CK, Humphries RL. *Current Emergency Diagnosis & Treatment*, 5th ed. New York: McGraw-Hill, 2004: 1055.)

- **Tx:** Nebulized epinephrine, albuterol, and $O_2$. Admit for low $O_2$ saturation, prematurity, age < 3 months, or toxic appearance. High-risk infants (premature infants and those with preexisting lung or heart disease) should receive palivizumab (Synagis), a monoclonal antibody, to ↓ the risk of contracting RSV.
- **Cx:** Mortality from bronchiolitis has ↓ with improved hospital care. There is a possible connection between bronchiolitis in infancy and the subsequent development of reactive airway disease, but the physiology is unclear.
- **Asthma:**
  - **Sx/Exam:** Expiratory wheezing and shortness of breath. Inability to speak, cyanosis, accessory muscle use, pulsus paradoxus, or signs of infection may indicate more serious disease.
  - **Tx:** Same as outpatient treatment, but consider IV or PO steroids. Intubation is necessary in severe cases.
- **Pneumonia:**
  - Common causative organisms are as follows:
    - **Newborns:** GBS, gram-⊖ enteric bacteria, CMV, *Listeria monocytogenes.*
    - **Infants:** *Chlamydia trachomatis,* RSV, *S. pneumoniae, S. aureus.*
    - **Toddlers:** Viruses, *S. pneumoniae,* nontypable *H. influenzae.*
    - **Children (4–14):** *Mycoplasma pneumoniae, Pneumococcus, Chlamydia pneumoniae.*
  - **Sx/Exam:** Presents with fever and respiratory findings (crackles, egophony, dullness to percussion).
  - **Dx:** CXR shows evidence of parenchymal infiltrates.
  - **Tx:** Antibiotics; hospitalize if the patient is unable to maintain an $O_2$ saturation > 92% on room air. Some patients may respond to bronchodilators.

## Fever

### FEVER IN NEONATES (< 3 MONTHS)

- Rectal temperature > 38°C.
- Respiratory and GI disorders are the most common sources. Also consider late onset of congenitally acquired illnesses such as rubella and CMV, or infections acquired at birth, such as GBS, *E. coli*, and *Listeria*. Early infection may also be the first sign of a congenital abnormality (e.g., in the GU system).
- **Dx:** CBC with differential, blood culture, UA, urine culture, LP. LP is occasionally omitted if the infant is > 30 days old and is felt to be low risk, and good follow-up is available. Also consider CXR, stool culture, and viral culture.
- **Tx:**
  - Admit if the infant is < 30 days old, if there is any abnormality on blood tests, or if the patient is at risk for lack of follow-up.
  - Treat with antibiotics while awaiting culture results.
    - Give ampicillin plus a third-generation cephalosporin or gentamicin if the child is < 30 days old.
    - Administer a third-generation cephalosporin if the child is 30–60 days old and treatment is indicated by laboratory or clinical findings. Add ampicillin if the child appears toxic.
    - Antibiotics may be discontinued at 48 hours if all cultures are ⊖ and the infant is clinically stable.

### FEVER IN INFANTS AND TODDLERS (3–36 MONTHS)

*The use of the pneumococcal conjugate vaccine and the Hib vaccine have dramatically ↓ the number of cases of invasive disease seen from Pneumococcus and H. influenzae type B infections.*

- Rectal temp > 39°C.
- Etiologies include viral infection, pneumonia, UTI, meningitis, and occult bacteremia. The source of the fever is more readily identifiable in this group than in younger children.
- **Dx:** In the absence of an obvious source of infection (e.g., otitis media, infectious diarrhea), diagnose as follows:
  - **Fully immunized females:** Check UA and urine culture if the child is < 24 months old.
  - **Fully immunized males:** Check UA and urine culture if the child is circumcised and < 6 months or uncircumcised and < 24 months.
  - If the child has not received a complete vaccination series, check CBC, blood cultures, UA, and urine culture. Also consider LP and CXR based on clinical presentation.
- **Tx:** Children who appear well or have a presentation consistent with a viral syndrome may be discharged with close follow-up. Empiric IV or IM antibiotics may be given while awaiting cultures in children who appear ill and in whom no obvious source is identified.

### FEVER IN CHILDREN (> 36 MONTHS)

The risk of occult bacteremia is lower in this age group, and a source of fever is generally identifiable and treated as needed. In children < 5 years of age with persistent fever, consider Kawasaki disease.

## Acute Otitis Media

- Commonly caused by *S. pneumoniae*, *H. influenzae*, and *Moraxella catarrhalis*.
- **Sx/Exam:** Presents with pain, fever, and hearing loss. May be preceded by a URI. Exam reveals a bulging tympanic membrane with loss of visual landmarks. Loss of movement of the tympanic membrane is both sensitive and specific.
- **Tx:** First-line treatment is amoxicillin. If children are high risk or have been treated in the last 30 days, consider amoxicillin-clavulanate. Recurrent infections may be an indication for referral to ENT for placement of tympanotomy tubes. In an effort to curb antibiotic resistance, some practitioners choose not to treat acute otitis media with antibiotics. This is appropriate only in children over the age of two years for whom close follow-up can be certain.
- **Cx:** Mastoiditis, hearing loss.

## Diarrhea

- Rotavirus is the most common cause of acute diarrhea, particularly in the winter months. Additional causes include other viruses, food poisoning, traveler's diarrhea, or diarrhea related to recent antibiotic use. Chronic diarrhea may be a sign of IBD, IBS, or celiac disease.
- **Dx:**
    - The history and physical are important in identifying signs of dehydration. Ask about the number of wet diapers and the presence of tears when crying.
    - Fecal leukocytes and stool cultures are not always necessary but may be helpful when a child has bloody diarrhea or appears significantly ill. The serum WBC count is generally higher in bacterial than in viral infection.
    - A chem 7 can help identify the degree of dehydration.
    - The combination of bloody diarrhea and acute renal failure should raise suspicion of hemolytic-uremic syndrome (HUS) triggered by Shiga toxin–producing *E. coli* O157:H7.
- **Tx:** The most important intervention is rehydration. This can usually be done with oral intake, but significant dehydration should be treated with IV fluids and occasionally with hospitalization. Most cases of infectious diarrhea will resolve without treatment, but antibiotics may speed recovery.

*Rotavirus accounts for as many as 50% of cases of acute diarrhea in winter. Enteric adenoviruses (serotypes 40 and 41) are the second most common viral pathogen in infants. In summer, most cases of diarrhea are caused by bacteria (including E. coli, Salmonella, and Shigella).*

---

A mother brings her eight-month-old son to the emergency department. He has been having episodes of inconsolable crying during which he pulls his knees to his chest. Between episodes he is lethargic, and he has vomited twice. As you go in to examine him, the nurse tells you that he has just had an episode of bloody diarrhea. How do you proceed? This presentation raises concern for intussusception. If the child does not appear toxic, a barium enema may be both diagnostic and therapeutic. If there is suspicion of necrotic bowel or perforation, air insufflation may be attempted or the child may need surgery.

## Vomiting

- In infants and children, common causes of vomiting include gastroenteritis (may precede diarrhea by a few days), intussusception, appendicitis, Reye's syndrome, or hepatitis.
- **Dx:** Consider CBC, electrolytes, and LFTs as indicated clinically. Evaluate for dehydration, and consider imaging for underlying causes. "Currant jelly" stools are the classic sign of intussusception and point to the need for a barium enema.

## Abdominal Pain

- The most likely etiologies of abdominal pain vary by age group:
  - **Infants:** Colic, constipation, gastroenteritis, intussusception, viral syndrome, volvulus.
  - **Younger children:** Appendicitis, constipation, gastroenteritis, pneumonia, UTI, viral syndromes.
  - **School-aged children:** Appendicitis, pregnancy, gastroenteritis, pneumonia, peptic ulcer, PID.
- Rare causes include pancreatitis, Henoch-Schönlein purpura, and HUS.
- **Dx:** Obtain CBC and electrolytes if the child appears ill. Obtain imaging as indicated by clinical presentation:
  - **AXR** (flat and upright or lateral): Helps identify free air (an indication of perforation) or air-fluid levels (an indication of obstruction).
  - **CXR:** To identify lower lobe pneumonia.
  - **Ultrasound or abdominal CT with IV and PO contrast:** To identify appendicitis.
  - **Testicular ultrasound:** To identify torsion.
  - **Barium enema:** To look for volvulus or intussusception.

## Meckel's Diverticulum

> *Meckel's diverticulum rule of 2's:*
>
> **2** inches long
> **2** feet from the ileocecal valve
> **2** types of tissue
> Peak incidence at age **2**

- An ileal diverticulum that may contain ectopic gastric tissue and therefore → painless bleeding. Males are affected more often than females.
- **Dx:** A technetium scan can identify ectopic gastric tissue.
- **Tx:** Surgical resection of symptomatic lesions (asymptomatic diverticulum do not need to be removed).

## Head Trauma

Can be due to direct impact or from acceleration/deceleration injuries. Direct injury to brain tissue and injury from pressure due to expanding hematomas or edema can be serious. The goals of evaluation and treatment are to promptly identify serious conditions and to monitor and treat sequelae, including seizures, altered mental status, ↑ ICP, and SIADH. Subtypes are as follows:

- **Concussion:** A brief loss or alteration of consciousness due to head trauma followed by a return to normal. Brain tissue is not damaged, and there are no focal findings. Amnesia, vomiting, confusion, dizziness, and sleep disturbances may be seen. A postconcussive syndrome may last for weeks to months. Children should not be put at risk for another event (e.g., competitive sports) until they have remained asymptomatic for at least one week.
- **Contusion:** A bruise of the brain matter. The child's level of consciousness ↓, and focal findings correspond to the area of the brain that is injured. Obtain a head CT and admit for observation.

- **Diffuse axonal injury:** Characterized by coma without focal signs on neurologic exam. There may be no external signs of trauma. The initial CT scan is normal or may demonstrate only small, scattered areas of cerebral contusion and areas of low density. Prolonged disability may follow diffuse axonal injury.
- **ICP elevation with or without herniation:** May be seen in traumatic injury, spontaneous intracranial hemorrhage, CNS infection, hydrocephalus, ruptured AVM, metabolic derangement (e.g., DKA), ventriculoperitoneal shunt obstruction, or tumor. Symptoms include headache, vision changes, vomiting, gait difficulties, and a progressively decreasing level of consciousness. Other signs may include stiff neck, cranial nerve palsies, and progressive hemiparesis. Cushing's triad (bradycardia, hypertension, and irregular respirations) is a late and prearrest finding. Papilledema is also a late finding.

### DIAGNOSIS

- **Infants:** Neurologic exam may be normal. Consider CT based on the mechanism of injury; the presence of physical findings such as scalp injury, hematoma, or skull fracture; a history of loss of consciousness; focal neurologic findings; or vomiting > 5 times or for > 5 hours.
- **Children:** A CT scan should be obtained in children with persistent vomiting (as defined above) or an abnormal or lateralizing neurologic examination, including an abnormal mental status that does not quickly return to normal. Loss of consciousness or seizure immediately following the event does not require imaging unless one of the other conditions has been met.

*In infants with head trauma, consider CT based on mechanism; in children, make this decision on the basis of the history and exam.*

## Abuse

### PHYSICAL ABUSE

- Physical indicators of abuse include the following:
    - Injuries that do not match the history.
    - Specific pathognomonic injuries (e.g., looped wire marks, cigarette burns, rib fractures, spiral fractures).
    - Multiple injuries in varying stages of healing.
    - Different types of injuries or disease (e.g., burns and fractures).
    - Overall evidence of poor care.
    - Evidence of FTT.
- Infants who are severely shaken can present with sudden onset of seizure or coma with no signs of head trauma. Infants who are severely shaken will typically have bilateral retinal hemorrhages and may have bilateral subdural hemorrhages on CT scan.
- When suspicious of abuse, document all injuries, consider a skeletal survey, and discuss the case with Child Protective Services prior to discharge.

*Abuse may be physical, sexual, emotional, or by neglect. In early childhood, FTT may be the first indicator.*

### SEXUAL ABUSE

- Behavioral changes may be an indicator of sexual abuse.
    - Preschool children may present with fear states (e.g., fear of adult males), nightmares, precocious sexual behavior, enuresis, encopresis, or behavior regression.

- School-aged children may exhibit sexual behavior, sexual aggression toward other children, cross-dressing, school failure, truancy, running away, or depression.
  - Adolescents may also develop problems with drugs, promiscuity, or prostitution.
- A careful vaginal exam of a young girl is sometimes needed and is best performed with the child in the knee-chest position.

## Seizures

### STATUS EPILEPTICUS

- Continuous seizure activity for 30 minutes or recurrent seizures without intervening return of consciousness.
- Children < 3 years of age are more likely to have an underlying cause such as CNS infection, vascular disorders, anoxia, trauma, intoxication, fever, or metabolic abnormalities. These conditions are often treatable.
- In older children, status epilepticus is more often the result of a chronic seizure disorder.
- **DDx:** Look for an underlying condition with a rapid blood glucose level, CBC, chemistry panel, LFTs, ammonia level, and toxicology screen.
- **Tx:** ABCs, anticonvulsants (benzodiazepines, phenytoin, barbiturates).

### FEBRILE SEIZURES

- May be simple or complex.
  - **Simple febrile seizure:** Typically occurs as a generalized, self-limited tonic-clonic seizure of several minutes' duration.
  - **Complex febrile seizure:** Denotes a seizure with high-risk features lasting > 15 minutes.
- Peak age is 8–20 months, although seizures may occur in children from approximately six months to six years of age.
- Often, underlying diseases are simply URIs or gastroenteritis. The seizure seems to be more the result of a rapid change in temperature than absolute temperature and is independent of the underlying condition.
- **DDx:** Syncope, hysteria, breath holding, night terrors. Also exclude head trauma and alcohol or drug intoxication.
- **Tx:** Simple febrile seizures are usually benign and require no therapy. Acetaminophen may be given orally or rectally as needed to address the fever. If a child is having recurrent seizures, consider loading with phenobarbital; chronic antiepileptic medication is needed only rarely. In some children who are prone to febrile seizure, diazepam is used at the onset of a febrile illness and repeated as necessary until the fever resolves.
- **Cx:** Children presenting with high-risk features are at greater risk for recurrent afebrile seizures.

## Meningitis

- Occurs following invasion of the subarachnoid space by a pathogenic organism. The most common route is by hematogenous spread, but it may also occur by direct extension from a contiguous focus of infection such as sinusitis or mastoiditis.

**TABLE 13.7.** **Etiologies and Treatment of Childhood Meningitis**

| AGE | COMMON CAUSES | ANTIBIOTIC | OTHER CAUSES |
|---|---|---|---|
| Preterm to < 1 month | GBS, *E. coli, Listeria* | Ampicillin plus cefotaxime or gentamicin | Enterovirus, *Candida albicans* |
| 1–3 months | GBS, *E. coli, Listeria, S. pneumoniae, N. meningitidis, H. influenzae* type B (rare) | Vancomycin plus cefotaxime or ceftriaxone | Enterovirus |
| 3 months – 6 years | *S. pneumoniae, N. meningitidis, H. influenzae* type B (rare) | Vancomycin plus cefotaxime or ceftriaxone | Enterovirus, mumps, *Mycobacterium tuberculosis* |
| > 6 years | *S. pneumoniae, N. meningitidis* | Vancomycin plus cefotaxime or ceftriaxone | Enterovirus, mumps, *M. tuberculosis* |

Adapted, with permission, from Stone CK, Humphries RL. *Current Emergency Diagnosis & Treatment,* 5th ed. New York: McGraw-Hill, 2004: 1068.

- Sx/Exam:
    - **Infants:** Clinical findings may be nonspecific and may include restlessness, irritability, poor feeding, emesis, diarrhea, lethargy, ↓ tone, respiratory distress, full fontanelle (late finding), and seizures. Obvious neck stiffness or other signs of meningeal irritation (e.g., Kernig's or Brudzinski's signs) are not reliably present in infants < 18 months of age.
    - **Children > 18 months:** Neck stiffness, headache, nausea, vomiting, focal neurologic signs, fever, lethargy, and photophobia are common. Infants and children with *Neisseria meningitidis* infection often present with a petechial rash.
- **Dx:** LP with analysis of protein and glucose as well as viral and bacterial cultures.
- **Tx:** Table 13.7 outlines treatment options.

## Poisoning

- **Prevention is key.** Families should be counseled early to store medications and chemicals in areas inaccessible to children.
- **Tx:** Includes induced vomiting (generally not indicated), gastric lavage, activated charcoal, urinary alkalinization, and dialysis. Poison control centers can offer guidance on treatment.

## Rash

Table 13.8 outlines the presentation, diagnosis, and treatment of common viral and bacterial causes of rash in infants in children.

**TABLE 13.8.** Common Causes of Rash in the Pediatric Population

| DISEASE | USUAL AGE | PRODROME | MORPHOLOGY/ DISTRIBUTION | ASSOCIATED FINDINGS | DIAGNOSIS | SPECIAL MANAGEMENT |
|---|---|---|---|---|---|---|
| Measles (rubeola virus) | Infants to young adults | High fever, symptoms of URI, conjunctivitis. | Erythematous macules and papules become confluent (see Figure 13.10). Begins on the face and moves centrifugally. | Koplik's spots, "toxic" appearance, photophobia, cough, adenopathy, high fever. | Usually clinical; acute/ convalescent hemagglutinin (HAI) serologic test. | Report to public health; give immunoglobulin within six days of exposure. |
| Rubella (rubella virus) | Adolescents/ young adults | Absent or low-grade fever, malaise, upper respiratory symptoms. | Rose-pink maculopapules; not confluent. Begins on the face and moves downward rapidly. | Postauricular and occipital adenopathy; headache, malaise, mild pruritus. | Rubella IgM or acute/ convalescent HAI serologic test. | Report to public health; check for exposure to pregnant women. |
| Erythema infectiosum (parvovirus B19) | 3–12 years | Usually none. | Slapped cheeks; reticular erythema or maculopapular rash (see Figure 13.11). Usually affects the arms and legs, but may be generalized. | Waxes and wanes for several weeks; occasionally presents with arthritis, headache, and malaise. | Usually clinical; acute/ convalescent serologic test. | Carries the potential complication of aplastic crisis. |
| Enteroviral exanthems (coxsackie-virus, echovirus, other enteroviruses) | Young children | Fever (occasionally). | Extremely variable; may be maculopapular, petechial, purpuric, or vesicular. Usually generalized, but may be acral. | Low-grade fever, occasional myocarditis, aseptic meningitis, pleurodynia. | Usually clinical; viral throat culture; rectal swabs in selected cases. | In the presence of petechiae or purpura, **meningococcemia must be considered.** |
| Hand-foot-mouth syndrome (several coxsackie-viruses) | Young children | Fever (occasional), sore mouth. | Gray-white vesicles 3–7 mm in size on a normal or erythematous base. The hands and feet are most commonly affected, but may affect the diaper area and is occasionally generalized. | Oral ulcers, occasional fever, adenopathy. | Same as for enteroviral exanthems. | |

**TABLE 13.8.** Common Causes of Rash in the Pediatric Population (continued)

| Disease | Usual Age | Prodrome | Morphology/ Distribution | Associated Findings | Diagnosis | Special Management |
|---|---|---|---|---|---|---|
| Adenovirus exanthems (adenoviruses) | Young children | Fever; symptoms of URI. | Rubelliform, morbilliform, roseola-like rash. Generalized. | Fever; symptoms of URI; occasionally pneumonia. | Viral isolation or acute/ convalescent seroconversion. | |
| Chickenpox (VZV) | 1–14 years | Fever, headache, and malaise 48 hours prior to exanthem. | Macules and papules rapidly become vesicles on an erythematous base, followed by crusts. Often begins on the scalp or face; more profuse on the trunk than on the extremities. | Pruritus, fever, oral and genital lesions, occasional malaise. | Usually clinical; Tzanck preparation or direct immuno-fluorescence. | Antihistamines for itching; aspirin is contraindicated (Reye's syndrome). |
| Roseola (may be linked to HHV-6) | < 3 years | High fever for 3–5 days prior to exanthem. | A maculopapular rash in rosettes appears **after** fever declines. Affects the trunk and neck but may be generalized. Lasts hour to days. | Cervical and postauricular adenopathy. | Clinical. | |
| Kawasaki disease | < 5 years | High fever, irritability. | Polymorphous—papular, vesicobullous, or morbilliform; erythema with desquamation. Generalized, often with perineal accentuation and desquamation. | Conjunctivitis, cheilitis, glossitis, peripheral edema, adenopathy, strawberry tongue. | Clinical. | Admit to the hospital for IVIG and salicylates. |
| Scarlet fever (group A streptococcus) | School age | Acute onset with fever, sore throat. | Diffuse erythema with sandpaper texture. Facial flushing with circumoral pallor; linear erythema in skin folds. | Exudative pharyngitis, palatal petechiae, abdominal pain. | Throat cultures. | IM penicillin or oral erythromycin. |

**TABLE 13.8.** Common Causes of Rash in the Pediatric Population (continued)

| DISEASE | USUAL AGE | PRODROME | MORPHOLOGY/ DISTRIBUTION | ASSOCIATED FINDINGS | DIAGNOSIS | SPECIAL MANAGEMENT |
|---|---|---|---|---|---|---|
| Staphylococcal scalded skin syndrome (*S. aureus* epidermolytic toxin) | < 5 years | None. | Abrupt onset, with tender erythroderma. Eruption with intensification in the neck, face, axillae, and groin. | Fever, conjunctivitis, rhinitis. | Clinical: culture of *S. aureus* from systemic site (not skin). | Neonate; if blistering is present, hospitalize for IV antibiotics and fluid/electrolyte therapy. |
| Henoch-Schönlein purpura | 4–7 years | Possibly abdominal pain. | Palpable purpuric or petechial rash. Begins on the malleoli and extends to the buttocks. | Arthralgia, nausea, vomiting, diarrhea, GI bleeding. | Clinical. | Consider Rocky Mountain spotted fever or meningococcemia; steroids for severe cases. |

Adapted, with permission, from Stone CK, Humphries RL. *Current Emergency Diagnosis & Treatment,* 5th ed. New York: McGraw-Hill, 2004: 1082.

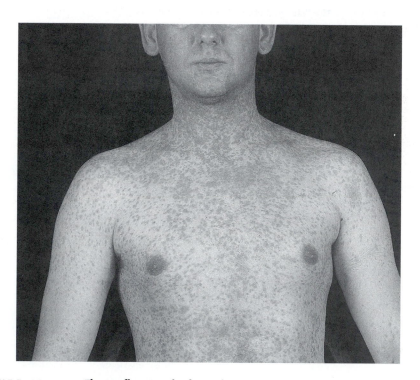

**FIGURE 13.10.** The confluent rash of measles.

(Reproduced, with permission, from Wolff K et al. *Fitzpatrick's Color Atlas & Synopsis of Clinical Dermatology,* 5th ed. New York: McGraw-Hill, 2005: 788.) (Also see Color Insert.)

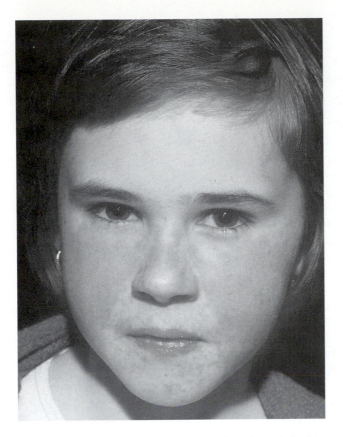

**FIGURE 13.11.** The "slapped cheek" appearance of erythema infectiosum.

(Reproduced, with permission, from Wolff K et al. *Fitzpatrick's Color Atlas & Synopsis of Clinical Dermatology*, 5th ed. New York: McGraw-Hill, 2005: 793.) (Also see Color Insert.)

## CARDIOLOGY

You are seeing a three-year-old girl for a routine well-child check. Her mother notes she is now fully potty trained and about to start preschool. On exam you note that her height and weight have been stable at the 50th percentile and that her developmental milestones are also appropriate for her age. On exam, you note that she has a quiet precordium, a regular rate, and normal S1 and S2 with a 2/6 systolic ejection murmur that is louder when she is supine. There is no radiation of the murmur to the neck, axillae, or back. What is your next step in management? Reassure the parents that the murmur is innocent, and observe the patient.

### Evaluation of a Murmur

The most common cardiovascular finding → a cardiology referral. Innocent heart murmurs (also known as functional murmurs) are extremely common. Between 40% and 45% of children have an innocent murmur at some time during childhood.

### SYMPTOMS

Symptoms of **pathologic murmurs** include FTT, exercise intolerance, dyspnea with exertion/diaphoresis, syncope, dizziness, cyanosis, loss of consciousness, and tachypnea with feeds or activity.

### EXAM

Assess the following:

- **Location:** Left upper sternal border, right upper sternal border, left lower sternal border, apex.
- **Radiation:** Neck, back, axillae.
- **Relationship to cardiac cycle and duration:**
  - **Systolic ejection:** Immediately following S1 with a crescendo/decrescendo change in intensity.
  - **Pansystolic:** Occurring throughout most of systole and of constant intensity.
  - Diastolic.
  - Continuous.
- **Intensity:**
  - **Grade I:** Soft and heard with difficulty.
  - **Grade II:** Soft but easily heard.
  - **Grade III:** Loud but without a thrill.
  - **Grade IV:** Loud and associated with a precordial thrill.
  - **Grade V:** Loud with thrill, and audible with the edge of the stethoscope.
  - **Grade VI:** Very loud and audible with the stethoscope off the chest.
- **Quality:** Harsh, musical, or rough; high, medium, or low in pitch.
- **Variation with position:** Whether audible when the patient is supine, sitting, standing, or squatting.

### DIAGNOSIS

**Indications of pathologic murmurs** include the following (see also Table 13.9):

- Cyanotic, symptomatic (FTT, tachypnea).
- Grade III or more.
- Diastolic murmur.
- Abnormal CXR or ECG.
- The patient has a syndrome with a high incidence of heart defects (e.g., Down, Turner's, Marfan's, Williams', Noonan's syndromes).

### TREATMENT

Refer pathologic murmurs to a pediatric cardiologist; observe benign murmurs.

## Atrial Septal Defect (ASD)

A through-and-through communication between the atria at the septal level. Oxygenated blood from the higher-pressure left atrium passes into the right atrium, increasing right ventricular output and pulmonary blood flow. Right-to-left shunting and cyanosis (Eisenmenger's syndrome) are found in 15% of cases. ASD takes **three forms:**

- Persistent ostium secundum (midseptum) (80% of cases)
- Persistent ostium primum (low septum)
- Sinus venosus defect (upper septum)

---

> **Features of innocent murmurs—**
>
> **the 8 S's**
>
> **S**oft
> **S**ystolic
> **S**hort
> **S**ounds (S1 and S2) normal
> **S**ymptomless
> **S**pecial tests (x-ray, ECG) normal
> **S**tanding/**S**itting (vary with position)
> **S**ternal depression (pectus excavatum)

> Eisenmenger's syndrome *is a general term applied to pulmonary hypertension and shunt reversal in the presence of a congenital defect.*

**TABLE 13.9.** Types of Murmurs Based on Location of Loudest Intensity

| LOCATION/DIAGNOSIS | UNIQUE FEATURES |
|---|---|
| **Right upper sternal border** | |
| Venous hum | **Continuous;** disappears when the jugular vein is compressed, when the patient's head is turned, or when the patient is supine. Benign. |
| Aortic stenosis | Systolic ejection quality (with audible S1 and S2); radiates to the neck; presents with thrill in the suprasternal notch. Often associated with a valve click. |
| **Left upper sternal border** | |
| Peripheral pulmonary stenosis | Systolic ejection quality; usually seen in infants; often louder in the axillae than over the precordium. Benign. |
| Pulmonary stenosis | Systolic ejection quality; radiates to the back and axillae; may be associated with a valve click. |
| PDA | Continuous; **"machinery"** quality; bounding pulses. |
| ASD | Systolic; fixed, split S2. |
| Coarctation of the aorta | Systolic; radiation to the back; weak, delayed femoral pulses. |
| **Left lower sternal border** | |
| Still's murmur | **"Vibratory"** systolic ejection quality; no radiation; louder when the patient is supine. Benign. |
| VSD | Holosystolic; harsh quality; often radiates all over the precordium; often louder as the defect gets smaller. |
| Hypertrophic obstructive cardiomyopathy | Systolic ejection quality; gets louder when the patient is upright; often radiates to the apex; may be heard in patients who have chest pain with activity. |
| **Apex** | |
| Mitral regurgitation | Holosystolic, decrescendo, **"cooing dove"** quality. |

Reproduced, with permission, from Le T et al. *First Aid for the Pediatric Boards,* 1st ed. New York: McGraw-Hill, 2006: 61.

## SYMPTOMS

A young child with an uncorrected ASD and normal pulmonary arterial pressures is usually asymptomatic, with normal or minimally diminished exercise tolerance. With advancing age in the third decade of life, exertional dyspnea and atypical chest pain ↑ in frequency. Pulmonary hypertension can be associated with arrhythmias, syncope, and heart failure.

## EXAM

- A moderately loud systolic ejection murmur is heard in the second and third interspaces.
- S2 is widely split and does not vary with breathing.
- Prominent right ventricular and pulmonary artery pulsations.

## DIAGNOSIS

- **Echocardiography:** Usually diagnostic.
- **ECG:** Shows incomplete or complete RBBB, right axis deviation, and RVH.
- **CXR:** Demonstrates large pulmonary arteries, ↑ pulmonary vascularity, and an enlarged right atrium and ventricle.

- Saline bubble contrast and Doppler flow can demonstrate shunting
- **Transesophageal echocardiography:** Superior sensitivity for small shunts and patent foramen ovale.
- **Cardiac catheterization:** Can show an ↑ in $O_2$ saturation between the vena cava and the right ventricle; can also quantify the shunt and measure pulmonary vascular resistance.

### TREATMENT

- Although there is no evidence of benefit from closure of small shunts, large shunts generally require closure.
- Surgery is contraindicated with pulmonary hypertension.
- Percutaneous closure devices are now available.
- There is no risk of infective endocarditis unless mitral regurgitation is present as well, so antibiotic prophylaxis is recommended only in these cases.

### COMPLICATIONS

- **Eisenmenger's syndrome:** Pulmonary hypertension resulting from systemic-to-pulmonary communication and associated with cyanosis.
- Paradoxical emboli.
- ↑ risk of complications with scuba diving and high altitudes.

## Ventricular Septal Defect (VSD)

The most common congenital heart malformation, accounting for about 30% of all cases of congenital heart disease. Defects in the ventricular septum occur both in the membranous portion of the septum (most common) and in the muscular portion, permitting blood in the high-pressure left ventricle to shunt into the low-pressure right ventricle. Shunt reversal occurs in roughly 25% of cases, with subsequent elevated pulmonary artery pressures resulting in Eisenmenger's syndrome.

### SYMPTOMS

- **Small to moderate shunts:** Often asymptomatic and acyanotic.
- **Moderate shunts:** May → pulmonary vascular disease and right-sided failure.
- **Large left-to-right shunts:**
    - Patients are ill early in infancy (with frequent upper and lower respiratory infections), growing and gaining weight slowly.
    - Dyspnea, exercise intolerance, and fatigue are common. CHF develops between one and six months of age.
    - With severe pulmonary hypertension, cyanosis is present.

### EXAM

- A systolic thrill is heard.
- **Small to moderate-size defects:** A loud, grade II–IV/VI pansystolic murmur is heard that is maximal along the lower left sternal border. Occasionally, a mid-diastolic flow murmur is heard. P2 is not accentuated.
- **Large defects:** Right ventricular volume and pressure overload may → pulmonary hypertension, CHF, and cyanosis. A grade II–IV/VI pansystolic murmur is maximal at the lower left sternal border. P2 is usually accentuated.

### DIFFERENTIAL

Mitral regurgitation; mitral valve prolapse.

### DIAGNOSIS

- **ECG:** LVH and/or RVH if the shunt is reversed.
- **CXR:** ↑ pulmonary vascularity.
- **Echocardiography:** Doppler is diagnostic and can assess the magnitude of the shunt as well as pulmonary arterial pressure.
- **Cardiac CT and MRI:** Can visualize the defect and other anatomic abnormalities.
- **Cardiac catheterization:** Reserved for those with at least moderate shunting; can measure pulmonary vascular resistance and the degree of pulmonary hypertension.

### TREATMENT

- Small shunts do not require closure in asymptomatic patients
- Symptomatic children should be managed with hypercaloric feeds, diuretics, and ACEIs.
- If symptoms persist despite maximal medical therapy or if there is ↑ pulmonary vascular resistance (affects approximately 50% of patients), the defect should be surgically or percutaneously repaired. Surgery is contraindicated in Eisenmenger's syndrome.
- Children who do not have surgery should be followed to assess for spontaneous closure of the defect or for the development of complications.
- Because infections can worsen heart failure, all children > 6 months of age should receive the influenza vaccine, and all children < 2 years of age should receive RSV prophylaxis.
- Endocarditis occurs more often with smaller shunts; antibiotic prophylaxis is mandatory for all patients.

### COMPLICATIONS

Endocarditis; pulmonary hypertension/Eisenmenger's syndrome. Surgical mortality is 2–3% but ↑ to ≥ 50% if pulmonary hypertension is present.

---

A two-year-old girl from Mexico is brought to the ER after a spell of intractable crying and irritability. Her mother mentions that she has a heart problem and that whenever doctors examine her, they hear a loud murmur. Pulse oximetry reveals an $O_2$ saturation of 62%. On auscultation, you hear a 1/6 murmur in systole at the left upper sternal border. What is your therapeutic strategy? You recognize that this girl is likely having a hypercyanotic spell associated with tetralogy of Fallot. You bring her knees up to her chest and administer a single dose of IV morphine, and her saturations rapidly improve to 92%.

---

## Cyanotic Heart Disease

The most common causes of cyanotic heart disease in the newborn period are transposition of the great vessels, total anomalous pulmonary venous return, truncus arteriosus (some types), tricuspid atresia, and pulmonary atresia or

**Causes of cyanotic heart disease—**

**5 terrible T's**

**T**ransposition of the great vessels
**T**otal anomalous pulmonary venous return
**T**etralogy of Fallot
**T**runcus arteriosus
**T**ricuspid atresia

critical pulmonary stenosis. Infants with these disorders present with early cyanosis. The hallmark of many of these lesions is cyanosis in an infant without associated respiratory distress.

## SYMPTOMS/EXAM

Table 13.10 outlines the common causes of cyanotic heart disease along with their clinical presentation and treatment.

## DIAGNOSIS

Differentiate between cardiac and noncardiac causes:

- **Hyperoxia test:** Obtain an ABG; then place the patient on 100% $O_2$ for 10 minutes and perform a repeat ABG. If the cause of cyanosis is pulmonary, the $PaO_2$ should ↑ by 30 mmHg. If the cause is cardiac, there should be minimal improvement in $PaO_2$.

**TABLE 13.10.** Causes of Cyanotic Heart Disease

| | DEFINITION | SYMPTOMS/EXAM | TREATMENT |
|---|---|---|---|
| Tetralogy of Fallot | Includes VSD, pulmonary stenosis, overriding aorta, and RVH. | Cyanosis, dyspnea, loud pulmonary stenosis murmur; a VSD (holosystolic) murmur may also be heard. Variable degree of cyanosis depending on the amount of right-to-left shunting. | Surgical repair through placement of a transannular patch across the pulmonary valve. |
| Tricuspid atresia/ hypoplastic right heart | Complete or partial agenesis of the right ventricular cavity in which the left ventricle provides pulmonary blood flow through the ductus arteriosus. | Tachypnea, dyspnea, anoxic spells, and evidence of right heart failure; cyanosis; a grade II–VI harsh blowing murmur heard best at the lower left sternal border. | Anticongestive therapy. The Fontan procedure (connection of the systemic venous return to the pulmonary artery) is performed when increasing cyanosis occurs. |
| Transposition of the great vessels | Connection of the left ventricle to the pulmonary artery and the right ventricle to the aorta, causing the systemic and pulmonary circulations to operate in parallel. | Cyanosis; a single S2 and no murmur. | Early corrective surgery is recommended through an arterial switch operation of the great vessels. |
| Total anomalous pulmonary venous return | All pulmonary veins terminate in a systemic vein or the right atrium. | Tachypnea, feeding difficulties, and heart failure; widely fixed, split S2 and grade II–III/VI ejection-type systolic murmur. | Surgery is always required. |
| Truncus arteriosus | A single arterial trunk arises from the ventricles and divides into the aorta and pulmonary arteries. | Mild or no cyanosis, early CHF, systolic ejection click, wide pulse pressure. | Anticongestive treatment and surgical repair. |

- **CXR:** Vasculature on CXR provides information about pulmonary blood flow.
- **ECG:** Provides information about rhythm and, grossly, ventricular size. Examine both the axis and the magnitude of the deflections. Remember that right axis deviation is normal for a neonate.
- **Echocardiography:** The gold standard of diagnosis, as well as a noninvasive means of assessing the cardiac anatomy.

### TREATMENT

For cyanotic heart disease in which circulation is ductus dependant (requiring a patent ductus arteriosus), immediate treatment with prostaglandins, which delay closing of the ductus, may be lifesaving while the child is transported to a facility in which cardiac surgery may be undertaken.

A five-year-old boy presents to your clinic with a five- to six-day history of persistent high fever and irritability. Three days ago he was given antibiotics for presumed acute otitis media, but his fever did not resolve. On exam, he is found to have an erythematous rash, cracked lips, and a "strawberry tongue." He refuses to stand on both feet and cries with each attempt to walk. Both ear canals appear red, which you attribute to the child's excessive crying. Do you continue the course of antibiotics? Recognizing that this child has Kawasaki disease, you discontinue antibiotics and admit the boy to the hospital for appropriate therapy.

## Kawasaki Disease

Previously called mucocutaneous lymph node syndrome, Kawasaki disease is an acute febrile vasculitis of childhood involving small and medium-size arteries, with characteristic involvement of the coronary arteries. The cause is unclear, and no specific diagnostic test is available. Eighty percent of affected patients are < 5 years of age, and the male-to-female ratio is 1.5:1.

### SYMPTOMS/EXAM

The condition is defined by the presence of fever for > 5 days and at least four of the following features (see also Figure 13.12):

- Bilateral, painless, nonexudative conjunctivitis.
- Lip or oral cavity changes (e.g., lip cracking and fissuring, strawberry tongue, inflammation of the oral mucosa).
- Cervical lymphadenopathy (≥ 1.5 cm in diameter and usually unilateral).
- Polymorphous exanthema.
- Extremity changes (redness and swelling of the hands and feet with subsequent desquamation).

### DIFFERENTIAL

JRA, infectious mononucleosis, viral exanthems, leptospirosis, Rocky Mountain spotted fever, toxic shock syndrome, staphylococcal scalded-skin syndrome, erythema multiforme, serum sickness, SLE, Reiter's syndrome.

> *Diagnosis of Kawasaki disease—*
>
> **FEAR ME**
>
> **F**ever
> **E**ye—perilimbic sparing, conjunctival injection
> **A**denopathy—usually cervical
> **R**ash
> **M**outh—red lips
> **E**xtremities—red hands and feet

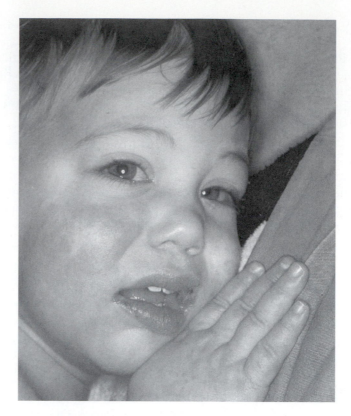

**FIGURE 13.12.  Kawasaki disease.**

Cherry-red lips with hemorrhagic fissures in a boy with prolonged high fever. This child also had a generalized morbilliform eruption, infected conjunctivae, and strawberry tongue (not shown). Note erythema and edema of the fingertips. (Reproduced, with permission, from Wolff K et al. *Fitzpatrick's Color Atlas & Synopsis of Clinical Dermatology*, 5th ed. New York: McGraw-Hill, 2005: 425.) (Also see Color Insert.)

### DIAGNOSIS

- Patients often have pyuria, transaminitis, normocytic anemia, and reactive thrombocytosis.
- Hyponatremia can be associated with an ↑ risk of cardiac complications.
- Echocardiography or angiography for coronary artery aneurysms.

### TREATMENT

- High-dose aspirin; IVIG.
- Warfarin for coronary artery aneurysms > 8 mm in diameter.
- Corticosteroids are controversial, as they may be associated with an ↑ incidence of aneurysms.

### COMPLICATIONS

- **Coronary artery lesions:** Range from mild transient dilation of a coronary artery to large aneurysm formation. Untreated patients have a 25% risk of developing an aneurysm of the coronary arteries. Those at greatest risk of aneurysm formation are males, young children (< 6 months), and those not treated with IVIG.
- **Other:** Also associated with myocarditis, pericarditis, and valvular heart disease (usually mitral or aortic regurgitation).

## Cystic Fibrosis (CF)

The most common lethal genetic disease in the United States, with an incidence of 1 in 3000 to 1 in 4000 among Caucasians, CF is a major cause of pulmonary and GI morbidity in children and is a leading cause of death in early adulthood. It is characterized by abnormalities in the hepatic, GI, and male reproductive systems. The most common mutation is the **delta F508**, a deletion of three base pairs at position 508 in the gene. These gene mutations → defects or deficiencies that cause cells to produce abnormally thick mucus. Life expectancy has ↑ from four years to 35 years owing to advances in therapy.

### SYMPTOMS/EXAM

- **GI:**
  - Abdominal distention and discomfort; bulky, greasy stools; ↑ flatulence 2° to exocrine pancreatic insufficiency and malabsorption.
  - Meconium ileus (15%) at birth.
  - Intestinal obstruction (meconium in the terminal ilium).
  - Hypoalbuminemia, anemia, edema, and hepatomegaly.
  - FTT (50%).
- **Pulmonary:**
  - Cough, tachypnea, rales, wheezing, clubbing, difficulty breathing, ↑ sputum production, ↓ exercise tolerance.
  - RSV infections (associated with added morbidity in early infancy).
  - Hemoptysis due to bronchiectasis; cor pulmonale.

### DIFFERENTIAL

Foreign body, carcinoma, broncholith, pneumonia, sinusitis, COPD, asthma, $\alpha_1$-antitrypsin deficiency, bronchiolitis, celiac sprue.

### DIAGNOSIS

- PFTs show an obstructive pattern.
- Lungs are colonized with *S. aureus* or *Pseudomonas*.
- CXR findings are consistent with bronchiectasis.
- Sweat chloride levels are > 60 mmol/L.
- Mutated CFTR gene (most labs test for the 20–30 most common defects).
- Newborn screen for elevated blood levels of immunoreactive trypsin.
- Pulmonary (recurrent respiratory infections), GI (meconium ileus, FTT), or hepatic dysfunction.

### TREATMENT

- **General:** Attention to nutritional status and psychosocial situation.
- **GI symptoms:** Pancreatic enzyme supplementation; cathartics and enemas for obstructive symptoms.
- **Pulmonary symptoms:**
  - Airway clearance therapy and aggressive antibiotic use.
  - Inhaled recombinant human DNase (Pulmozyme) and inhaled tobramycin.
  - Bronchodilators and anti-inflammatory therapies.
  - Corticosteroids (adverse effects include glucose intolerance, frank diabetes, and ↓ linear growth)
  - Lung transplant for end-stage disease.

---

*Presentation of cystic fibrosis—*

**CF PANCREAS**

**C**hronic cough and wheezing
**F**ailure to thrive
**P**ancreatic insufficiency (symptoms of malabsorption such as steatorrhea)
**A**lkalosis and hypotonic dehydration
**N**eonatal intestinal obstruction (meconium ileus)/**N**asal polyps
**C**lubbing of fingers/**C**hest radiograph with characteristic changes
**R**ectal prolapse
**E**lectrolyte elevation in sweat; salty skin
**A**bsence or congenital atresia of the vas deferens
**S**putum with *Staphylococcus* or *Pseudomonas* (mucoid)

---

### COMPLICATIONS

- Intussusception.
- Liver cirrhosis, portal hypertension, esophageal varices, GI bleed, hypersplenism.
- Infertility in > 95% of males (due to lack of development of the vas deferens).
- Spontaneous pneumothorax and hemoptysis.
- Progressive pulmonary disease (the cause of death in 95% of cases).

## Bronchopulmonary Dysplasia (BPD)

Defined as acute respiratory distress in the first week of life, BPD remains one of the most significant sequelae of acute respiratory distress in the NICU, with an incidence of about 30% for infants with a birth weight of < 1000 g. BPD represents the consequences of lung injury caused by $O_2$ toxicity, barotrauma, and inflammation superimposed on a susceptible, generally immature lung. Although neonates with BPD have an ↑ risk of mortality, most survivors have normalization of their lung function in early childhood.

### SYMPTOMS/EXAM

- Patients present with dyspnea, wheezing, tachypnea, cyanosis, and hypoxia.
- Exam reveals hypoxia with ↑ $O_2$ requirement.

### DIFFERENTIAL

Meconium aspiration syndrome, persistent pulmonary hypertension, congenital infection (e.g., CMV), cystic adenomatoid malformation, recurrent aspiration, congenital heart disease, overhydration, idiopathic pulmonary fibrosis.

### TREATMENT

- Inhaled corticosteroids together with occasional use of β-adrenergic agonists.
- Chest physiotherapy is used for the thick secretions that may contribute to airway obstruction or recurrent atelectasis.
- Fluid restriction with attention to adequate nutrition.
- Diuretics as needed.
- RSV prophylaxis.
- Comprehensive interdisciplinary planning on discharge to ensure adequate follow-up.

### COMPLICATIONS

Pulmonary hypertension, recurrent respiratory infections, cor pulmonale, exercise intolerance, ↑ risk for COPD, neurodevelopmental problems.

## HEMATOLOGY/ONCOLOGY

## Rhabdomyosarcoma

The most common soft tissue sarcoma occurring in childhood; can occur anywhere in the body. Accounts for 10% of solid tumors in childhood. The peak incidence is at 2–5 years of age; 70% of children are diagnosed before age 10. A second, smaller peak is seen in adolescents with extremity tumors. Males are affected more often than females.

### SYMPTOMS/EXAM

- Presenting symptoms and signs of rhabdomyosarcoma result from disturbances of normal body function due to tumor growth.
- Presents with a painless, progressively enlarging mass.
- Orbital invasion may cause proptosis; mucosal invasion may cause chronic drainage (nasal, aural, sinus, vaginal). Cranial nerve palsies are also seen.
- Bowel or bladder invasion may cause urinary obstruction, constipation, and hematuria.

### DIAGNOSIS

- Biopsy of the mass.
- When rhabdomyosarcoma imitates striated muscle and cross-striations are seen on light microscopy, the diagnosis is straightforward. Immunohistochemistry, electron microscopy, or chromosomal analysis is sometimes necessary to make the diagnosis.
- A plain radiograph and a CT or MRI can determine the extent of the 1° tumor and assess regional lymph nodes.
- A lung CT can rule out pulmonary metastasis, the most common site of metastatic disease at diagnosis.
- A skeletal survey and a bone scan are obtained to rule out bony metastases.

### TREATMENT

- Combined-modality therapy.
- Tumors should be excised if possible.
- Chemotherapy and radiation are appropriate for all patients and can shrink large tumors before surgery is attempted.

## Wilms' Tumor

A tumor of the kidney consisting of a variety of embryonic tissues, such as abortive tubules and glomeruli, smooth and skeletal muscle fibers, spindle cells, cartilage, and bone. Seventy-five percent of children affected are < 5 years of age; the peak incidence is at 2–3 years of age. The constellation of Wilms' tumor, aniridia, GU anomalies, and mental retardation (WAGR syndrome) is associated with deletion of 11p13.

*Most children with Wilms' tumor present with an increasingly large abdomen or with an asymptomatic abdominal mass incidentally discovered by a parent.*

### SYMPTOMS/EXAM

- Presents with abdominal enlargement with or without pain, hematuria, malaise, weakness, anorexia, weight loss, and fever.
- Hypertension is noted in more than half of patients.
- An abdominal mass, palpable in almost all cases, can be large, firm, and smooth and does not ordinarily extend across the midline.

### DIFFERENTIAL

Abdominal masses, including hydronephrosis, multicystic or duplicated kidneys, neuroblastoma, teratoma, hepatoma, and rhabdomyosarcoma.

### DIAGNOSIS

- Abdominal ultrasound to assess for venous invasion.
- CT is required to determine the extent of the mass as well as to assess for bilateral disease, venous invasion, and metastases.

### TREATMENT

- Surgical excision to completely remove the tumor (nephrectomy) and ureter.
- Very large tumors may be treated preoperatively with radiation therapy and chemotherapy to ↓ their size.
- Metastatic foci in the lung or liver may be resected or treated with radiation therapy.
- Overall survival is 85%.

## Liver Neoplasms

Uncommon in childhood, accounting for 2% of all pediatric malignancies. More than 70% of pediatric liver masses are malignant. The majority of hepatic malignancies are of epithelial origin, while most benign lesions are vascular in nature.

### HEPATOBLASTOMA

Hepatoblastoma accounts for nearly 50% of all liver masses in children and approximately two-thirds of malignant tumors, and it is the most common asymptomatic abdominal mass seen in healthy-appearing children. Most masses are seen in children < 4 years of age, and two-thirds are noted in children < 2 years of age. Beckwith-Wiedemann syndrome, fetal alcohol syndrome, and parenteral nutrition administration in infancy all ↑ the risk.

### SYMPTOMS/EXAM

- Presents with obstructive GI symptoms 2° to compression of the stomach or duodenum or with acute pain 2° to hemorrhage into the tumor.
- Advanced tumors present with weight loss, ascites, and FTT.
- Exam reveals a nontender, firm mass in the RUQ or midline that moves with respiration.

### DIFFERENTIAL

Hepatic adenoma, focal nodular hyperplasia (nonencapsulated nodular liver mass), mesenchymal hamartoma.

### DIAGNOSIS

- Tissue biopsy.
- **Labs:** Reveal nonspecifically elevated LFTs and mild anemia. Thrombocytosis is also seen, and AFP is significantly ↑ in 90–95% of cases.
- **Imaging:** Abdominal CT with IV contrast is useful both for diagnosis and for planning therapy. The typical CT appearance is that of a solid solitary mass with lower attenuation levels than those of the surrounding liver.

### TREATMENT

- Complete surgical resection.
- Lobectomy or extended lobectomy (trisegmentectomy).
- Chemotherapy.
- The overall survival rate for all children with hepatoblastoma is approximately 50%.

## HEPATOCELLULAR CARCINOMA

Less common than hepatoblastoma, typically presenting in older children and adolescents (median age 10 years). Associated with preexisting chronic hepatitis, cirrhosis due to HBV, and other causes of childhood cirrhosis (tyrosinemia, biliary cirrhosis, $\alpha_1$-antitrypsin deficiency, type 1 glycogen storage disease, long-term parenteral nutrition). Table 13.11 contrasts the clinical presentation of hepatocellular carcinoma with that of hepatoblastoma.

### SYMPTOMS/EXAM

- Presents with abdominal pain, weight loss, anorexia, and jaundice.
- Exam reveals an abdominal mass or diffuse abdominal swelling.

### DIAGNOSIS

- Biopsy.
- **Labs:** Serum AFP level is ↑ in 50% of patients.
- **Imaging:** Abdominal CT.

### TREATMENT

- As a result of multicentricity, bilobar involvement, portal vein invasion, and lymphatic metastases, only 15–20% of hepatocellular carcinomas are resectable.
- Overall long-term survival is poor (15%) even for resectable disease.

## LIVER HEMANGIOMA

The most common benign pediatric hepatic lesion. Tumors may be solitary (cavernous hemangioma) or multiple (infantile hemangioendothelioma) and

**TABLE 13.11.  Hepatoblastoma vs. Hepatocellular Carcinoma**

|  | HEPATOBLASTOMA | HEPATOCELLULAR CARCINOMA |
|---|---|---|
| **Median age at presentation** | 1 year (0–3 years) | 12 years (5–18 years) |
| **Male-to-female ratio** | 1.7:1 | 1.4:1 |
| **Pathologic features** | Fetal or embryonal cells; mesenchymal component (30%) | Large pleomorphic tumor cells and tumor giant cells |
| **Solitary hepatic lesion** | 80% | 20–50% |
| **Unique features at diagnosis** | Osteopenia (20–30%), isosexual precocity (3%) | Hemoperitoneum, polycythemia |
| **Laboratory features:** |  |  |
| Hyperbilirubinemia | 5% | 25% |
| Elevated AFP | 90% | 50% |
| Abnormal LFTs | 15–30% | 30–50% |

Adapted, with permission, from Hay WW et al. *Current Diagnosis & Treatment in Pediatrics,* 18th ed. New York: McGraw-Hill, 2007: 910.

involve the bulk of the liver. Isolated cavernous hemangiomas are not often associated with cutaneous hemangiomas, whereas infantile hemangioendotheliomas are commonly associated with hemangiomas in other parts of the body.

*Hemangiomas are the most common benign liver tumors and are often asymptomatic vascular lesions.*

### SYMPTOMS/EXAM

- **Solitary hemangioma:** Frequently asymptomatic or presents with a mass.
- **Hemangioendothelioma:** Commonly presents with massive hepatomegaly and high-output cardiac failure.

### DIAGNOSIS

- RBC-labeled radionuclide scan, abdominal CT.
- Percutaneous biopsy is contraindicated.

### TREATMENT

- No treatment is necessary in an asymptomatic child.
- Patients with CHF or thrombocytopenia are treated with corticosteroids, digoxin, and diuretics.
- Indications for surgery include ruptured lesions with hemorrhage, masses with uncertain diagnoses, symptomatic lesions, and disease limited to one lobe.

## Neuroblastoma

The third most common pediatric malignancy, accounting for approximately 10% of all childhood cancers. Overall survival is < 30%. More than 80% of cases present before the age of four, and the peak incidence is at two years of age. Neuroblastomas arise from the neural crest cells and show different levels of differentiation. The tumor most frequently originates in the adrenal glands, posterior mediastinum, neck, or pelvis but can arise in any sympathetic ganglion.

*Neuroblastoma is an extremely malignant neoplasm. Most patients do not present with symptoms of the 1° lesion but with complications of metastatic disease.*

### SYMPTOMS/EXAM

- Can present with an asymptomatic abdominal mass or with pain from the tumor mass.
- Bone pain results from metastases.
- Tumor can invade the spinal cord → muscle weakness or sensory changes.
- The majority of patients already show signs of metastatic disease at presentation.
- The tumor/abdominal mass may cross the midline.

### DIAGNOSIS

The minimum criterion for diagnosis is based on one of the following findings:

- An unequivocal pathologic diagnosis made from tumor tissue examined by light microscopy with or without immunohistology, electron microscopy, or ↑ levels of serum catecholamines or urinary catecholamine metabolites.
- A combination of bone marrow aspirate or biopsy containing unequivocal tumor cells and ↑ levels of serum catecholamines or urinary catecholamine metabolites.

### TREATMENT

- Preoperative chemotherapy.
- Complete surgical resection of tumor.

# ADOLESCENT MEDICINE

## Normal Growth and Development

Adolescents often feel uncomfortable, clumsy, and self-conscious by virtue of the rapid changes taking place in their bodies. They must adapt to a new physical identity that includes hormonal changes, menstruation, unpredictable spontaneous erections, nocturnal ejaculations ("wet dreams"), growth of pubic and axillary hair, and even the odors from maturing apocrine glands, which necessitate deodorant use. Stages of normal growth and development are as follows (see also Table 13.12):

- **Early adolescence:** Occurs between 11 and 13 years of age and merges with midadolescence at 14–15 years.
- **Midadolescence:** Begins around 14–15 years of age and blends into late adolescence at about 17 years.
- **Late adolescence:** Begins at approximately 17–21 years of age. The upper end is particularly variable and is dependent on cultural, economic, and educational factors.

## Tanner Staging

Describes the development of pubic hair and breasts for girls and pubic hair and genitalia for boys. Progression through the five stages is predictable. Lack of this predictable progression can be an indication of a pubertal disorder and may require further examination and possible referral to an endocrinologist. Stages are as follows:

- **Tanner staging for males:**
  - **Stage 1:** Onset of physical development between 9 and 13 years of age.
  - **Stages 3 and 4:** Peak height velocity, with an average height gain of 5–7 inches. First ejaculations typically occur during stage 3.
  - **Stages 4 and 5:** Strength peaks.
- **Tanner staging for females:**
  - **Stage 1:** Prepubertal; onset between 8 and 13 years of age.
  - **Stage 2:** Growth spurt with an average height gain of 4 inches. Development of breast buds.
  - **Stages 3:** Continued breast development; acne is common.
  - **Stage 4:** Menarche average age 12. Two-mound breast development.
  - **Stage 5:** Adult breast contour.

**TABLE 13.12.    Stages of Adolescence**

|  | EARLY ADOLESCENCE | MIDADOLESCENCE | LATE ADOLESCENCE |
|---|---|---|---|
| Characteristics | 2° sexual characteristics have begun to appear. | 2° sexual characteristics are well advanced. | Physically mature; statural and reproductive growth are virtually complete. |
| Growth | Growth rapidly accelerating; reaches peak velocity. | Growth decelerating; stature reaches 95% of adult height. |  |

## Cognitive/Psychosocial Development

Table 13.13 outlines milestones in adolescents' nonphysical development.

**TABLE 13.13.    Cognitive and Psychosocial Milestones of Adolescence**

| CHARACTERISTICS | EARLY ADOLESCENCE (11–13) | MIDADOLESCENCE (14–15) | LATE ADOLESCENCE (17–21) |
|---|---|---|---|
| Cognition | Concrete thought dominant. | Rapidly gaining competence in abstract thought. | Established abstract thought processes. |
| | Existential orientation; often narcissistic with focus on self and bodily changes. | Capable of perceiving future implications of current acts and decisions but variably applied. | Future oriented. |
| | Cannot perceive long-range implications of current decisions and acts. | Reverts to concrete operations under stress. | Capable of perceiving and acting on long-range options. |
| Psychosocial self | Preoccupation with rapid body change. | Reestablishes body images as growth decelerates and stabilizes. | Emancipation or individuation completed. |
| | Former body image disrupted. | Preoccupation with fantasy and idealism in exploring expanded cognition and future options. | Intellectual and functional identity established. |
| | | Development of a sense of omnipotence and invincibility. | May experience "crisis of 21" when facing societal demands for autonomy. |
| Family | Defining independence-dependence boundaries. | Major conflicts over control may occur. | Transposition of child-parent dependency relationship to the adult-adult model. |
| | No major conflicts over parental control. | Struggle for emancipation. | |
| Peer group | Seeks peer affiliation to counter instability generated by rapid change. | Strong need for identification to affirm self-image. | Recedes in importance in favor of individual friendships. |
| | Compares own normality and acceptance with same sex/age mates. | Looks to peer group to define behavioral code during emancipation process. | |
| Sexuality | Self-exploration and evaluation. Limited dating. | Multiple plural relationships. Heightened sexual activity. | Forms stable relationships. |
| | | | Capable of mutuality and reciprocity in caring for another rather than former narcissistic orientation. |
| | Limited intimacy. | Testing ability to attract sexual partners and parameters of masculinity or femininity. | Plans for future in thinking of partners, long-term relationships, family. Sexual identity secured. |
| | | Preoccupation with romantic fantasy. | Intimacy involves commitment rather than exploration and romanticism. |

## Routine Screening

Guidelines for routine screening of adolescents are as follows:

- **All adolescents:**
  - Measure BP.
  - Conduct subjective hearing tests at every well-child visit; conduct objective tests at 8, 10, 12, 15 and 18 years.
  - Visual acuity—conduct a Snellen test.
  - Calculate BMI.
- **High-risk or symptomatic adolescents:** TB, anemia, visual screening, cholesterol.

## Laboratory Tests

Often not necessary in the asymptomatic teenager, screening laboratory tests should be kept to a minimum.

- General guidelines:
  - **Hemoglobin or hematocrit:** Anemia screening is recommended at the first encounter or at the end of puberty.
  - **UA:** Obtain at the first encounter or at the end of puberty.
  - **Sickle cell screening:** Obtain at the first visit with African-American adolescents.
  - **Cholesterol and fasting triglyceride testing:** Indicated in teens with heart disease, hypertension, and DM (or a strong family history of hyperlipidemia).
- Sexually active adolescents:
  - **Females:** Patients should receive a Pap smear after three years of first sexual intercourse or by age 21. Frequent gonorrhea/chlamydia testing (every 6–12 months) is recommended in high-risk youth, as are syphilis testing and a vaginal wet mount.
  - **Males:** Gonorrhea, chlamydia, annual syphilis serology.
  - **Males who have sex with males:** Annual syphilis, gonorrhea, chlamydia, and HBV screening.

## Immunizations

- **Diphtheria, tetanus:** A booster of tetanus toxoid, reduced diphtheria toxoid, and acellular pertussis (Tdap) is recommended 10 years after the initial series.
- **Meningococcal conjugate vaccine:** Administer to unvaccinated adolescents at high school entry (15 years of age). All college freshmen living in dormitories should be vaccinated as well.
- **Influenza vaccine:** Recommended for adolescents with certain risk factors that can compromise respiratory function or handling of respiratory secretions.
- **Hepatitis A and B:** Administer if vaccines were not received during childhood.
- **Pneumococcal vaccine:** Indicated in adolescents with chronic illnesses (sickle cell disease, HIV, asplenia, B-cell immune deficiency) and, in particular, to those with cardiovascular or pulmonary disease.
- **HPV vaccine:** Provisional recommendations are that all females 11–12 years of age should receive the three-dose series.

## HEADSS Assessment

Adolescence is generally a period of extremely good physiologic health and well-being. Underlying psychosocial issues may thus have more significance than physical problems in patients within this age group. The areas of sex, school performance, family, peer group, identity, and future should all be explored. The **HEADSS** assessment provides a systematic approach to addressing these issues.

## Safety

Injuries are the most significant health problem of adolescents. A strong need for peer approval and lack of ability to appreciate consequences may lead youths to participate in a variety of risk-taking behaviors. Providing safety guidelines for teens is thus crucial in decreasing mortality from high-risk behavior. Guidelines are as follows (see also the mnemonic **SAFE TEENS**):

- **Motor vehicle safety:** Focus on the roles of driver, passenger, and pedestrian as well as on the influence of substance abuse and the importance of using seat belts.
- **Sexual activity:** Offer education regarding contraception, teen pregnancy, STI, unwanted intercourse, sexual readiness, sexual abuse, and sex with older partners.
- **Recreational athletic activities:** Counsel with regard to the use of adequate equipment, protective gear and clothing, helmets, safe facilities, proper rules of safe play, and rational approaches toward activities requiring advanced skill levels.
- **Substance use:** Instruct patients of the potential dangers (including sudden death) that may occur not only with regular substance abuse but also with experimental use of drugs and alcohol. Include a discussion of nicotine and steroids.
- **Firearms:** Adolescents with firearms in the home need to learn proper use, safety, and legal issues associated with guns.

## Anticipatory Guidance

Adolescents should receive health guidance annually, but information shared with them should be kept confidential. Recommendations for health guidance are designed to help adolescents approach development with greater knowledge and understanding, particularly as they develop cognitively and psychologically. Goals of anticipatory guidance should include the following:

- To promote a better understanding of physical growth, psychosocial and psychosexual development, and the importance of becoming actively involved in health care decisions.
- To promote the reduction of injuries, wearing helmets, use of seat belts, and sunscreen use.
- To provide information regarding dietary habits, the benefits of a healthy diet, and ways to achieve a healthy diet and safe weight management.
- To provide information about the benefits of physical activity.
- To offer information regarding responsible sexual behaviors.
- To promote avoidance of illicit substances.

## Consent and Confidentiality

Adolescents may fail to seek or delay seeking health care for a number of reasons. In addition to lack of access, finances, and awareness of clinical services, they may have concerns about confidentiality. Adolescents are more likely to seek care about sensitive issues if they feel that the health provider will not disclose that information to their parents. Laws about confidentiality vary from state to state.

- Mature minors have a right to give informed consent to health care. Laws deal with circumstances in which minors are not required to have parental consent (reproductive health care, treatment of STIs, rape or incest, health-risk behaviors, and emergency health care).
- Other laws are based on emancipation status, such as whether a minor is a parent, is or has been married, lives away from home, is in the armed forces, is a high school graduate, or is mature as determined by age.
- In most states age of maturity is considered to be 18, although in a few states it is younger (14 in Alabama, 15 in Oregon, and 16 in South Carolina except for surgery). In Nebraska the age of consent is 19.

Issues of confidentiality and consent are best managed in the context of a long-term physician-family relationship. Consent and confidentiality issues do not bind the physician to provide care that may violate the physician's own moral code. Teens should be aware of the physician's legal responsibility to report situations in which patients are at risk for suicide or homicide or are victims of sexual or physical abuse.

## SEXUALITY

Adolescence is a time of significant physical and emotional turmoil. At the same time, differing family values, cultural values, and personal experiences may give rise to varying sex education needs, which may include understanding body functions, exploring personal values, and setting sexual limits with partners. However, parents as well as many clinicians may be ill prepared to discuss sex-related health issues with adolescents. Additionally, teens may be uncomfortable discussing sexual issues with their peers and with adults. At the same time, a lack of comprehensive sex education programs as well as differences in cognitive and physical maturity put adolescents at ↑ risk for unwanted or unhealthy consequences of sexual activity.

### Sexual Development

Table 13.14 outlines the stages of sexual development by time period.

#### TREATMENT

- Provide information to parents and adolescents, both together and separately. Emphasize the healthy expression of sexuality.
- Issues to discuss include timing of the initiation of sexual activity, abstinence resources (sex education, family planning clinics, professional education), contraception, education on STIs, and violence prevention.
- Discuss the use of latex condoms to prevent STIs, including HIV infection.

#### COMPLICATIONS

Teen pregnancy, STIs, unwanted sexual experiences such as sexual abuse or exploitation.

**TABLE 13.14.** Stages of Sexual Development in Adolescence

| STAGE | CHARACTERISTICS |
| --- | --- |
| Preadolescence | Low investment in sexuality. |
| | Information with regard to sexuality comes from friends, school, and family. |
| | Physical appearance is prepubertal. |
| Early adolescence | Physical maturation begins. |
| | Curiosity with regard to one's own body persists. |
| | Sexual fantasies are common. |
| | Masturbation begins. |
| | Sexual activities are often nonphysical (e.g., phone calls, e-mail). |
| Late adolescence | Full physical maturation. |
| | Sexual behavior and thoughts are more expressive. |
| | Intimate physical and sharing relationships may develop. |
| | Sexual behavior can include masturbation, petting, oral sex, anal intercourse, and vaginal intercourse. |

## COMMON MEDICAL PROBLEMS

### Abdominal Pain

*Functional pain is most often the cause of recurrent abdominal pain in teen girls.*

A common primary care problem, especially among females, that is most often benign but can be related to serious diagnoses. Functional pain is the most common recurrent form of pain. Generally a diagnosis of exclusion, it is defined as nonorganic pain related to everyday stress. School, peer, and family problems are commonly associated stressors. Abdominal pain can be related to school absenteeism and may be a sign of depression. Organic etiologies are varied but include the following:

- **GI/GU conditions:** Appendicitis, IBD, PUD, GI infections, lactose intolerance, bowel obstruction, biliary tract obstruction/gallstones, kidney stones, pancreatitis, testicular torsion.
- **Gynecologic conditions:** PID, ectopic pregnancy, endometriosis, torsion or ruptured ovarian cyst.
- **Musculoskeletal pain:** Costochondritis, abdominal wall muscle strain.
- **Systemic conditions:** DKA, sickle cell crisis, lead intoxication, porphyria.

#### SYMPTOMS

Symptoms of functional abdominal pain include the following:

- Crampy and dull pain located in the periumbilical area.
- May be accompanied by nausea and vomiting, headache, fatigue, dizziness, or diarrhea.

#### EXAM

- Obtain a thorough history, including information on home, school, sexual behaviors, menstrual history, trauma, and substance use.
- Abdominal exam; pelvic and speculum exam when indicated.

- Functional abdominal pain presents with normal findings on exam or with mild midepigastric tenderness without rebound.

### DIAGNOSIS

- Based on a guided history.
- Order a CBC, a chemistry profile with LFTs, ESR, UA, urine hCG, stool studies, and plain films of the abdomen.
- Functional pain is likely when serious diagnoses have been ruled out.

### TREATMENT

- Treat the underlying cause when it has been identified.
- For functional abdominal pain, offer counseling for stress reduction, and encourage dietary changes for normal bowel movements.

## Chest Pain

A common complaint among adolescents, but rarely a sign of a serious problem. As many as 650,000 cases of chest pain occur each year in patients 10–21 years of age. The most common causes in teens are idiopathic factors, anxiety, and musculoskeletal problems (e.g., costochondritis). Other etiologies include the following:

*Cardiac disease is a rare cause of chest pain, but if misdiagnosed it may be life-threatening. The most common cause of chest pain (30% of children) is inflammation of musculoskeletal structures of the chest wall.*

- **Cardiac chest pain:**
    - MI rarely occurs in healthy children. Youth with underlying illnesses such as DM, chronic anemia, or an anomalous left coronary artery may be at ↑ risk for ischemia.
    - **Arrhythmias:** Supraventricular tachycardia, atrial flutter/fibrillation, premature ventricular contractions.
    - **Structural lesions that cause chest pain:** Aortic stenosis, pulmonary stenosis, mitral valve prolapse.
    - **Other:** Dilated cardiomyopathy, hypertrophic obstructive cardiomyopathy, myocarditis, rheumatic fever, aortic dissection, pericarditis.
- **Noncardiac chest pain:**
    - **Respiratory:** May be due to illness, reactive airway disease, pneumonia, pneumothorax, or pulmonary embolism.
    - **GI:** Reflux, esophagitis, foreign body.

### SYMPTOMS

Presentation varies depending on the type of chest pain.

- **Musculoskeletal:** Reproducible pain with palpation.
- **Respiratory:** Pain with inspiration.
- **Cardiac:** Dull, aching pain.

### EXAM

- **History:**
    - Obtain a detailed past medical history. Inquire about Kawasaki disease, since such patients are at risk for cardiac sequelae (MI 2° to thrombosis of coronary aneurysms, cardiac arrhythmias, or sudden death).
    - Obtain a social history to identify psychosocial stressors and cigarette smoke exposure.

- The duration, location, intensity, frequency, and radiation of the pain should be documented, and possible triggering events preceding the pain should be explored.
- **Respiratory exam:** Wheezing and diminished breath sounds may suggest a pulmonary cause.
- **Cardiac exam:** Focus on heart sounds, murmurs, and rate.
- **Musculoskeletal exam:** Reproducible pain suggests a muscular origin or recent trauma.

### DIAGNOSIS

- Rarely is there a need for laboratory tests or further evaluation by a specialist.
- Chest pain following exertion may warrant a more elaborate evaluation for a cardiac disorder.
- If a cardiac origin is suspected, a pediatric cardiologist should be consulted. $\oplus$ cardiac findings on initial evaluation should be followed with ECG, CXR, echocardiogram, Holter monitor, serum troponin, and CK assays.
- If the timing of the pain is in relation to meals, it may point to a GI cause.
- CXR and pulse oximetry if clues suggest a respiratory cause.

### TREATMENT

Guided by underlying disorders.

- **Cardiac:** Patients with known heart disease or chest pain with exertion, syncope, or palpitations should be referred to a cardiologist.
- **Musculoskeletal:** NSAIDs, rest.
- **GI (dyspepsia, GERD):** Dietary modifications; $H_2$ blockers if indicated.
- **Pulmonary:** Treat the underlying disorder; refer to a pulmonologist if indicated.

*Persistent headaches in teens may be 2° to stress, anxiety, and depression.*

## Headaches

A common problem in adolescents, accounting for numerous office visits and lost days of school. Recurrent headaches are generally not associated with severe intracranial pathology but are more often 2° to stress, anxiety, and depression. Chronic headaches can also be related to migraine or tension. The single acute headache in an adolescent without a prior headache history may be due to CNS or systemic disease

### SYMPTOMS/EXAM

- **Tension headache:** Presents with a bandlike throbbing pain that worsens with stress at the end of the day. Can be associated with TMJ syndrome.
- **Migraine:** Aura or sensory disturbances, photophobia, and phonophobia. Lateralized pain is common.
- **Cluster headache:** Tends to occur at the same time each day or night. Lateralized pain is common, as is ocular pain. Horner's syndrome may occur ipsilaterally during an attack.
- **Pseudotumor cerebri** (benign intracranial hypertension): Presents with papilledema, dull pain, and visual obscuration (transient dimming or loss of vision with straining); associated with excessive vitamin A or D intake.
- **Depressive headaches:** "All day all the time; no relief." Associated with excessive disability (school absenteeism, social isolation).

- **Intracranial mass–related headache:** Characterized by dull or steady pain that is worse in the morning.

### DIFFERENTIAL

Severe hypertension, otitis media, acute periodontal disease, head injury, carbon monoxide poisoning, meningitis; withdrawal from caffeine, alcohol, or drugs; depression.

### DIAGNOSIS

- Identify onset, pattern, chronology, precipitants of specific episodes (stress, foods, medications, drugs), substance abuse, and depressive mood disorders.
- Determine precipitating factors, such as recent sinusitis, dental surgery, and head injury.
- CSF examination if a meningeal infection is suspected.
- Cranial MRI or CT to exclude an intracranial mass in patients with a progressive headache disorder, symptoms of SAH, headaches that disturb sleep or are related to exertion, and headaches associated with neurologic symptoms.

### TREATMENT

- **Recurrent headaches:** Encourage a headache diary in which diet, stressors, substance use, and sleep patterns are noted.
- **Tension headache:** Massage, NSAIDs, acetaminophen.
- **Migraine headaches:** NSAIDs, acetaminophen, antiemetics, ergotamines, triptans. Prophylaxis with β-blockers, TCAs, and calcium channel blockers.

### COMPLICATIONS

School absenteeism; functional limitations (sports, social activities).

## Acne Vulgaris

An inflammatory disease of the pilosebaceous unit (sebaceous glands and their associated small hairs) that often begins during puberty and is typically caused by blockage of the pilosebaceous unit with sebum and desquamated cells. Exacerbating factors include genetic factors, androgens, stress, excessive friction on the skin, cosmetics, and medications (including OCPs).

*Open and closed comedones are the hallmark of acne vulgaris.*

### SYMPTOMS/EXAM

- Presents with redness, dry skin, pruritus, and nodules (see Figure 13.13).
- Lesions occur mainly over the face, neck, upper chest, back, and shoulders and may take the form of open comedones (blackheads), closed comedones (whiteheads), papules, pustules, nodules, or cysts.

### DIFFERENTIAL

Acne rosacea, tinea, eosinophilic folliculitis, miliaria (heat rash), pseudofolliculitis barbae (ingrown beard hairs), bacterial folliculitis.

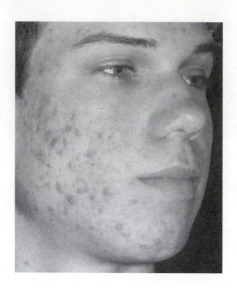

**FIGURE 13.13. Acne vulgaris.**

A spectrum of lesions is seen: comedones, papules, pustules, and erythematous macules and scars at site of resolving lesions. (Reproduced, with permission, from Wollf K et al. *Fitzpatrick's Color Atlas & Synopsis of Clinical Dermatology*, 5th ed. New York: McGraw-Hill, 2005: 5.)

### TREATMENT

- **Comedonal acne:** Benzoyl peroxide; topical retinoids (tretinoin, adapalene, tazarotene).
- **Papular inflammatory acne:** Topical or oral antibiotics are the mainstay of treatment.
    - **Mild acne:** Treat with a combination of erythromycin or clindamycin with benzoyl peroxide topical gel. Tretinoin used at night enhances the efficacy of treatment.
    - **Moderate acne:**
        - Tetracycline, erythromycin, doxycycline, and minocycline 50–100 mg BID. Tetracycline, minocycline, and doxycycline are contraindicated in pregnancy.
        - OCPs or spironolactone may be added as an antiandrogen in women with antibiotic-resistant acne.
    - **Severe cystic acne:**
        - Isotretinoin (Accutane), a vitamin A analog, should be used before significant scarring occurs or if symptoms are not promptly controlled by antibiotics.
        - The drug is teratogenic and must not be used in pregnancy; in females, check two serum pregnancy tests before starting the drug and every month thereafter. Two forms of effective contraception must be used during treatment.
        - Side effects of dry skin and mucous membranes occur in most patients; at higher dosages, an ↑ in cholesterol and triglycerides and a ↓ in HDL can occur. Minor elevations of LFTs and fasting blood sugar may also be seen, and moderate to severe myalgias necessitate decreasing the dosage or stopping the drug.

### COMPLICATIONS

- Severe scarring, cyst formation, hypo-/hyperpigmentation.
- Social concerns with regard to physical appearance/self-image.

# Obesity

Excess adipose tissue → a BMI > 30. Upper body obesity (obesity of the abdomen and flank) is of greater health consequence than lower body obesity (affecting the buttocks and thighs). Physical inactivity has played a major role in the staggering rise of obesity among children and adolescents. During adolescence, levels of spontaneous physical activity ↓ precipitously from childhood levels. Obesity is associated with a significant ↑ in morbidity and mortality.

### SYMPTOMS/EXAM

Fatigue; sedentary lifestyle; poor nutritional status; excessive overeating.

### DIFFERENTIAL

- ↑ caloric intake.
- **Fluid retention:** Nephrotic syndrome, heart failure.
- **Hormonal abnormalities:** Cushing's disease, hypothyroidism.

### DIAGNOSIS

- Determine BMI.
- Measure abdominal circumference (waist/hip ratio).
- Obtain TSH level.
- Assess for medical consequences and metabolic syndrome by measuring BP and fasting glucose, cholesterol, and triglyceride levels.
- Food diary.

### TREATMENT

- A multidisciplinary approach consisting of ↓ caloric intake, behavior modification, aerobic exercise, and social support is most effective.
- **Medications:** Orlistat ↓ fat absorption in the GI tract by inhibiting intestinal lipase. Side effects include diarrhea, gas, cramping, and possible ↓ absorption of fat-soluble vitamins.
- **Surgery** (Roux-en-Y gastric bypass, vertical banded gastroplasty, gastric banding): Consider only for patients with a BMI > 40 or in those with a BMI > 35 and obesity-related comorbidities.

### COMPLICATIONS

Type 2 DM, hypertension, hyperlipidemia, obstructive sleep apnea, psychosocial disability, thromboembolic disorders, degenerative joint disease, CAD.

## MENTAL HEALTH

# Depression

An often unrecognized characteristic of teens who are acting out or are out of control. The intensity of feelings and emotions during this time period makes it difficult to differentiate severe depression from normal sadness. In less severe depression, sadness or unhappiness associated with problems of everyday life is generally short-lived, with symptoms usually resulting in only minor impairment in school performance, social activities, and relationships with others. These symptoms, even if they seem minor, must be evaluated and may respond to support and reassurance. Depression is the precursor to suicide attempts. With more severe forms of depression, psychological help may be useful.

*As with adults, depression in teens is often marked by a disturbance of self-esteem with a sense of guilt and worthlessness.*

### SYMPTOMS/EXAM

- Serious depressive symptoms in adolescence may be similar to those in adults, with vegetative signs such as depressed mood.
- May also present with the following:
  - A sense of emptiness and meaninglessness.
  - $\ominus$ expectations of oneself and the environment.
  - Isolation.
  - Persistent psychosomatic complaints (abdominal pain, chest pain, headache, lethargy, weight loss, dizziness, syncope).
- Other behavioral manifestations (depressive equivalents) of masked depression include truancy, running away from home, defiance of authority, self-destructive behavior, vandalism, drug and alcohol abuse, sexual acting out, and delinquency.

### DIFFERENTIAL

- Eating disorders.
- **Organic CNS disorders:** Tumors, vascular lesions, closed head trauma, subdural hematomas.
- **Metabolic and endocrinologic disorders:** SLE, hypothyroidism, hyperthyroidism, Wilson's disease, hyperparathyroidism, Cushing's syndrome, Addison's disease, PMS.
- **Infections:** Infectious mononucleosis, syphilis.
- **Other:** Drug use or withdrawal; other mental health disorders such as schizophrenia; a family history of depression, suicide, or bipolar affective disorder.

### DIAGNOSIS

If an underlying medical condition is suspected, consider TSH, CBC, ESR, VDRL or RPR, and liver enzymes.

### TREATMENT

- Counsel adolescents and parents if depression is mild or results from an acute personal loss or frustration.
- For depressive disorder, suicidal thoughts, or psychotic thinking, psychological referral is necessary.
- SSRIs may be prescribed for patients who will be closely followed. Most SSRIs are activating and should be given in the mornings. Some patients may experience sedation with paroxetine, fluvoxamine, and mirtazapine. Clinical response varies from two to six weeks.
- In 2004, the FDA issued a black-box warning regarding the risk of ↑ suicidality in children and adolescents prescribed antidepressant medications.

## Suicidality

With the normal mood swings of adolescence, short periods of depression are common, and a teenager may have thoughts of suicide. Suicide is the third leading cause of mortality among adolescents. The suicide rate of teen males is five times higher than that of females, and white males have the highest rate. The incidence of unsuccessful suicide attempts is three times higher in females than in males. Firearms account for the majority of suicide deaths in both males and females.

### SYMPTOMS/EXAM

Inability to keep up with schoolwork; social withdrawal; symptoms of depression; anger; a history of a previous suicide attempt.

### DIAGNOSIS

Determine the extent of the patient's depression and assess the risk of inflicting self-harm. The history should include the medical, social, emotional, and academic background. Inquire about the following:

- Common signs of depression.
- Recent stressful events.
- Evidence of long-standing problems in the home, at school, or with peers.
- Drug or substance use and abuse.
- Signs of psychotic thinking, such as delusions or hallucinations.
- Evidence of masked depression, such as rebellious behavior, running away from home, reckless driving, or other acting-out behavior.

### TREATMENT

- Medical therapy should be aimed at treating medical complications of the suicide attempt.
- Physical protection is needed to avoid harm to self if a plan is in place.
- Provide emergency psychological consultation for any teenager who is severely depressed, psychotic, or acutely suicidal.
- Contract with the patient about increasing suicidal ideation or plans.

---

A 17-year-old high school senior is brought to your clinic because her mother is concerned about her daughter's abnormal eating habits. The girl denies that she has a problem, stating that she is just picky with her food and is attempting to become a vegetarian. She has lost 18 pounds over the past six months, and her periods have stopped. What is your advice for her anxious mother? Interview the girl alone and look for signs and symptoms of an eating disorder.

---

## Eating Disorders

Teenagers and younger children continue to develop eating disorders at an alarming rate. The spectrum of eating disorders includes anorexia nervosa, bulimia nervosa, eating disorders not otherwise specified, and binge-eating disorder. The relationship between biology and environment in the development of eating disorders is complex. Contributing factors appear to include growing influence by the media (television, magazines, movies, videos), in which thin young woman are often depicted as the norm. Anorexia and bulimia are distinguished as follows:

*The commonalities among the eating disorders include disturbance in body image as well as a drive for thinness.*

- **Anorexia nervosa:** Diagnosis requires four diagnostic criteria as defined in the DSM-IV:
    - Refusal to maintain weight within a normal range for height and age (more than 15% below ideal body weight).
    - Fear of weight gain.
    - Severe body image disturbance (body image is the predominant measure of self-worth, along with denial of the seriousness of the illness).
    - In postmenarchal females, absence of the menstrual cycle, or amenorrhea (> 3 cycles).
- **Bulimia:** Defined as episodic and uncontrolled ingestion of large quantities of food followed by recurrent inappropriate compensatory behavior to prevent weight gain, such as self-induced vomiting, diuretic or cathartic use, strict dieting, or vigorous exercise.

### SYMPTOMS

- **Anorexia:** Amenorrhea, depression, fatigue, weakness, hair loss, bone pain, constipation, abdominal pain.
- **Bulimia:** Normal or near-normal body weight, mouth sores, dental caries, heartburn, muscle cramps and fainting, hair loss, easy bruising, intolerance to cold, menstrual irregularity, abuse of diuretics and laxatives, misuse of diet pills (→ palpitations and anxiety), frequent vomiting (resulting in throat irritation and pharyngeal trauma).

### EXAM

- Assess vitals to evaluate for bradycardia, hypotension, or orthostatic hypotension.
- Perform a detailed physical and dental exam, including height, weight, and BMI.
    - **Anorexia:** Signs include brittle hair and nails; dry, scaly skin; loss of subcutaneous fat; fine facial and body hair (lanugo hair); and breast and vaginal atrophy.
    - **Bulimia:** Signs include a callused finger (Russell's sign; results when the finger is used to induce vomiting), dry skin, periodontal disease, and sialadenosis (swelling of the parotid glands).
- Obtain a psychiatric history to assess for substance abuse and mood/anxiety/personality disorders.
- Ask about suicidal ideation.

### DIAGNOSIS

- Explore body image, exercise regimen, eating habits, sexual history, current and past medication use, diuretic and laxative use, binging and purging behavior, and substance use.
- Obtain electrolytes, CBC, LFTs, and ECG to evaluate for arrhythmias and electrolyte disturbance.

### TREATMENT

- The goal is restoration of normal body weight and eating habits along with resolution of psychological difficulties.
    - **Behavioral therapy:** Intensive psychotherapy and family therapy.
    - **Pharmacotherapy:** TCAs, SSRIs, lithium carbonate.
- Enteral or parenteral feeding in patients with severe malnutrition.
- Hospitalization as indicated in cases of severe malnutrition or failed outpatient therapy.

## COMPLICATIONS

Severe malnutrition, cardiac arrhythmias, suicide attempt, osteopenia, heart failure, dental disease.

> A 16-year-old girl comes to your clinic for 2° amenorrhea. She tells you that she feels better than ever after joining her neighborhood gym. The girl is sexually active and uses condoms for contraception. You obtain a urine pregnancy test, which is ⊖. How do you work up her amenorrhea? Obtaining a better history about the type and amount of exercise is important in determining the cause of amenorrhea in a young female.

## Female Athlete Triad

Many young women engage in exercise to control body weight and improve exercise capacity. The consequences of excessive exercise can include amenorrhea, infertility, and delay of puberty and menarche. The likelihood of amenorrhea varies with the type and amount of exercise as well as with the rapidity of ↑ in exercise. Activities that are associated with low body weight and amenorrhea include running, ballet dancing, and figure skating. Gradual increases in exercise are less likely to → amenorrhea than acute increases. Amenorrhea occurs only when there is relative caloric deficiency due to inadequate nutritional intake for the amount of energy expended.

### TREATMENT

- Educate patients on the need for adequate caloric intake to match energy expenditure.
- Take an interdisciplinary approach with sports coaches, family, school, and school counselors.
- Estrogen replacement for women with amenorrhea (OCPs).
- Patients should be encouraged to take 1200–1500 mg of calcium daily along with supplemental vitamin D (400 IU daily).

*The "female athlete triad" consists of an eating disorder, amenorrhea, and osteoporosis.*

### COMPLICATIONS

Exercise-induced amenorrhea; loss of bone density.

## Substance Use and Abuse

Use of substances during adolescence may compromise physical, cognitive, and psychosocial aspects of adolescent development and can be a risk factor for substance abuse later in life. Commonly used substances include alcohol, marijuana, opioids, cocaine, amphetamines, sedative-hypnotics, hallucinogens, inhalants, nicotine, anabolic steroids, γ-hydroxybutyrate (GHB), and 3,4-methylenedioxymethamphetamine (Ecstasy). When discussing substance use with adolescents, physicians must be aware of confidentiality laws in their state.

### SYMPTOMS/EXAM

Substance abuse is defined as follows (see also Tables 13.15 and 13.16):

**TABLE 13.15.** Presentation of Substance Use and Abuse

| VARIABLE | PRESENTATION |
|---|---|
| Physical | Fatigue, insomnia or hypersomnia, runny nose, shortness of breath, injected eyes, pinpoint pupils. |
| Emotional | Personality change, sudden mood changes, irritability, irresponsible behavior, low self-esteem, poor judgment, depression, withdrawal, general lack of interest. |
| Family | Breaking rules or withdrawing from the family; high family conflict; lack of bonding. |
| School | Truancy, academic failure, lack of commitment to school and education, early persistent behavioral problems. |
| Social/behavioral | Peer group involvement with drugs and alcohol; problems with the law. |

- A maladaptive pattern of substance use → clinically significant impairment or distress, as manifested by one or more of the following occurring within a 12-month period:
    - Recurrent substance use → failure to fulfill major role obligations at work, school, or home (e.g., repeated absences or poor work performance related to substance use; substance-related absences, suspensions, or expulsions from school; neglect of children or household).
    - Recurrent substance use in situations in which it is physically hazardous (e.g., driving an automobile or operating a machine when impaired by substance use).
    - Recurrent substance-related legal problems (arrests for substance-related disorderly conduct).
    - Continued substance use despite having persistent or recurrent social or interpersonal problems caused or exacerbated by the effects of the substance (e.g., arguments with spouse about consequences of intoxication, physical fights).
- The symptoms have never met the criteria for substance dependence for this class of substance.

### DIAGNOSIS

Clinical history, specific physical examination findings (see Table 13.16), and a drug screen if drug abuse is suspected.

### TREATMENT

- Counsel about the dangers of substance use and abuse.
- Family therapy.
- **Smoking:** Nicotine patches, gum.
- **Alcohol:** Recommend participation in Alcoholics Anonymous.
- **Illicit drug use:** Recommend drug rehabilitation programs.

### COMPLICATIONS

Death and injury (from motor vehicle accidents, other unintentional injuries, homicide, and suicide); physical and sexual abuse; ↑ sexual activity (teen pregnancy, STIs); alterations in mood, sleep, and appetite; frank psychosis indistinguishable from schizophrenia; irreversible cardiomyopathy; noncardiogenic pulmonary edema; pulmonary hypertension; drug overdose with multiorgan system failure.

**TABLE 13.16.    Physiologic Effects of Common Illicit Substances**

| SYMPTOM | SUBSTANCE |
|---|---|
| **Eyes/pupils** | |
| Mydriasis | Amphetamines, MDMA or other stimulants, cocaine, jimsonweed, LSD; withdrawal from alcohol or opioids. |
| Miosis | Alcohol, barbiturates, benzodiazepines, opioids, PCP. |
| Nystagmus | Alcohol, barbiturates, benzodiazepines, inhalants, PCP. |
| Conjunctival injection | LSD, marijuana. |
| Lacrimation | Inhalants, LSD; withdrawal from opioids. |
| **Cardiovascular** | |
| Tachycardia/hypertension | Amphetamines, MDMA, cocaine, LSD, marijuana, PCP;. withdrawal from alcohol, barbiturates, or benzodiazepines. |
| Hypotension | Barbiturates, opioids; withdrawal from depressants. Orthostatic hypotension—marijuana. |
| Arrhythmia | Amphetamines, MDMA, cocaine, inhalants, opioids, PCP. |
| **Respiratory** | |
| Depression | Opioids, depressants, GHB. |
| Pulmonary edema | Opioids, stimulants. |
| **Core body temperature** | |
| Elevated | Amphetamines, MDMA, cocaine, PCP; withdrawal from alcohol, barbiturates, benzodiazepines, or opioids. |
| Decreased | Alcohol, barbiturates, benzodiazepines, opioids, GHB. |
| **PNS response** | |
| Hyperreflexia | Amphetamines, MDMA, cocaine, LSD, marijuana, PCP; withdrawal from alcohol or benzodiazepines. |
| Hyporeflexia | Alcohol, benzodiazepines, inhalants, opioids. |
| Tremor | Amphetamines, cocaine, LSD; withdrawal from alcohol, benzodiazepines, or cocaine. |
| Ataxia | Alcohol, amphetamines, MDMA, benzodiazepines, inhalants, LSD, PCP, GHB. |
| **CNS response** | |
| Hyperalertness | Amphetamines, MDMA, cocaine. |
| Sedation/somnolence | Alcohol, benzodiazepines, inhalants, marijuana, opioids, GHB. |
| Seizures | Alcohol, amphetamines, MDMA, cocaine, inhalants, opioids; withdrawal from alcohol or benzodiazepines. |
| Hallucinations | Amphetamines, MDMA, cocaine, inhalants, LSD, marijuana, PCP; withdrawal from alcohol or benzodiazepines. |
| **Gastrointestinal** | |
| Nausea/vomiting | Alcohol, amphetamines or other stimulants, cocaine, inhalants, LSD, opioids, peyote, GHB; withdrawal from alcohol, benzodiazepines, cocaine, or opioids. |

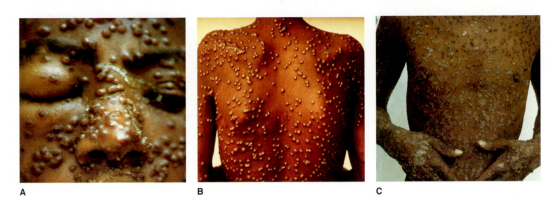

A            B            C

**FIGURE 2.2.**    **Smallpox lesions.**

(Reproduced, with permission, from Wolff K et al. *Fitzpatrick's Color Atlas & Synopsis of Clinical Dermatology*, 5th ed. New York: McGraw-Hill, 2005: 771.)

## HEMATOLOGY/ONCOLOGY

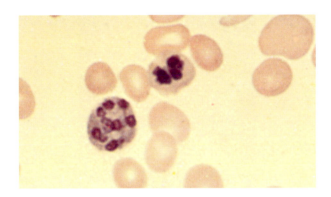

**FIGURE 7.2.**    **Megaloblastic anemia.**

(Reproduced, with permission, from Kasper DL et al [eds]. *Harrison's Principles of Internal Medicine*, 16th ed. New York: McGraw-Hill, 2005: 605.)

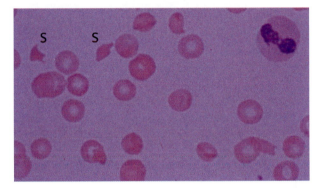

**FIGURE 7.3.**    **Thrombotic thrombocytopenic purpura.**

(Courtesy of Dr. Peter McPhedran, Yale Department of Hematology.)

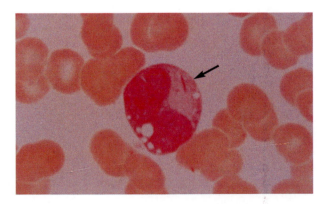

**FIGURE 7.4.**    **Auer rod in acute myelocytic leukemia.**

(Courtesy of Dr. Peter McPhedran, Yale Department of Hematology.)

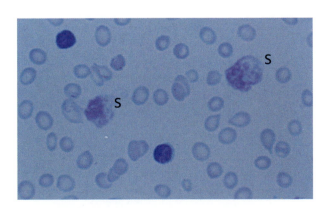

**FIGURE 7.5.**    **Chronic lymphocytic leukemia.**

(Courtesy of Dr. Peter McPhedran, Yale Department of Hematology.)

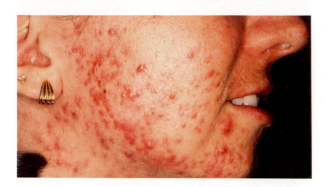

**FIGURE 10.1.** Severe inflammatory acne with pustules and comedones.

(Reproduced, with permission, from Kasper DL et al. *Harrison's Principles of Internal Medicine*, 16th ed. New York: McGraw-Hill, 2005: 295.)

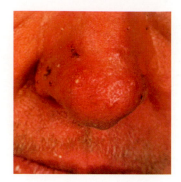

**FIGURE 10.2.** Rhinophyma and pustules on a male with rosacea.

(Reproduced, with permission, from Wolff K, Johnson RA, Suurmond D. *Fitzpatrick's Color Atlas & Synopsis of Clinical Dermatology*, 5th edition, Online Picture Gallery. New York: McGraw-Hill, 2007: Figure 1e-R5.)

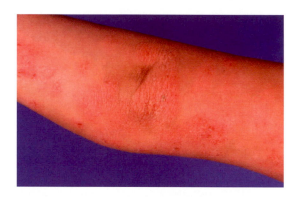

**FIGURE 10.3.** Atopic dermatitis in the antecubital region of a child.

(Reproduced, with permission, from Wolff K et al. *Fitzpatrick's Color Atlas & Synopsis of Clinical Dermatology*, 5th ed. New York: McGraw-Hill, 2005: Figure 2e-AD12.)

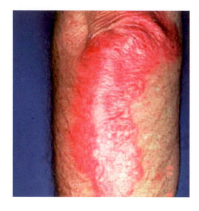

**FIGURE 10.4.** Erythematous plaque of psoriasis.

(Reproduced, with permission, from Bondi EE et al. *Dermatology: Diagnosis & Therapy*, 1st ed. Stamford, CT: Appleton & Lange, 1991.)

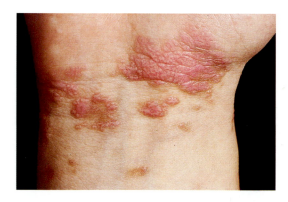

**FIGURE 10.6.** Lesions of lichen planus.

(Reproduced, with permission, from Wolff K et al. *Fitzpatrick's Color Atlas & Synopsis of Clinical Dermatology*, 5th ed. New York: McGraw-Hill, 2005: 125.)

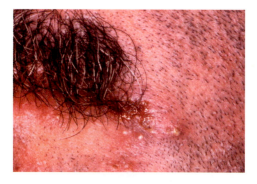

**FIGURE 10.8.** Folliculitis in the beard area with impetigo at the corner of the mouth.

(Reproduced, with permission, from Wolff K et al. *Fitzpatrick's Color Atlas & Synopsis of Clinical Dermatology*, 5th ed. New York: McGraw-Hill, 2005: 980.)

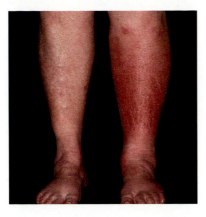

**FIGURE 10.9.** Cellulitis of the lower extremity.

(Reproduced, with permission, from Knoop KJ et al. *Atlas of Emergency Medicine*, 2nd ed. New York: McGraw-Hill, 2002: 348.)

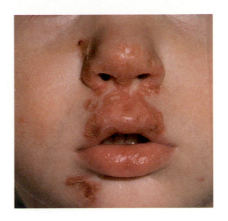

**FIGURE 10.10.** Lesions of impetigo.

(Reproduced, with permission, from Wolff K et al. *Fitzpatrick's Color Atlas & Synopsis of Clinical Dermatology*, 5th ed. New York: McGraw-Hill, 2005: 589.)

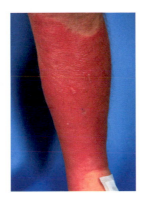

**FIGURE 10.11.** Erysipelas.

(Reproduced, with permission, from Wolff K et al. *Fitzpatrick's Color Atlas & Synopsis of Clinical Dermatology*, 5th ed. New York: McGraw-Hill, 2005: 607.)

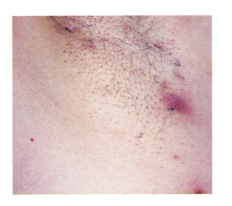

**FIGURE 10.12.** Hidradenitis suppurativa.

(Reproduced, with permission, from Wolff K et al. *Fitzpatrick's Color Atlas & Synopsis of Clinical Dermatology*, 5th ed. New York: McGraw-Hill, 2005: 15.)

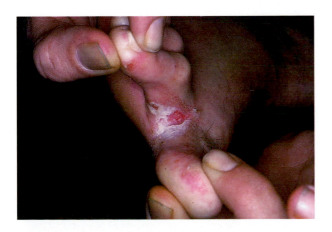

**FIGURE 10.13.** Interdigital tinea pedis.

(Reproduced, with permission, from Knoop KJ et al. *Atlas of Emergency Medicine*, 2nd ed. New York: McGraw-Hill, 2002: 402.)

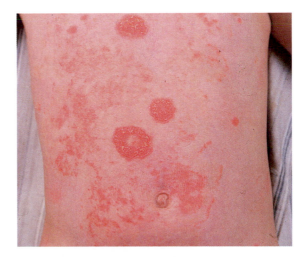

**FIGURE 10.14.** Tinea corporis.

(Reproduced, with permission, from Wolff K et al. *Fitzpatrick's Color Atlas & Synopsis of Clinical Dermatology*, 5th ed. New York: McGraw-Hill, 2005: 702.)

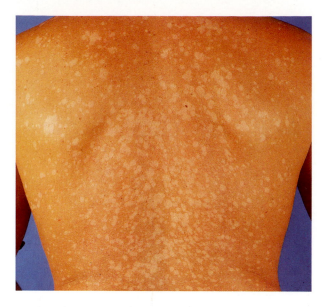

**FIGURE 10.15.** **Tinea versicolor.**

(Reproduced, with permission, from Wolff K et al. *Fitzpatrick's Color Atlas & Synopsis of Clinical Dermatology,* 5th ed. New York: McGraw-Hill, 2005: 731.)

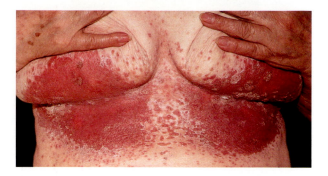

**FIGURE 10.16.** **Cutaneous candidiasis—intertrigo.**

(Reproduced, with permission, from Wolff K et al. *Fitzpatrick's Color Atlas & Synopsis of Clinical Dermatology,* 5th ed. New York: McGraw-Hill, 2005: 719.)

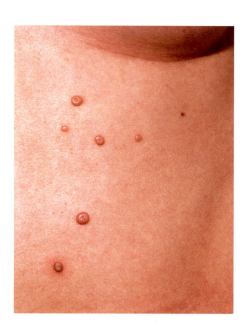

**FIGURE 10.17.** **Molluscum contagiosum on the chest of a female.**

(Reproduced, with permission, from Wolff K et al. *Fitzpatrick's Color Atlas & Synopsis of Clinical Dermatology,* 5th ed. New York: McGraw-Hill, 2005: 763.)

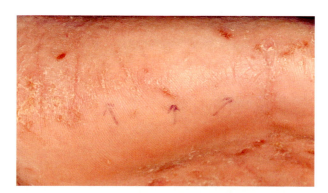

**FIGURE 10.18.** **Linear burrows of infection caused by scabies.**

(Reproduced, with permission, from Wolff K et al. *Fitzpatrick's Color Atlas & Synopsis of Clinical Dermatology,* 5th ed. New York: McGraw-Hill, 2005: 857.)

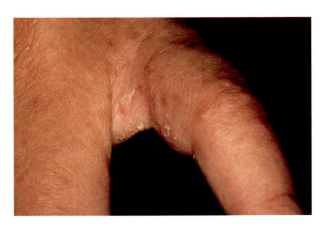

**FIGURE 10.19.** Burrows of the scabies mite in the web spaces of the hands.

(Reproduced, with permission, from Wolff K et al. *Fitzpatrick's Color Atlas & Synopsis of Clinical Dermatology*, 5th ed. New York: McGraw-Hill, 2005: 855.)

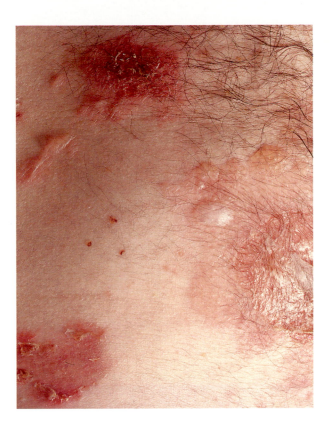

**FIGURE 10.22.** Characteristic lesions of pemphigus.

(Reproduced, with permission, from Wolff K et al. *Fitzpatrick's Color Atlas & Synopsis of Clinical Dermatology*, 5th ed. New York: McGraw-Hill, 2005: 104.)

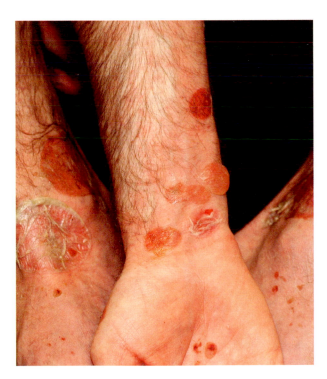

**FIGURE 10.23.** Characteristic lesions of bullous pemphigoid.

(Reproduced, with permission, from Wolff K et al. *Fitzpatrick's Color Atlas & Synopsis of Clinical Dermatology*, 5th ed. New York: McGraw-Hill, 2005: 108.)

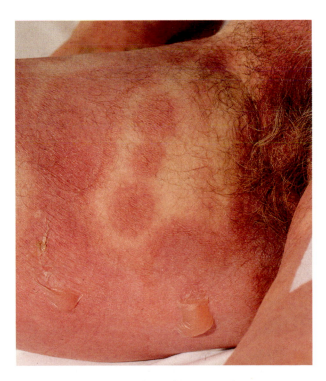

**FIGURE 10.24.** Lesions of Stevens-Johnson syndrome.

(Reproduced, with permission, from Wolff K et al. *Fitzpatrick's Color Atlas & Synopsis of Clinical Dermatology*, 5th ed. New York: McGraw-Hill, 2005: 145.)

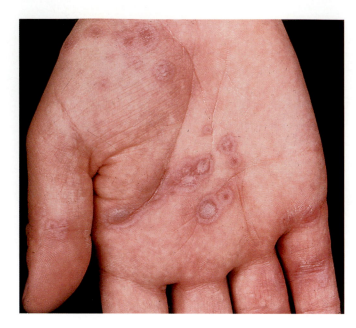

**FIGURE 10.25.** Lesions of erythema multiforme.

(Reproduced, with permission, from Wolff K et al. *Fitzpatrick's Color Atlas & Synopsis of Clinical Dermatology*, 5th ed. New York: McGraw-Hill, 2005: 141.)

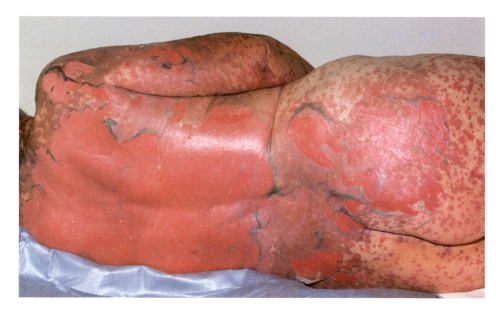

**FIGURE 10.26.** Lesions of toxic epidermal necrolysis.

(Reproduced, with permission, from Wolff K et al. *Fitzpatrick's Color Atlas & Synopsis of Clinical Dermatology*, 5th ed. New York: McGraw-Hill, 2005: 147.)

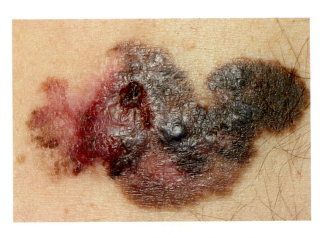

**FIGURE 10.27.** Superficial spreading melanoma.

(Reproduced, with permission, from Wolff K et al. *Fitzpatrick's Color Atlas & Synopsis of Clinical Dermatology,* 5th ed. New York: McGraw-Hill, 2005: 318.)

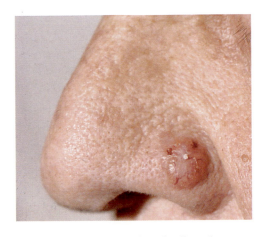

**FIGURE 10.28.** Nodular basal cell carcinoma.

(Reproduced, with permission, from Wolff K et al. *Fitzpatrick's Color Atlas & Synopsis of Clinical Dermatology,* 5th ed. New York: McGraw-Hill, 2005: 283.)

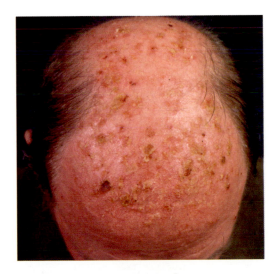

**FIGURE 10.29.** Actinic keratosis.

(Reproduced, with permission, from Wolff K et al. *Fitzpatrick's Color Atlas & Synopsis of Clinical Dermatology,* 5th ed. New York: McGraw-Hill, 2005: 263.)

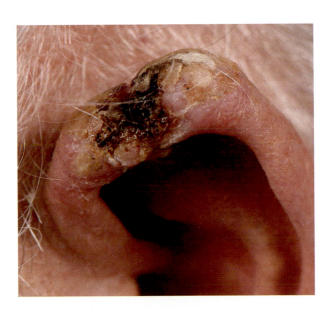

**FIGURE 10.30.** Squamous cell carcinoma.

(Reproduced, with permission, from Wolff K et al. *Fitzpatrick's Color Atlas & Synopsis of Clinical Dermatology,* 5th ed. New York: McGraw-Hill, 2005: 279.)

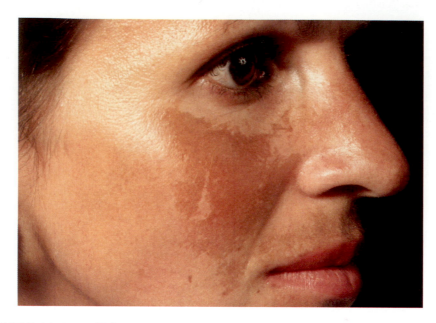

**FIGURE 10.31.    Melasma.**

(Reproduced, with permission, from Wolff K et al. *Fitzpatrick's Color Atlas & Synopsis of Clinical Dermatology*, 5th ed. New York: McGraw-Hill, 2005: 349.)

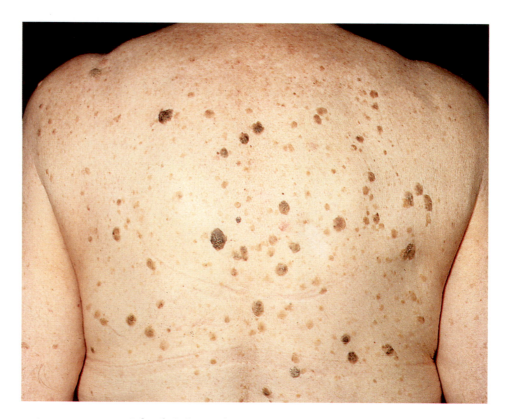

**FIGURE 10.32.    Seborrheic keratosis.**

(Reproduced, with permission, from Wolff K et al. *Fitzpatrick's Color Atlas & Synopsis of Clinical Dermatology*, 5th ed. New York: McGraw-Hill, 2005: 207.)

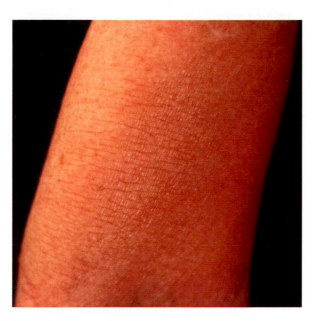

**FIGURE 13.5.** **Atopic dermatitis.**

(Reproduced, with permission, from Wolff K et al. *Fitzpatrick's Color Atlas & Synopsis of Clinical Dermatology*, 5th ed. New York: McGraw-Hill, 2005: 39.)

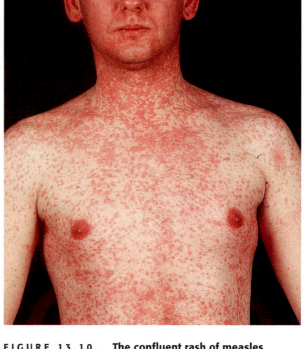

**FIGURE 13.10.** **The confluent rash of measles.**

(Reproduced, with permission, from Wolff K et al. *Fitzpatrick's Color Atlas & Synopsis of Clinical Dermatology*, 5th ed. New York: McGraw-Hill, 2005: 788.)

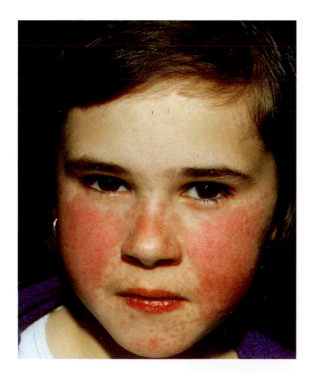

**FIGURE 13.11.** **The "slapped cheek" appearance of erythema infectiosum.**

(Reproduced, with permission, from Wolff K et al. *Fitzpatrick's Color Atlas & Synopsis of Clinical Dermatology*, 5th ed. New York: McGraw-Hill, 2005: 793.)

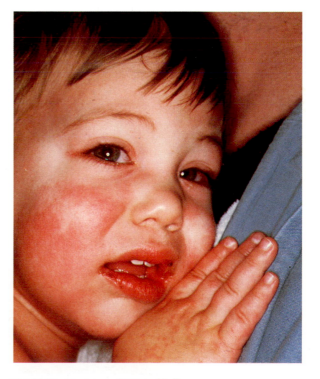

**FIGURE 13.12.** **Kawasaki disease.**

(Reproduced, with permission, from Wolff K et al. *Fitzpatrick's Color Atlas & Synopsis of Clinical Dermatology*, 5th ed. New York: McGraw-Hill, 2005: 425.)

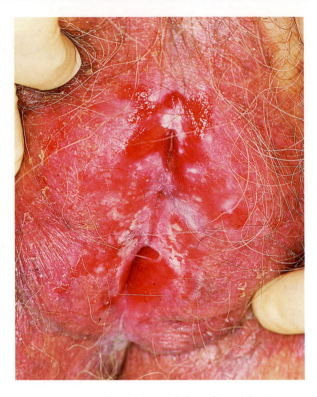

**FIGURE 16.16.** **Squamous cell carcinoma of the vulva arising in an area of lichen sclerosus.**

(Reproduced, with permission, from Wolff K et al. *Fitzpatrick's Color Atlas & Synopsis of Clinical Dermatology,* 5th ed. New York: McGraw Hill, 2005: 1047.)

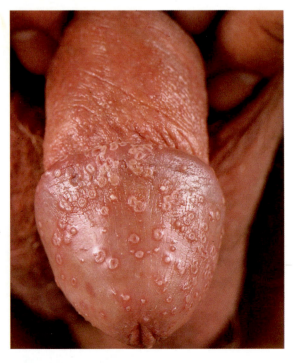

**FIGURE 16.18.** **Candidal balanitis.**

(Reproduced, with permission, from Wolff K et al. *Fitzpatrick's Color Atlas & Synopsis of Clinical Dermatology,* 5th ed. New York: McGraw-Hill, 2005: 727.)

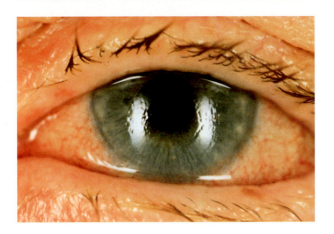

**FIGURE 18.8.** **Angle-closure glaucoma.**

(Reproduced, with permission, from Knoop KJ et al. *Atlas of Emergency Medicine*, 2nd ed. New York: McGraw-Hill, 2002: 49.)

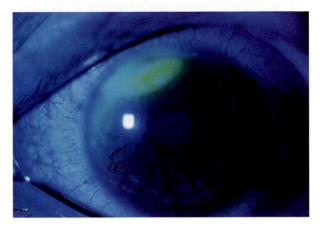

**FIGURE 18.9.** **Corneal abrasion.**

(Reproduced, with permission, from Knoop KJ et al. *Atlas of Emergency Medicine*, 2nd ed. New York: McGraw-Hill, 2002: 98.)

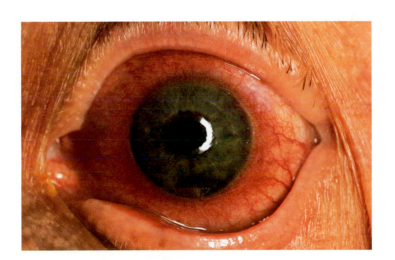

**FIGURE 18.10.** **Acute uveitis.**

(Reproduced, with permission, from Knoop KJ et al. *Atlas of Emergency Medicine*, 2nd ed. New York: McGraw-Hill, 2002: 52.)

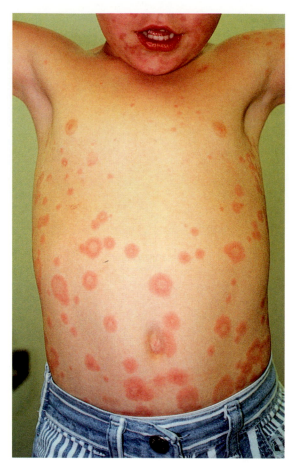

**FIGURE 18.14.** **Erythema multiforme.**

(Reproduced, with permission, from Knoop KJ et al. *Atlas of Emergency Medicine*, 2nd ed. New York: McGraw-Hill, 2002: 378.)

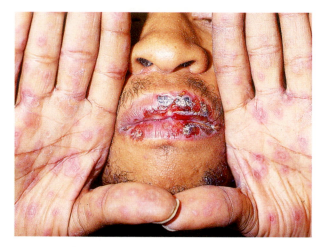

**FIGURE 18.15.** **Stevens-Johnson syndrome.**

(Reproduced, with permission, from Knoop KJ et al. *Atlas of Emergency Medicine*, 2nd ed. New York: McGraw-Hill, 2002: 379.)

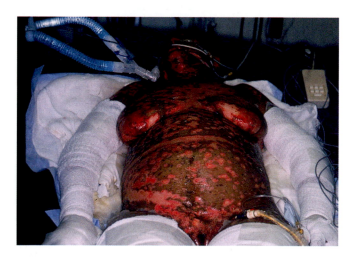

**FIGURE 18.16.** **Toxic epidermal necrolysis.**

(Reproduced, with permission, from Knoop KJ et al. *Atlas of Emergency Medicine*, 2nd ed. New York: McGraw-Hill, 2002: 380.)

# CHAPTER 14

# Psychiatry and Behavioral Science

Shira Shavit, MD

## Communication

Good communication is key to strong patient-physician and family-physician relationships. Focusing on communication skills enhances these relationships and → **higher adherence** as well as to **greater patient satisfaction.** Components of a good communication style include the following:

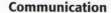

- **Eye contact** and exchanging pleasantries (shaking hands).
- **Avoiding interruptions** while keeping patients on track.
- Making extra effort to build **trust.**
- Not appearing rushed.
- **Managing expectations** by asking patients what their expectations may be.
- **Empowering patients** to ask questions and make decisions that → to a more balanced patient-physician relationship.
- **Respecting confidentiality,** including remembering not to disclose information to family members who may also be under your care (especially important to remember with patients in their teens).
- **Providing information** (reviewing medication dosages; using patient handouts).

*An exception to the general requirement for confidentiality may be made when physicians feel that patients may be at risk of hurting themselves or others.*

## Cultural Competence

Although it may not be realistic for physicians to be familiar with all of their patients' cultural backgrounds, it is important for clinicians to understand how culture affects the patient-physician relationship and hence treatment outcomes. Above all, physicians must take care **not to apply stereotypes** or prejudices to patients whose gender, race, ethnicity, sexual orientation, or culture may differ from their own. Providers should be aware of their own feelings, biases, and prejudices prior to their interaction with patients. Factors that may influence the patient-physician relationship include the following:

- Cultural beliefs (e.g., in Hmong culture, seizure disorders are thought to result from possession by a spirit).
- Cultural expectations of care (e.g., because questioning does not play a significant role in traditional Navajo healing, some Navajo patients are unfamiliar with conventional history taking).
- Traditional or alternative treatments, language barriers, and family systems (e.g., in China, some families expect physicians not to tell patients that they are terminally ill but to inform their children instead).

*Harm reduction is a method by which physicians can find a middle ground between what they feel is best and the patient's wishes. This method helps the patient modify his or her behaviors to reduce the harm they may be causing themselves (e.g., cutting down on smoking vs. smoking cessation; using clean needles vs. quitting heroin).*

Techniques to **minimize cultural misunderstandings** include the following:

- Be respectful (address all patients as Ms. or Mr.).
- Where feasible, use competent interpreters who are not only bilingual but bicultural.
- Spend more time with the patient if needed.
- Anticipate that patients may have had ⊖ interactions with the medical system in the past.
- Review treatment plans carefully, and have patients demonstrate an understanding of these plans.
- Be nonjudgmental and accepting of patients' cultural differences.
- Be attentive to nonverbal forms of communication.

## Patient Preferences

All patients have their own preferences for treatment, many of which are shaped by their expectations, cultural beliefs, and understanding of their illness. Often, however, patients' preferences may be at odds with the provider's treatment plan. For this reason, it is important for physicians to inquire about patients' treatment preferences as well as to ascertain the source of these preferences. By this means, gaps in a patient's understanding of a given disease may be identified, or, alternatively, a physician may recognize the need to modify a treatment plan in accordance with the patient's needs. Above all, it is essential that the physician understand and respect the patient's wishes, as such understanding will foster a stronger relationship while also increasing the likelihood of adherence.

## Abuse

It is essential that physicians understand the role they play in the recognition and reporting of abuse of any kind. Guidelines are as follows:

- **Child abuse:** Mandatory reporting laws exist for all suspected cases of child abuse or neglect, and physicians are required to report all such cases.
- **Domestic violence:** Reporting laws with regard to domestic violence vary from state to state, with few states requiring reporting. Nonetheless, domestic violence should by no means be considered a "private matter," and although reporting it may not be mandatory, physicians must screen for it in 1° care visits. In this context, physicians should not judge their success on the basis of whether a patient leaves his or her partner, but they should let the victim know that the abuse is not their fault; that they do not merit such treatment; and that the violence they are confronting is unacceptable.
- **Elder abuse:** Approximately 1–2 million older Americans are victims of abuse or neglect by their 1° caretakers. Physicians are **mandatory reporters** of elder abuse and neglect.

*When victims of domestic violence leave their abusers, they have a 75% ↑ risk of being murdered.*

*One in seven women in outpatient visits is a victim of domestic violence.*

> **Guidelines for domestic violence surveillance—**
>
> **RADAR**
>
> **R**emember to ask about partner violence.
> **A**sk directly about violence.
> **D**ocument information in the patient's chart.
> **A**ssess the patient's safety.
> **R**efer the patient to outside resources (e.g., legal services, support groups, shelters).

## MOOD DISORDERS

### Dysthymia

Defined as **depressed mood** occurring on most days and lasting **at least two years.** Although **less severe** than major depression, dysthymia significantly impairs work and social functioning by virtue of its chronicity. Its prevalence in the United States is approximately 6%.

#### SYMPTOMS

Diagnostic criteria are as follows:

- **Two** of the following symptoms must be present, most of the day, more days than not, for at least **two** years:
    - Poor appetite or overeating
    - Insomnia or hypersomnia
    - Low energy, fatigue
    - Poor concentration
    - Low self-esteem
    - Hopelessness

*Dysthymia is a "low-grade" depression commonly encountered in the 1° care setting that lasts several years with few symptom-free periods.*

- During a two-year period, affected patients must **not have had a symptom-free period** for **> 2 months.**
- Symptoms must → significant impairment in daily functioning.

### DIFFERENTIAL

- **Major depression:** A more severe form of depression.
- **Depression due to a medical condition:** Depressive symptoms may be similar to those of dysthymia but are caused by a medical condition (e.g., hypothyroidism, anemia).
- **Bipolar disorder:** Characterized by periods of mania or hypomania in addition to the depressive symptoms.
- **Substance abuse disorders:** Presentation is often similar to that of dysthymia, but symptoms are precipitated by the use of or withdrawal from alcohol or an illicit substance.

### TREATMENT

- **Behavioral:** Various forms of individual and group psychotherapy may be of benefit.
- **Pharmacologic:** SSRIs; other classes of antidepressants.

## Major Depressive Disorder (MDD)

Defined as **severe depression** that has a significant effect on a patient's ability to function. Has a variable age of onset. Its prevalence in men is about 10% and in women about 20%, and there is a two- to threefold ↑ risk in first-degree family members. MDD is increasing in prevalence and is occurring at earlier ages. Full recovery from an episode is achieved within six months in half of all cases.

### SYMPTOMS

Characterized by one or more episodes of **depressed mood** or **anhedonia** (loss of interest or pleasure) for **at least two weeks,** as well as by at least five of the following symptoms: sleep disturbance, anhedonia, guilt, lack of energy, poor concentration, change in appetite, suicidality, and psychomotor changes.

### DIFFERENTIAL

- **Adjustment disorder with depressed mood:** A reaction to a specific incident or psychosocial stressor → depressed mood.
- **Bereavement:** After the loss of a loved one, depressive symptoms consistent with major depression may occur but should not last > 2 months or have suicidality or psychosis as features.
- **Mood disorder due to a medical condition:** May occur 2° to a variety of disorders (e.g., anemia, hypothyroidism, pancreatic cancer, Parkinson's disease) or as a result of medications taken for a medical condition, such as thiazide diuretics, β-blockers, digoxin, cyclosporine, and metoclopramide.
- **Substance abuse mood disorder:** Major depressive symptoms due to use of or withdrawal from an abused substance.
- **Bipolar disorder:** Episodes of major depressive symptoms accompanied by manic periods.
- **Schizoaffective disorder:** Predominantly a psychotic disorder with accompanying mood symptoms.

*Symptoms of depression—*

**SIG E CAPS**

**S**leep—hypersomnia/ insomnia
**I**nterest—loss of interest or pleasure in activities
**G**uilt—a feeling of worthlessness or inappropriate guilt
**E**nergy—low energy
**C**oncentration—poor concentration
**A**ppetite—↑ or ↓ appetite
**P**sychomotor agitation or retardation
**S**uicidal ideation

## TREATMENT

- **Behavioral:** Many forms of individual and group psychotherapy are appropriate, including cognitive behavioral therapy (CBT) and interpersonal psychotherapy.
- **Pharmacologic:** Antidepressants are associated with a response rate of 60–80%. The goal of the provider is to select the medication with the most tolerable side effect profile while maximizing efficacy in the individual patient.
    - **SSRIs** (e.g., paroxetine, fluoxetine, sertraline): Generally first line owing to their **lower side effect profile.**
    - **TCAs** and **MAOIs:** Have demonstrated a level of efficacy similar to that of SSRIs.
- **Electroconvulsive therapy (ECT):** Primarily used for patients who show a lack of response to several antidepressants, **severe depression** with psychosis, a high risk of suicide, or prior response to ECT. More effective than antidepressants (about 80%).

## COMPLICATIONS

- **Psychosis:** Patients with severe MDD can develop psychotic symptoms such as auditory hallucinations, paranoia, and delusions. In such cases, the response rate is 40% with antidepressants alone, 20% with antipsychotics alone, and 70% with both taken together.
- **Suicidality:** Severe untreated MDD can → suicidality. Women tend to attempt more suicides, whereas men tend to succeed more often. When presented with a patient with symptoms of MDD, clinicians **must assess** the risk of suicidality.
    - Factors that ↑ **suicidality risk** include prior attempts, degree of premeditation or plan, and access to a weapon or proposed plan.
    - If a high risk of suicidality is present, the clinician must hospitalize the patient to ensure his or her safety.

## Bipolar Disorder

A disorder characterized by **manic or hypomanic behaviors** that are sometimes accompanied by a depressive disorder. Lifetime prevalence is 1%, and the male-to-female ratio is 1:1. Individuals are at higher risk if family members are affected. There are two types of bipolar disorder: type I, which is characterized by at least one episode of mania, and type II, which consists of at least one hypomanic episode and one major depressive episode. The mean age of onset is around 19 years.

## SYMPTOMS

The symptoms of a manic episode of bipolar disorder are expressed in the mnemonic **DIG FAST:**

- **D**istractibility.
- **I**njudiciousness or **I**mpulsivity (poor judgment—e.g., spending sprees, sudden travel, sexual indiscretion, reckless driving).
- **G**randiosity (↑ self-esteem).
- **F**light of ideas (racing thoughts).
- **A**ctivities—psychomotor agitation; ↑ goal-directed activities (e.g., socializing, hypersexuality, ↑ productivity).
- **S**leep—↓ need for sleep.
- **T**alkativeness—pressured speech.

**Treatment phases of MDD:**

- **Acute phase:** About 12 weeks.
- **Continuation phase:** Full remission of symptoms, but at high risk for relapsing within the next 4–6 months. Continue antidepressant treatment at acute-phase doses and eventually taper down.
- **Maintenance phase:** For patients with a high risk of relapsing (e.g., those with a history of three or more episodes of MDD, who will have a recurrence 80% of the time), continue antidepressant treatment at acute-phase doses for prevention.

**Types of bipolar disorder:**

**Type I:** Has at least one manic episode with or without major depression.

**Type II:** Characterized by at least one hypomanic episode with a major depressive episode.

To qualify as mania, symptoms **must last 4–7 days** and must produce social or occupational dysfunction. If there is no social or occupational dysfunction, the symptoms qualify as **hypomania**.

### DIFFERENTIAL

- **MDD:** Characterized by depressive symptoms without manic or hypomanic episodes.
- **Schizophrenia:** Although bipolar patients may exhibit signs of psychosis during a manic phase, schizophrenics do not experience mania.
- **Attention deficit disorder (ADD):** Distractibility and impulsivity are components of bipolar disorder, but ADD patients do not exhibit other manic symptoms.
- **Cyclothymia:** Consists of mood swings between dysthymia and hypomania.
- **Medical conditions → manic symptoms:** Include use of illicit substances (methamphetamines, cocaine), thyroid disorders, Cushing's syndrome, HIV or HSV encephalitis, antidepressant treatment, steroid treatment, and neurologic disorders such as MS, frontal lobe syndromes, and temporal epilepsy.

### TREATMENT

- **Pharmacologic: Mood stabilizers** (lithium, valproic acid, carbamazepine, lamotrigine, atypical antipsychotics) **treat at least one phase** of bipolar disorder (mania or depression) **without worsening the other phase.** Therefore, antidepressants are not mood stabilizers, since they are known to precipitate mania.
- **Behavioral:** Individual therapy, CBT, and interpersonal therapy are useful in the treatment of bipolar patients. Establishing a therapeutic alliance is also key.

### COMPLICATIONS

- Associated with a high rate of **completed suicides** (up to 15%).
- Although bipolar disorder is not associated with a downward drift of socioeconomic status, patients have high divorce rates, multiple jobs, and a high incidence of achievement followed by decline.
- Bipolar disorder is associated with several **comorbid conditions;** 60% have **substance abuse,** and 50% have **anxiety disorders.**

## Premenstrual Dysphoric Disorder (PMDD)

A severe form of premenstrual syndrome (PMS) defined by nonspecific psychological, behavioral, and somatic symptoms occurring only during the luteal phase of the menstrual cycle. Affects 3–5% of menstruating women, and is often superseded by PMS in late adolescence or the early 20s. The condition tends to remain stable over time, with the majority of women seeking care in their 30s.

### SYMPTOMS

- Presents with depressed mood, feelings of hopelessness, self-deprecating thoughts, anxiety, tension, ↑ emotional lability, persistent and significant anger or irritability, anhedonia, lethargy, appetite changes, poor concentration, sleep disturbances, and a sense of being overwhelmed.
- Physical symptoms include bloating, breast tenderness, hot flashes, headache, and joint pain.

*Hypomania consists of manic symptoms that do not → social or occupational dysfunction.*

*Even if patients experience only one manic episode, they are diagnosed with bipolar disorder. The diagnosis is made regardless of the number of manic episodes experienced.*

*In cyclothymia, depressive symptoms are not of sufficient severity to warrant a diagnosis of MDD, and manic symptoms do not reach the threshold sufficient for a manic episode.*

### DIFFERENTIAL

- **PMS:** Characterized by mild luteal symptoms that do not interfere with performance or interpersonal relationships.
- **Mood disorders:** Symptoms do not resolve with menses.
- **Medical conditions:** Include dysmenorrhea, migraine, IBS, fibrocystic breast disease, and hypothyroidism.

### DIAGNOSIS

- Specified symptoms must be present and limited to the luteal phase.
- Must → significant impairment in one or more areas of daily life.
- Rule out medical etiologies or other psychiatric conditions.

### TREATMENT

- Recommend lifestyle changes such as aerobic exercise, dietary changes, ↓ caffeine, ↓ sodium intake, and a diet rich in complex carbohydrates.
- Stress reduction, anger management, and individual and group therapy may be of benefit.
- Nutritional supplementation with vitamin $B_6$, vitamin E, calcium carbonate, magnesium, and tryptophan.
- Pharmacologic treatment with antidepressants or anxiolytics.
- Ovulation suppression with GnRH agonists; danazol for severe symptoms refractory to other treatments.
- Bilateral oophorectomy should be used only in the most severe and refractory cases.

*Antidepressants → rapid cycling, in which patients have more manic-depressive episodes. It is therefore important to have a history that is ⊖ for manic episodes before starting a depressed patient on antidepressants.*

*PMDD is distinguished from PMS by the severity of its symptoms and by its disruption of performance and interference with interpersonal relationships.*

## Postpartum Major Depression (PMD)

A major depressive episode associated with childbirth. Affects one in ten childbearing women. Onset can begin 24 hours to several months after delivery, lasting several months to the second year postpartum.

### SYMPTOMS

Presents with depressed mood, anhedonia, sleep disturbance, ↓ energy, weight loss, a sense of hopelessness or guilt, ↓ concentration, thoughts of suicide or death, and thoughts of harming the infant.

### DIFFERENTIAL

- Normal physiologic response to childbirth.
- **"Baby blues":** Characterized by mild symptoms that usually peak after postpartum day 4 or 5 and resolve by postpartum day 10. Affects 30–80% of childbearing women.
- Preexisting psychiatric disorders.
- Medical conditions such as thyroid dysfunction and anemia.
- **Puerperal psychosis:** Affects 0.2% of postpartum women. Constitutes a psychiatric emergency.

### TREATMENT

- **Behavioral:** Individual or group therapy; couples therapy if indicated.
- **Pharmacologic:** Used in patients with moderate to severe PMD; treatment is the same as that for major depression (SSRIs, TCAs). There is no evidence of morbidity in breast-fed infants with SSRIs and TCAs, but the

*The mainstay of treatment for severe PMDD consists of SSRIs.*

*"Baby blues" typically peaks four or five days after delivery and resolves after ten days.*

*Postpartum psychosis is a psychiatric emergency.*

drugs and their metabolites have been found in breast milk. Weigh the risks and benefits, and discuss options with the patient.

- **Referral:** Any woman with suicidal/infanticidal ideation, no response to antidepressant therapy, or psychotic symptoms should be referred to a psychiatrist.

### PREVENTION

Identify those at risk prior to delivery (e.g., those with poor family support, stressful life events, a history of a mood disorder, or previous PMD).

### COMPLICATIONS

- Long-term use of fluoxetine during pregnancy and postpartum can → drug accumulation in the infant. Check infant blood levels after six weeks of breast-feeding.
- Check blood levels in infants exposed to antidepressants who have unexplained or persistent irritability.
- Untreated PMD can have serious adverse effects on the mother and can also adversely affect the emotional and psychological development of the child.

## ANXIETY DISORDERS

### Generalized Anxiety Disorder

Defined as excessive worrying that is out of proportion to the situation and lasts **at least six months.** There is a 2:1 female predominance, usually beginning in childhood or adolescence, and the prevalence is about 5%. The condition is generally **chronic** but has flares of worsening severity.

### SYMPTOMS

Presents with **excessive worrying and anxiety** about a variety of subjects more days than not, with difficulty controlling the worry. Three of the following must be present: restlessness, easy fatigability, poor concentration, muscle tension, insomnia, and irritability. Associated with significant functional impairment.

### DIFFERENTIAL

- **Post-traumatic stress disorder (PTSD):** Must have a precipitating traumatic event.
- **Major depression:** Accompanied by depressive symptoms.
- **Panic disorder:** Consists of discrete, short-lived panic attacks.
- **OCD:** Anxiety that is due to obsessions and is relieved by compulsions.

### DIAGNOSIS

Rule out medical causes (e.g., hyperthyroidism, substance abuse).

### TREATMENT

- **Behavioral:** CBT.
- **Pharmacologic:** Antidepressants, buspirone, and long-acting benzodiazepines (e.g., clonazepam).

## Panic Disorder

Characterized by **recurrent unexpected** panic attacks, with fear of additional ones occurring. Prevalence is up to 3.5% with a 2:1 female-to-male predominance. Onset is from late adolescence through the third decade of life.

### SYMPTOMS

- Characterized by episodes of **abrupt anxiety** that peak after 10 minutes and are associated with several features of **autonomic arousal.**
- Must include at least four of the following features of autonomic arousal: **palpitations,** tachycardia, chest discomfort, **shortness of breath,** nausea, a choking sensation, trembling, dizziness, **paresthesias,** sweating, chills, hot flashes, dissociation, and **fear of losing control or dying.**

### DIFFERENTIAL

- **Psychiatric:**
  - **PTSD:** Must have a precipitating traumatic event.
  - **Generalized anxiety disorder:** Characterized by continuous anxiety but no discrete attacks.
- **Medical:**
  - **Endocrine:** Hypoglycemia, hyperthyroidism, pheochromocytoma.
  - **Cardiac:** Arrhythmia, MI.
  - **Pulmonary:** COPD, asthma, pulmonary embolus.
- **Pharmacologic:** Side effects of medications (e.g., SSRIs, albuterol); acute intoxication.

### DIAGNOSIS

Rule out medical causes first (e.g., ECG, CXR, metabolic panel).

### TREATMENT

- **Behavioral:** CBT.
- **Pharmacologic:** SSRIs (fluoxetine, sertraline, paroxetine), benzodiazepines.

## Obsessive-Compulsive Disorder (OCD)

A chronic syndrome of intrusive, recurrent, undesired thoughts (**obsessions**) and/or uncontrollable repetitive behaviors or rituals (**compulsions**) that → significant distress in a patient's daily life. Prevalence is 2–3%, with a mean onset in the second decade. Rarely presents after age 35.

### SYMPTOMS

- **Obsessions: Recurrent** and persistent ideas, impulses, thoughts, or images that are perceived to be intrusive and meaningless and → anxiety or grief. Not anxieties about real-life problems.
- **Compulsions: Uncontrollable** repetitive behaviors or rituals. May temporarily relieve anxiety.

### DIFFERENTIAL

- **Obsessive-compulsive personality disorder:** Generally lacks the obsessions and compulsive behaviors and rituals common to OCD. Patients are perfectionists, with inflexibility and obsessive attention paid to detail.

*Agoraphobia, which is sometimes a complication of panic disorder, is fear of being in a place from which escape would be difficult, or where it might be difficult to get help if a panic attack were to occur.*

*Panic attacks come "out of the blue," whereas PTSD is caused by a precipitating traumatic event.*

*Long-acting benzodiazepines such as clonazepam are used to prevent panic attacks; short-acting benzodiazepines such as alprazolam are used to relieve attacks.*

Patients typically are not disturbed by their symptoms, whereas in OCD they often are.

- **Generalized anxiety disorder:** Anxiety tends to be generalized to all areas of the patient's life, and the patient does not present with ritual behaviors to relieve anxiety.
- **Schizophrenia:** The patient is typically unaware that the obsessions are a product of his or her own mind and will have other symptoms characteristic of schizophrenia, such as psychotic and ⊖ symptoms.

*Patients with OCD recognize that their obsessions are the product of their own minds.*

### DIAGNOSIS

The following criteria must be met to characterize a disorder as OCD:

- The presence of obsessions or compulsions.
- The patient is able to recognize that the obsessions or compulsions are to the **point of excess or unreason.**
- The obsessions or compulsions **interfere with daily living,** cause anguish, or are significantly time-consuming (> 1 hour in one day)

### TREATMENT

- **Behavioral:** Begin with CBT with the goal of stopping intrusive thoughts and behaviors.
- **Pharmacologic:** Generally, medications should be started once the patient has failed behavioral treatment. SSRIs are indicated and may need to be titrated to higher doses than those used to treat depression or other anxiety disorders. Clomipramine (a TCA) is also indicated in the treatment of OCD.

### COMPLICATIONS

Can → depression if untreated. Can also → significant impairment in one's life, such as loss of income, family stressors, and substance abuse.

## Post-traumatic Stress Disorder (PTSD)

Avoidance, hyperarousal, and **re-experiencing** of a traumatic, life-threatening event that overwhelms the person's coping mechanisms. Prevalence in the general population is 8% but is higher among those exposed to trauma (e.g., combat veterans). Risk factors include young age, a history of prior trauma, a history of mental illness, low intelligence, and minimal social support.

### SYMPTOMS

- **Re-experiencing:** The patient experiences frequent intrusive memories of the event. He or she feels as if the event were occurring again and also has sensations of reliving the event, flashbacks, hallucinations, and nightmares.
- **Avoidance/numbing:** The patient avoids any reminder of the event, such as conversations, people, and places. For example, a patient who has experienced combat may avoid all films about war. He or she may also feel detached from others, feel emotionally restricted, and have little hope for the future.
- **Hypervigilance:** The patient experiences hyperarousal, may be easily startled, and has a persistently elevated autonomic response characterized by difficulty sleeping, irritability, anger, and difficulty concentrating.

## DIFFERENTIAL

- **Acute stress disorder:** Similar to PTSD, but lasts < 1 month.
- **Adjustment disorder:** May have symptoms similar to those of PTSD, but not caused by a life-threatening, severely traumatic event.
- **OCD:** The patient experiences recurrent intrusive thoughts, but they are not the result of a severe trauma.

## DIAGNOSIS

- Patients must have witnessed or **experienced a life-threatening or severe injury-threatening event** that elicited a response of intense horror, hopelessness, and fear.
- Avoidance symptoms must be present.
- Re-experiencing symptoms must be present.
- ↑ arousal symptoms must be present.
- Symptoms must last > 1 month.
- Symptoms must → severe impairment and significant distress in the patient's life.

## TREATMENT

- **Behavioral:**
  - **CBT:** Effective, as is psychotherapy geared toward reducing survivor guilt, hopelessness, and anger.
  - **Family therapy:** May be helpful in reducing the ⊖ effects of PTSD on family members who may not understand or be aware of the trauma inflicted on the patient.
- **Eye movement and desensitization reprocessing (EMDR):** A technique used to ↓ ⊖ responses to trauma with rapid eye movements. The method of action is not well understood, and opinions vary as to its efficacy.
- **Pharmacologic:**
  - SSRIs (fluoxetine) or TCAs (desipramine, amitriptyline) can be used to treat depression.
  - For mood swings, mood stabilizers such as carbamazepine or valproic acid are effective. β-blockers such as propranolol can help ↓ hypervigilance, and benzodiazepines (alprazolam, clonazepam) can be used for anxiety.

## COMPLICATIONS

Comorbid conditions associated with PTSD include alcohol and substance abuse, MDD, somatoform disorders, dissociative disorders, other anxiety disorders, and ongoing trauma.

> Acute stress disorder is diagnosed when symptoms occur within one month of the event but do not last > 1 month. In PTSD, symptoms last > 1 month.

## Specific Phobias

Involve persistent and notable **fear of a specific thing or situation** → marked anxiety and avoidance that impair the patient's life. Has a prevalence of 10%. Fear of animals or natural environments (e.g., snakes, heights, water) and of blood and injections usually starts in childhood, whereas fear of situations (e.g., flying, small spaces) starts in childhood or in the second decade of life.

## SYMPTOMS

- Presents with persistent, marked fear that is **excessive** and unreasonable in relation to the object and situation.

*Fear is a normal reaction to an actual threat or danger. A phobia is an excessive and unreasonable reaction to a certain situation or object.*

- Exposure to the fear → **extreme** anxiety and panic.
- The patient recognizes that the fear is unreasonable.
- The object or situation is avoided or dreaded.

### DIFFERENTIAL

- **Panic disorder:** Panic attacks are not related to fear of a specific object or situation.
- **PTSD:** Panic symptoms are triggered by severe trauma.
- **Generalized anxiety disorder:** Anxiety is generalized and not related to a specific situation or object.

### TREATMENT

- **Behavioral:** CBT is geared toward extinguishing the anxiety response to the specific situation. This is done through **desensitization** or repeated exposures to the inciting agent.
- **Pharmacologic:** Antianxiety medications such as benzodiazepines can help ↓ anxiety and ↑ exposure to the offending object/situation.

## PSYCHOTIC DISORDERS

## Delusional Disorder

A chronic disorder of delusions (**fixed false beliefs**) that form a coherent system characterized by a certain level of plausibility. An uncommon disorder, with a prevalence of 0.01–0.05%.

### SYMPTOMS

- Presents with highly specific delusions forming a coherent belief system that seems somewhat plausible.
- Patients are otherwise normal and maintain a high level of functioning.

### DIFFERENTIAL

- **Schizophrenia:** Associated with more functional impairment, auditory hallucinations, and thought disorders.
- **Substance-induced delusions:** Seen primarily with CNS stimulants such as cannabis and amphetamines.
- **Medical conditions:** Include thyroid disorders, Huntington's disease, Parkinson's disease, Alzheimer's disease, CVAs, metabolic causes (uremia, hepatic encephalopathy, hypercalcemia), alcohol withdrawal, and other causes of delirium.

### TREATMENT

- Patients are often resistant to treatment or medications.
- The first goal is to create a strong physician-patient alliance. Avoid directly challenging the patient's beliefs, but do not pretend to be in full acceptance of the delusions.
- Low-dose **antipsychotics** are indicated (atypicals such as olanzapine or risperidone are preferred). **Antidepressants,** especially clomipramine, may be helpful.
- The goal of medications is to help the patient avoid acting on the delusion.

## Schizophrenia

A **chronic** disorder characterized by **delusions, hallucinations, behavioral disturbances,** and **impaired social function** (without any mental status changes). Prevalence is 1%, manifesting earlier (18–25) and more severely in males and later (26–45) in females, with an equal male-to-female ratio (1:1). **Prevalence is higher** in the presence of a ⊕ **family history** (10% if there is a sibling or parent with schizophrenia).

### SYMPTOMS

- Patients must have at least a **six-month period** of continuous symptoms.
- Symptoms include the following:
    - **Hallucinations:** Mostly auditory.
    - **Delusions:** Fixed false beliefs that are not shared by others in the same culture and that persist despite evidence to the contrary.
    - **Disorganized speech.**
    - **Catatonic** or bizarre behavior.
    - **Negative symptoms:** Flat affect, alogia (poverty of speech), avolition, lack of purposeful action.

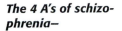

**The 4 A's of schizo-phrenia—**

**A**ffective flattening
**A**sociality
**A**uditory hallucinations
**A**logia (poverty of speech)

### DIFFERENTIAL

- **Mood disorders:**
    - **Bipolar affective disorder:** Psychotic symptoms tend to occur during manic or depressive episodes.
    - **Schizoaffective disorder:** Predominantly a mood disorder (mania or depression) with psychotic symptoms (lasting at least two weeks) during normal mood.
    - **Depression with psychotic features:** Depression predominates with superimposed psychotic features. Patients are not psychotic when depression improves or resolves.
    - **Delusional disorder:** Delusions tend not to be bizarre, and there are no associated symptoms such as hallucinations, thought disorders, or negative symptoms.
- **Drug-induced psychosis:** Amphetamines or cocaine can → paranoia and hallucinations. LSD, PCP, ketamine, and MDMA (Ecstasy) can all → psychosis. Typically accompanied by other signs of substance abuse.
- **Organic causes:** Include medical conditions such as neurosyphilis, dementia, delirium, complex partial seizures, Huntington's disease, heavy metal exposure, neoplasms, and medications (e.g., prednisone).
- **Negative symptoms:** If the patient has negative symptoms only, other disorders should be ruled out, including Parkinson's disease, depression, hypothyroidism, frontal lobe injury, PTSD, and substance abuse.

*Schizophrenia often starts with negative symptoms without the delusions or hallucinations (positive symptoms). This is called the* **prodromal or residual** *phase.*

### DIAGNOSIS

- Diagnosis is made by the history. Patients must have either bizarre delusions or hallucinations or two or more of the above symptoms (thought disorder, disorganized speech, catatonia, negative symptoms).
- Initially, **medical causes must be ruled out.** Consider BMP, calcium, CBC, TFTs, LFTs, VDRL, vitamin $B_{12}$, folate, HIV, a toxicology screen, brain imaging (CT or MRI), and EEG (if clinically indicated).

### TREATMENT

- Antipsychotics are the treatment of choice. **Atypical neuroleptics,** or second-generation antipsychotics, are **often first-line agents** (e.g., olanzapine,

*Atypical antipsychotics treat negative symptoms more effectively than typical or first-generation antipsychotics.*

quetiapine, risperidone), but typical or first-generation antipsychotics (e.g., haloperidol, fluphenazine, chlorpromazine) can be effective as well.

- Acutely, the goal of therapy is to **minimize symptoms and side effects** and, once the patient is stable, to titrate to the lowest effective dose that will maintain maximal functioning and prevent recurrence.
- Since 25–50% of schizophrenics continue to have residual symptoms and impaired functioning, psychosocial treatment is a component of therapy and includes **CBT, individual therapy, group therapy, family therapy,** and **social skills training.** In more severe cases, a **multidisciplinary team** (case manager, nurse, and physician) is often needed to prevent hospitalization.

### COMPLICATIONS

- Without treatment, patients with schizophrenia may experience "**downward drift**" in socioeconomic class.
- **Tardive dyskinesia** (involuntary movements of the tongue, lips, face, trunk, and extremities) can be caused by long-term treatment with typical antipsychotics such as haloperidol. This complication can be minimized through use of atypical antipsychotics or by adding benztropine concurrently with typical antipsychotic medication.
- Individuals with schizophrenia have an ↑ **rate of violence** that is seen more often with uncontrolled paranoia and disorganized symptoms.

## SUBSTANCE ABUSE DISORDERS

A 55-year-old man was admitted to your service for cellulitis two days ago and now complains of nausea, vomiting, and diarrhea. He appears feverish and diaphoretic and is yawning repeatedly. Exam reveals no abdominal tenderness, rebound, or guarding. You note that his eyes and nose are watering, and his pupils are unusually dilated. On further questioning, you find that the patient takes oxycodone, which he buys from a friend. What treatment do you give him to relieve his symptoms? Daily methadone.

**CAGE** *questionnaire for alcohol abuse:*

**C:** Have you ever felt the need to **C**ut down on your drinking?

**A:** Do you get **A**nnoyed when people talk to you about your drinking?

**G:** Do you feel **G**uilty or bad about your drinking?

**E:** Do you ever have an **E**ye opener (a drink first thing in the morning)?

*Substance abuse can be characterized either by brief episodes or by more chronic patterns. Substance dependence is recurrent despite the ⊖ results.*

The compulsion to use substances persists despite adverse consequences. Substance abuse disorders range from abuse to dependence (physical and emotional reliance on the substance). Commonly abused substances include the following:

- **Alcohol:**
    - The prevalence of alcoholism is 6% in women and 12% in men. Alcohol-related deaths are the **third leading cause of preventable deaths** in the United States. Some 49% of cases of alcoholism are family related.
    - In **men,** "safe" levels of alcohol consumption equal **two drinks per day**; in **women,** "safe" levels of alcohol consumption equal **one drink per day.**
- **Opiates:** The prevalence of opiate abuse is 6%, with a male-to-female ratio of 3:1. The age of onset is generally in the teens, with the death rate among opioid abusers 20 times greater than that in the nonusing population.
- **Stimulants:** Some 12% of people have used cocaine at least once in their lifetimes, 3% in the last year and 1% in the last month.

## SYMPTOMS/EXAM

Table 14.1 outlines the presentation and treatment of common substance abuse disorders.

## DIAGNOSIS

- All patients should be screened for substance abuse disorders. Questions should be asked in a **nonjudgmental** manner and in a **confidential** environment to ensure the most open responses. The **CAGE questionnaire** is an example of a tool used to screen for alcohol abuse disorders.
- **Substance abuse** requires at least **one** of the following criteria, in addition to not meeting the criteria for dependence:
  - Continued use in **physically dangerous** situations (e.g., drinking and driving).
  - **Legal problems** due to use.
  - Continual **failure to complete important obligations.**
  - Persistent use despite ⊖ social or interpersonal impact.

*The majority of people who abuse alcohol have a comorbid psychiatric disorder.*

**TABLE 14.1.  Presentation and Treatment of Substance Abuse Disorders**

| DRUG | MEDICAL COMPLICATIONS | WITHDRAWAL SYMPTOMS | TREATMENT |
|---|---|---|---|
| Alcohol | **General:** Cirrhosis, pancreatitis, ataxia, delirium, GI bleed, hepatitis, hypertension, cardiomyopathy, sexual dysfunction, depression, peripheral neuropathy, memory loss, depression, ↑ risk of cancer (esophageal, stomach, lung, colon). **In pregnancy:** Fetal alcohol syndrome. | **Early** (eight hours after last drink): Sweating, flushing, sleep disturbances, hallucinations, seizures, mild mental status changes. **Late** (48 hours after last drink): DTs (tremor, hallucinations, delirium, ↑ autonomic tone). | **Withdrawal: Benzodiazepines (long-acting, e.g., chlordiazepoxide).** **Long-term treatment:** **Naltrexone:** ↓ cravings and relapse. **Disulfiram:** → flushing, nausea, and vomiting when mixed with alcohol. **SSRIs:** ↓ cravings. |
| Cocaine | **General:** Hypertension, tachycardia, arrhythmias, vasospasm of coronary arteries (MI) and cerebral arteries (CVA), hemoptysis, chest pain, nasal septum necrosis, dehydration, malnutrition, weight loss. **In pregnancy:** Fetal hypoxia and placental abruption. | Depressed mood, fatigue, disturbing dreams, ↑ appetite, insomnia or hypersomnia, agitation or retardation. | No specific treatment for withdrawal; no pharmacologic treatments for dependence. |
| Opiates | **IV use:** Endocarditis, HIV, HBV/HCV, cellulitis, abscesses, septic arthritis, osteomyelitis, pneumonia, meningitis, pulmonary emboli, nephrotic syndrome. **In pregnancy:** Infant withdrawal. | Depressed mood, nausea, vomiting, diarrhea, yawning, insomnia, myalgias, runny nose, watering eyes, dilated pupils, sweating, fever. | **Withdrawal:** Methadone, clonidine, buprenorphine, clonidine-naltrexone. **Long-term treatment:** Methadone maintenance, buprenorphine, naltrexone. |

*The stages of behavioral change are precontemplation, contemplation, preparation, action, maintenance, and relapse.*

- **Substance dependence** requires **three or more** of the following criteria:
  - Physiologic **tolerance** or **withdrawal.**
  - Repeated **attempts to cut down** or stop using.
  - Use for a **longer amount of time** than was originally intended.
  - Main activities are **centered on the substance** (e.g., intoxication or obtaining drugs).
  - **Giving up important activities** for drugs (e.g., work).
  - **Persistent use** regardless of the knowledge that continued use can → physical or psychological problems.

### TREATMENT

- Before formulating an approach toward substance abuse, it is important for the clinician to understand what **phase of behavioral change** the patient is in. It is also crucial to recognize that substance abuse has a **relapsing and remitting pattern.**
- **Psychotherapy:** Methods include the following:
  - **Individual therapy:** Includes CBT, harm reduction (minimizing ⊖ effects of behaviors), and psychoeducation.
  - **Family support/education:** Essential in the treatment of abusers, since family members are strongly affected by ⊖ behaviors. Education (e.g., Al-Anon) helps families recognize what to expect and how best to be supportive.
  - **Group therapy:** Includes self-help organizations such as Alcoholics Anonymous. Such groups tend to focus on relapse prevention and maintenance of sobriety. Users are supported by peer mentors who have maintained abstinence.
  - **Therapeutic communities:** Residential treatment centers. Treatment duration is generally 6–18 months; communities tend to have strict limits and are highly structured. Associated with high dropout rates, but successful for highly motivated individuals.

## BEHAVIORAL DISORDERS

A 35-year-old woman comes to your office for an initial visit. Her chart is thick and shows multiple 1° care providers, numerous ER visits for self-mutilation, and a history of alcohol abuse. The woman states that she was referred to you by a friend, and throughout the visit she continually praises you, saying that you are not like the other doctors, who were just interested in prescribing pills and making a cut from the drug companies. On further questioning, the patient tells you that she hasn't had any stable partners because they all turned out to be shallow, empty users who didn't care about her. As she tells you more about herself, you begin to remember complaints about this patient and her inappropriate behavior in the waiting room. You suspect a personality disorder. What personality disorder does the patient have? Borderline personality disorder.

## Personality Disorders

Distinguished by **persistently inadequate adaptive capacities** and patterns of behavior → significant impairment in areas such as social relationships and occupational performance. Disorders start in **early childhood** and persist through adulthood. They are **always coded on Axis II.**

496

## SYMPTOMS

Personality disorders are classified into three clusters that share characteristics:

1. **Cluster A** (odd and eccentric):
   - Paranoid
   - Schizoid
   - Schizotypal
2. **Cluster B** (dramatic, emotional, and erratic):
   - Antisocial
   - Borderline
   - Histrionic
   - Narcissistic
3. **Cluster C (anxious and fearful):**
   - Avoidant
   - Dependent
   - Obsessive-compulsive

*Personality disorders are classified into three clusters: cluster A ("weird"–odd and eccentric), cluster B ("wild"– dramatic, emotional, and erratic), and cluster C ("wimpy"–anxious and fearful).*

## DIFFERENTIAL

- Distinguish from personality changes caused by a medical condition, mental retardation, and other Axis I disorders.
- Differentiating can sometimes be difficult, but personality disorders have an early-childhood onset and possess characteristics not found in Axis I disorders, such as intact reality testing, normal abstracting ability, and the absence of formal thought disorders.

## DIAGNOSIS

The diagnosis is made after several visits, when the persistent patterns of behavior become apparent.

## TREATMENT

- Because personality disorders are deeply ingrained, patients are often **resistant to treatment.**
- **Psychoanalysis** and psychodynamic psychotherapy help the patient recognize and change maladaptive behavior patterns.
- Although of limited utility, **pharmacologic treatments** are used in some cases. In **antisocial** and **borderline** personality disorder, mood stabilizers such as lithium and carbamazepine are sometimes used; in **paranoid** and **schizotypal personality disorder,** low-dose **antipsychotics** have been given.

## SOMATOFORM DISORDERS

A 22-year-old woman is brought to the office by her mother. She complains of sudden onset of bilateral blindness. She denies any trauma. Her mother states, "I can't believe this is happening. First her father is dying of cancer, and now this." As the patient moves toward the exam table, you are struck by how easily she avoids all obstacles that lie between her and the table. On exam, you note normal bilateral pupillary responses, and you are surprised that she has none of the expected bruises or scrapes. You order a visual evoked potential, and it comes back normal. What is the most likely explanation for your patient's symptoms? Conversion disorder.

A group of psychiatric disorders that share the common feature of **overimportance of physical symptoms (with no clear medical etiology)** in a patient's life. This often → a feeling of being misunderstood by health providers. Somatization can → inappropriate workups, hospitalizations, and procedures (up to $30 billion per year).

### SYMPTOMS

Generally categorized as follows:

- **Somatization disorder:** A **chronic** disorder characterized by **multiple clinically significant symptoms** that vary over time and are **not explained by medical findings.** Patients usually have an extensive treatment history with age of onset < 30. Has a higher prevalence in women.
- **Conversion disorder:** Usually characterized by self-limited symptoms that affect voluntary motor or sensory systems and **suggest a neurologic disorder** but are **not consistent with anatomic structures.** Age of onset is 10–40. **Preceded by stress.**
- **Hypochondriasis:** A chronic preoccupation with or **fear of having a serious medical disease** that is not relieved by appropriate evaluation or reassurance. Usually begins in early adulthood.
- **Body dysmorphic disorder:** Chronic preoccupation with **an imagined defect in physical appearance;** usually begins in adolescence.
- **Chronic pain syndrome:** An often chronic condition in which **pain without an identified organic cause** is the central feature.

### DIFFERENTIAL

- **Malingering:** Motivated by external gain; symptoms are intentional with poor cooperation in evaluation.
- **Factitious disorder:** Motivated by assumption of the sick role, in which symptoms are fabricated or self-inflicted. Histories are often vague, and patients go from hospital to hospital seeking care.

### DIAGNOSIS

A careful assessment and evaluation should be performed using standard medical workups, with an emphasis on avoiding exhaustive and unnecessary testing.

### TREATMENT

- Stress empathy along with the importance of establishing and maintaining a strong 1° care relationship.
- Avoid stratifying the diagnosis as mental or physical; address in "stress" terms or emphasize the mind-body connection.
- Co-morbid psychiatric disorders should be addressed and treated.
- Consider a psychiatry referral to provide a framework for treatment (not to take the place of the 1° care provider).
- Individual or group therapy may be of benefit, as may stress identification and reduction.
- Prevent iatrogenesis by limiting workup and treatments to objective findings (not complaints).

*Somatoform disorders are motivated by inner psychic gain; symptoms are unintentional or involuntary and are precipitated by stress.*

## Adverse Effects of Therapeutic Drugs

Table 14.2 outlines both common and potentially serious adverse effects associated with psychiatric drugs.

**TABLE 14-2.** Adverse Effects of Commonly Administered Psychiatric Drugs

| CLASS | EXAMPLES | COMMON SIDE EFFECTS | MEDICALLY SERIOUS SIDE EFFECTS |
|---|---|---|---|
| SSRIs | Paroxetine (Paxil), fluoxetine (Prozac), sertraline (Zoloft), citalopram (Celexa), fluvoxamine (Luvox), others | Sedation, weight gain, GI discomfort, sexual dysfunction. | Serotonin syndrome (tachycardia, hypertension, fever, hyperthermia, myoclonus, convulsions, coma). |
| Antidepressants | Bupropion (Wellbutrin) Venlafaxine (Effexor) | Insomnia, "jitteriness." Constipation, dizziness. | Lowered seizure threshold. Lowered seizure threshold, hypertension. |
| Mood stabilizers | Lithium | Cognitive dulling, tremor, sedation, nausea, diarrhea, T-wave flattening. | Lithium toxicity, **hypo**thyroidism (in long-term use), nephrogenic diabetes insipidus (DI). |
| Mood stabilizers/ anticonvulsants | Valproic acid (Depakote) Carbamazepine (Tegretol) | Weight gain, sedation, cognitive dulling. | Thrombocytopenia. SIADH, agranulocytosis, Stevens-Johnson rash. |
| Typical high-potency antipsychotics | Haloperidol (Haldol), fluphenazine (Prolixin) | Sedation. | Acute dystonic reactions, neuroleptic malignant syndrome, tardive dyskinesia (in long-term use). |
| Typical midpotency antipsychotics | Thioridazine (Mellaril), chlorpromazine (Thorazine) | Sedation, anticholinergic side effects (dry mouth, constipation, urinary retention, tachycardia). | Acute dystonic reactions, neuroleptic malignant syndrome, tardive dyskinesia (in long-term use). |
| Typical low-potency antipsychotics | Thiothixene (Navane), perphenazine (Trilafon), trifluoperazine (Stelazine) | Orthostatic hypotension. | Acute dystonic reactions, neuroleptic malignant syndrome, tardive dyskinesia (in long-term use). |
| Atypical antipsychotics | Olanzapine (Zyprexa) | Weight gain, sedation. | Hypercholesterolemia, possible diabetes mellitus. |
| | Risperidone (Risperdal) | Weight gain. | Hyperprolactinemia; side effects of typical antipsychotics (when used in high doses). |
| | Quetiapine (Seroquel) | | Cataracts. |
| | Clozapine (Clozaril) | Drooling. | Agranulocytosis. |

Reproduced, with permission, from Le T et al. *First Aid for the Internal Medicine Boards,* 1st ed. New York: McGraw-Hill, 2006: 550.

Handwritten note: *Paroxetine - C/I in pregnancy. fluoxetine - Safe in pregnancy*

## Psychotropic Medications During Pregnancy and Breast-feeding

Women and their physicians tend to **overestimate the teratogenic risk** of psychotropic medications during pregnancy and to **underestimate the risk of untreated maternal mental illness.** To prevent unnecessary terminations of pregnancy or untreated mental conditions, it is important to familiarize patients with both the benefits and the risks of psychotropic medicines in pregnancy.

- Antidepressants:
    - **TCAs: Not** associated with **major congenital malformations.** Reports do exist linking TCA use to postpartum irritability, shakiness, and urinary and bowel obstruction.
    - **SSRIs:** Extensive research has shown **no** association between **major congenital malformations** and **fluoxetine,** but preliminary studies show a possible increase in persistent pulmonary hypertension in the newborn (PPH) when SSRIs are given after 20 weeks' gestation. **Paroxetine** is contraindicated in pregnancy in the wake of recent studies showing an association with cardiac malformations. Other SSRIs have not been researched as extensively. However, case reports exist linking their use with perinatal irritability, hypoglycemia, and shakiness.
    - Both medications have also been shown **not to have neurobehavioral toxicity,** and children exposed in utero have been found to develop normally. In contrast, studies have shown that untreated depression does have a $\ominus$ effect on children's development.
- Mood stabilizers:
    - **Carbamazepine and valproic acid:** Both have a **well-established risk** of **neural tube defects** (1% and 5%, respectively). Carbamazepine may also ↑ the risk of neonatal hemorrhage.
    - **Lithium:**
        - Lithium use during the first trimester is associated with a **10–20% higher risk of Ebstein's anomaly** (tricuspid valve malformation). However, the **overall risk is still low (0.1%),** since the incidence of this anomaly is low to begin with.
        - Lithium remains the preferred medication for the treatment of pregnant patients with severe bipolar disease, as treatment in such cases can be considered to outweigh the risks.
        - In other patients, it may be safer to discontinue the medication in the first trimester and resume it in the second or third trimester.
        - In the perinatal period, hypotonia, cyanosis, and DI have generally been reported to be rare and self-limited.
- Antipsychotics:
    - **High-potency neuroleptics** are considered **safe** in pregnancy. By contrast, study data are limited with regard to the atypical antipsychotics (olanzapine, risperidone, quetiapine).
    - **Perinatal toxicities** (tremor, restlessness, dystonia) have been reported but tend to resolve within weeks. Limited data exist regarding the neurobehavioral effects of these agents.
    - Again, the **benefits** (such as ↓ substance abuse and continuity with prenatal care) must be **weighed against the above risks.**
- **ECT:** Considered safe and effective during pregnancy.
- **Medication use and breast-feeding:**
    - All psychotropic medications are **secreted in breast milk.** Therefore, infants of mothers taking such medications must be **monitored for behavioral changes.** In infants with symptoms, drug levels should be checked.

*Patients who do stay on lithium during their pregnancy should have a second-trimester level II ultrasound to screen for congenital anomalies.*

*Breast-feeding while taking lithium is considered a relative contraindication in light of the ↑ risk of lithium toxicity in dehydrated infants.*

- Carbamazepine and **valproic acid** are **not** contraindicated in breast-feeding but are associated with infant **thrombocytopenia** and **anemia**.

### Drug-Drug Interactions

The following psychotropic drugs can potentially interact with other medications:

- **Lithium:**
  - ↑ **lithium levels:** Thiazide diuretics, ACEIs, NSAIDs, metronidazole.
  - ↓ **lithium levels:** Theophylline, urinary alkalization (sodium bicarbonate).
  - **Cause neurotoxicity (rare):** Antipsychotics, carbamazepine, methyldopa, calcium channel blockers.
  - **Cause serotonin syndrome (rare):** SSRIs, TCAs.
- **Valproic acid:**
  - ↑ **valproic acid levels:** Aspirin, erythromycin, ibuprofen.
  - ↓ **valproic acid levels:** Phenobarbital, phenytoin, carbamazepine.
  - ↓ **efficacy of other agents:** AZT, warfarin, many benzodiazepines.
- **Carbamazepine:**
  - ↑ **carbamazepine levels:** Valproic acid, antifungals, calcium channel blockers, INH, protease inhibitors, grapefruit juice.
  - ↓ **carbamazepine levels:** Phenytoin, phenobarbital.
  - ↓ **efficacy of other agents:** Warfarin, benzodiazepines, many anticonvulsants, antidepressants, antipsychotics, OCPs.
- **SSRIs:**
  - ↑ **risk of serotonin syndrome:** MAOIs (contraindicated), lithium, serotonergic agents.

*Serotonin syndrome is a rare but sometimes fatal syndrome that presents as nausea, hyperthermia, hyperreflexia, agitation, autonomic dysfunction, muscle rigidity, delirium, and coma.*

PSYCHIATRY AND BEHAVIORAL SCIENCE

# Geriatric Medicine

Cynthia L. Salinas, MD

### Cataracts

- Opacity of the lens that ↓ visual acuity. Due to oxidative damage to the lens → deposition of insoluble proteins in otherwise transparent tissue. Risk factors include smoking, diabetes, atopic dermatitis, and cortico-steroid therapy.
- **Sx/Exam:** Presents with painless blurred vision. Symptoms are progressive, developing over months or years. Lens opacities can be grossly visible or seen as a diminished red reflex.
- **Dx:** Diagnosed with slit-lamp biomicroscopy during ophthalmologic exam.
- **Tx:**
  - The decision to treat is based on the degree of functional impairment imposed by the cataracts.
  - Surgery consists of removal of the cataract and placement of an intraocular lens.
  - Constitutes one of the most successful surgical procedures, improving visual acuity in 95% of cases.

A 79-year-old Caucasian ex-smoker presents to your office with several months of deteriorating eyesight. On further questioning he describes his bilateral vision as blurred and notes ↓ ability to read fine print. He also finds it difficult to discriminate features when he looks at objects straight on but reports intact peripheral vision. His visual impairment has not affected his driving. On exam you find opaque deposits on both retinas. What is the most likely diagnosis? Age-related macular degeneration is the leading cause of permanent visual loss in the elderly. Its exact cause is unknown, but the risk factors include age > 50, Caucasian ethnicity, female gender, family history, and a history of cigarette smoking.

### Age-Related Macular Degeneration (MD)

Deterioration of the macula → **bilateral central vision loss.** The leading cause of permanent legal blindness in the elderly. May be **atrophic** (dry) or **exudative** (wet); atrophic MD is the **most common** type.

#### SYMPTOMS

- Blurred vision is the earliest symptom of atrophic MD, whereas the classic early symptom of exudative MD consists of straight lines appearing bent or crooked.
- Reading vision is lost, whereas peripheral vision is often maintained (e.g., patients have difficulty with reading but less difficulty with driving).

#### EXAM

Small yellow-white deposits called **drusen** appear underneath the retina.

### TREATMENT

- Limited treatment exists for the **atrophic** type.
- Early laser photocoagulation surgery may delay or reverse visual loss in the **exudative** type.

## Glaucoma

A group of disorders characterized by ↑ intraocular pressure → irreversible damage to the optic nerve. Two forms are most relevant to geriatrics: open-angle and angle-closure glaucoma.

### OPEN-ANGLE GLAUCOMA

↑ intraocular pressure due to abnormal aqueous drainage through the trabecular meshwork of the eye. The **most common** form of glaucoma, accounting for > 90% of cases. There is an ↑ prevalence in first-degree relatives of affected individuals and in diabetics. May also develop after uveitis or trauma. Those at **high risk** include patients with a family history of glaucoma, African-Americans, patients > 65 years of age, and diabetics.

#### SYMPTOMS

- Insidious onset; patients are often asymptomatic until vision is seriously compromised.
- Characterized by bilateral peripheral vision loss → tunnel vision.
- Patients may also complain of "halos around lights."

#### DIAGNOSIS

- Diagnosis is made through visualization of an anatomically normal or "open" anterior chamber angle and through excavation or "cupping" of the optic nerve in the setting of ↑ intraocular pressure.
- Periodic ophthalmologic exams are the best way to diagnose the disease, especially in **high-risk** individuals.

#### TREATMENT

- Avoid anticholinergics that can worsen glaucoma.
- **Medications** include the following:
    - **β-blockers:** Timolol is an effective antiglaucoma agent and should be used to ↓ intraocular pressure and thus prevent irreversible optic nerve damage and loss of peripheral visual fields regardless of whether the patient has symptoms.
    - **Cholinergic agonists:** Pilocarpine is less effective as monotherapy than β-blockers. May cause myopia.
    - **Cholinesterase inhibitors:** Neostigmine is shorter acting.
    - **Carbonic anhydrase inhibitors:** Acetazolamide and dorzolamide can be used as adjunctive therapy. Long-term use may induce kidney stones or acidosis in predisposed patients.
    - **Prostaglandin analogs:** Latanoprost appears to be as effective as timolol.
    - **Osmotic diuretics:** Glycerin or mannitol is usually used for acute angle closure.
- **Surgical treatments:** Surgical trabeculectomy is recommended in patients whose intraocular pressure remains ↑ despite medical therapy.

## ANGLE-CLOSURE GLAUCOMA

An ophthalmologic emergency due to a closed anterior chamber angle. The only type of glaucoma that is curable. Accounts for roughly 10% of glaucoma cases in the United States. More prevalent among Asians.

### SYMPTOMS

- Rapid onset; usually unilateral.
- Presents with severe pain and profound vision loss.
- As intraocular pressure ↑, patients may experience nausea, vomiting, and abdominal pain that may be mistaken for an acute abdomen.

### EXAM

- Exam reveals a red, tender globe that may be firm to touch.
- A steamy or hazy cornea and a nonreactive, dilated pupil may be seen.
- Tonometry or palpation of the globe reveals ↑ intraocular pressure.

### DIFFERENTIAL

Angle-closure glaucoma must be differentiated from acute conjunctivitis, uveitis, and corneal disorders.

### TREATMENT

- Constitutes a **medical emergency,** requiring immediate referral to an ophthalmologist. Delayed treatment can → irreversible vision loss.
- Therapy for 1° acute angle-closure glaucoma consists of immediate intraocular pressure lowering via IV acetazolamide in conjunction with a topical agent followed by laser peripheral iridotomy. Usually → permanent cure.


## Retinal Detachment

Results from separation of the sensory portion of the retina from its pigment epithelium. Most often occurs in people > 50 years of age. Risk factors include aging, myopia, cataract surgery, trauma, and a family history of retinal detachment.

### SYMPTOMS

- Presents with unilateral blurred vision described by patients as a "curtain coming down over my eye."
- Marked by flashes of light and a shower of floaters.

### EXAM/DIAGNOSIS

- Exam reveals the retina hanging in the vitreous like a gray cloud.
- Diagnosis is based on an ophthalmoscopic exam in addition to the **clinical triad of eye flashes, floaters,** and a **visual field defect.**

### TREATMENT

Retinal detachments require immediate referral to an ophthalmologist. Treatment is surgical and is directed at closing retinal tears via cryotherapy or laser photocoagulation. Roughly 80% of uncomplicated cases can be cured with a single surgery.

A new patient arrives at your practice in tears. She is 76 years old, and her companion states that except for some minor arthritis pain, she is in excellent health and usually very lively. However, over the past year she no longer participates in social activities at their independent living community due to her embarrassment at being unable to understand her peers. She often perceives that others are mumbling, and she dreads the idea of needing a hearing aid, stating that it will make her feel old. Her last complete physical was three years ago. What is the most likely diagnosis? Sensorineural hearing loss. A thorough exam to rule out easily treated causes of conductive hearing loss (e.g., cerumen impaction) and referral for audiometry is warranted. Timely screening may have prevented this patient's isolation.

## Sensorineural Hearing Loss

Disease of the cochlea or the eighth cranial nerve (CN VIII) → bilateral hearing loss. Affects almost half of those > 75 years of age, making it the most common disability among the elderly. Timely treatment can help prevent social isolation, depression, and functional dependence on caregivers.

### SYMPTOMS

- Presents with bilateral, gradual, and usually symmetric hearing loss.
- Loss of speech discrimination is seen in noisy environments.
- Patients have ↓ ability to hear high-frequency (> 4000-Hz) sounds.

### EXAM

- Otoscopic exam may reveal findings that suggest conductive hearing loss (e.g., cerumen occlusion) or anomalies of the ear canal or tympanic membrane (e.g., otitis media, tumors, tympanosclerosis, perforation).
- Tuning fork tests such as the Rinne and Weber tests can be performed, but these yield limited information and should not be relied on for diagnosis.

TABLE 15.1.  **General Guidelines for the Interpretation of Audiometric Findings**

| DECIBEL MEASURE | AUDIOMETRIC FINDING |
|---|---|
| 0–25 dB | Hearing within normal limits. |
| 26–50 dB | Mild hearing loss. Patients will have trouble with soft sounds, with background noise, and when at a distance from the source of the sound. |
| 51–70 dB | Moderate hearing loss. Patients will have significant difficulties with normal conversational-level speech and will rely on visual cues. |
| 71–90 dB | Severe hearing loss. Patients cannot hear conversational speech and miss all speech sounds; however, they can hear environmental sounds, such as dogs barking and loud music. |
| 91+ dB | Profound hearing loss. Patients can hear only loud environmental sounds, such as jackhammers, airplane engines, and firecrackers. |

**GERIATRIC MEDICINE**

### DIFFERENTIAL

Metabolic derangements (e.g., diabetes, hypothyroidism, dyslipidemia, renal failure), infections (e.g., measles, mumps, syphilis), and radiation therapy are less common but potentially reversible causes of sensory hearing loss.

### DIAGNOSIS

- Audiometry is a standardized tool for recording hearing thresholds at different frequencies (see Table 15.1 and Figure 15.1).
- Frequencies **most important** for human speech are in the 250- to 6000-Hz range.
- Hearing loss accompanied by pulsatile tinnitus may signify a serious vascular abnormality such as carotid vaso-occlusive disease, aneurysm, AVM, or glomus tumor, warranting workup via MRA to establish the diagnosis.

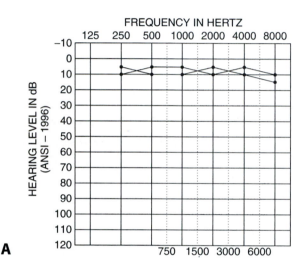

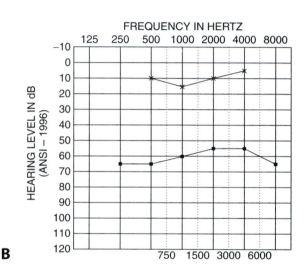

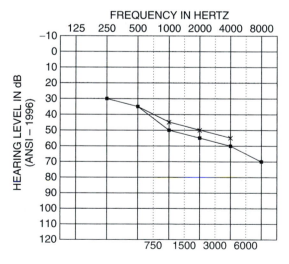

**FIGURE 15.1. Common audiograms.**

Examples of audiograms: A. Normal audiogram. B. Conductive hearing loss. C. Sensorineural hearing loss. * = bone conduction. ■ = air conduction. (Reproduced, with permission, from Lalwani A et al. *Current Otolaryngology—Head and Neck Surgery,* 1st ed. New York: McGraw-Hill, 2004: Figure 44-2.)

- **Hearing aids:** The 1° treatment for presbycusis; however, < 50% of elderly patients who might benefit from hearing aids actually wear them.
  - **Behind-the-ear aids:** The most powerful ear-level units; easier to see and manipulate.
  - **In-the-canal aids:** Smaller and more expensive; the best choice for patients with mild to moderate hearing loss.
- **Aural rehabilitation:** Most patients benefit from this treatment, which includes practical advice on how to optimize communication.

## Conductive Hearing Loss

Hearing loss that occurs when sound is not conducted efficiently through the ear canal, tympanic membrane, or ossicles of the middle ear. This type of hearing loss can often be medically or surgically corrected.

### SYMPTOMS/EXAM

- May present with painless sudden or gradual loss of hearing.
- Exam may reveal **obstruction** (e.g., cerumen impaction), **mass loading** (e.g., middle ear effusion), **stiffness** (e.g., otosclerosis), and **discontinuity** (e.g., ossicular disruption).

### DIAGNOSIS

*Sensorineural hearing loss is the most common type of hearing loss in the elderly.*

Tuning forks can be useful in differentiating conductive from sensorineural losses:

- **Weber test:** A tuning fork is placed on the forehead. In conductive losses, the sound appears louder in the poorer hearing ear, whereas in sensorineural losses it radiates to the better side.
- **Rinne test:** A tuning fork is placed alternately on the mastoid bone and in front of the ear canal. In conductive losses, bone conduction exceeds air conduction; in sensorineural losses, the opposite is true.

### TREATMENT

Treatment is geared toward correcting the underlying cause.

## DEMENTIA

An acquired **progressive impairment of memory** and **at least one** other domain of cognition, such as **abstraction, language, problem-solving ability, calculation, insight,** or **judgment,** that → a decline of activities of daily living (ADLs). Clinically significant impairment occurs in approximately 5–10% of those ≥ 65 years of age and in 20% of those > 80 years of age. Of the dementia types, Alzheimer's makes up 50–60% and vascular dementia 10–20% of cases; mixed Alzheimer's and vascular dementia constitute 20–30% of cases. Risk factors are listed in Table 15.2.

### SYMPTOMS/EXAM

- Presents with gradual, steadily progressive memory loss.
- Early on, social graces may give the impression of preserved intellectual function.
- Word-finding and concentration problems are common.

**TABLE 15.2.** Risk Factors for Dementia

| Strong Risk Factors | Additional Risk Factors |
|---|---|
| Age (especially for Alzheimer's type) | Head trauma |
| A family history of first-degree relatives | A history of depression |
| Apolipoprotein E e4 genotype | Low educational achievement |
| DM | Female gender (for Alzheimer's) |
| Hyperlipidemia | |
| Hypertension | |

- Difficulty with dressing, cooking, and balancing the checkbook occur.
- Late disease is characterized by severe memory loss, disorientation, and social withdrawal.
- Subtypes are distinguished clinically as follows:
  - **Alzheimer's dementia:** Characterized by visuospatial disturbances such as getting lost in familiar surroundings. Emotional lability and uncharacteristic behavior are also seen. A diagnosis of exclusion.
  - **Vascular/multi-infarct dementia:** Usually marked by a stepwise decline and by abrupt decreases in cognitive function alternating with periods of stabilization. More common in men; associated with a history of hypertension and stroke.

### DIAGNOSIS

- Obtain a complete history, physical, and mood assessment.
- The Mini-Mental Status Exam is the **best instrument** for screening for dementia. Remember that accuracy depends on age and educational level.
- **Labs:** Order a screening set of labs to rule out reversible causes of cognitive dysfunction, including CBC, serum glucose, electrolytes and creatinine, albumin, calcium, LFTs, TSH, vitamin $B_{12}$, and UA. Consider a VDRL in older patients suspected of having 3° syphilis.
- **Imaging:** Routine brain imaging is controversial. If imaging is obtained, a noncontrast CT is usually adequate and can help identify rare but potentially reversible causes of structural abnormalities such as subdural hematomas, hydrocephalus, and brain tumors.

### TREATMENT

- Discontinue nonessential medications, especially sedatives and hypnotics.
- Identify and treat coexisting depression, malnutrition, thyroid dysfunction, and occult infections. Eliminate home hazards and minimize social isolation. Provide emotional support to the family.
- **Medications:**
  - **Cholinesterase inhibitors** (donepezil, galantamine, rivastigmine) may temporarily extend independence, but studies suggest only a small benefit.
  - **N-methyl-D-aspartate (NMDA) antagonists** (e.g., memantine) with or without acetylcholinesterase inhibitors have been shown to have a statistical benefit in patients with advanced disease.
  - Vitamin E may slow progression of Alzheimer's.
  - Estrogen and NSAIDs have shown no benefits.

An acute fluctuation of mental status marked by inattention, inability to concentrate, and fluctuating levels of consciousness. Occurs commonly in elderly patients, and its incidence ↑ with hospitalization and/or surgical procedures. **Risk factors** include advanced old age, underlying dementia, functional impairment, and medical comorbidity and its treatments.

### SYMPTOMS/EXAM

- Presents with a ↓ ability to focus, sustain, or shift attention.
- Characterized by rapid onset with a fluctuating course.
- Disorganized thinking is manifested by rambling, irrelevant, or incoherent speech.
- Level of arousal may be ↑, as seen with the following:
    - **Hyperactive delirium:** Agitation is prominent; can be misdiagnosed as anxiety → inappropriate administration of sedatives, potentially delaying proper workup.
    - **Hypoactive delirium:** Psychomotor activity is ↓; frequently misdiagnosed as depression.

### DIAGNOSIS

- Obtain a thorough history from a caregiver or family physician to determine the frequency and duration of mental status changes.
- Perform a complete physical exam with assessment of vital signs and $O_2$ saturation.
- **Labs:** CBC, serum glucose and electrolytes, UA, and blood cultures are the most useful tests.
- **Imaging:** Head CT and LP are indicated for patients who are high risk (e.g., those with head trauma or focal neurologic findings) or when the physical exam does not confirm the etiology. ECG and CXR can reveal cardiac and pulmonary causes of delirium.

### TREATMENT

- Identify and treat any underlying disorders.
- Avoid physical and chemical restraints. Always provide clocks and/or calendars to orient patients.
- Patients who need eyeglasses and hearing aids should be encouraged to wear them.
- The presence of family members or caregivers who are known to patients can help reorient them.
- **Medications:**
    - **Low-dose antipsychotics** (haloperidol or risperidone): **Preferred treatments** for hyperactive delirium. Risperidone may have slightly fewer extrapyramidal effects than haloperidol. Start low and go slow.
    - **Benzodiazepines:** Last-line therapy to treat agitation. Frequent assessment of symptoms and patient response is key.

### COMPLICATIONS

- Hospitalized patients with delirium are at ↑ risk for deconditioning, pressure ulcers, atelectasis, and malnutrition → longer hospitalization and higher mortality.
- Although delirium is usually reversible, cognitive deficits may take weeks or even months to abate following resolution of acute illness.

---

*Delirium precipitating factors—*

**DELIRIUM**

**D**rugs—especially when a drug is introduced or changed

**E**lectrolyte and physiologic abnormality—hyponatremia, hypoxemia, acidosis

**L**ack of medication—withdrawal

**I**nfection—UTI, respiratory infection, sepsis

**R**educed sensory input—blindness, deafness, isolation, change of surroundings

**I**ntracranial problems—hemorrhage, meningitis, stroke, seizures

**U**rinary retention and fecal impaction

**M**yocardial problems—MI, arrhythmia, CHF

GERIATRIC MEDICINE

511

A syndrome characterized by **resting tremor, bradykinesia, muscular rigidity,** and **loss of postural reflexes.** A common disorder in those > 60 years of age; affects both sexes and all ethnic groups. Results from the depletion of dopamine in the **substantia nigra** → unopposed cholinergic activity.

### SYMPTOMS/EXAM

- Presents with resting tremor or "pill rolling" that is less severe during voluntary movement.
- Bradykinesia is often manifested as ↓ arm swinging while walking.
- Rigidity is usually evident during passive movement of limbs—e.g., "cogwheeling."
- Shuffling gait and impaired postural reflexes are seen.
- Masklike facial expressions and infrequent eye blinking are characteristic.
- Seborrhea of the scalp and face is common.

### DIAGNOSIS/TREATMENT

- Diagnosis is made on the basis of symptoms and neurologic exam (see Table 15.3).
- Discontinue drugs that can worsen parkinsonism (e.g., antipsychotics).
- **Nonpharmacologic treatment:** Regular exercise and physical therapy may help restore confidence and maintain balance; occupational therapy may be indicated to help patients learn strategies for carrying out ADLs and using adaptive equipment.
- Medications:
  - **Levodopa/carbidopa: First-line** treatment that has been shown to improve all major features of parkinsonism. Levodopa, a precursor of

**TABLE 15.3.** **Clinical Features of Parkinson-Plus Syndromes**

| SYNDROME | KEY FEATURES |
|---|---|
| **Dementia with Lewy bodies** | Cognitive decline, **visual hallucinations, misidentifications** of family/friends, marked **daily fluctuations** in mental status. |
| **Progressive supranuclear palsy** | Cognitive decline. Extraocular abnormalities, especially **vertical gaze.** Prominent **rigidity of the entire body,** leading to frequent **falls** and a **characteristic facial appearance** ("wide-eyed," scared expression). |
| **Corticobasal degeneration** | Cognitive decline; **"alien limb"** phenomenon; **limb apraxia;** inability to perform learned motor tasks (e.g., brush teeth, salute). |
| **Multiple-system atrophy** | Encompasses a group of Parkinson-plus syndromes. |
| Shy-Drager syndrome | **Autonomic dysfunction,** especially orthostatic hypotension. |
| Olivopontocerebellar atrophy | **Ataxia;** incoordination with mild parkinsonism. |
| Striatonigral degeneration | **Isolated parkinsonism;** no tremor; **no response to levodopa.** |

Reproduced, with permission, from Le T et al. *First Aid for the Internal Medicine Boards,* 1st ed. New York: McGraw-Hill, 2005: 486.

dopamine, is administered with carbidopa, a decarboxylase inhibitor that inhibits the peripheral conversion of dopamine, thereby reducing the amount of levodopa required for treatment while lowering the risk of side effects.

- **MAOIs:** Selegiline may be used as an adjunctive treatment to levodopa. It inhibits the degradation of levodopa and is sometimes used to improve declining response to levodopa.
- **Dopamine agonists:** Pramipexole and ropinirole are newer agents that are more selective than older agents and have fewer side effects. Effective in early and advanced disease.
- **Catechol-*O*-methyltransferase (COMT) inhibitors:** Tolcapone ↑ dopamine levels.
- **Surgical measures:** Thalamotomy or pallidotomy may be helpful for patients who become unresponsive to medical treatment or have intolerable side effects with medicines.

A disorder characterized by the unintentional loss of urine. Causes are multifactorial. **Transient factors** include inadequate mobility, motivation, or dexterity; confusion; and medications. **Established factors** include detrusor overactivity/underactivity or urethral obstruction. Left untreated, incontinence can → decubitus ulcers, UTI, sepsis, renal failure, and ↑ mortality. Social implications include loss of self-esteem, restriction of social activities, isolation, depression, and dependence on caregivers.

### Urge Incontinence

The **most common** type of incontinence in geriatric patients. Due to an overactive bladder.

#### SYMPTOMS/EXAM

- Patients feel the urge to urinate but cannot get to the toilet in time. Nocturnal incontinence may occur.
- Physical exam may reveal atrophic vaginitis and urethritis.

#### DIFFERENTIAL

Mixed, overflow, or stress incontinence vs. the diuretic effect of caffeine or medications.

#### DIAGNOSIS

- Postvoid residual (PVR) is the single most important test; if PVR is > 200, proceed to ultrasound.
- UA with cytology to rule out UTI.
- Cystoscopy in patients with hematuria to rule out irritative processes such as stones or cancer.

*Always check PVR before giving anticholinergics, as these drugs can → worsening incontinence in patients with a distended bladder.*

### TREATMENT

- **Nonpharmacologic:**
    - Pelvic muscle-strengthening exercises (e.g., Kegel exercises).
    - Bladder training such as urge suppression exercises and timed/prompted voiding.
    - Behavior modification, such as reducing caffeine intake, avoiding late-night fluid intake, and scheduling timed voids every two hours when awake.
- **Pharmacologic: Anticholinergics** antagonize acetylcholine at muscarinic receptors → bladder smooth muscle relaxation.
    - **Oxybutynin:** Can cause dry mouth.
    - **Tolterodine:** Efficacy is similar to that of oxybutynin, but with ↓ dry mouth symptoms. More expensive.
    - **Nortriptyline:** Has the fewest anticholinergic and orthostatic side effects of the TCAs. Check ECG first, as nortriptyline may worsen QT-interval prolongation.
    - Topical estrogen helps ↓ vaginal/urethral atrophy that may → urge incontinence.

## Stress Incontinence

Instantaneous loss of urine during a stress maneuver (e.g., sneezing, coughing, laughing) due to weak pelvic floor muscles or an internal urethral sphincter deficit.

### SYMPTOMS/EXAM

- Pelvic exam may reveal pelvic prolapse, but exam is often normal.
- **Rare in men,** but can develop after prostate surgery.
- Nocturnal symptoms are uncommon.

### DIAGNOSIS

Look for evidence of pelvic prolapse and causes of intrinsic sphincter deficiency such as use of α-adrenergic antagonists (e.g., terazosin), radiation, or surgical trauma.

### TREATMENT

- Kegel exercises to strengthen pelvic muscles. Reinforce, as patients often give up too early.
- α-adrenergic agonists (e.g., pseudoephedrine/imipramine) to contract the internal sphincter.
- Pessaries provide support to the vaginal walls and pelvic organs.
- Surgery is an effective treatment for women with pelvic prolapse and has a cure rate of 75–85%.

## Overflow Incontinence

Unpredictable dribbling of urine or weak urine stream due to underactive bladder. The **second most common** cause of incontinence in older men. Underactive bladder may be due to medications (e.g., calcium channel blockers/anticholinergics) or to detrusor denervation or injury (seen in diabetic neuropathy, tumors, radiation or surgery, or BPH).

Thorough history and exam.

### DIAGNOSIS

- **Check UA:** Do not assume that BPH is the only cause of a male patient's incontinence.
- PVR > 450 distinguishes overflow incontinence from stress/urge incontinence.
- **Urodynamic testing:** To differentiate overflow incontinence from urethral obstruction in men.

### TREATMENT

- Acute urinary retention and acontractile bladders require indwelling or intermittent catheterization.
- Prazosin or terazosin are $\alpha$-blockers that induce internal sphincter relaxation.
- Discontinue anticholinergics and narcotics that may $\rightarrow$ bladder relaxation; stop decongestants such as pseudoephedrine that may $\uparrow$ sphincter tone.

## Urethral Obstruction

Postvoid dribbling/urge incontinence from detrusor overactivity or overflow incontinence due to urinary retention. May be caused by BPH, prostate/bladder cancer, or urethral stricture.

### SYMPTOMS/EXAM

Thorough history and exam.

### DIAGNOSIS

- UA with cytology and PVR.
- Urodynamic testing to confirm obstruction prior to surgery.

### TREATMENT

- Surgical decompression is the most effective treatment for obstruction.
- Nonoperative candidates with urinary retention require intermittent or indwelling catheterization.
- $\alpha$-adrenergic antagonists such as terazosin may relieve retention associated with BPH.
- $5\alpha$-reductase inhibitors such as finasteride may partially relieve symptoms, but the onset of effect requires months.

## Mixed Incontinence

- A combination of stress and urge incontinence.
- **Sx/Exam:** The external sphincter is weak and the detrusor muscle is overactive.
- **Tx:** Geared toward the type of incontinence symptoms that predominate.

## Functional Incontinence

Involuntary loss of urine despite normal bladder and urethral function.

GERIATRIC MEDICINE

515

### SYMPTOMS/EXAM

■ Exam may reveal slow gait or difficulty undressing due to ↓ dexterity and/or cognitive impairment.
■ Sicca, Sjögren's syndrome, and anticholinergics can cause dry mouth → polydipsia and ↑ urine production and incontinence.

### TREATMENT

■ Redistribution of edema from CHF or stasis can → nocturia. Compression stockings may help ↓ accumulation of edema during the day and thus ↓ urinary incontinence at night.
■ Improving gait and dexterity can help functional incontinence.
■ A bedside commode or urinal can help accommodate functional impairments.

## OSTEOPOROSIS

An 83-year-old female patient with a history of hypertension presents with sudden onset of severe left-sided back pain that radiates to her left buttock. Her symptoms occurred when she bent over to pick up a laundry basket. She denies a loss of urine but reports numbness in her left leg. On exam you find a short, overweight woman in obvious pain, especially when sitting. You are unable to perform a straight-leg test due to her discomfort. What is the diagnosis? This patient has a vertebral fracture secondary to osteoporosis. Her age and sudden onset of back pain are core features of symptomatic disease. Although osteoporosis affects > 10 million individuals in the United States, only a small proportion are properly diagnosed and treated.

Age-related decline in bone mass → bone fragility and ↑ fracture risk. **Risk factors** include smoking, excessive alcohol consumption, a sedentary lifestyle, estrogen deficiency, female gender, Caucasian or Asian ethnicity, and prolonged corticosteroid use.

### SYMPTOMS

■ Typically asymptomatic until fractures occur.
■ Patients may complain of "getting fat," loss of waistline, and hip and neck pain.
■ Sudden acute back pain while performing routine activities such as lifting or bending may herald the first symptoms of osteoporosis and is usually due to vertebral fractures.

### EXAM

Classic findings include ↑ thoracic kyphosis and loss of height in a thin-habitus woman.

### DIFFERENTIAL

Osteomalacia, hyperthyroidism, hyperparathyroidism, Cushing's syndrome, multiple myeloma.

- CBC, chem 7, and TSH help exclude other correctable causes of bone loss.
- **Dual-energy x-ray absorptiometry (DEXA):** Measures loss of bone mineral density (BMD); the **most accurate and precise method** to diagnose osteoporosis.
- **T-scores:** Compare values to normal and healthy bones of young adults. Osteoporosis represents a T-score of −2.5 (i.e., a BMD that is 2.5 SDs below normal).
- **Z-scores:** Compare a patient's BMD with those of age- and sex-matched controls. Used to track accelerated osteoporosis and treatment response.

*TREATMENT*

- **Nondrug therapy:**
  - **Diet:** Should include adequate protein, calcium, and vitamin D. The goal calcium intake is 1500 mg/day along with 800 IU of daily vitamin D.
  - **Exercise:** Weight-bearing exercise such as walking can help strengthen bones.
  - **Smoking cessation:** Lifelong smoking is known to accelerate bone loss. Encouraging smoking cessation will help ↓ the risk of osteoporosis.
- **Medical therapy:**
  - **Bisphosphonates:** Alendronate and risedronate are first-line treatments that ↑ bone mass and ↓ the incidence of vertebral and nonvertebral fractures. Effective in women with established osteoporotic fractures.
  - **Selective estrogen receptor modulators (SERMs):** Raloxifene ↑ BMD and ↓ total LDL cholesterol concentrations while reducing the incidence of vertebral fractures. Less effective than bisphosphonates.
  - **PTH:** Teriparatide is recombinant human PTH that stimulates bone formation. It is a good choice for high-risk patients who have failed previous treatment. Drawbacks include high cost, daily injection, and risk of osteosarcoma. Contraindicated in patients with Paget's disease.
  - **Calcitonin:** Second-line therapy for the treatment of osteoporosis, but can be used for its analgesic effects in patients who have substantial pain from an acute osteoporotic fracture. Drawbacks include high cost and poor adherence due to the intranasal and SQ route of administration.
  - **Thiazides:** For postmenopausal women who also have hypertension, treatment with a thiazide diuretic modestly attenuates bone loss via its hypocalciuric effects.

## CONSTIPATION

Attributable partly to normal physiologic changes such as ↑ rectal compliance, impaired rectal sensation, and weak pelvic floor and abdominal muscles. Often exacerbated by underlying medical and surgical conditions.

*SYMPTOMS*

- Characterized by ↓ stool frequency, difficult passage of feces, and/or a feeling of incomplete evacuation.
- Severe fecal impaction can → symptoms of intestinal obstruction, colonic ulceration, overflow fecal incontinence, and paradoxical diarrhea.

### EXAM

- An enlarged rectum is seen with fecal impaction.
- Hemorrhoids, anal fissures, and rectal prolapse result from excessive straining

### DIAGNOSIS

- Identify misperceptions about normal bowel movement frequency.
- Screen for depression and anxiety to uncover contributing factors.
- Review the physical exam to exclude anal or rectal masses.
- Chem 7 and TSH to exclude metabolic factors; abdominal x-ray to identify the distribution of stool and findings that warrant surgical consultation.
- Colonoscopy to evaluate for structural lesions.

### TREATMENT

- **Dietary** and **behavioral changes** constitute the **first-line** approach to correcting constipation.
- Include the following:
    - ↑ hydration and foods high in fiber with fiber supplementation if needed.
    - ↑ exercise to strengthen abdominal muscles important in defecation.
    - Laxatives are third-line therapy and include lactulose and sorbitol for chronic constipation. Stool softeners (e.g., docusate) are helpful for patients who are on opiates or who are bedridden. Stimulant laxatives (e.g., senna, cascara) augment the effect of stool softeners and are best reserved for short-term use.
    - Enemas are best employed when fecal impaction is present.

## FALLS

Falls are a major cause of morbidity and mortality, especially for women. More than 50% of community-dwelling seniors > 80 years of age fall each year, and falls are the sixth leading cause of death in the elderly. Table 15.4 lists common causes of falls and their appropriate interventions.

### COMPLICATIONS

Falls can lead to fractures of the wrist, vertebrae, and hip. The mortality rate is 20% in one year in elderly women with hip fractures.

TABLE 15.4. **Causes and Treatment of Falls**

| | INTERVENTIONS | |
| RISK FACTORS | MEDICAL | REHABILITATIVE/ENVIRONMENTAL |
| --- | --- | --- |
| ↓ visual acuity | Corrective lenses; cataract extraction. | Home safety assessment. |
| ↓ hearing | Cerumen removal; audiologic evaluation. | Hearing aid. |
| Vestibular dysfunction | Avoid drugs affecting the vestibular system; ENT evaluation. | Physical therapy for habituation. |
| Proprioceptive dysfunction | Screen for cervical spondylosis and vitamin $B_{12}$ deficiency. | Gait and balance exercises. |
| Dementia | Avoid sedative drugs. | Gait and balance exercises. |
| Postural hypotension and syncope | Assess medications and consider carotid and cardiac ultrasounds to assess for carotid artery and aortic valve stenosis; rehydration. | |
| Medication assessment | ↓ polypharmacy; select the least centrally acting drugs; prescribe the lowest effective dose. Frequent reassessment of risks and benefits. | |

Adapted, with permission, from Tierney LM et al. *Current Medical Diagnosis & Treatment,* 40th ed. New York: McGraw-Hill, 2000: 60.

## PRESSURE ULCERS

Skin breakdown often attributable to ↓ subcutaneous fat, poor nutrition, and poor circulation in the setting of prolonged pressure and friction over bony prominences such as the hip and sacrum. Immobilization and incontinence are major risk factors for the development of pressure ulcers.

### SYMPTOMS/EXAM

Staging is as follows:

- **Stage 1:** Nonblanchable erythema of intact skin.
- **Stage 2:** Partial-thickness superficial skin loss up to subcutaneous tissue.
- **Stage 3:** Full-thickness skin loss through subcutaneous tissue.
- **Stage 4:** Tissue loss down to the level of muscle, tendon, or bone.

### DIFFERENTIAL

Infectious ulcers (actinomycotic or herpetic ulcer), thermal burns, malignant ulcers (cutaneous lymphoma, basal cell carcinoma or squamous cell carcinoma), rectocutaneous fistula.

### TREATMENT

- ↓ pressure, friction, and shearing forces via frequent repositioning and employment of protective devices such as pillows, foam or sheepskin, and special beds.
- ↓ moisture by treating bladder and bowel incontinence, and provide adequate nursing care to keep affected areas clean.

GERIATRIC MEDICINE

- Evaluate nutritional status and consider zinc supplementation.
- Mobilize the patient as soon as possible.

## INSOMNIA

Impaired ability to fall and stay asleep. Up to 50% of elderly people report sleep problems. Factors that contribute to sleep disorders include the following:

- **Psychiatric:** Bereavement, social isolation, anxiety, depression.
- **Neurologic:** Dementia → nocturnal agitation.
- **Medication:** Includes sedative-hypnotics, bronchodilators, diuretics, decongestants, and caffeine.
- **Pain syndromes:** Neuropathic pain, arthritic pain, malignancy syndromes.
- **Respiratory:** Dyspnea from cardiac and pulmonary conditions.

Sleep consists of two types of sleep: nonrapid eye movement (NREM) and rapid eye movement (REM). Sleep is a cyclical phenomenon with alternating NREM and REM sleep. A majority of time is spent in NREM sleep. NREM sleep has four stages: stages 1 and 2, defined as light sleep, and stages 3 and 4, consisting of deep restorative sleep. Age-related changes in normal sleep include an unchanging percentage of REM sleep and a marked ↓ in stage 3 and 4 NREM sleep.

### SYMPTOMS/EXAM

Presents with difficulty falling asleep, intermittent wakefulness during the night, early-morning awakening, and daytime sleepiness.

### DIAGNOSIS/TREATMENT

- Evaluate for stress, depressed mood, level of physical activity, and dietary habits.
- Consider sleep apnea and/or restless leg syndrome in the patient and/or the partner.
- Identify sleep hygiene patterns that may worsen insomnia and recommend the following:
  - Adherence to regular sleep time and morning rise time.
  - Limitation of daytime napping.
  - Avoidance of caffeine, alcohol, and nicotine in the evening.
  - Limitation of nighttime fluid intake.
  - Limitation of noise, uncomfortable beds, and inappropriate temperature settings.
  - Avoidance of benzodiazepines and antihistamines that ↑ the likelihood of falls and hip fractures.

## POSTHERPETIC NEURALGIA (PHN)

- Exquisite pain that persists after the initial rash of herpes zoster has healed. Can occur at any age, but has a peak incidence in patients 50–70 years of age. The duration and severity of PHN ↑ sharply with age.
- **Sx/Exam:** Symptoms vary but can include constant pain; deep aching, burning pain; spontaneous intermittent lancing pain; or hyperesthesia. Pain is unilateral. There are no specific exam findings.

- **Dx:** Diagnosis is made by a history of a vesicular rash that resolves and is followed by the pain syndrome.
- **Tx:**
  - Once established, PHN is difficult to treat. The most effective treatment is prevention with early and aggressive antiviral therapy.
  - Capsaicin ointment, lidocaine patches, gabapentin, pregabalin and TCAs are helpful. Regional anesthetic blocks with or without steroids can also be considered for resistant cases. Narcotics should be avoided.
  - A new live attenuated varicella-virus vaccine (Zostavax) has been shown to ↓ the occurrence of herpes zoster, and consequently the frequency of PHN, in patients 70 years and older.

## POLYPHARMACY

Defined as problems that can occur when patients are taking more medications than are actually needed, rendering them prone to dosage errors and adverse drug reactions. Changes in physiologic function and pharmacokinetics promote ↑ sensitivity to medications, increasing the possibility of iatrogenic illness. Such factors include the following:

- **Distribution:**
  - ↓ total body water → more concentrated water-soluble drugs.
  - ↑ in body fat → longer half-lives of fat-soluble drugs.
  - ↓ albumin levels ↓ protein binding of some drugs (e.g., warfarin, phenytoin), leaving the more active drug available.
- **Metabolism:**
  - **Phase I:** Hepatic enzyme activity (e.g., cytochrome P-450) is ↓ and thus affects the metabolism of drugs with high first-pass metabolism (e.g., propranolol).
  - **Phase II:** Conjugation by acetylation, glucuronidation, or sulfation is not affected by aging.
- **Excretion:** ↓ GFR → ↓ excretion of drugs.

### SYMPTOMS/EXAM

May present with delirium, nausea, anorexia, weight loss, hypotension, and ARF.

### DIAGNOSIS

- Adverse drug reactions must be considered as a potential cause of ill presentations in the elderly.
- Obtain a thorough history of both prescribed and OTC medications, including cold pills containing antihistamines that can → anticholinergic effects.

### TREATMENT

- Ensure that the symptom requiring treatment is not itself due to another drug.
- Use drug therapy only after nonpharmacologic methods have been tried.
- Start with less than the usual adult dosage and ↑ slowly.
- Simplify dosage schedule and number of pills, and avoid frequent medication changes.

You have assigned the care of a patient with end-stage metastatic prostate cancer to your second-year resident. While on call your resident finds herself paged to the patient's bedside every hour to address inadequate pain control, and each time she diligently assesses the patient. She writes another order to increase IV hydromorphone and goes to her call room to catch some sleep prior to morning rounds. Shortly thereafter you receive a frantic call from your resident stating that she is afraid that she has killed the patient. She feels terrible and believes she should quit medicine. How should you respond? End-of-life care can present very challenging ethical issues. The doctrine of double effect argues that the potential to hasten imminent death is acceptable if it comes as an unintended consequence of a 1° intention to provide comfort and relieve suffering.

End-of-life care focuses on care of the whole person who is approaching death rather than on curing the underlying disease. Central to end-of-life care is the physician's responsibility to help the patient understand that his or her life is ending; that treatment of physical pain and reversible illness will continue; and that emotional, psychological, social, and spiritual needs will be valued. Physicians must also appreciate the central role played by the family and help them come to terms with the imminent loss of a loved one.

## Ethical and Legal Issues

End-of-life care is guided by the same ethical principles that inform other types of medical care. In addition, there are three unique ethical considerations that are relevant to end-of-life care:

- **Medical futility:** A unilateral decision by the physician to forgo futile interventions. May create conflict between the physician and the patient or family, but such conflict can usually be resolved through timely, frequent, and consistent communication.
- **Withdrawal of care:** The concept that the patient has the right to stop unwanted treatments once begun, as well as to refuse those treatments before they are started.
- **Doctrine of double effect:** Argues that the potential to hasten imminent death is acceptable if it comes as an unintended consequence of a 1° intention to provide comfort and relieve suffering.

### DECISION-MAKING CAPACITY

Considered intact when a patient can communicate a choice that takes into account the risks, benefits, and consequences of that choice. Must be consistent with the patient's values and goals.

## INFORMED CONSENT

A process in which a patient is given information about the nature of the intervention, the expected risks and benefits, the likely consequences, and the alternatives to the interventions.

## ADVANCE DIRECTIVES

Oral or written statements that allow patients to express their preferences and values to guide care if they can no longer make informed decisions. Valid only for futile care or terminal illness. Include the following:

- **Living will:** Patients direct their physicians to withhold or withdraw life-sustaining treatment if they develop a terminal condition or enter a persistent vegetative state.
- **Durable power of attorney for health care:** Patients designate a surrogate to make proxy decisions when they themselves are unable to communicate their wishes **or** lose decision-making capacity. Applies to all health situations, not just terminal illness.
- **Do not resuscitate (DNR) orders:**
    - Only 15% of all patients who undergo CPR in the hospital survive to hospital discharge.
    - Patients should be informed of mortality outcomes as well as the potential $\ominus$ consequences of surviving CPR (e.g., neurologic disability, damage to internal organs, likelihood of requiring other aggressive interventions).

## Hospice Care

- Focuses on the patient and family rather than on the disease; emphasizes the provision of comfort and pain relief rather than treating illness and prolonging life.
- Only 15% of all patients who die receive hospice care despite evidence that hospice ↑ family satisfaction and ↓ anxiety.
- Requires physicians to estimate the patient's probability of survival as < 6 months.

## Symptom Management

The following tasks are aimed at maximizing quality of life:

- **Pain:**
    - Very common, but often inadequately treated.
    - Assess pain via numeric and visual facial pain scales.
    - Allow the patient to set goals of pain management.
    - Regularly assess and treat side effects of opioids such as nausea and constipation.
    - There is no maximum allowable dosage for opioids such as morphine sulfate.
- **Dyspnea:**
    - A sensation of dyspnea is common among dying patients.
    - Identify treatable causes (e.g., pneumonia, pleural effusion).
    - Buccal morphine sulfate is highly effective; benzodiazepines may help anxiety.
    - Consider supplemental $O_2$ or open windows for fresh air.

- **Nausea and vomiting:**
  - If opioid related, consider substituting an equianalgesic dose of another opioid or a sustained-release formulation, or add a dopamine antagonist antiemetic (e.g., haloperidol) to block the chemoreceptor trigger zone.
  - If due to an intra-abdominal process such as constipation, gastroparesis, or gastric outlet obstruction, consider NG suction, laxatives, prokinetic agents, high-dose corticosteroids, and ondansetron.
  - Around-the-clock dosing of antiemetics and as-needed benzodiazepines are also highly effective.
- **Constipation:**
  - Opioids, poor dietary intake, and physical inactivity make constipation common among the dying.
  - Anticipating and preventing constipation via prophylactic bowel regimens of stool softeners and stimulants should be started when opioid treatment is begun.
  - Consider simple considerations such as privacy, undisturbed toilet time, and a bedside commode in appropriate patients.
- **Delirium and agitation:**
  - Many terminally ill patients experience delirium before death.
  - Nonpharmacologic strategies to help orient patients may be sufficient to ↓ delirium when no other reversible causes are identified.
  - Haloperidol or risperidone can be highly effective.
  - It may be acceptable to do nothing if the delirium does not negatively affect the family or patient.

### Nutrition and Hydration

- Individuals at the end of life have the right to refuse nutrition and hydration.
- Eating without hunger and artificial nutrition can → potential complications such as nausea, vomiting, choking, and aspiration.
- Starvation is associated with ketonemia, which can → a sense of well-being, analgesia, and mild euphoria.
- Allow the family to express concerns, and remind them that withholding nutrition at the end of life engenders little hunger or distress.

### Withdrawal of Support

- Requests for withdrawal of care from informed and competent patients or their surrogates must be respected.
- Physicians may determine medical futility and cease further medical intervention.
- Educate the patient and family on the expected course of events and the difficulty involved in determining the precise timing of death after withdrawal of support.

### Psychological, Social, and Spiritual Issues

- Invest time in family meetings to allow patients and families to raise concerns, to share memories, and to grieve and let go.
- Dying may intensify the need for the patient to feel cared for by their doctor, highlighting the physician's obligation to provide compassion and empathy.

- Remain attentive to patients' spiritual need to understand the underlying meaning of their lives and their experience in the world.
- Attempt to understand how cultural beliefs and ethnic traditions can affect the experience of dying.

## ELDER ABUSE

An intentional or unintentional act that → harm to an elderly person. According to the best available estimates, between one and two million elderly Americans are abused each year. These types of abuse include both verbal and physical abuse as well as neglect and financial exploitation. This abuse often goes unreported. Domestic and institutional **risk factors** for abuse include isolation, poverty, lack of community resources, a low staff-to-patient ratio, low compensation, and staff burnout. Table 15.5 outlines the characteristics of victims and their abusers; Table 15.6 lists the types of elder abuse and their clinical presentation.

*Elder abuse is widespread but often goes unreported.*

### SYMPTOMS/EXAM

- Symptoms are wide-ranging and may include unexplained withdrawal from normal activities, depressed mood, or a strained or tense relationship with the caregiver or spouse.
- Exam may reveal findings of poor hygiene, unusual weight loss, or bedsores, bruises, pressure marks, broken bones, and abrasions.

### DIAGNOSIS

Ask screening questions **while the patient is alone.** Inquire about perceived safety and violence in the family. Ask about the patient's dependency on caregivers, friends, and family.

### TREATMENT

- Document the type, frequency, and severity of abuse. Assess the decision-making capacity of the victim.
- Health care providers are mandated by law to report suspected elder mistreatment. Reports should be given to the state or county division of Adult Protective Services. In the absence of such services, the reporter should contact the county or state extension office of Child and Family Services.
- If the patient has the capacity to make decisions and refuses intervention:
  - Educate the patient about the incidence of mistreatment of the elderly and the tendency for mistreatment to ↑ in frequency and severity over time.
  - Provide written information about emergency assistance numbers.

*Elder abuse rarely resolves spontaneously. It tends to escalate in the same way as spousal abuse.*

**TABLE 15.5. Characteristics of Elder Abuse Victims and Abusers**

| CHARACTERISTICS OF VICTIMS | CHARACTERISTICS OF ABUSERS |
|---|---|
| Physical and emotional dependence on caregiver | Related to the victim |
| | Often substance abusers |
| > 75 years of age | Dependent on the victim for money and housing |
| Recent deterioration of health | |
| History of family violence | Long duration of care for the victim |

**TABLE 15.6.** **Types and Characteristics of Elder Abuse**

| TYPE | DESCRIPTION |
| --- | --- |
| Domestic | Maltreatment of an older adult living at home or in a caregiver's home. |
| Institutional | Maltreatment of an older adult living in a residential facility. |
| Self-neglect | Behavior of an older adult who lives alone that threatens his or her own health or safety. |
| Physical abuse | Intentional infliction of physical pain or injury. |
| Financial abuse | Improper or illegal use of the resources of an older person without his/her consent, benefiting a person other than the older adult. |
| Psychological abuse | Infliction of mental anguish (e.g., humiliating, intimidating, threatening). |
| Neglect | Failure to fulfill a caretaking obligation to provide goods or services (e.g., abandonment; denial of food or health-related services). |
| Abandonment | Desertion of an elderly person by someone who has assumed responsibility for providing care to that person. |
| Sexual abuse | Nonconsensual sexual contact of any kind. |

Reproduced, with permission, from Le T et al. *First Aid for the Internal Medicine Boards,* 1st ed. New York: McGraw-Hill, 2005: 298.

- Develop and review a safety plan.
- Refer the patient to agencies that provide respite care, support for personal care, and transportation.
- If the patient **does not** have the capacity to make decisions, the physician should initiate the process of separating the victim from the perpetrator while arranging supportive services for the whole family, including the abuser.

# CHAPTER 16

# Reproductive Health

Sarah-Anne Schumann, MD

Jessica Stanton, MD

Debra Stulberg, MD

REPRODUCTIVE HEALTH

# OBSTETRICS

Given that some 40% of pregnancies are unplanned, any medical visit with a female patient of childbearing age should be considered an opportunity to offer basic prepregnancy counseling, regardless of the patient's pregnancy plans. Preconception risk assessment and counseling specifically reduces neonatal morbidity and mortality in women with medical disorders (especially metabolic and autoimmune diseases), nutritional deficiencies, and teratogen exposure (e.g., recreational drugs, cigarettes, EtOH, warfarin, isotretinoin).

## Preconception Risk Assessment

A thorough preconception risk assessment should include the following elements:

- **Past medical history:** See above.
- **Dietary habits:** Determine body mass index (BMI), food restrictions, and diabetic risk; ascertain if caffeine intake is > 250 mg daily.
- **Medication history:** Ask about prescription drugs, OTC medications, and herbal supplements.
- **Substance abuse:** Inquire about EtOH and illicit drug use.
- **Environmental exposures:** Determine if the patient has a history of exposure to toxins (e.g., organic solvents or lead), radiation, or infectious agents (e.g., toxoplasmosis, rubella, parvovirus).
- **Age and reproductive history:** Ask about past gynecologic or pregnancy complications and DES exposure.
- **Family history:** Ask about CF, thalassemia, sickle cell anemia, birth defects, endocrine disorders, thromboembolic disease, and multiple gestation.
- **Psychosocial history:** Inquire about domestic violence, financial stability, emotional support, and barriers to care.

## Preconception Lab Workup

- **Routine prenatal labs:** Labs should include CBC, ABO/Rh, rubella titer, hepatitis B antigen, RPR, Pap smear, chlamydia screening in women < 25 years of age or at risk, gonorrhea in women at risk, and HIV testing.
- Other labs should be obtained in accordance with the following guidelines:
  - **Varicella titer:** If patients have no history of varicella vaccination or disease.
  - **Hepatitis C antibody:** If patients are at high risk for HCV (e.g., if they have a history of IV drug use, have tattoos, or received blood products before 1992).
  - **Fasting blood glucose:** If patients are at high risk for diabetes (e.g., if they are obese; have a strong family history of diabetes; or have a prior history of gestational diabetes, macrosomic infant, or fetal demise/structural anomalies).
  - **PPD +/− CXR:** For patients who are at high risk for TB (e.g., immigrants and those with known exposure).
  - **Toxoplasmosis titer:** For patients who are exposed to cat feces or undercooked meat.

- **CMV/parvovirus titer:** For patients at risk (e.g., those who work at day care centers).
- **Genetic carrier testing:** For familial heritable diseases if indicated (e.g., Tay-Sachs disease, sickle cell anemia).

## Preconception Interventions

The goal of preconception medical care is to minimize risk, thereby ensuring a healthy outcome for both mother and baby. Recommended interventions include the following:

- Discontinue teratogenic medications.
- Control medical conditions (obtain specialty consultation if indicated).
- Provide dietary and/or substance abuse counseling where applicable.
- Vaccinate against teratogenic illnesses (patients should wait one month to attempt conception after receiving live attenuated rubella or varicella vaccines).
- Refer for genetic counseling if indicated (e.g., advanced maternal age; family or individual history of congenital problems or heritable diseases).

## FIRST-TRIMESTER ISSUES

### Diagnosis of Pregnancy

Approximately 80–85% of women present to care within the first trimester; however, many women present with symptoms of pregnancy even before they have noticed any abnormality in their menstrual cycle. Common symptoms include breast tenderness, fatigue, and nausea or vomiting. Signs on physical exam in the early first trimester include Chadwick's sign (blue cervix) or Goodell's sign (cervical softening) and uterine enlargement.

- Definitive diagnosis of pregnancy is made by urine qualitative hCG assay (approximately 98% sensitive seven days after implantation), serum quantitative β-hCG assay (sensitive 4–5 days after implantation), or pelvic ultrasound (a gestational sac is usually visible four weeks after the last menstrual period, or LMP).
- Accurate assessment of the gestational age of a pregnancy is important for tracking growth and fetal development; for the timing of routine screening and interventions; and for risk assessment in the event of preterm labor or delivery. The estimated date of delivery can be established by several methods:
  - LMP + 40 weeks, adjusting for cycle length if ≠ 28 days.
  - Uterine size.
  - The presence of fetal heart tones on Doppler ultrasound (audible after 9–12 weeks).
  - The presence of fetal movement (felt by the mother by 16–20 weeks).
  - Pelvic ultrasound (the most reliable method):
    - Gestational sac diameter (in millimeters) + 30 = gestational age (in days) **or**
    - Crown-rump length (in millimeters) + 42 = gestational age (in days) (most accurate at 9–12 weeks) **or**
    - Biparietal diameter or femur length (most accurate at 12–15 weeks) **or**
    - Abdominal circumference (most accurate at > 15 weeks).

*Accuracy of ultrasound measurement:*

- ***First-trimester ultrasound:*** *Accurate to within approximately **one** week.*
- ***Second-trimester ultrasound:*** *Accurate to within approximately **two** weeks.*
- ***Third-trimester ultrasound:*** *Accurate to within approximately **three** weeks.*
- *The most accurate ultrasound measurement is a crown-rump length performed between 9 and 12 weeks, which is accurate to within 3–5 days.*

REPRODUCTIVE HEALTH

*Assessing gestational age by uterine bimanual exam during the first trimester:*

■ *At six weeks the uterus is the size of a large lemon.*

■ *At eight weeks it is the size of an orange.*

■ *At ten weeks it is the size of a grapefruit.*

## First-Trimester Routine Prenatal Care

The goals of the initial prenatal visit are fourfold: to identify patients with undesired pregnancies and refer for adoption counseling/abortion if applicable; to identify any major medical or psychosocial problems that merit immediate attention; to establish the gestational age of the pregnancy; and to begin patient education.

■ **Physical exam:** A full exam, including a thyroid, breast, and pelvic exam along with BP screening, should be performed within 1–2 weeks of the diagnosis. At this time, patients should also be counseled regarding the physiologic changes of pregnancy and normal fetal development. After 9–12 weeks of gestation, fetal heart tones should be auscultated at each visit with a Doppler ultrasound (or with a fetoscope after 18–20 weeks).

■ **Prenatal labs/studies** should include the following:
  ■ Preconception labs as above, if not already done.
  ■ A maternal serum antibody test (if Rh $\ominus$, give RhoGAM at 28 weeks and postpartum to prevent Rh isoimmunization).
  ■ A complete UA with culture.
  ■ A one-hour 50-g glucose challenge for diabetic screening in high-risk patients.
  ■ Pelvic ultrasound for dating if the LMP is unknown.
  ■ A urine dipstick at each visit to screen for proteinuria and glucosuria.

■ **Prenatal counseling:**
  ■ **Overview of prenatal care:** Patients should be counseled regarding the frequency of prenatal visits, routine pregnancy monitoring, how to reach after-hours care, and other resources that may be available (e.g., childbirth classes).
  ■ **Nutrition:** Patients should be advised to follow a healthy, balanced diet, aiming for a 25- to 35-pound total weight gain for a singleton pregnancy (10–15 pounds for a BMI > 26; 35–45 pounds for a BMI < 19.8). They should also be counseled to avoid uncooked food, unpasteurized dairy products, mercury-containing fish, and excess vitamin A. A daily prenatal vitamin with at least 400 μg of folic acid can help prevent neural tube defects.
  ■ **Drug/alcohol cessation:** Alcohol use is associated with growth retardation, small-for-gestational-age (SGA) babies, fetal alcohol syndrome, and fetal alcohol effects. Illicit drug use is also associated with ↑ neonatal morbidity and mortality and is primarily related to preterm birth, respiratory problems, mental retardation, and poor growth. Promptly refer patients to appropriate cessation programs where applicable.
  ■ **Tobacco cessation:** Smoking during pregnancy is associated with low birth weight, prematurity, and an ↑ risk of miscarriage and thromboembolic events. Nicotine patches or gum may be used to aid in tobacco cessation; the use of bupropion is not well studied in pregnancy.
  ■ **Safety:** Screen all patients for domestic violence. Patients should avoid trauma (no contact sports; use seatbelts), environmental toxins (organic solvents, lead, radiation), extremes of temperature (no hot tubs), and prolonged immobility. Toxoplasmosis and *Listeria* precautions should also be discussed (e.g., avoidance of raw meat/fish, unpasteurized dairy products, and cat litter), as should safe sex practices.
  ■ **Genetic counseling:** Offer counseling to any pregnant woman either of advanced maternal age (defined as age ≥ 35 years) or at risk for congenital problems or heritable diseases. Additional studies may include nuchal translucency to assess the risk of Down syndrome, chorionic villus sampling for fetal karyotyping, amniocentesis, or a detailed anatomic survey by ultrasound to detect congenital anomalies.

## First-Trimester Fetal Development

Milestones of first-trimester fetal development are outlined in Table 16.1.

## Common Problems of the First Trimester

### HYPEREMESIS GRAVIDARUM

Defined as persistent vomiting with weight loss and ketonuria, usually starting at < 10 weeks of gestation. It affects 1 in 200 pregnancies and is especially associated with molar pregnancies and multiple gestations. Advanced maternal age and nicotine use may be protective. A mild degree of nausea is seen in 50–90% of all pregnancies but is usually limited to the first trimester.

*Elevated β-hCG levels probably account for the ↑ incidence of hyperemesis gravidarum in molar and multiple-gestation pregnancies.*

### SYMPTOMS/EXAM

- Presents with persistent vomiting accompanied by weight loss > 5% of prepregnancy weight.
- Determine orthostatic BPs and fluid status.

### DIFFERENTIAL

Normal nausea of early pregnancy; GI disorders (gastroenteritis, hepatitis, appendicitis, biliary disease); metabolic disorders (DM, porphyria); pyelonephritis or other infections; neurologic or psychiatric disease; medication side effects; preeclampsia or HELLP syndrome if diagnosed after 20 weeks; fatty liver of pregnancy.

**TABLE 16.1.** **Fetal Development Milestones**

| WEEKS | MILESTONES |
|-------|-----------|
| 1–2 | Implantation with the beginning of placental development. |
| 3–4 | Gestational sac with distinct ectoderm, mesoderm, and endoderm layers. |
| 4–5 | Primitive brain. |
| 5–6 | Fetal pole with cardiac activity. |
| 4–8 | Primitive eyes, ears, abdominal organs, and limb buds. |
| 7 | Fetal movement is visible. |
| 8–9 | Spine/limb formation and organogenesis are complete. |
| 10 | The palate is formed. |
| 12 | Breathing, swallowing, sucking motions; the fetus is able to move the head, arms, hands, legs, and feet. Formation of fingernails and toenails. |
| 14 | Blinking, meconium accumulation, cardiac/digestive systems are fully functional. |

### DIAGNOSIS

- **Labs:** Obtain urine ketones, TSH/$T_4$, and serum electrolytes.
- **Imaging:** Ultrasound to rule out molar pregnancy or multiple gestation.

### TREATMENT

- Initial treatment consists of avoiding triggers; eating small, salty meals with clear fluids; ginger; and using Sea-Bands and acupressure.
- Antiemetics (e.g., vitamin $B_6$, doxylamine, $H_2$ blockers, promethazine, dolasetron) may be of benefit.
- Patients with severe dehydration and/or > 5% weight loss should be hospitalized with IV/enteral fluids and nutrition.
- Corticosteroids are the last resort for treatment.

### COMPLICATIONS

Hypokalemia, metabolic alkalosis, Wernicke's encephalopathy, Mallory-Weiss esophageal tears. Mild hyperthyroidism and hyperparathyroidism may also be associated with the condition.

### FIRST-TRIMESTER VAGINAL BLEEDING

Defined as any vaginal bleeding that occurs prior to 15 weeks of gestation, which can range from spotting to life-threatening hemorrhage (see Table 16.2). The immediate goals of management are to maintain maternal hemodynamic stability and to rule out ectopic pregnancy or trophoblastic disease. In the case of spontaneous, incomplete, or missed abortion, uterine evacuation may be performed if the patient desires or if bleeding does not resolve spontaneously or with the administration of misoprostol.

> A 20-year-old woman with a recent history of chlamydial cervicitis presents to your clinic with several days of increasing right lower abdominal pain. Her last menstrual period was > 6 weeks ago, and her urine pregnancy test is ⊕. Pelvic ultrasound reveals an empty uterus and an ectopic tubal pregnancy with a visible fetal pole, a tubal mass size of 2.0 cm, and no cardiac activity. How should she be treated? Appropriate management of this patient would include treatment of her chlamydial infection and a dose of methotrexate with serial serum β-hCG levels (to ensure resolution of the tubal pregnancy) or surgical intervention to remove the tubal pregnancy. If methotrexate administration is unsuccessful or there are signs of hemodynamic instability, immediate surgical intervention is indicated.

### ECTOPIC PREGNANCY

A pathologic condition in which an otherwise normal embryo implants outside of the uterus, most frequently in one of the fallopian tubes but on rare occasions in the peritoneal cavity. Tubal pregnancies never survive to term and if left untreated will → rupture of the fallopian tube, which is considered an **obstetric emergency.** Risk factors for ectopic pregnancy include the following:

---

**Causes of recurrent miscarriage—**

**RIBCAGE**

**R**adiation
**I**mmune reaction
**B**ugs (infection)
**C**ervical incompetence
**A**natomic anomalies (e.g., uterine septum)
**G**enetic (e.g., aneuploidy, balanced translocation)
**E**ndocrine

*Any patient who has had > 2–3 SABs should be worked up for thromboembolic disorders and chromosomal anomalies.*

*Most ectopic pregnancies present between six and eight weeks of gestation.*

**Risk factors for ectopic pregnancy—**

**PID**

**P**rior ectopic pregnancy/**P**rior abdominal or gynecologic surgery
**I**UD/**I**nfection
**D**ES exposure in utero/**D**amaged tubes

| Cause | Definition/Presentation | Treatment |
|---|---|---|
| Physiologic bleeding | Vaginal spotting in the early first trimester without any other cause; does not present with cramping or other symptoms. A closed cervix is seen on pelvic exam. | Pelvic exam; ultrasound for prolonged spotting; expectant management. The differential includes threatened SAB, ectopic pregnancy, and gynecologic pathology. |
| Spontaneous abortion (SAB) | The most common complication of early pregnancy (occurs in roughly 20% of recognized pregnancies). Defined as expulsion of an embryo/fetus < 500 g (usually at < 20–22 weeks). Generally presents with moderate bleeding, cramping, and passage of tissue. An open cervix is seen on pelvic exam. | Pelvic exam; ultrasound with serial serum $\beta$-hCG if the history of tissue passage is uncertain; D&C for prolonged or heavy bleeding. Risk factors include advanced maternal age, prior SAB, multiparity, toxin/teratogen exposure, and invasive intrauterine procedures. |
| Threatened abortion | Vaginal bleeding with a closed cervix but no passage of tissue. Cramping is variable. Fetal cardiac activity is present, and uterine size is appropriate for gestational age. | Pelvic exam; ultrasound and/or $\beta$-hCG; expectant management. The differential includes SAB, physiologic bleeding, gynecologic pathology, and ectopic pregnancy. Most threatened abortions do **not** result in loss of pregnancy. |
| Inevitable abortion | Usually painful uterine cramps, increasing bleeding, and a dilated cervix with gestational tissue often visible at the cervical os. | Pelvic exam; removal of tissue at the os may stop bleeding. D&C is indicated for significant cramping or blood loss; otherwise treat with expectant management. |
| Incomplete abortion | Embryonic demise with partial passage of tissue. Cramping/bleeding is variable; uterine size is less than dates; retained placental tissue may be visible. Usually occurs at > 12 weeks. | Expectant or medication management can be offered. D&C indicated for significant cramping or blood loss or for retention of gestational products for a prolonged period. |
| Septic abortion | Uterine infection. Presents with fever, chills, pelvic pain, bleeding, purulent vaginal discharge, a boggy and tender uterus with a dilated cervix, and signs of sepsis. | Stabilize with IV fluids; broad-spectrum antibiotics; D&C. Usually a complication of nonsterile elective abortion or other invasive procedures. |
| Missed abortion ("blighted ovum") | Embryonic/fetal demise prior to 20 weeks or anembryonic pregnancy with retention of pregnancy. Presents with inadequate growth and absent fetal heart tones on routine monitoring. | Ultrasound to confirm diagnosis; may choose between expectant management × 2 weeks (15–75% will pass spontaneously), medical management with misoprostol, or D&C/D&E for prolonged retention/unsuccessful medical management/patient preference. |

- Previous ectopic pregnancy
- Current use of an IUD
- Prior abdominal/gynecologic surgery or invasive procedures
- A prior history of PID
- In utero DES exposure
- Tubal/uterine pathology or unusual anatomy

REPRODUCTIVE HEALTH

*The absence of an adnexal mass on ultrasound does not necessarily rule out an ectopic pregnancy.*

### SYMPTOMS/EXAM

Presents with pelvic pain, vaginal bleeding (variable), and nausea/vomiting.

### DIAGNOSIS

- **Imaging:** Ultrasound reveals an enlarged adnexal mass and an empty uterus.
- **Labs:** ⊕ qualitative or ↑ quantitative β-hCG (+/− abnormal doubling time for β-hCG in early pregnancy).

### TREATMENT

- Give IM methotrexate if the ectopic is small (< 3 cm) and unruptured with no fetal cardiac activity and if the patient is stable and likely to be compliant. Follow with serial β-hCG measurements to ensure resolution. Methotrexate treatment may be repeated in one week in cases of incomplete resolution.
- Laparoscopic injection of methotrexate is appropriate if the patient is unstable and/or unlikely to be compliant.
- Surgical removal is necessary if the ectopic is ruptured or if medical treatment is not indicated or is unsuccessful.

## HYDATIDIFORM MOLAR PREGNANCY

A nonmalignant subtype of gestational trophoblastic disease in which an abnormal fertilization event → a tumor of fetal origin. Gestational trophoblastic disease must be ruled out in any patient with a ⊕ pregnancy test and significant vaginal bleeding. Malignant variants (gestational trophoblastic neoplasia) are covered elsewhere, but it is important to recognize that a malignant variant may arise after an otherwise "normal" molar pregnancy. Molar pregnancies can be complete (no normal fetal tissue is present) or partial (some fetal tissue is present). Risk factors include nulliparity, a history of prior gestational trophoblastic disease, and extremes of maternal age (< 20 or > 35 years).

*The presence of fetal cardiac activity is insufficient to rule out the presence of a hydatidiform molar pregnancy.*

### SYMPTOMS/EXAM

Presents with vaginal bleeding +/− anemia; pelvic pressure or pain; hyperemesis gravidarum; hyperthyroidism; and early-onset preeclampsia.

### DIAGNOSIS

- **Imaging:** Ultrasound reveals enlarged ovaries with theca-lutein cysts and an enlarged uterus with a heterogeneous mass with anechoic areas.
- **Labs:** CBC reveals anemia; β-hCG is ↑. Tissue pathology confirms the diagnosis.

### TREATMENT

Hemodynamic stabilization; expeditious uterine evacuation; serial β-hCG measurements to ensure resolution; CXR. Consider a repeat pelvic ultrasound.

## SECOND- AND THIRD-TRIMESTER ISSUES

### Second- and Third-Trimester Routine Prenatal Care

Because the second trimester is the time of most rapid fetal growth, continued self-care and good nutrition are key to ensuring a healthy pregnancy. The third trimester is often characterized by the most maternal discomfort and anxiety regarding labor and delivery; therefore, visits should be used as an opportunity to continue patient education as well as to address any medical or psychosocial problems that may arise.

## PHYSICAL EXAM DURING THE SECOND AND THIRD TRIMESTERS

The second- and third-trimester physical exam should include the following elements at each visit:

- **Fundal height measurement:** By 20 weeks, the uterine fundus should be palpable at the umbilicus. After 20 weeks, fundal height (in centimeters) should correspond to gestational age (in weeks) +/– 2 cm until the fetus descends into the pelvis at 34–36 weeks.
- **Other:**
    - BP screening; fetal heart rate auscultation (normal is 120–160 bpm); examine for the presence of edema.
    - Additional measures include Leopold maneuvers (see Figure 16.1) to determine fetal position after 36 weeks and/or a digital cervical exam to determine the extent of cervical ripening if an induction is planned.

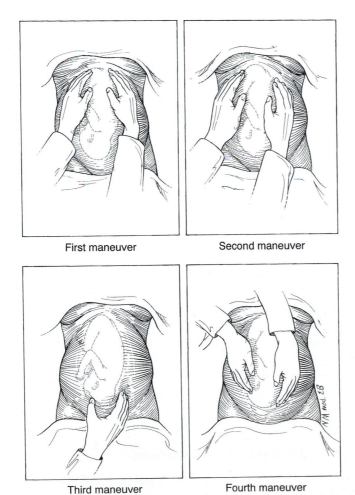

First maneuver        Second maneuver

Third maneuver        Fourth maneuver

**FIGURE 16.1.** **Leopold maneuvers for palpation of fetal position.**

(Reproduced, with permission, from Cunningham FG et al. *Williams Obstetrics*, 22nd ed. New York: McGraw-Hill, 2005: 416.)

### Second- and Third-Trimester Labs/Studies

Labs to obtain include the following:

- Obtain a urine dipstick for glucosuria and proteinuria at each visit.
- Perform a "quadruple screen" at 15–18 weeks to measure maternal serum α-fetoprotein, hCG, unconjugated estriol, and inhibin A levels (helps predict the risk of Down syndrome, neural tube defects, and trisomy 18).
- Obtain a one-hour 50-g glucose challenge test at 26–28 weeks.
- Check hematocrit; treat with iron if anemic.
- Where applicable, obtain a test of cure for UTIs or genital tract infections; repeat gonorrhea/chlamydia screen in high-risk patients.
- Periodic urine toxicology screens are necessary for high-risk patients.
- Perform colposcopy as indicated for patients with an abnormal Pap smear.
- Ultrasound for routine anatomic survey is recommended by many providers, although there is no evidence that this measure has any effect on morbidity or mortality.
- Obtain a vaginal/rectal swab for group B streptococcus (GBS) at 36 weeks.

### Second- and Third-Trimester Counseling

> **The ABCs of second- and third-trimester prenatal visits:**
>
> **A**mniotic fluid leakage?
> **B**leeding vaginally?
> **C**ontractions?
> **D**ysuria?
> **E**dema?
> **F**etal movement?

- Second trimester:
  - Continue to discuss nutrition, weight gain, and exercise recommendations.
  - Recommend Kegel exercises for pelvic strengthening.
  - Conduct ongoing screening for domestic violence.
  - Offer education on maternal physiologic changes.
  - Administer influenza vaccine.
- Third trimester: As above, plus the following:
  - **Fetal kick counts:** To monitor fetal well-being.
  - **Travel:** Caution patients to avoid airline travel after 35–36 weeks.
  - **Sex:** Counsel patients that sexual activity may stimulate uterine contractions but is safe in uncomplicated pregnancies with intact membranes.
  - **Work:** Most women are eligible for disability or family leave for the last 3–4 weeks of pregnancy. Patients should also be cautioned to avoid excessive exertion.
  - **Labor plans:** Discuss emotional support (including plans for a doula if available), anesthesia options, fetal monitoring during labor, the labor process, and orientation to the hospital or birth center.
  - **Postpartum birth control:** Discuss options; obtain signed consent for tubal ligation if desired.
  - **Breast-feeding:** Encourage all patients to try breast-feeding; provide patients with information on the advantages of breast-feeding both for the infant and for the mother.
  - **Other postpartum measures:** Discuss routine postpartum and newborn care as well as postpartum follow-up.

### Second- and Third-Trimester Fetal Development

Table 16.3 lists significant milestones associated with second- and third-trimester fetal development.

TABLE 16.3. Second- and Third-Trimester Milestones

| WEEKS | MILESTONES |
|---|---|
| 18 | Sleep/wake cycles, hair growth, egg development in females, fully formed placenta. |
| 20 | Rapid brain and bone growth; testicular descent in males; thumb sucking. |
| 22 | Continuing growth; ability to hear maternal sounds. |
| 24 | Tooth buds; beginning of lung maturation. |
| 26 | Brain growth; eyes open. |
| 28 | Rhythmic breathing motions; disappearance of lanugo; fat accumulation. |
| 30 | Head hair develops; lack of space → "fetal position"; brain development. |
| 32 | Continued brain growth; immune system development. |
| 34 | Vertex position; lungs fully mature. |
| 36 | Descent into the maternal pelvis begins. |
| 38 | Vernix (sebaceous secretion protecting the skin from the amniotic fluid) is gone. |
| 40 | Term gestation. |

A 35-year-old G8P6 with no history of prenatal care in this pregnancy presents to labor and delivery complaining of heavy vaginal bleeding. Her BP is 90/60, pulse 115, and temperature 37°C; a fetal strip is nonreactive with ↓ variability and tachycardia. The patient has a scar from a prior C-section and has a steady flow of bright red blood from her vagina. How should she be treated? Initial management of this patient, who has a presumed diagnosis of placenta previa, includes placement of two large-bore IVs, typing and crossing of 2–4 units of blood, a call to anesthesia and obstetrics for a stat C-section, and expeditious ultrasound determination of placental position where possible.

## Common Problems of the Second and Third Trimesters

### THIRD-TRIMESTER BLEEDING

Third-trimester bleeding most commonly results from placenta previa, placental abruption, and vasa previa. Table 16.4 outlines the etiologies, presentation, and treatment of these conditions as well as the risk factors associated with each. Low-lying placentas (i.e., those in the lower uterine segment but not covering or immediately adjacent to the os) are also at ↑ risk of bleeding (see Figure 16.2).

**TABLE 16.4. Presentation and Management of Third-Trimester Bleeding**

| Cause | Definition | Presentation | Risk Factors | Management |
|---|---|---|---|---|
| Placenta previa | Placental tissue completely or partially covering the internal cervical os. Diagnosed by ultrasound. | Asymptomatic, or presents with generally painless vaginal bleeding late in the second or third trimester. Incidence is 1 in 4000 pregnancies. | Advanced maternal age, multiparity, multiple gestation, uterine anomalies, prior gynecologic surgery. May be complicated by placenta accreta (placenta ingrown into the uterine wall). | **If no bleeding:** Complete pelvic rest until resolution of the previa is confirmed on serial ultrasounds or until delivery. **If actively bleeding:** Admit and stabilize the mother; immediate C-section delivery if fetal/maternal status is nonreassuring. **If bleeding resolves:** Conservative inpatient management with bed rest, corticosteroids, and serial ultrasounds; C-section once fetal lung maturity is confirmed at approximately 34 weeks. |
| Placental abruption | Separation of the placenta prior to delivery of the infant. An **obstetric emergency;** second-trimester abruption is associated with an extremely poor fetal prognosis. | Constant severe uterine contractions +/− vaginal bleeding (80%); nonreassuring fetal heart tracing. Partial abruption may be difficult to distinguish from early labor. Diagnosis is clinical; ultrasound is insufficiently sensitive to rule out abruption. | Abdominal trauma, maternal hypertension, smoking, advanced maternal age, thrombophilic disease, increasing parity, cocaine use, polyhydramnios with sudden rupture of membranes (ROM), preterm premature rupture of membranes (PPROM), multiple gestation, previous abruption. | Stabilize the mother (IVs, type and cross, transfuse PRN); continuous internal fetal monitoring. **If nonreassuring maternal/fetal status:** Immediate C-section. **If term and stable:** May deliver vaginally in the OR. **If preterm and stable:** Inpatient conservative management. |
| Vasa previa | Amniotic blood vessels presenting in front of the fetal head. | Painless vaginal bleeding with ROM, often with fetal heart rate anomalies (a sinusoidal pattern is classic). | Low-lying or multilobed placentas; multiple gestations; in vitro fertilization. | **If term and/or unstable:** Immediate C-section. **If preterm and stable:** Inpatient conservative management; C-section when fetal lungs are mature. Transvaginal ultrasound with color Doppler and/or Apt/Kleihauer-Betke tests to determine the origin of bleeding if the diagnosis is unclear. Rule out DIC. |

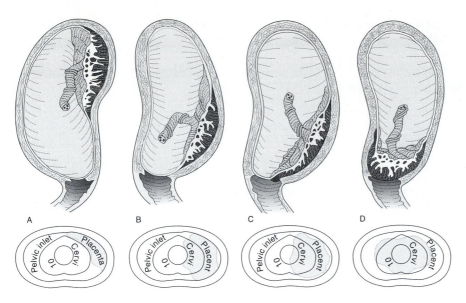

**FIGURE 16.2.** **Placental implantation.**

(Reproduced, with permission, from DeCherney AH et al. *Current Obstetrics & Gynecologic Diagnosis and Treatment*, 9th ed. New York: McGraw-Hill, 2003: Figure 20-3.)

## INTRAUTERINE GROWTH RETARDATION (IUGR)

Defined as fetal weight below the 10th percentile for gestational age, IUGR occurs in roughly 7% of pregnancies. Most SGA babies are simply constitutionally small; etiologies for true growth restriction are typically classified as fetal, maternal, or placental. Fetal factors include congenital anomalies, genetic syndromes, and multiple gestations; maternal factors include substance abuse, smoking, poor nutrition, hypoxemia, thrombotic and hypertensive disorders, and infections. Placental causes include abruption, hematoma, structural anomalies, and a two-vessel cord.

### SYMPTOMS/EXAM

Presents with uterine fundal measurements > 2 cm less than expected for gestational age; confirm with ultrasound. If dates are unknown, serial ultrasounds may be needed every two weeks for evaluation.

### DIAGNOSIS

- A detailed fetal anatomic survey by ultrasound can confirm the diagnosis, distinguish symmetric from asymmetric growth restriction, and evaluate the patient for placental causes of IUGR.
- Determine fetal karyotype, especially in severe cases and/or those associated with polyhydramnios.
- Obtain maternal serum infection titers if rubella, CMV, or syphilis is suspected.
- Doppler flow velocimetry of the umbilical artery can determine the systolic/diastolic ratio to rule out placental insufficiency.

### TREATMENT

- Give corticosteroids for lung maturity if the fetus is preterm; follow with antenatal testing.

REPRODUCTIVE HEALTH

541

■ Deliver by 40 weeks or sooner if there is evidence of placental insufficiency or nonreassuring antenatal testing.

## GESTATIONAL DIABETES MELLITUS (GDM)

Defined as glucose intolerance beginning or first recognized during pregnancy, GDM affects 1.4–14.0% of pregnancies. At particularly high risk are women with a family history of diabetes as well as those with a personal history of glucose intolerance, polycystic ovarian syndrome (PCOS), obesity, glucocorticoid use, or prior macrosomic infants. Hispanics, Native Americans, and African-Americans are also at ↑ risk. Universal preliminary screening with a one-hour 50-g glucose challenge should generally be performed at 24–28 weeks of gestation but should be done earlier in the presence of risk factors or suspicion of undiagnosed type 2 DM. If a one-hour glucose challenge test is ↑ (> 140 after one hour), a three-hour glucose tolerance test should be performed within one week to confirm the diagnosis.

*Any one of the diagnostic criteria for GDM is sufficient to make the diagnosis.*

### SYMPTOMS/EXAM

■ Often asymptomatic, or may present with polydipsia/polyuria or frequent infections, especially UTIs or yeast infections.
■ Obesity and acanthosis nigricans may also be seen.

### DIAGNOSIS

Diagnostic criteria are as follows:

■ Random blood glucose > 200 mg/dL on two separate occasions **or**
■ Fasting blood glucose > 126 mg/dL on two separate occasions **or**
■ A 100-g glucose challenge with two or more abnormal values: > 95 fasting, > 180 at one hour, > 155 at two hours, or > 140 at three hours.

### TREATMENT

*Cornerstones of GDM management—*

**DIABETIC**

**D**iet
**I**nformation
**A**ntenatal testing
**B**aby growth monitoring
**E**xercise
**T**est home blood glucose
**I**nsulin
**C**heck postpartum blood glucose

■ Offer nutritional counseling. Aim for 30 kcal/kg/day in women of normal weight, with carbohydrates making up no more than 40% of total caloric intake.
■ Encourage regular blood sugar monitoring and exercise regimens; offer diabetic education.
■ If fasting blood glucose is > 95 **or** postprandial glucose is > 130 on > 2 occasions, start insulin (bedtime NPH for high fasting glucose at a starting dose of 0.2 U/kg; mealtime regular/lispro for high postprandial glucose at a starting dose of 1.0–1.5 U/10 g of carbohydrates).
■ **Peripartum management:** IV saline, NPO, and hourly blood glucose monitoring should be initiated with a goal of 70–110 mg/dL. Most laboring diabetic patients do not require insulin.
■ **Postpartum management:** Continue diet and exercise counseling, weight control, and diabetic education, as women with GDM have a significantly ↑ risk of developing subsequent type 2 DM. Check a two-hour 75-g glucose tolerance test six weeks postpartum, and check fasting blood glucose yearly thereafter.

### COMPLICATIONS

Preeclampsia, polyhydramnios, fetal macrosomia with ↑ risk of birth trauma/operative delivery, neonatal metabolic complications and ↑ perinatal morbidity, subsequent maternal development of type 2 DM.

## MACROSOMIA

Defined as a fetal weight at term exceeding 4.5 kg. Incidence is roughly 9% in the United States. May be associated with maternal DM and congenital anomalies, although many cases of macrosomia are simply constitutionally large.

### SYMPTOMS/EXAM

Maternal impression of ↑ fetal weight; uterine fundal height > 2 cm greater than the number of weeks of gestation.

### DIAGNOSIS

Clinical assessment by Leopold's maneuvers; ultrasound (fetal abdominal circumference is the most accurate parameter).

### TREATMENT

- Maintain tight control of maternal diabetes if applicable.
- Induction or elective C-section at term should be considered only in severe cases.
- In the case of vaginal births, prepare for shoulder dystocia.

### COMPLICATIONS

Shoulder dystocia; maternal traumatic injury. ↑ morbidity is associated with a fetal weight > 4 kg.

*Maternal assessment is a more accurate measure of fetal weight than Leopold's maneuvers or ultrasound.*

## POLYHYDRAMNIOS

Defined as an accumulation of excess amniotic fluid. Affects 0.2–1.6% of pregnancies, with potential causes including fetal malformations (especially those that cause problems with fetal breathing or swallowing), fetal anemia, maternal DM, and multiple gestations.

### SYMPTOMS/EXAM

Presents with a uterine size measuring large for dates; may be accompanied by ↓ fetal movement.

*Most idiopathic cases of polyhydramnios resolve spontaneously.*

### DIAGNOSIS

- Ultrasound to evaluate amniotic fluid index (AFI), as well as fetal surveillance to look for fetal GI obstruction (e.g., esophageal or duodenal atresia or gastroschisis) or neurologic abnormalities.
- Glucose challenge test if one has not already been done.
- Kleihauer-Betke test to look for fetomaternal hemorrhage.
- Maternal serology for infectious agents and hereditary metabolic abnormalities; amniocentesis for karyotype analysis if severe.

### TREATMENT

- Monitor AFI every 1–3 weeks.
- Amnioreduction is appropriate for cases that are symptomatic and severe.
- Give indomethacin, especially if severe and/or preterm.

REPRODUCTIVE HEALTH

### COMPLICATIONS

Maternal respiratory compromise, preterm labor, PPROM, fetal malposition, umbilical cord accidents, postpartum hemorrhage.

### OLIGOHYDRAMNIOS

Defined as inadequate amniotic fluid; has an incidence of approximately 1 in 200 pregnancies. Oligohydramnios is usually idiopathic but can be associated with uteroplacental insufficiency (maternal hypertension, medications, placental abruption or infarction) as well as with fetal factors such as intrauterine fetal demise, chromosomal/congenital anomalies, and twin-twin transfusion. Postdate pregnancy and unrecognized rupture of amniotic membranes should also be considered.

### SYMPTOMS/EXAM

Presents with a uterine size less than dates and ↓ fetal movement.

### DIAGNOSIS

Inadequate AFI measured on ultrasound; consider amniocentesis for karyotype analysis.

### TREATMENT

- Maternal hydration; amnioinfusion if necessary for adequate ultrasound assessment of the fetus. Antepartum surveillance with biweekly AFI measurements.
- Labor induction is indicated at term or earlier if there is evidence of nonreassuring fetal status.

### COMPLICATIONS

Meconium aspiration, cord accidents, fetal growth restriction.

### PRETERM LABOR

Defined as uterine contractions → cervical change prior to 37 weeks of gestation. Approximately 10% of births in the United States are preterm. Preterm labor is the second leading cause of perinatal mortality (after congenital anomalies) and is the leading cause of perinatal morbidity. Risk factors are outlined in Table 16.5.

### DIAGNOSIS

- UA and culture to rule out pyelonephritis; sterile speculum exam to rule out PPROM (pooling/ferning/nitrazine).
- Obtain cervical swabs for gonorrhea, chlamydia, and bacterial vaginosis.
- Obtain a fetal fibronectin specimen between 24 and 35 weeks.
- Ultrasound to measure cervical length.
- Serial sterile vaginal exams if membranes are unruptured to evaluate cervical change.

### TREATMENT

- **Initial management of preterm contractions:** See Figure 16.3.
- **Active management of preterm labor:**

---

**Risk factors for preterm labor—**

**PIMS**

**P**lacental abruption/
    **P**olyhydramnios
**I**nfection/**I**nadequate
    cervix
**M**ultiple
    gestation/**M**ultiple
    years (advanced
    maternal age)
**S**ingle, **S**ad, or
    **S**tressed/**S**ubstance
    abuse

---

**TABLE 16.5.**    **Risk Factors for Preterm Labor**

| RISK CATEGORY | RISK FACTORS |
|---|---|
| Socioeconomic | Single, anxiety/depression, emotional stress, poor nutrition, maternal age > 40 or < 18, substance abuse, tobacco, African-American, extreme physical exertion. |
| Uterine/placental | Multiple gestation, polyhydramnios, uterine anomalies (especially those → uterine overdistention), cervical incompetence, placental abruption or placenta previa. |
| Infectious | Bacteriuria/pyelonephritis, STIs, bacterial vaginosis, periodontal disease. |
| Fetal | Congenital anomalies, growth restriction. |

- Give antibiotics to treat any UTI or genital infections as indicated; GBS prophylaxis.
- Administer corticosteroids (betamethasone 12 mg QD × 2; maximum benefit is derived 48 hours after the first dose) if prior to 34 weeks gestation.
- Bed rest (unproven benefit); tocolytics (see Table 16.6).

### PREMATURE RUPTURE OF MEMBRANES (PROM)

Defined as rupture of amniotic membranes before the onset of uterine contractions. Preterm premature rupture of membranes (PPROM) refers to PROM that occurs prior to 37 weeks of gestation. The incidence of PROM is one in ten pregnancies; most patients will enter labor spontaneously within 24 hours. Risk factors are similar to those for preterm labor and include genital tract infection, a prior history of PPROM, smoking, cervical incompetence, polyhydramnios, multiple gestation, and antepartum hemorrhage.

*Fetal fibronectin (fFN) is a protein that acts as a trophoblastic "glue" between the uterine lining and the chorionic membranes; its presence in the vagina between 24 and 34 weeks may indicate chorionic-decidual separation. If correctly performed, it has a 98% negative predictive value.*

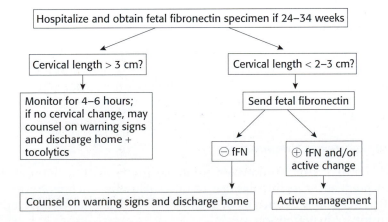

**FIGURE 16.3.**    **Algorithm for the treatment of preterm contractions.**

TABLE 16.6. Guidelines for Treatment with Tocolytics

| MEDICATION | CLASS | LOADING DOSE | MAINTENANCE DOSE | SIDE EFFECTS/COMPLICATIONS |
|---|---|---|---|---|
| Terbutaline | β-adrenergic agonist | 2.5–5.0 μg IV | Up to 25 μg/min or until contractions abate | Contraindicated in women with cardiac disease. |
| Magnesium sulfate | | 4–6 g IV | IV infusion 2–4 g/hr; monitor serum magnesium levels and DTRs | Magnesium toxicity (loss of DTRs, respiratory paralysis, cardiac arrest). No benefit over placebo. |
| Nifedipine | Calcium channel blocker | 30 mg PO | 20 mg q 4–8 h | Fewest side effects; no benefit over placebo. |
| Atosiban | Oxytocin receptor antagonist | Not available in the United States | Not available in the United States | Considered first-line treatment outside the United States owing to favorable side effects; efficacy is similar to that of terbutaline. |

### SYMPTOMS/EXAM

Presents with leaking or gushing of clear fluid from the vagina and pooling of amniotic fluid in the vaginal vault. Avoid a digital cervical exam until the patient is in labor!

### DIAGNOSIS

⊕ **nitrazine testing** (blood or semen may also turn nitrazine paper ⊕); **ferning** of amniotic fluid.

### TREATMENT

An algorithm for the treatment of PROM is outlined in Figure 16.4.

### COMPLICATIONS

Chorioamnionitis, endometritis, preterm delivery.

### HYPERTENSIVE DISORDERS OF PREGNANCY

A spectrum of complex multisystem diseases of uncertain etiology that complicate up to one in five pregnancies and are associated with greatly ↑ fetal and maternal morbidity and mortality. Milder forms (e.g., transient gestational hypertension) are often a precursor to more severe forms (e.g., preeclampsia).

### TRANSIENT GESTATIONAL HYPERTENSION

Defined as a BP ≥ 140/90 on two occasions six hours apart, with onset after 20 weeks of pregnancy, in the absence of other causative factors. Severe gestational hypertension is defined as BPs > 160/105. Risk factors include a prior or family history of hypertension.

---

**Contraindications to tocolysis—**

**OH SH\*\***

Pregnancy **O**ver (intrauterine fetal demise or lethal anomaly)
**H**ypertension (severe preeclampsia or eclampsia)
**S**mall baby (IUGR)
**H**emorrhage (especially with maternal hemodynamic instability)
**I**nfection (chorioamnionitis)
**T**roubled baby (nonreassuring fetal heart tracing)

---

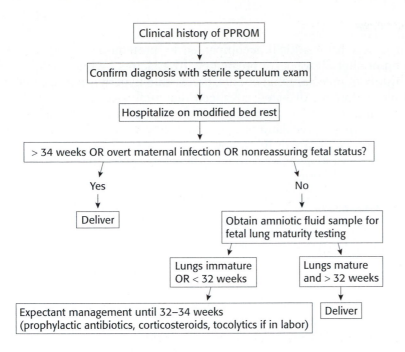

**FIGURE 16.4.** Treatment of premature rupture of membranes.

## DIAGNOSIS

- Elevated blood pressure as above.
- Obtain CMP, CBC, and urine dipsticks to test for proteinuria.

## TREATMENT

- Provide diet and exercise counseling.
- Labetalol or methyldopa to control BPs if persistently elevated.
- Antepartum surveillance.
- In severe cases, consider delivery by 38–39 weeks.

A 36-year-old G3P1 with a history of gestational hypertension presents to labor and delivery at 36 weeks of gestation with a complaint of intense frontal headaches, progressive pedal edema, and nausea over the past week. On initial evaluation, her BP is 176/92, her cervix is favorable, and her urine dip reveals 2+ proteinuria. External fetal monitoring shows a reactive strip. How should she be managed? Appropriate management of severe preeclampsia at term includes hospital admission, obstetrical consultation, initiation of a 24-hour urine collection and GBS swab if this has not previously been done, and induction of labor with IV magnesium for seizure prophylaxis.

## PREECLAMPSIA

Defined as a BP ≥ 140/90 accompanied by proteinuria > 300 mg/24 hours with onset after 20 weeks of pregnancy. Risk factors include primigravidity, a past history of preeclampsia, obesity, preexisting hypertension or renal disease, multiple gestations, diabetes, advanced maternal age, antiphospholipid antibody syndrome, chronic autoimmune disease, and a partner with a prior history of fathering a preeclamptic pregnancy. Severe preeclampsia is diagnosed in the presence of any of the following: BPs > 160/110, CNS or pulmonary symptoms, thrombocytopenia, IUGR, hepatic involvement, oliguria, or proteinuria > 5 g/24 hours.

### SYMPTOMS/EXAM

Patients may present with edema, blurry vision, epigastric pain, nausea, headache, and hyperactive DTRs.

### DIAGNOSIS

- Screen with a urine dipstick for proteinuria on each visit; obtain 24-hour urine protein if dipstick is elevated.
- LFTs, CBC with smear, creatinine, uric acid.

*Management of preeclamptic patients should include frequent assessment of DTRs and pulmonary status, as neurologic complications and pulmonary edema can progress rapidly.*

### TREATMENT

- **Mild preeclampsia:** Give labetalol, hydralazine, or nifedipine to control blood pressure; supplement with antepartum surveillance and frequent weight checks. Deliver at term; consider $MgSO_4$ for seizure prophylaxis.
- **Severe preeclampsia:**
    - Immediate delivery with continuous fetal monitoring; consider a 48-hour delay only to give steroids for fetal lung maturity.
    - Restrict fluids and monitor urine output; control BP with hydralazine or labetalol; give $MgSO_4$ for seizure prophylaxis; monitor magnesium q 4–6 h; repeat LFTs and creatinine. Aggressive furosemide treatment is appropriate in the presence of pulmonary edema.

### COMPLICATIONS

Pulmonary edema, neurologic deterioration, coma, stroke.

### ECLAMPSIA

- Onset of grand mal seizures in a preeclamptic patient in the absence of any other cause. Approximately 1 in 50 severely preeclamptic patients will progress to seizures.
- **Tx:** Check ABCs; stabilize the mother; administer $MgSO_4$ (6 g IV) for seizure control accompanied by fetal monitoring. If $MgSO_4$ is not effective, consider benzodiazepines.

### HELLP SYNDROME

A hypertensive disorder characterized by **H**emolysis, **E**levated **L**iver enzymes, and **L**ow **P**latelets. The pathogenesis is unknown but is thought to be due to vasospasm and/or coagulation defects. Its incidence is approximately 1 in 1000 pregnancies, and it develops in up to 10–20% of women with preeclampsia. HELLP syndrome is usually diagnosed during the third trimester but may present earlier or even postpartum.

### SYMPTOMS/EXAM

Patients may present with nausea/vomiting, edema, headache and blurry vision, and ↓ urine output.

### DIFFERENTIAL

Acute fatty liver of pregnancy; gastroenteritis or appendicitis; cholecystic or hepatic disease; HUS/TTP.

### DIAGNOSIS

- Look for the presence of preeclampsia.
- **Labs:** Hemolytic anemia, platelet count < 100,000, and either LDH > 600 and total bilirubin > 1.2 or AST > 70.
- **Imaging:** Obtain CT/MRI if hepatic infarction, rupture, or hematoma is suspected.

### TREATMENT

- Hospitalize and stabilize the mother; assess the fetus.
- Consider corticosteroids for fetal lung maturity if < 34 weeks.
- Hypertensive medications to control maternal BP; platelet transfusion if platelet count is < 20,000 or there is maternal bleeding.
- Expeditious delivery is indicated at > 34 weeks of gestation or in the setting of nonreassuring fetal status or severe maternal disease.

### COMPLICATIONS

Associated with a maternal morbidity rate of 1%. See also the **4 H's** mnemonic.

> **Complications of HELLP syndrome—**
>
> **The 4 H's**
>
> **H**epatic failure
> **H**epatic infarction
> **H**ematoma
> **H**epatic rupture

## CHOLESTASIS OF PREGNANCY

A syndrome of pruritus and ↑ serum bile acids that typically develops after 30 weeks of gestation. Cholestasis of pregnancy is associated with fetal prematurity and sudden intrauterine demise; its pathogenesis is unknown.

### SYMPTOMS/EXAM

- Presents with intolerable itching, especially on the palms and soles, that usually worsens at night.
- Exam reveals jaundice.

### DIAGNOSIS

↑ bile acids. Total bilirubin, alkaline phosphatase, and AST/ALT may also be high.

### TREATMENT

- Synthetic bile acids; cholestyramine; hydroxyzine for symptomatic relief.
- Deliver by 38 weeks or sooner if severe and fetal lung maturity is established.

## PRURITIC URTICARIAL PAPULES AND PLAQUES OF PREGNANCY (PUPPP)

The most common dermatosis of pregnancy, with an incidence of 1 in 160. The cause is unknown. Usual onset is in the late third trimester. There is no associated risk of ↑ fetal/maternal morbidity.

### Symptoms/Exam

- Presents with extreme pruritus, with erythematous papules coalescing to plaques within striae (see Figure 16.5).
- The rash usually starts on the abdomen and spreads to the extremities.

### Differential

Pemphigoid gestationis, viral syndromes, allergic reactions, cholestasis.

### Treatment

Topical steroids; antihistamines for symptomatic relief.

## Breech Presentation

Nonvertex presentation of the fetus occurs in 3–4% pregnancies at term, with the frequency decreasing as the pregnancy approaches term. Risk factors include placental or uterine anomalies, fetal anatomic anomalies, multiple gestation, poly- or oligohydramnios, and a short umbilical cord. Frank, complete, and footling breech presentations are illustrated in Figure 16.6.

### Symptoms/Exam

- The fetal head is not palpable on cervical exam.
- Breech position is found by Leopold's maneuvers.

### Diagnosis

Confirm the position with ultrasound.

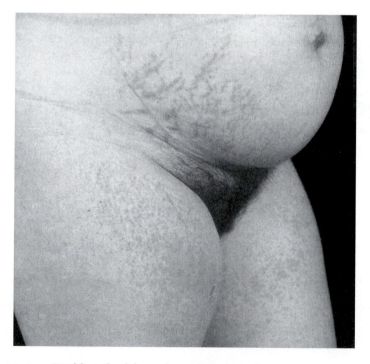

**FIGURE 16.5.** **Pruritic urticarial papules and plaques of pregnancy.**

(Reproduced, with permission, from Wolff K et al. *Fitzpatrick's Color Atlas & Synopsis of Clinical Dermatology,* 5th ed. New York: McGraw-Hill, 2005: 433.)

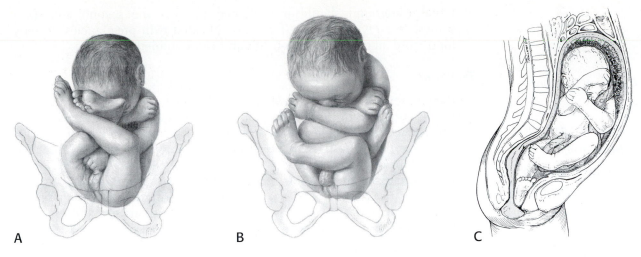

**FIGURE 16.6.** Breech presentations: (A) frank, (B) complete, and (C) footling presentations.

(Reproduced, with permission, from Cunningham FG et al. *Williams Obstetrics*, 22nd ed. New York: McGraw-Hill, 2005: 566 & 567.)

### TREATMENT

- **If diagnosed prior to onset of labor,** external cephalic version may be attempted at 36–39 weeks.
- **If cephalic version is unsuccessful,** schedule a C-section at 39–40 weeks.
- **If presentation is in active labor,** proceed to C-section.

### COMPLICATIONS

Labor dystocia; maternal and/or fetal birth trauma. External cephalic version is associated with a risk of placental abruption, cord accident, or fetal distress.

### MULTIPLE-GESTATION PREGNANCIES

Although the incidence of monozygotic (identical) twins has remained constant at roughly 1 in 250, dizygotic (fraternal) twinning varies from 1 in 30 to 1 in 100 depending on the population. Multiple gestations are becoming more common in the United States owing to an ↑ in assisted reproductive technology and maternal age; increasing parity and a family history of twins are additional risk factors. Associated with higher rates of all pregnancy complications except for post-term pregnancy and macrosomia, the most frequent complication of multiple gestation is preterm labor. Accurate dating of the pregnancy is thus critical, and patients with multiple-gestation pregnancies should ideally be managed in consultation with an obstetrician.

### SYMPTOMS/EXAM

- Presents with ↑ uterine size for dates and > 1 fetal heart tone heard on Doppler.
- Also associated with prolonged or more severe nausea than that associated with a singleton pregnancy.

### DIAGNOSIS

- Early ultrasound to establish amnionicity/chorionicity; level 2 ultrasound to detect congenital anomalies.

> **Complications of multiple-gestation pregnancies—**
>
> **PAPA PIG**
>
> **P**reterm labor
> **A**ntepartum hemorrhage
> **P**reeclampsia
> **A**bortion (intrauterine fetal demise)
> **P**olyhydramnios
> **I**UGR
> **G**estational diabetes

*If division of the embryo*

*occurs:*

- **Up to three days after fertilization:**

  *Diamniotic/dichorionic.*

- **Between 4 and 8 days:**

  *Diamniotic/monochorionic.*

- **Between 8 and 12 days:**

  *Monoamniotic/monochorionic (high risk for morbidity/mortality)*

- **After 13 days:** *Conjoined twins (extremely high risk; refer to a perinatologist).*

- Serial ultrasound should be obtained through the second and third trimesters every 4–6 weeks (for uncomplicated twin pregnancies) to look for discordant growth or twin-twin transfusion problems.

### TREATMENT

- Recommend an extra 300 kcal daily over singleton pregnancies and a 35- to 45-pound weight gain by term for uncomplicated twin pregnancies.
- Antepartum testing with biweekly **non-stress testing (NST)/AFI** after 36 weeks has not been shown to be effective but is nevertheless recommended by the American College of Obstetricians and Gynecologists (ACOG).
- Perform elective induction/C-section at 37–38 weeks if fetal lungs are mature; epidural anesthesia and continuous monitoring are recommended.
- The route of delivery depends on presentation, risk factors, and maternal preference. If twin A delivers vaginally, the position of twin B should be evaluated by ultrasound prior to delivery.

## PERIPARTUM ISSUES

## Normal Labor and Delivery

Labor is a physiologic process in which regular uterine contractions → cervical dilation and effacement and, ultimately, to expulsion of the fetus and placenta. Labor is separated into three stages, each with distinct management recommendations: cervical dilation and effacement, descent and delivery of the fetus, and delivery of the placenta. Initial assessment of a patient presenting in labor should include the following:

- A brief physical exam, including a sterile vaginal exam for cervical dilation and effacement (unless ROM is suspected).
- Assessment of fetal presentation, position, and station.
- Determination of amniotic membrane status (intact vs. ruptured); sterile speculum exam if ROM/PROM is suspected (defer the vaginal exam).
- Assessment of the quality and quantity of uterine contractions (an adequate number of uterine contractions in active labor is defined as 3–5 regular intense contractions every 10 minutes, each > 60 Montevideo units of pressure above baseline).
- Assessment of vaginal bleeding.
- Initial assessment of fetal heart rate tracing with NST.

### STAGE I: CERVICAL DILATION AND EFFACEMENT

Routine expectant management of normal stage I labor includes vaginal exams every 1–4 hours to monitor progress, intermittent fetal heart rate monitoring (every 15 minutes during active and transitional phases), and analgesia as needed. All labors should be plotted on a Friedman curve to monitor progress as well as to facilitate prompt recognition of a protraction or arrest disorder (see Figure 16.7). Phases within stage I are as follows:

- **Latent phase (cervical dilation 0–3 cm):** Characterized by loss of the cervical mucous plug ("bloody show") and by slow, irregular uterine contractions. May last up to 20 hours in nulliparous women and up to 14 hours in multiparous women.
- **Active phase (cervical dilation 3–9 cm):** Characterized by increasingly intense, regular uterine contractions, usually with spontaneous ROM. Cervical dilation should progress at a rate of ≥ 1 cm/hr in nulliparas and at ≥ 1.2 cm/hr in multiparas.

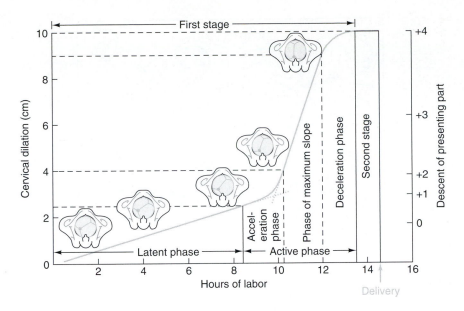

**FIGURE 16.7.** Friedman curve showing normal progression of stage I labor.

(Reproduced, with permission, from DeCherney AH et al. *Current Obstetric & Gynecologic Diagnosis & Treatment*, 8th ed. Stamford, CT: Appleton & Lange, 1994: 211.)

- **Transition (cervical dilation 9–10 cm):** Characterized by continued intense uterine contractions; cervical dilation may slow during this phase.

### STAGE II: DESCENT AND DELIVERY OF THE FETUS

Routine expectant management of a normal second stage of labor includes serial vaginal exams to monitor progress, more frequent fetal heart rate monitoring (every five minutes), analgesia as needed, and preparation for delivery of the fetus. The second stage is characterized by an ↑ in bloody show, continuing intense uterine contractions, intrapelvic pressure, and a maternal urge to push. Accurate assessment of fetal position and station is important for anticipation of potential problems during stage II. Additional considerations are as follows:

- **Duration:** Stage II should last no longer than one hour in multiparas and two hours in nulliparas, although the presence of epidural/spinal anesthesia may prolong the second stage. Assessment of fetal station (3+, 3, 2, 1, 0, −1, −2, −3) refers to the relative position of the fetal head and maternal ischial spines in centimeters (0 = fetal head level with ischial spines).
- **Assessment of fetal position:** The fetus undergoes a series of position changes during the end of stage I and stage II in order to pass through the birth canal (see Figures 16.8 and 16.9). Most babies are born either right or left occiput anterior (ROA or LOA). Occiput posterior (OP) babies are associated with protracted labors and with an ↑ likelihood of maternal birth trauma. The key to determining position lies in palpation of the sutures of the fetal head.

### STAGE III: DELIVERY OF THE PLACENTA

Signs of imminent placental delivery include cord lengthening, a gush of blood indicating placental separation, and a ↓ in uterine fundal height. The

*The cardinal movements of labor—how to get engaged:*

**Descend** to the floor.
**Flex** your knee.
**Look down** (internal rotation) at the ring you are about to give your beloved.
**Extend** your hand to give your beloved the ring.
**Look up** (external rotation) to see what the answer will be.
**Straighten up** (restitute) when the answer is yes!

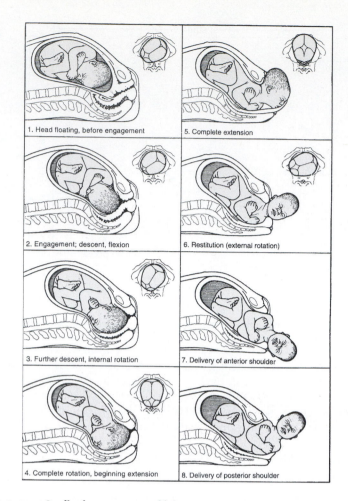

**FIGURE 16.8.** **Cardinal movements of labor.**

Cardinal movements consist of engagement, descent, flexion, internal rotation, extension, external rotation, restitution, and expulsion. (Reproduced, with permission, from Cunningham FG et al. *Williams Obstetrics*, 22nd ed. New York: McGraw-Hill, 2005: 418.)

third stage of labor should last no longer than 30 minutes. Active management is associated with ↓ rates of postpartum hemorrhage and includes oxytocin administration prior to placental delivery, early cord clamping, and controlled traction. Collecting cord blood prior to placental delivery provides a sample of fetal blood if needed for testing.

## Fetal Monitoring

### FETAL HEART RATE ASSESSMENT

Assessment of fetal heart rate during labor is a controversial practice but has nonetheless become accepted as the standard of care. Initially developed in an attempt to ↓ the rate of cerebral palsy and hypoxic birth injury, continuous electronic fetal monitoring has not been shown to be of benefit, and in uncomplicated labor it is associated with ↑ risk of operative delivery. Nonetheless, the practice is unlikely to be abandoned in the near future, as intermittent monitoring is nursing-intensive, and most clinicians have become dependent on the reassurance provided by a normal fetal heart rate tracing.

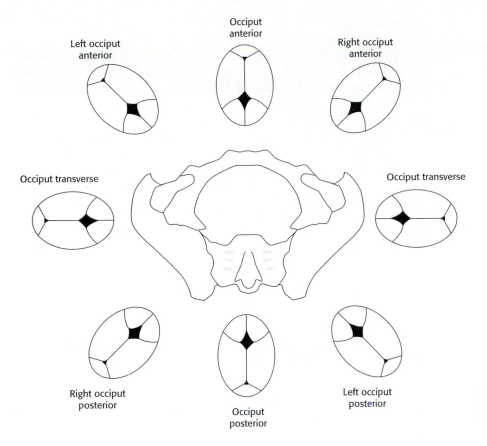

**Left occiput anterior**

**Occiput anterior**

**Right occiput anterior**

**Occiput transverse**

**Occiput transverse**

**Right occiput posterior**

**Occiput posterior**

**Left occiput posterior**

FIGURE 16.9. **Fetal positions with head sutures visible.**

- **Monitoring techniques:** Performed with an external ultrasound monitor or internal placement of fetal scalp electrodes (more accurate, but more invasive and requires ROM).
- **Monitoring recommendations:**
  - **Intermittent auscultation or external fetal monitoring:** Appropriate for uncomplicated labors; performed every 15 minutes in the active phase of stage I and every five minutes in stage II.
  - **Continuous external fetal monitoring:** Indicated if the mother is receiving IV pitocin for labor induction or augmentation or with conditions known to be associated with ↑ fetal morbidity/mortality.
  - **Continuous internal fetal monitoring:** Use if fetal heart rate tracing cannot be consistently followed with external monitoring or if fetal heart rate tracing is not reassuring.
- **Criteria for reassuring fetal heart tracing:** A baseline pulse of 120–160; no decelerations; accelerations above baseline appropriate for gestational age; normal heart rate variability.

## ANTENATAL TESTING

Methods and indications for antenatal testing are as follows:

- **Biophysical profile (BPP):** The BPP is a series of biophysical variables measured by ultrasound that, taken together, can help predict fetal well-being. These variables include the following:
  - Fetal tone.

REPRODUCTIVE HEALTH

555

- Fetal movements.
- Fetal breathing motions.
- NST assessment of fetal heart rate. For term pregnancies, a "reactive" NST is defined as at least two accelerations ≥ 15 seconds in duration and ≥ 15 bpm over a baseline of 120–160 bpm, with no decelerations during a 20-minute period.
- Measurement of AFI.
- **Modified BPP:** Consists of NST and AFI; currently indicated on a bi-weekly basis after 36–37 weeks of gestation for pregnancies complicated by gestational diabetes, a hypertensive disorder, multiple gestation, cholestasis of pregnancy, poly- or oligohydramnios, preeclampsia, or other serious medical or obstetrical conditions.
    - An abnormal NST/AFI should be followed by a full BPP.
    - If the BPP is normal (10/10), the NST/AFI should be repeated in 2–3 days; if the BPP is 8/10 due to inadequate fluid, rule out ruptured membranes, hydrate, and repeat the NST/AFI in 2–3 days.
    - A BPP < 8/10 with adequate amniotic fluid indicates a pregnancy at risk for fetal asphyxia; the patient should be admitted for observation, a BPP should be repeated, and a contraction stress test should be conducted (see below).
- **Contraction stress test (CST):** A CST is performed to evaluate fetal ability to tolerate labor. External fetal heart monitors are placed, and either nipple stimulation or IV pitocin is used to stimulate uterine contractions until either three strong uterine contractions occur in 10 minutes with no decelerations in fetal heart rate **or** ≥ 2 fetal heart rate decelerations occur.
    - One fetal heart rate deceleration associated with uterine contraction is considered an equivocal test and should be repeated.
    - A ⊕ CST is a contraindication to labor, and operative delivery should be considered.

## Labor Arrest and Protraction Disorders

A protraction disorder is defined as slower-than-normal labor; complete cessation of progress is termed *arrest of labor*.

### MANAGEMENT OF STAGE I PROTRACTION/ARREST

- Assess maternal/fetal well-being.
- Perform a digital cervical exam every 1–2 hours.
- Amniotomy if membranes are still intact.
- Oxytocin administration is indicated if uterine contractions are inadequate; titrate the dose to effect.
    - An intrauterine pressure catheter (IUPC) is recommended for greater accuracy of oxytocin titration.
    - Adequate uterine contractions are typically defined as at least three contractions every 10 minutes, each ≥ 60 Montevideo units above baseline and lasting ≥ 10 seconds (200 Montevideo units in a 10-minute period).
- A C-section should be performed in the setting of complete arrest despite four hours of adequate uterine contractions.

### MANAGEMENT OF STAGE II PROTRACTION/ARREST

- Observation is adequate as long as maternal/fetal status is reassuring and some progress has been made.
- Oxytocin administration with IUPC as above is appropriate in the presence of inadequate uterine forces.
- Attempt operative vaginal delivery (see below).
- A C-section should be performed if complete arrest is diagnosed and/or operative vaginal delivery is unsuccessful or contraindicated.

## Nonreassuring Fetal Heart Rate

A continuum of abnormal fetal heart rate tracings that may be indicative of fetal hypoxia or asphyxia. Types of nonreassuring fetal heart rate tracings include the following:

- **Absent variability:** May be due to fetal sleep cycle, anesthetic medications, or fetal acidosis.
- **Variable decelerations:** Slowing of the fetal heart rate in association with uterine contractions; may be due to cord compression or other vagal response.
- **Late decelerations:** Start after the uterine contraction has begun and conclude after the contraction has ended; indicative of impending fetal acidosis (see Figure 16.10).
- **Sinusoidal heart rate:** Thought to be a response to hypoxemia in cases of severe fetal anemia.
- **Saltatory pattern:** Excessive variability; indicative of mild hypoxia.
- **Prolonged bradycardia:** A fetal heart rate < 100 for several minutes; an ominous sign of fetal acidosis.
- **Tachycardia with diminished variability:** Often a response to maternal fever; rule out fetal arrhythmia.

Management of a nonreassuring fetal heart rate tracing consists of IV fluid, moving the mother onto her left side, oxygen administration, discontinuation of exogenous pitocin, and treatment of underlying conditions. An internal fetal scalp electrode should be placed for continuous accurate monitoring. Consider terbutaline administration to stop contractions. Prolonged or severe nonreassuring fetal status (as in Figure 16.10B) is an indication for immediate delivery.

## Pain Control during Labor and Delivery

Labor pain is caused primarily by distention of mechanoreceptors in the uterus and cervix during stage I and by stretching and/or tearing of the birth canal and pelvic ligaments during stage II. Fetal malpresentation and nulliparity are physiologic risk factors for ↑ pain, but fear or emotional distress can exacerbate pain as well. A feeling of control over the labor process can greatly improve patients' experience of labor; thus, early education about the labor process and pain control options, along with encouragement of maternal involvement in the decision-making process, is key. Treatment options are as follows:

- **Nonpharmacologic options:** Presence of a doula/labor support person; acupuncture; hypnosis.

---

*Causes of protraction and arrest disorders—*

*The 3 P's*

**P**ower: Hypocontractile uterine activity, epidural anesthesia, chorioamnionitis.
**P**assenger: Fetal macrosomia, malposition (especially occiput posterior fetus), postdate pregnancy.
**P**elvis: Pelvic contraction, cephalopelvic disproportion, short maternal stature, obesity.

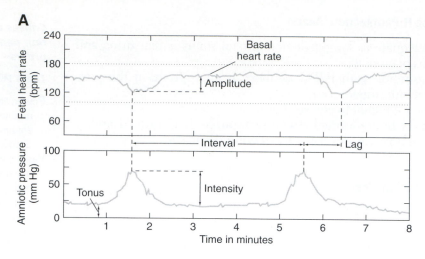

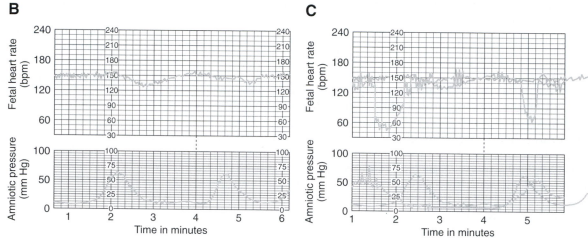

**FIGURE 16.10.** **A. Schematic fetal heart rate tracing. B. Late decelerations. C. Variable decelerations.**

(Reproduced, with permission, from DeCherney AH et al. *Current Obstetric & Gynecologic Diagnosis & Treatment*, 8th ed. Stamford, CT: Appleton & Lange, 1994: 301.)

---

> ***Contraindications to spinal/epidural–***
>
> **BK PAIN**
>
> **B**lood pressure too low (uncorrected hypovolemia)
> **K**oagulopathy (bleeding disorder)
> **P**ressure (↑ ICP)
> **A**natomic back problems
> **I**nfection of the soft tissue overlying the epidural injection site
> **N**o (the patient refuses)

- **Pharmacologic options:** Vary according to stage.
  - **Stage I:**
    - Nalbuphine IV 10–20 mg q 3–4 h.
    - Fentanyl 25–100 μg IV/IM q 1–2 h.
    - Epidural anesthesia (continuous drip of local anesthetic and opiate, e.g., bupivacaine and fentanyl). Requires bed rest, urinary catheter placement, and continuous fetal monitoring.
    - Spinal anesthesia (opioid injection alone during early labor, or combination opioid/local anesthetic later in labor and/or for C-section). Requires bed rest, urinary catheter placement, and continuous fetal monitoring.
  - **Stage II:**
    - Pudendal block (10 mL 1% lidocaine injected posterior to both ischial spines).
    - Local anesthetic into the perineum, especially if an episiotomy is to be performed.
    - Epidural/spinal anesthesia may be initiated during the second stage (see above) but is less desirable given the prolonged latency of medications and the potential for fetal respiratory depression.

## Induction of Labor

Indicated when prolonging the pregnancy puts the mother, the fetus, or both at risk. The most common indication is for post-term pregnancy (≥ 42 weeks); however, induction may be necessary at any gestational age. If possible, fetal lung maturity should be established either by accurate pregnancy dating or by amniocentesis, and if necessary, corticosteroids should be administered for fetal lung maturity. The method of induction depends on the extent of cervical ripening as assessed by the Bishop score (see Table 16.7). Once determined, Bishop scores are interpreted as follows:

- **Bishop score > 6:** Associated with a higher chance of success. IV pitocin may be started without the need for cervical ripening agents until uterine contractions achieve a satisfactory level.
- **Bishop score < 6:**
  - The failure rate is 10–50%, and a cervical ripening agent such as misoprostol (25–50 µg PV q 4 h) may be used.
  - An alternative method involves insertion of a Foley catheter into the internal os and gentle traction.
  - Continuous fetal monitoring should be employed throughout any induction attempt.

## Peripartum Complications

### GROUP B STREPTOCOCCUS (GBS) INFECTION

Prior to the development of screening and prophylaxis protocols, this component of normal vaginal flora was the most common cause of neonatal sepsis. Transmission to the fetus occurs during passage through the birth canal, with the main risk factors consisting of preterm delivery and prolonged ROM. Universal prenatal screening should be performed at 35–37 weeks (or sooner if an earlier delivery is planned). The only exceptions are women with GBS bacteriuria at any time during pregnancy as well as those with a history of a previous infant with invasive GBS disease, who should be treated as if they were confirmed as GBS ⊕. Women who are planning an elective C-section should be screened as well but do not require treatment in the absence of labor or ruptured membranes. Figure 16.11 and Table 16.8 outline further guidelines.

In the presence of threatened preterm labor, if a GBS screen has not previously been performed, collect cultures and initiate prophylaxis for 48 hours

**TABLE 16.7. The Bishop Scoring System**

| CERVIX | SCORE | | | |
|---|---|---|---|---|
| | 0 | 1 | 2 | 3 |
| Position | Posterior | Midposition | Anterior | – |
| Consistency | Firm | Medium | Soft | – |
| Effacement | 0–30 | 40–50 | 60–70 | ≥ 80 |
| Dilation | Closed | 1–2 | 3–4 | ≥ 5 |
| Station | –3 | –2 | –1, 0 | +1, +2 |

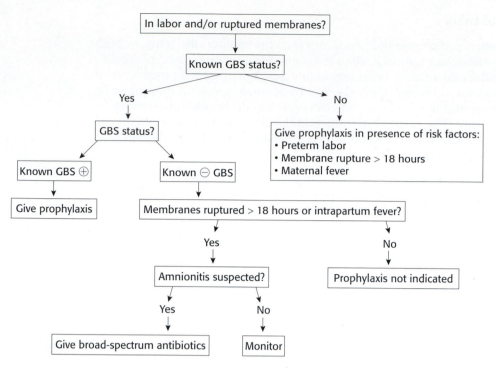

**FIGURE 16.11.** **Antibiotic prophylaxis for GBS infection.**

during tocolysis. If the patient is GBS ⊖, discontinue prophylaxis at the discretion of the provider after 48 hours, and rescreen for GBS at 35–37 weeks.

### SHOULDER DYSTOCIA

Defined as failure of the fetal shoulders to deliver spontaneously one minute after the delivery of the baby's head, usually because the baby's anterior shoulder is stuck behind the maternal pubic bone. **Considered an obstetrical emergency,** shoulder dystocia occurs in 0.5–2.9% of deliveries, with most cases affecting babies weighing > 4 kg. Other risk factors include maternal obesity, maternal diabetes, and vacuum or forceps delivery. A dystocia should be anticipated if there is prolonged fetal descent and/or "turtling" of the fetal

**TABLE 16.8.** **GBS Prophylaxis Regimens**

| | MEDICATION | INITIAL DOSE | MAINTENANCE DOSE |
|---|---|---|---|
| Preferred regimen | Penicillin G | 5M U IV | 2.5 MU IV q 4 h until delivery |
| Alternative regimen | Ampicillin | 2 g IV | 1 g IV q 4 h until delivery |
| Penicillin-allergic patients with low risk of anaphylaxis | Cefazolin | 2 g IV | 1 g q 8 h until delivery |
| Penicillin-allergic patients with high risk of anaphylaxis | Clindamycin | 900 mg IV | 900 mg IV q 8 h until delivery |

head. Complications include fetal hypoxia, fetal clavicular fracture, Erb's palsy, and maternal perineal laceration.

### GENITAL TRACT LACERATIONS

Injury to the birth canal during vaginal delivery is the one of the most common obstetrical complications. Perineal midline tears are most common, but periurethral, labial, and cervical lacerations also occur frequently. Risk factors include primiparity, precipitous delivery, fetal macrosomia or malpresentation, operative vaginal delivery, and maternal connective tissue disorders.

### SYMPTOMS/EXAM

Categorized according to the extent of injury as follows:

- **First degree:** Laceration of the vaginal mucosa only.
- **Second degree:** Extension of the laceration into the vaginal deep tissue.
- **Third degree:** Extension of the laceration into the external rectal sphincter muscle.
- **Fourth degree:** Extension of the laceration through the rectal mucosa.

### TREATMENT

Surgical repair or, if minor, healing by 2° intention.

### COMPLICATIONS

Postpartum hemorrhage, urinary or fecal incontinence, fistula formation.

### CHORIOAMNIONITIS

Infection of the amniotic membranes; also known as amnionitis or intrapartum fever. The most commonly implicated pathogens are gram-$\ominus$ rods and anaerobes (*Bacteroides, Mycoplasma, Ureaplasma, Gardnerella*, GBS). Risk factors include nulliparity, preterm or prolonged ROM, genital tract infections, internal monitoring, digital cervical exams in women with ruptured membranes, and meconium-stained amniotic fluid.

### SYMPTOMS/EXAM

- Presents with maternal fever > 38°C (100.4°F), uterine tenderness, and foul-smelling amniotic fluid.
- Exam reveals maternal and/or fetal tachycardia.

### DIAGNOSIS

CBC; culture of amniotic fluid.

### TREATMENT

Treat with broad-spectrum antibiotics (ampicillin and gentamicin) along with continuous fetal monitoring.

### COMPLICATIONS

Fetal sepsis, fetal neurologic damage, ↑ C-section rate, wound infection, endomyometritis, postpartum hemorrhage.

---

**Management of shoulder dystocia—**

**HELPER**

**H**elp (ask for help)
**E**pisiotomy
**L**egs up (perform McRoberts' maneuver)
**P**ressure (suprapubic)
**E**nter the vagina to rotate with Wood's screw maneuver
**R**eturn the fetal head to the pelvis for C-section (Zavanelli maneuver)

*Operative vaginal delivery should **not** be undertaken unless the provider is willing to abandon the attempt should it prove unsuccessful.*

***Maternal indications for operative vaginal delivery:***

- *Mother **can't** push (e.g., inability to push effectively due to epidural anesthesia)*
- *Mother **won't** push (e.g., maternal exhaustion)*
- *Mother **shouldn't** push (e.g., cardiac disease, ↑ ICP)*

---

***Procedure for vacuum delivery—***

**CONEHEAD**

**C**onsent obtained?
**0** station or lower?
**N**o contraindications (e.g., preterm or macrosomia/shoulder dystocia suspected)?
**E**nter vagina with vacuum cup
**H**ead placement correct (over sagittal suture, 3 cm above the anterior fontanelle)?
**E**dges of cervix clear?
**A**pply pressure (roughly 500 mmHg)
**D**ownward pull with next contraction (3–5 pulls with a maximum of three pop-offs)

## OPERATIVE VAGINAL DELIVERY

Refers to application of a vacuum or forceps to assist in vaginal delivery in cases of a prolonged or arrested second stage with nonreassuring fetal status. Criteria for operative delivery include a completely dilated cervix and a term fetus in vertex position and **at least 0 station,** with no shoulder dystocia anticipated. Before operative delivery is attempted, the bladder and bowel should ideally be emptied and adequate anesthesia established. Complications include maternal birth trauma, fetal cephalohematoma, subgaleal hematoma, fetal retinal hemorrhage, and fetal intracranial hemorrhage.

## CESAREAN SECTION

Defined as operative removal of the fetus through an abdominal incision. C-sections are indicated for a variety of reasons, classified as either fetal indications (malpresentation, intolerance of labor, fetal congenital anomalies; consider for estimated fetal weight > 4.5 kg) or maternal indications (failure to progress, placenta or vasa previa, 1° HSV infection, medical contraindications to labor, uterine/cervical abnormalities). Approximately 20-25% of babies in the United States are delivered via C-section. Preoperative preparation includes the following:

- Informed consent (with tubal ligation consent if desired)
- Placement of a Foley catheter
- Spinal/epidural anesthesia (general anesthesia if emergent)
- Removal of fetal monitors
- Sterile prep/drape

Complications of C-section include bleeding; infection; damage to the abdominal organs, especially the uterus, ureters, and bladder; prolonged maternal recovery time; anesthesia risks; and neonatal injury or respiratory depression.

## VAGINAL BIRTH AFTER C-SECTION (VBAC)

VBAC has undergone considerable scrutiny over the last two decades, primarily because of concerns over uterine rupture, risk factors for which include prior uterine incision extending into the fundus and prior uterine rupture. The current recommendation is to confine VBAC deliveries to hospitals with 24-hour onsite anesthesia and obstetric services only, and to patients with a history of no more than one low transverse or low vertical uterine incision, as the risk of uterine rupture ↑ with the number of prior C-sections.

### SYMPTOMS/EXAM

Symptoms and signs of uterine rupture include fetal bradycardia, constant severe abdominal pain, vaginal bleeding, loss of uterine tone, a change in uterine shape, and hypovolemia.

### TREATMENT

The management of VBACs includes continuous monitoring, avoidance of prostaglandin cervical ripening agents, and very close monitoring if oxytocin augmentation is used.

REPRODUCTIVE HEALTH

## Meconium-Stained Amniotic Fluid

Occurring in roughly 14% of deliveries, meconium-stained amniotic fluid is associated with neonatal meconium aspiration syndrome. Risk factors include postdate gestation and nonreassuring fetal status.

### Diagnosis

Diagnosed clinically by the characteristic thick, "pea soup" appearance of amniotic fluid on ROM.

### Treatment

- Consider warm saline amnioinfusion for variable decelerations on fetal heart tracing.
- If there is no spontaneous cry at delivery, attempt intubation with a meconium suction device × 2 before initiating the Neonatal Advanced Life Support (NALS) protocol (see Figure 16.12).

## Placental Pathology

The placenta is an organ that supports fetal growth in utero. Composed of fetal tissue, it is a unique interface of maternal and fetal nutrient exchange and, as such, contains many clues to intrauterine pathology. The basic placental

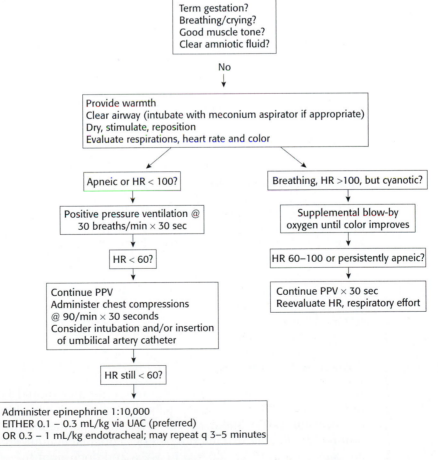

**FIGURE 16.12.   Neonatal Advanced Life Support protocol.**

exam should thus include an assessment of the weight/appearance of placental parenchyma and membranes, cord length, and number of vessels. Indications for a full pathology exam include abnormal placental appearance; preterm or post-term birth; stillbirth; fetal infection, hydrops, or congenital anomalies; oligo- or polyhydramnios; antepartum hemorrhage; or severe hypertensive disorders. Abnormalities include the following:

- **Cord abnormalities:**
  - **Hypo- or hypercoiled cord/short cord:** Associated with poor fetal growth.
  - **Long cord:** Presents with a knotted or compressed cord.
  - **Abnormal cord insertion** (e.g., marginal or velamentous): Associated with cord trauma or thrombi.
  - **Abnormal number of vessels:** Associated with congenital anomalies and IUGR.
- **Membrane abnormalities:**
  - **Abnormal color:** Associated with infection, meconium, or hemorrhage.
  - **Abnormal membrane insertion:** May be circummarginate (in which membranes originate from the inside margin of the placental disk) or circumvallate (in which membranes are grooved from abnormally deep implantation in the disk).
- **Parenchymal abnormalities:**
  - **Small placenta:** Associated with inadequate placental perfusion.
  - **Missing lobe:** Presents with retained placental tissue in the uterus.
  - **Calcified placenta:** Associated with post-term pregnancy.
  - **Placenta succenturiata:** An additional lobe; associated with a retained placental lobe or with placenta or vasa previa.
  - **Duplex placenta:** Complete separation into two lobes; associated with velamentous cord insertion.
  - **Circumvallate placenta:** A small chorionic plate with growth of extrachorial placental tissue; associated with premature separation and second-trimester bleeding.

## POSTPARTUM ISSUES

### Routine Postpartum Care

Although the average length of hospitalization for an uncomplicated vaginal delivery is 1–3 days, the postpartum period is currently defined as lasting until six weeks after delivery. The main focus of routine care during this period consists of mother-baby bonding, establishing breast-feeding, and education regarding routine newborn and self-care. While most obstetrical problems resolve after delivery, the clinician must also be aware of the possibility of continuing gestational diabetes, eclampsia, venous thromboembolism, infection, or hemorrhage.

#### POSTPARTUM PHYSICAL EXAM

Immediate postpartum examination of the mother should include an evaluation of the extent of bleeding, palpation of the uterine fundus for size and firmness, and assessment of the cervix and perineum for the presence of trauma (see the discussion on repair of vaginal lacerations). Prior to discharge, an exam should be conducted to assess and document the quantity and quality of continuing lochia, lower extremity edema, and any uterine tenderness

---

*Postpartum physical exam assessment–*

**BUBBLES**

**B**reast
**U**terus
**B**owel
**B**ladder
**L**ochia
**E**pisiotomy
**S**urgical site (for cesarean section)

or breast/nipple abnormalities. A complete physical, including a pelvic exam, should be conducted at approximately six weeks postpartum.

### POSTPARTUM LABS

- Recheck hematocrit the day after delivery or sooner in the presence of postpartum hemorrhage.
- A fasting blood glucose should be obtained the day after delivery and a two-hour 75-g glucose challenge obtained at six weeks after delivery to ensure resolution of GDM if applicable.

### POSTPARTUM COUNSELING

- Ask about common discomforts (e.g., urinary retention, constipation, perineal care).
- Determine the frequency of breast-feeding and commonly encountered problems.
- Counsel patients with regard to routine newborn care, including how to take the baby's temperature, anticipate URIs, use car safety seats, and perform jaundice checks.
- Offer information about postpartum depression, family support, and emotional self-care.
- Counsel patients with regard to birth control methods (estrogen-containing methods can potentially ↓ the quantity of breast milk and/or pass to the baby).
- Discuss the duration of normal bleeding, and recommend pelvic rest for six weeks.

## Postpartum Complications

### POSTPARTUM ENDOMETRITIS

Defined as uterine infection after delivery, usually caused by *Bacteroides, Enterobacter*, group A or B streptococcus, or *Chlamydia trachomatis* (late endometritis). Its incidence after a vaginal birth is < 3% but is higher after a C-section; risk factors include operative delivery, prolonged ROM, and amnionitis.

### SYMPTOMS/EXAM

Presents with fever, abdominal pain, and uterine tenderness without any other identifiable cause.

### DIFFERENTIAL

UTI, retained placental products, wound/episiotomy infection, pelvic abscess, septic pelvic thrombophlebitis, drug fever, pulmonary embolism.

### DIAGNOSIS

- CBC; UA and urine culture.
- Consider CXR and ultrasound.

### TREATMENT

- Ampicillin, gentamicin, and clindamycin **or** ticarcillin/clavulanate.
- Continue antibiotics until the patient is afebrile for 24–48 hours.

> ***Causes of postpartum hemorrhage—***
>
> ***The 4 T's***
>
> **T**issue (retained placenta)
> **T**one (uterine atony)
> **T**rauma (traumatic delivery, episiotomy)
> **T**hrombin (coagulation disorders, DIC)

> ***Treatment of uterine atony—***
>
> **Arm Pits Help Me Pack Blood In**
>
> **Arm** (bimanual pressure)
> **Pits** (pitocin; may be given IV or IM)
> **Help** (call for help) and **He**mabate (250 μg IM q 1.5–3.5 h unless asthmatic)
> **Me**thergine (200 μg IM unless hypertensive)
> **Pack** (the uterus)
> **Blood** (type and cross; transfusion PRN)
> **In**to the OR for emergent uterine ligation/hysterectomy; **In**terventional radiology for embolization.

## POSTPARTUM HEMORRHAGE

Defined as ≥ 500 mL of blood loss 0–24 hours after delivery or blood loss sufficient to make the patient symptomatic (e.g., lightheadedness, dizziness, tachycardia). Risk factors include prolonged or very rapid labor, large baby, multiple gestations, nulliparity or grand multiparity, use of endogenous oxytocin, uterine infection, retained placenta, or lacerations of the cervix and vagina. The most common causes are uterine atony and retained tissue or blood clot.

### *SYMPTOMS*

Patients present with continued vaginal bleeding.

### *EXAM*

- Perform a cervical and perineal exam for lacerations; do a bimanual exam to assess uterine tone.
- A placental exam, uterine sweep, and ultrasound can assess for clots/retained tissue.

### *DIAGNOSIS*

Diagnosed through accurate assessment of blood loss postpartum (providers consistently **underestimate** blood loss for vaginal and cesarean deliveries).

### *TREATMENT*

- **Retained placental tissue:** Evacuation or curettage.
- **Genital tract laceration:** Expeditious repair!
- **Uterine inversion** (see Figure 16.13): Give terbutaline to relax the uterus; then replace the uterus in the pelvis. Do **not** remove the placenta while the uterus is inverted!
- **Uterine atony:** See the mnemonic "**Arm Pits Help Me Pack Blood In.**"

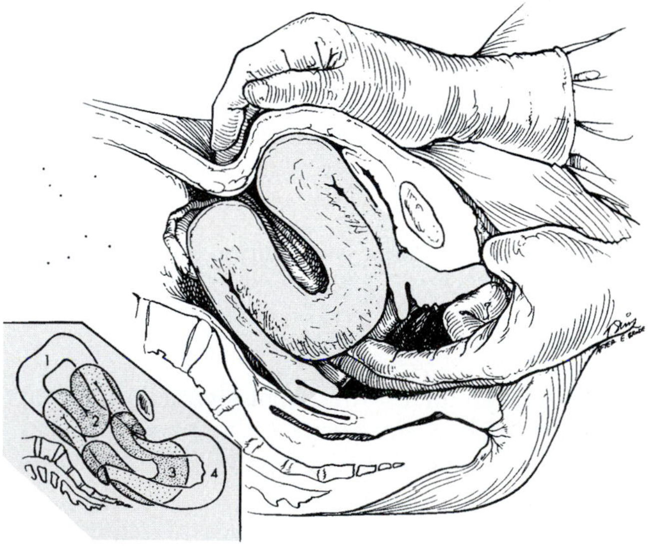


**FIGURE 16.13. Partial uterine inversion.**

(Reproduced, with permission, from Cunningham FG et al. *Williams Obstetrics*, 22nd ed. New York: McGraw-Hill, 2005: 833.)

REPRODUCTIVE HEALTH

### RETAINED PLACENTA

Diagnosed when the third stage of labor lasts > 30 minutes or when the placental exam confirms retention of placental tissue. Occurs in 1–2% of deliveries and is associated with uterine abnormalities and placenta accreta.

#### DIAGNOSIS

Ultrasound to determine whether the placenta is detached from the uterine wall.

#### TREATMENT

- **If the placenta is completely detached:** Manual traction on the umbilical cord.
- **If the placenta is partially or completely adherent:** Attempt manual removal.
- May require general anesthesia in the OR.

#### COMPLICATIONS

Postpartum hemorrhage, intrauterine infection.

### BREAST-FEEDING ISSUES

Breast-feeding imparts passive immunity and complete nutrition to the newborn and promotes mother-baby bonding. Exclusive breast-feeding is recommended for the first six months of life and partial breast-feeding thereafter for the first year. Breast-feeding should be continued as long as mutually desired. Common problems encountered include the following:

- **Engorgement:** Treat with frequent and complete feeds along with cool compresses.
- **Plugged ducts:** Presents with a palpable tender lump. Treat with frequent feeds; aspiration may be required.
- **Mastitis:** Presents with a hard, red, tender area associated with fevers, chills, and malaise. Treat with frequent feeds along with dicloxacillin × 10–14 days.
- **Poor latch:** Improper seal of the infant's lips around the nipple. Address with a lactation consult.
- **Nipple soreness/trauma:** Keep nipples clean with water and saline; air dry; use lanolin cream and/or mupirocin (Bactroban) ointment for refractory cracking or soreness.

## INFECTIONS IN PREGNANCY

A 27-year-old G3P2 with poorly controlled gestational diabetes presents to the ER at 30 weeks of gestation with a complaint of 12 hours of lower abdominal pain radiating to the back accompanied by fever, chills, nausea, and vomiting. Her urine is cloudy with 25–50 WBCs/hpf. How should she be treated? Appropriate management of pyelonephritis includes hospital admission, IV fluid administration, fetal monitoring, and IV antibiotics until the patient has been afebrile for 24 hours. Urine should be sent for culture, and antibiotic treatment should be adjusted according to culture and sensitivity results.

## Urinary Tract Infections and Asymptomatic Bacteriuria

Caused by the same pathogens as those that affect nonpregnant patients, UTIs complicate roughly 5% of pregnancies. Risk factors include bladder/kidney anomalies, gestational diabetes, and multiparity. Rapid progression to pyelonephritis is the main risk of UTIs in pregnancy.

### DIAGNOSIS

Obtain a clean-catch urine culture; perform routine screening at the first prenatal visit.

### TREATMENT

- Treat with a short course of antibiotics (nitrofurantoin, amoxicillin, cephalosporins, or sulfisoxazole); adjust treatment in accordance with culture and sensitivity.
- Obtain follow-up urine cultures.
- Hospitalize for IV antibiotics if pyelonephritis is suspected.
- GBS bacteriuria requires intrapartum antibiotic prophylaxis.

### COMPLICATIONS

Pyelonephritis. Bacteriuria is also associated with an ↑ risk of preterm birth and perinatal mortality.

## Bacterial Vaginosis

Overgrowth of normal vaginal bacterial flora. Occurs in 10–25% of pregnant women and is nearly always asymptomatic.

### SYMPTOMS/EXAM

Patients are generally asymptomatic; exam reveals a vaginal discharge with a fishy odor.

### DIAGNOSIS

- ⊕ KOH "whiff test"; clue cells on wet mount.
- Vaginal discharge with pH > 4.5.

### TREATMENT

Oral metronidazole. Treatment does not appear to ↓ the complication rate.

### COMPLICATIONS

Higher incidence of PPROM; spontaneous abortion; preterm birth.

## HIV Infection in Pregnancy

### DIAGNOSIS

- Perform routine screening of all pregnant women at the first prenatal visit.
- If the patient has had no prenatal care, obtain a rapid HIV test at the time the patient presents to the hospital in labor.

### TREATMENT

- Consultation with an HIV specialist.
- Offer mental health and drug abuse resources as well as behavioral interventions as applicable.
- Assess current disease status with a CD4 cell count and viral load.
- Initiate antiretroviral treatment during pregnancy.
- Give antibiotic prophylaxis as indicated for opportunistic infections (as with nonpregnant patients).
- Consider elective C-section in the presence of a high viral load.
- Intrapartum antiretroviral prophylaxis.
- Avoid fetal scalp electrode, episiotomy, or artificial ROM.
- Wash the baby **immediately** after birth.
- Counsel to avoid breast-feeding.

## Genital Herpes Simplex Infection

See the STI discussion for signs, symptoms, and diagnosis.

### TREATMENT

- During pregnancy, treat genital HSV outbreaks with acyclovir (400 mg PO BID-TID) or valacyclovir (500 mg PO QD) × 7–14 days for the first outbreak.
- Begin suppressive therapy at 36 weeks.
- A C-section should be performed if a 1° genital HSV outbreak occurs during labor.
- Consider C-section for any patient with active genital lesions.

### COMPLICATIONS

Systemic neonatal herpetic infection from passage through the birth canal. Neonatal herpes has a 50% mortality rate.

## Varicella-Zoster Infection

Infection with varicella zoster, or "chickenpox," affects 1–5 in 10,000 pregnancies and is caused by respiratory transmission of VZV.

### SYMPTOMS/EXAM

Normal symptoms of fever, malaise, myalgias, and vesicular rash may be more severe in pregnant women.

### DIAGNOSIS

Diagnosed by viral titer.

### TREATMENT

- Administer VZIG to neonates at risk and to nonimmune pregnant women who have been exposed to VZV.
- Avoid varicella vaccination during pregnancy.

Maternal varicella pneumonia (40% mortality), congenital varicella syndrome, neonatal varicella infection.

## Syphilis

Given that perinatal transmission in mothers with 1° or 2° syphilis is 50%, universal screening for serology (RPR or VDRL) is recommended at the first prenatal visit.

### TREATMENT

Penicillin. Desensitization to penicillin is recommended in penicillin-allergic patients.

### COMPLICATIONS

Perinatal death, preterm birth (especially in the setting of a Jarisch-Herxheimer reaction), congenital anomalies, IUGR.

## Gonorrhea and Chlamydia

Cervical infection with either *Neisseria gonorrhoeae* or *Chlamydia trachomatis* is associated with an ↑ risk of PROM and preterm labor, chorioamnionitis, endometritis, and neonatal ophthalmologic infection. The incidence of gonorrheal infection is < 1%; chlamydial infections are more common, complicating roughly 5% of pregnancies.

### DIAGNOSIS

- Perform routine screening of all pregnant women at the first prenatal visit.
- Consider retesting later in pregnancy for patients at high risk.

### TREATMENT

- Treat with ceftriaxone 125 mg IM × 1 and azithromycin 1 g PO × 1.
- Public health reporting is mandatory for confirmed diagnosis of either pathogen.
- A test of cure should be obtained after treatment.

## OTHER MEDICAL ISSUES IN PREGNANCY

## Depression in Pregnancy/Postpartum Depression

Some 3–5% of pregnant women and 1–5% of postpartum women experience major depression. Risk factors include a prior or family history of depression.

### DIFFERENTIAL

Bipolar disorder, hypothyroidism, generalized anxiety disorder, recreational substance use.

### DIAGNOSIS

CBC, TSH, CMP; urine toxicology screen.

- Counseling; family support; SSRIs (fluoxetine and sertraline are the best studied).
- Hospitalization may be necessary if the depression is severe and/or associated with psychosis.

### COMPLICATIONS

- Noncompliance with medical care; impaired maternal-infant bonding; poor nutrition; suicidal/homicidal ideation and attempts; postpartum psychosis.
- Use of SSRIs may be associated with "neonatal behavioral syndrome," which consists of self-limited tremors, mild tachypnea, and, rarely, seizures. Recent reports have also linked SSRI use with persistent pulmonary hypertension of the newborn.
- Paroxetine is contraindicated because of its association with fetal cardiac abnormalities.

## Thromboembolic Disease

Pregnancy is considered a hypercoagulable state, and DVT or pulmonary embolism occurs in 0.2% of pregnancies. Risk factors include inherited thrombophilia, C-section, preterm delivery, and multiple births.

### SYMPTOMS/EXAM

- **DVT:** Presents with lower extremity swelling or pain.
- **Pulmonary embolism:** Presents with dyspnea or cough.

### DIAGNOSIS

- D-dimer has excellent negative predictive value.
- Lower extremity Doppler ultrasound for suspected DVT; V/Q scan for pulmonary embolism.

### TREATMENT

- Anticoagulation with low-molecular-weight or unfractionated heparin up to 4–6 weeks postpartum.
- May switch to warfarin postpartum; titrate to an INR of 1.5–2.5.
- IVC filter for patients in whom anticoagulation is contraindicated.

## Medications in Pregnancy

Medications are categorized according to their safety in pregnancy as well as in lactation. Accepted categories are as follows:

- **Pharmaceutical pregnancy categories:**
    - **A:** Safety established using human studies.
    - **B:** Presumed safety based on animal studies.
    - **C:** Uncertain safety; no human/animal studies to date show an adverse effect.
    - **D:** Unsafe; risk may be justifiable in certain clinical circumstances.
    - **X:** Highly unsafe; the risk of use outweighs all possible benefits.
- **Pharmaceutical lactation categories:**
    - ⊕: Generally accepted as safe.

TABLE 16.9.    Medications Not Contraindicated in Pregnancy

| Category | Examples |
|---|---|
| Analgesics | Acetaminophen, narcotics (except if used on a long-term basis or in high doses at term). |
| Antimicrobials | Penicillin, cephalosporin, erythromycin, azithromycin, nystatin, clotrimazole, metronidazole, nitrofurantoin. |
| Cardiovascular | Labetalol, methyldopa, hydralazine, heparin. |
| Dermatologic | Erythromycin, clindamycin, benzoyl peroxide. |
| Endocrinologic | Insulin, levothyroxine, glyburide. |
| ENT | Chlorpheniramine, diphenhydramine, dextromethorphan, guaifenesin, intranasal steroids. |
| GI | Antacids, simethicone, $H_2$ blockers, metoclopramide, docusate, doxylamine. |
| Psychiatric | Fluoxetine, desipramine, doxepin. |
| Pulmonary | Albuterol, cromolyn, inhaled steroids, short-term prednisone. |

- ▪ ?: Safety is unknown or controversial.
- ▪ ⊖: Generally regarded as unsafe.
- ▪ Medications generally accepted as safe for use in pregnancy are outlined in Table 16.9.

# GYNECOLOGY

## FAMILY PLANNING

A 31-year-old woman presents to your office five weeks after the birth of her first baby. Breast-feeding is going well, and she occasionally supplements with formula. She and her partner had planned to remain abstinent until her six-week postpartum checkup, but last night they had sex on the "spur of the moment" without a condom or any birth control. She feels strongly that they are not yet ready to have another baby. How would you counsel her? Since she is not breast-feeding exclusively, she should not rely on lactational amenorrhea to prevent pregnancy. You can offer her several options for emergency contraception that are safe during breast-feeding and are available in the office. After that, she may choose from any number of maintenance birth control methods that will be safe both for her and for the baby. She should take a urine pregnancy test in 2–3 weeks.

## Contraception

Planning when and if to have children is an important part of overall health maintenance for men, women, and adolescents. Whether through abstinence, natural family planning, or one of the many contraceptive options available, the goal of birth control is to prevent unintended pregnancy so that people may have children when they are ready to be parents.

### EMERGENCY CONTRACEPTION

- Defined as postcoital contraception that ↓ the chance of pregnancy if used after unprotected sex or method failure (e.g., a condom slips off).
- All methods of emergency contraception are more effective the sooner after intercourse they are used.
- Emergency contraception does not interrupt or terminate an established pregnancy. Like other hormonal birth control methods, its 1° mechanism of action lies in preventing ovulation. It may also prevent fertilization or implantation.
- Emergency contraception may be most needed at night or on weekends, when clinics are closed. In order to prevent delay in obtaining such contraception, consider providing patients with advance prescriptions (and refills) at routine office visits. Advance provision has been found to be safe and effective and does not ↑ high-risk sexual behavior.
- Plan B is the only product on the U.S. market approved specifically as emergency contraception. If Plan B is not available, correct doses can be obtained from combined or progestin-only OCPs.
- Plan B is labeled for patients to take two pills 12 hours apart, but it is equally effective if both pills are taken together.
- Plan B has proven efficacy up to five days after intercourse.
- There are no evidence-based contraindications to Plan B.
- Table 16.10 outlines options for emergency contraception along with their indications and effectiveness.
- Plan B is FDA approved for over-the-counter sales to people 18 years and older. Patients under 18 still need a prescription.

### COMBINED HORMONAL METHODS

- OCPs, the weekly patch (Ortho Evra), and the monthly ring (NuvaRing) all work by releasing estrogen and progestin into the bloodstream.
- With > 99% effectiveness for perfect use and 92% for typical use, these contraceptives are among the most effective available and have also demonstrated good safety and tolerability.

**TABLE 16.10. Emergency Contraception Options**

| | PROGESTIN ONLY (PLAN B) | COMBINED HORMONAL ("YUZPE METHOD") | COPPER IUD (PARAGARD) |
|---|---|---|---|
| How supplied | Two pills of Plan B (0.75 mg of levonorgestrel) or 40 pills of Ovrette (norgestrel). | Multiple pills from OCP pack (each dose is equivalent to 100–120 μg of ethinyl estradiol and 0.50-0.75 mg of levonorgestrel). | Inserted by provider. |
| Effective if used | In five days | In five days | In 5–8 days |
| Pregnancy rate following use | 1–4% | 1–4% | < 1% |

- Conditions that contraindicate the use of combined hormonal methods include the following:
    - DVT, thrombophlebitis, or a thromboembolic disorder.
    - Uncontrolled hypertension, especially if > 160/100.
    - A history of MI, CVA, CAD, or valvular heart disease with thrombogenic complications.
    - Diabetes of > 20 years' duration or with vascular involvement.
    - Heavy tobacco use (≥ 15 cigarettes per day) in patients > 35 years of age. Use caution in all smokers > 35 years of age.
    - Breast cancer.
    - Migraines with aura, or any migraines in patients > 35 years of age.
    - Hepatic adenoma, hepatic carcinoma, or acute or chronic hepatocellular disease with abnormal liver function.
    - Planned surgery with prolonged immobilization.
- Caution should also be exercised with breast-feeding mothers in the first six weeks postpartum and in all women in the first three weeks postpartum (in view of ↑ DVT risk).
- Noncontraceptive benefits include reduction in ovarian and endometrial cancer risk and treatment of acne, dysmenorrhea, PMS, irregular or heavy menses, endometriosis, menstrual migraines, and ovarian cysts.
- Combined hormonal contraceptives may be safely used continuously—skipping the withdrawal bleed—for the treatment of menses-related conditions or for convenience. This may ↑ the rate of breakthrough bleeding.
- Methods may be started on any day of the menstrual cycle. For convenience, the first day of menses or the first Sunday after the beginning of menses has traditionally been recommended.
- If starting on the first day of a regular menstrual cycle, no backup method is needed. All others should use a barrier method or abstain for seven days.
- The Quick Start method, in which the patient takes her first dose during the visit with her provider, has been proven to ↑ adherence. While the provider should be reasonably sure that the patient is not pregnant, there is no proven risk to an established pregnancy of exposure to hormonal contraception.
- Serious complications—including MI, CVA, and DVT—are exceedingly rare.

### PROGESTIN-ONLY METHODS

- Available as medroxyprogesterone injected every three months (Depo-Provera IM or Depo-SubQ Provera 104) or as progestin-only pills ("mini-pills") taken daily.
- Associated with an effectiveness of > 99% with perfect use, vs. 92% (for pills) and 97% (for injections) with typical use.
- Safe for breast-feeding mothers and their babies.
- Current breast cancer is the only absolute contraindication. Use caution if patients have a history of the following conditions:
    - Multiple risk factors for cardiovascular disease.
    - Uncontrolled severe hypertension (≥ 160/110).
    - Current DVT or pulmonary embolism.
    - Ischemic heart disease or CVA.
    - Migraine with focal neurologic symptoms.
    - Unexplained vaginal bleeding prior to evaluation.
    - Past breast cancer.
    - Hepatic adenoma, hepatic carcinoma, active hepatitis, or severe cirrhosis.
    - Postpartum < 6 weeks and breast-feeding.

- Irregular spotting and amenorrhea are common.
- Depo-Provera users may have more weight gain than with other methods.
- Long-term use of Depo-Provera (> 2 years), especially in teens, may → ↓ bone mineral density (BMD) in a manner similar to that seen during pregnancy and lactation. Although extensive international experience shows no ↑ in osteoporosis or fractures, long-term risk is unknown. An FDA warning advises long-term use only if other birth control methods are unacceptable. Encourage all users to take adequate calcium and vitamin D and to engage in weight-bearing exercise.
- Progestin-only pills must be taken at the same time every day to maintain their effectiveness.

### INTRAUTERINE DEVICE (IUD)

- Copper-T (ParaGard) and levonorgestrel-releasing (Mirena) IUDs are now available in the United States.
- Associated with an effectiveness of > 99% with perfect use and > 99% with typical use.
- Mirena is approved for use up to five years, with newer evidence suggesting that its effectiveness lasts seven years. Paragard is approved for use up to 10 years, with evidence of effectiveness extending to 12 years. If a device is removed or spontaneously expelled at any time, fertility returns to baseline.
- Counsel patients to use condoms if they are at risk for STIs. IUDs do not ↑ the risk of acquiring STIs or PID. With monofilament strings, modern IUDs do not cause the ascending infection that older devices are known for. Mirena ↓ risk of PID through its effect on cervical mucus.
- Contraindications include the following:
  - Pregnancy.
  - Active infection (endometritis, PID, cervicitis).
  - Anatomic abnormalities or fibroids that distort the uterine cavity enough to make insertion difficult (most fibroids **are** compatible with IUD insertion).
  - Current gynecologic cancer.
  - Breast cancer (Mirena only).
  - Unexplained vaginal bleeding prior to evaluation.
  - For Mirena, all the cautions of progestin-only methods apply.
- IUDs ↓ the overall risk of ectopic pregnancy and are not contraindicated for women with a history of ectopic pregnancy or PID. If a pregnancy occurs, there is an ↑ likelihood that it will be ectopic if an IUD is in place.
- Light or absent menses are common with Mirena, making it a good treatment for menorrhagia and dysmenorrhea. Irregular spotting, especially in the first six months, is not uncommon.
- Heavier menses and cramps are expected with the Paragard.

*Past use of an IUD does not ↑ the risk of an ectopic pregnancy. Current use of an IUD reduces the risk of pregnancy in general, including an ectopic pregnancy. However, if a pregnancy does occur in a woman with an IUD, it is more likely to be an ectopic pregnancy.*

### MALE CONDOMS

- When used alone, latex condoms provide 98% effectiveness with perfect use and 85% with typical use. All condom types have similar contraceptive effectiveness, but animal-skin condoms do not protect against STIs (see Table 16.11).
- Educate patients about proper condom use and emergency (postcoital) contraception as a backup method.
- Disadvantages include lack of control by the female partner and possible diminishing of sexual pleasure for one or both partners.

TABLE 16.11. **Condom Choices**

| | LATEX | SYNTHETIC | ANIMAL SKIN |
|---|---|---|---|
| Acceptable for latex-allergic users | No | Yes | Yes |
| Effective pregnancy prevention | Yes | Yes | Yes |
| Effective STI prevention | Yes | Yes | No |
| Acceptable lubricant | Water based | Any | Any |

## VAGINAL BARRIERS

- Women have a variety of choices if they wish to use a barrier method that is inserted prior to sexual contact (see Table 16.12).
- All vaginal barrier methods confer some degree of protection against STIs, but only the female condom provides protection equivalent to or better than the male condom.
- Educate patients about proper use, cleaning, and storage, as well as the use of emergency (postcoital) contraception as a backup method.

## VAGINAL SPERMICIDES

- Sold as foams, creams, jellies, films, or suppositories.
- When used alone, they are 82% effective with perfect use and 71% with typical use.

TABLE 16.12. **Vaginal Barrier Choices**

| | DIAPHRAGM | FEMALE CONDOM | SPONGE | CERVICAL BARRIERS[a] |
|---|---|---|---|---|
| Acceptable for latex-allergic users | No | Yes | Yes | Yes |
| Acceptable lubricant | Water based | Any | Any | Any |
| Effectiveness (perfect use) | 94%[b] | 95% | 91% nulliparous; 80% parous | Estimated 91–98% |
| Effectiveness (typical use) | 80%[b] | 79% | 84% nulliparous; 68% parous | Data not available |
| STI prevention | +/– | + | +/– | +/– |
| How to obtain | Fitted and prescribed by provider | OTC | OTC | Fitted and prescribed by provider |

[a] The two products currently distributed in the United States are Lea's Shield and FemCap.
[b] When used as recommended with spermicidal jelly.

## IMPLANTS

- Implanon is a matchstick-sized single-rod implant that releases progestin slowly, providing up to three years of contraception. It is now available from providers trained in insertion and removal technique.
- Effectiveness (with both perfect and typical use) is > 99%.
- Norplant, a progestin-releasing method that involved six implanted rods, is no longer distributed.

## STERILIZATION

- Female sterilization can be accomplished by tubal interruption surgery or by transcervical fallopian tube coil insertion (Essure). Both have an effectiveness of > 99%.
- Male sterilization is by vasectomy and is also > 99% effective.
- Sterilization is considered permanent. Patients should be sure they do not want to have children in the future, as reversal procedures are not reliable.

## ABSTINENCE

- The only way to absolutely guarantee against pregnancy is the complete avoidance of penile-vaginal contact.
- Most currently abstinent patients will become sexually active in the future and may still wish for information about other family planning methods.
- Those choosing abstinence can still be at risk for nonconsensual intercourse and should be aware of the availability of emergency (postcoital) contraception.

## FERTILITY AWARENESS

- Defined as methods that chart fertility based on menstrual cycle timing or physical signs (cervical mucus, basal body temperature, breast and other body changes). The information thus derived can be used to plan a pregnancy or to prevent pregnancy through use of barrier methods or abstinence during fertile periods.
- With perfect use, fertility awareness methods are 91–99% effective at preventing pregnancy. With typical use, they are 75% effective.

## LACTATION

- Women who are nursing their infants frequently and exclusively, and who remain amenorrheic, may rely on breast-feeding (effectiveness with perfect use is > 98%) for the first six months of breast-feeding or until their menses return.
- Pumping and supplementing both ↓ the contraceptive effectiveness of breast-feeding.
- Nonhormonal and progestin-only methods are safe for breast-feeding mothers and their infants.
- The estrogen in combined hormonal contraceptives (pills, ring, patch) may ↓ milk production. For nursing mothers who choose an estrogen-containing method, it may be best to delay initiation until six weeks postpartum in order to establish optimal breast-feeding.

### WITHDRAWAL

- Coitus interruptus, in which the male partner withdraws his penis from his partner's vagina prior to ejaculating, ↓ the risk of pregnancy but does not prevent STIs.
- Provides approximately 96% effectiveness with perfect use and 73% with typical use.
- Disadvantages include lack of control by the female partner and possible diminishing of sexual pleasure for one or both partners.
- Educate patients about emergency (postcoital) contraception as a backup method.

## Abortion

*Contrary to popular myth, abortion does not ↑ a woman's risk of breast cancer or future pregnancy complications.*

When the diagnosis of pregnancy is made, a woman should be offered all options—continuing the pregnancy and parenting, continuing the pregnancy and placing the baby for adoption, or terminating the pregnancy. Half of all pregnancies in the United States are unintended, and half of these are electively terminated. It is estimated that up to 40% of women have an abortion in their lifetimes. Up to 24 weeks' gestation, abortion is legally protected; when performed by a trained provider, it is extremely safe, with overall complication rates < 1%.

### FIRST-TRIMESTER ABORTION WITH ASPIRATION

- Dilation followed by aspiration, with or without sharp curettage, is the most common abortion procedure up to approximately 12 weeks' gestation, and can be performed by electric suction or with a handheld manual vacuum aspirator (MVA).
- Analgesia includes local paracervical block plus the option of systemic agents such as NSAIDs, benzodiazepines, and/or narcotics.
- Perioperative antibiotics ↓ the risk of infection.
- The most common complications are incomplete abortion (continued pregnancy or retained tissue) and infection (combined < 1%). Perforation and the need for hospitalization are extremely rare (< 0.1%). Mortality is < 1 in 100,000.

A 40-year-old mother comes to your rural family medicine practice concerned because her period is late. Since the birth of their third child six years ago, she and her husband have been practicing natural family planning. Her period, which she reports comes every 28 days "like clockwork," is five days late. She has mild breast tenderness and nausea but otherwise feels well, with no cramping or bleeding. A sensitive urine pregnancy test is ⊕. A pelvic exam is normal, with a small uterus consistent with a five-week pregnancy. Upon learning she is pregnant, the patient is distraught. You provide supportive counseling and discuss her options, and several days later she returns with her husband. They have decided to terminate the pregnancy medically. What medical regimen do you offer her, and what, if any, further testing is needed? Since her history and exam provide reliable pregnancy dating and there are no signs or symptoms of ectopic pregnancy, you can offer this patient medical termination

> with either methotrexate or mifepristone followed by misoprostol. You can follow with history, exam as needed, and serial quantitative β-hCG levels or ultrasound to confirm completion of the abortion.

*Approximately 88% of abortions in the United States are obtained in the first trimester.*

### FIRST-TRIMESTER ABORTION WITH MEDICATION

- A regimen of mifepristone (formerly RU-486) followed by misoprostol is FDA approved for pregnancy termination up to seven weeks' (post-LMP) gestation. It is commonly used, based on abundant evidence of effectiveness and safety, up to nine weeks.
- In commonly used evidence-based regimens, the patient takes mifepristone in the provider's office and is then given misoprostol to take at home. Heavy cramping and bleeding follow the misoprostol, and the patient typically passes the pregnancy within several hours.
- Methotrexate followed by misoprostol is also safe and effective for pregnancy termination up to 7–8 weeks' gestation.
- Oral NSAIDs and acetaminophen-narcotic combinations are offered as analgesia.
- Prophylactic antibiotics have shown no benefit and are not routinely used.
- Complications include continuing pregnancy (1–4%), infection, and heavy bleeding. Fatal toxic shock syndrome following mifepristone abortion has occurred but is extremely rare. Medication abortion remains a very safe option for women.
- In the United States, mifepristone can be dispensed by or under the supervision of any physician who certifies that he or she can accurately assess gestational age, diagnose ectopic pregnancy, and offer access to a surgical provider if needed. Ultrasound capability is not required.

*With an early abortion, keep in mind the possibility of an ectopic or heterotopic pregnancy. Neither uterine aspiration nor mifepristone treats an ectopic pregnancy!*

### SECOND-TRIMESTER ABORTION

- Dilation and evacuation (D&E), which combines vacuum aspiration with forceps extraction, is the safest and most commonly used procedure.
- Analgesia is usually with IV sedation or general anesthesia, but oral analgesics (plus local cervical block) may be adequate for early second-trimester procedures.
- After the first trimester, maternal morbidity and mortality associated with abortion ↑ with gestational age. Second-trimester abortion nonetheless remains very safe, with mortality (approximately 3 per 100,000) lower than that associated with childbirth.

*All abortion patients with Rh- ⊖ blood type should receive Rh(D) immune globulin (RhoGAM). Use 50 μg for women who are < 12 weeks' pregnant and 300 μg for those ≥ 12 weeks.*

### POSTABORTION CARE

- Pelvic rest (no intercourse, tampons, or douching) is recommended for two weeks following an abortion, although there are no data indicating that this is necessary.
- Postabortion bleeding usually abates with time and may continue for up to 2–4 weeks. Patients with excessive bleeding should be assessed for retained products of conception. Monitor for anemia.
- Menses usually return to normal within 4–6 weeks of the abortion.
- Routine follow-up two weeks after an uncomplicated abortion is encouraged. At this visit, the provider should address contraceptive needs, offer

*Hormonal contraceptive methods can be started at the time of or immediately following an abortion procedure. IUDs can be placed at the conclusion of an aspiration procedure.*

**REPRODUCTIVE HEALTH**

testing and treatment for STIs, and discuss general social support issues, including patients' remaining questions or sentiments about the abortion.

## SEXUALLY TRANSMITTED INFECTIONS (STIs)

*In patients diagnosed with gonorrhea, treat presumptively for chlamydia unless you can definitively rule it out.*

*Gonorrhea has developed resistance to fluoroquinolones in many parts of the world, especially the Pacific. In 2007 the CDC issued guidelines recommended this class of antibiotics not be used to treat gonorrhea.*

A 23-year-old woman presents for a routine checkup and Pap smear. She is sexually active only with her boyfriend of one year and uses OCPs. She expresses concern about several small, painless growths on her labia. Her external genital exam reveals multiple nontender, cauliflower-like, skin-colored papules. Speculum and bimanual exams are unremarkable. What is the most likely diagnosis? HPV-associated genital warts (see Figure 16.14). You offer the patient treatment options of topical medications or cryotherapy as well as testing for other STIs.

The most common STIs are usually asymptomatic in women, so it is important to consider who is at risk and offer testing where appropriate. Routine screening for STIs is recommended for pregnant women as well as for women or men who are at high risk on the basis of the following risk factors:

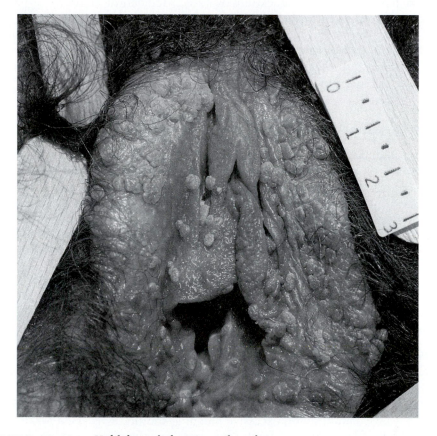

**FIGURE 16.14.** **Multiple genital warts on the vulva.**

(Reproduced, with permission, from Wolff K et al. *Fitzpatrick's Color Atlas & Synopsis of Clinical Dermatology*, 5th ed. New York: McGraw Hill, 2005: 888.)

- A history of a prior STI or a current diagnosis of another STI.
- New or multiple sex partners, or a partner with multiple partners.
- Age under 25.
- Inconsistent use of barrier contraceptives.

### SYMPTOMS/EXAM

- Evaluation of all patients of reproductive age should include a sexual history. Any patient with a history of any STI, current risk factors, or current symptoms of any STI should be offered testing for all STIs, including HIV.
- The specific symptoms, signs, and diagnostic tests for each STI are listed in Table 16.13.

### TREATMENT

Patients diagnosed with any STI should make sure their sexual partners are also treated to prevent reinfection. Disease-specific treatments are outlined in Table 16.13.

*The chancre of syphilis is painless. With painful genital ulceration, think herpes or chancroid.*

**TABLE 16.13. Presentation, Diagnosis, and Treatment of Common STIs**

| STI | SYMPTOMS | EXAM | DIAGNOSIS | TREATMENT |
|-----|----------|------|-----------|-----------|
| Gonorrhea (GC) (*Neisseria gonorrhoeae*) | Usually asymptomatic in women, or may present with purulent discharge. | Exam reveals **mucopurulent discharge** and a friable cervix. | Test sample from urine or cervical swab using nucleic acid amplification tests, genetic probe, or culture. | Ceftriaxone, cefixime. Consider treating presumptively for chlamydia. |
| Chlamydia (*Chlamydia trachomatis*) | Usually asymptomatic in women, or may present with purulent discharge. | Exam reveals **mucopurulent discharge** and a friable cervix. | Test sample from urine or cervical swab using nucleic acid amplification tests, genetic probe, or culture. | Azithromycin 1 g PO × 1. Doxycycline 100 mg PO BID × 7 days (avoid in pregnancy). |
| Trichomoniasis (*Trichomonas vaginalis*, a protozoan) | Presents with a copious greenish-yellow vaginal discharge. | Exam reveals a frothy greenish-yellow fluid in the vagina. | Wet mount reveals motile trichomonads. | Metronidazole 2 g PO × 1. Alternatively, metronidazole 500 mg PO BID × 7 days. |
| Pelvic inflammatory disease (PID) (polymicrobial, including *C. trachomatis* and *N. gonorrhoeae*) | Presents with lower abdominal pain +/− fever +/− nausea and anorexia. | Exam reveals abdominal tenderness with possible rebound along with cervical motion tenderness. | Diagnosis is clinical. GC and chlamydia cultures may or may not be ⊕. | Consider inpatient IV treatment. Broad-spectrum antibiotics, including coverage for GC, chlamydia, and anaerobes. |

| STI | SYMPTOMS | EXAM | DIAGNOSIS | TREATMENT |
|---|---|---|---|---|
| Genital herpes (HSV-1 or -2) | Presents with painful vesicles (pain may precede eruption) +/– systemic symptoms (fever, myalgia) +/– vaginal discharge. May also be asymptomatic or present with non-specific symptoms. | Exam reveals tender grouped vesicles on an erythematous base. Ruptured vesicles appear as shallow ulcers or abrasions. Inguinal lymphadenopathy is also seen. | Diagnosis is mainly clinical. Consider viral culture or Tzanck smear from vesicular fluid. | Oral acyclovir, valacyclovir, or famciclovir. Treatment resolves lesions but does not cure HSV; recurrence is common. Suppressive therapy for frequent outbreaks or during pregnancy. |
| Genital warts (HPV) | Presents with painless growths on the genitals, anus, or perineum (see Figure 16.14). | Exam reveals fleshy, skin-colored "cauliflower" papules or plaques on the vulva, vagina, or cervix. | Diagnosis is clinical. Rarely may need biopsy. | Treatment resolves lesions but does not cure HPV; recurrence is common. Treatment options include topical imiquimod or podofilox applied by the patient; podophyllin; cryotherapy; trichloroacetic acid; electrocautery; or excision. |
| Syphilis (*Treponema pallidum*) | 1°: Painless genital ulcer. 2°: Fever, malaise, diffuse rash. **Latent:** Asymptomatic. 3°: Aortic aneurysm rupture, CNS symptoms. | 1°: Nontender **chancre.** 2°: Nonspecific maculopapular rash; **condylomata lata.** **Early latent (< 1 year):** Fourfold ↑ in titer. **Late latent (> 1 year or unknown):** Serology remains ⊕. 3°: Aortitis, gummas, meningitis, encephalitis, tabes dorsalis, Argyll Robertson pupil. | Start with nonspecific RPR or VRDL (may be false ⊕). FTA-ABS or darkfield microscopy to confirm; LP if neurosyphilis is suspected. | Penicillin 2.4 MU IM × 1 for new infections; × 3 for infections of > 1 year's duration. In penicillin-allergic patients, consider desensitization. For neurosyphilis, IV penicillin G (3–4 MU IV q 4 h × 10–14 days). |
| Chancroid (*Haemophilus ducreyi*) | Presents as a painful genital ulcer. | Exam reveals a tender papule, pustule, or ulcer with an erythematous edge. Tender inguinal lymphadenopathy is also seen. | Diagnosis is largely clinical. Gram stain may help. Rule out HSV and syphilis. | Azithromycin, ceftriaxone, ciprofloxacin (avoid in pregnancy). |

| STI | SYMPTOMS | EXAM | DIAGNOSIS | TREATMENT |
|---|---|---|---|---|
| HIV/AIDS | Acute retroviral syndrome 3–6 weeks after infection; opportunistic infections. | Exam findings vary depending on the cause of presentation. | Serology: ELISA and Western blot. Rapid test is available. | HAART; appropriate prophylaxis (see the Infectious Diseases chapter). |
| Hepatitis B (HBV) | Presents as acute hepatitis with flulike symptoms and jaundice. | Exam reveals acute hepatitis with jaundice and hepatomegaly. | HBsAg (may be used alone for screening). | See the Infectious Diseases chapter. |
| Pubic lice or "crabs" (*Phthirus pubis*) | Presents with an itch in the pubic hair. May also affect the axillae and other hair-covered areas. | Tiny white nits are attached to hair. Adult lice may be seen. | Diagnosis is clinical. Lice may be viewed under the microscope. | Topical permethrin, malathion, or lindane; decontaminate bedding and clothing. |
| Molluscum contagiosum | Presents with multiple small bumps that are painless and nonpruritic. | Dome-shaped pearly papules with central umbilication are seen. | Diagnosis is clinical. Giemsa stain of material expressed from the lesion contains inclusion bodies. | Most resolve spontaneously and do not require treatment. Treatment options include imiquimod, cryotherapy, curettage, and electrodesiccation. |

## PREVENTION

- Complete sexual abstinence is the only way to ensure prevention of STIs.
- For patients who are sexually active, consistent use of latex condoms offers the best protection against STIs.
- All children, as well as adults with risk factors, should be vaccinated against HBV.
- Vaccination against HPV is recommended for all girls by age 12, and for young women up to age 26. The three-dose vaccine Gardasil protects against virus strains that cause most cervical cancer (types 16 and 18) and genital warts (types 6 and 11). It is more effective if given before the patient initiates sexual activity.

## COMPLICATIONS

- Even without frank PID, gonorrhea and chlamydia infections ↑ the risk for tubal scarring, which can → infertility and ectopic pregnancy.
- PID can → multiorgan systemic illness and even death.
- Untreated syphilis and HIV are fatal.
- Untreated STIs in pregnant women can be transmitted to newborn.

---

**Complications of PID—**

**I FACE PID**

**I**nfertility
**F**itz-Hugh–Curtis syndrome
**A**bscesses
**C**hronic pelvic pain
**E**ctopic pregnancy
**P**eritonitis
**I**ntestinal obstruction
**D**isseminated—sepsis, endocarditis, arthritis, meningitis

---

583

A 19-year-old woman complains of one week of yellow-gray vaginal discharge with a fishy odor. She has no urinary symptoms or vaginal itching or burning. She has tried douching with a vinegar preparation but finds that the symptoms return. She is not currently sexually active and denies a history of STIs. Speculum exam reveals copious discharge but an otherwise normal vulva, vagina, and cervix. Bimanual exam is unremarkable. Litmus paper applied to the discharge shows a pH of 5. Saline wet mount reveals epithelial cells with peripheral stippling. KOH applied to the slide releases a strong amine "fishy" odor. KOH prep is ⊖ for hyphae. What is the mostly likely diagnosis? Bacterial vaginosis based on the presentation, the presence of "clue cells" on microscopy (see Figure 16.15), and a ⊕ "whiff test." You offer the patient treatment with metronidazole and advise against douching.

With the exception of trichomoniasis, the causes of vulvovaginitis are normal flora that have overgrown rather than STIs. Therefore, patients' partners generally do not require treatment.

### SYMPTOMS/EXAM

The specific presentation of each cause of vulvovaginitis is given in Table 16.14. In general, the diagnosis should be considered for any of the following:

- Unusual vaginal discharge
- Unusual vaginal/vulvar odor
- Vaginal/vulvar itch or irritation

### PREVENTION

- Douching is associated with an ↑ risk of bacterial vaginosis and should be discouraged.
- Patients with bacterial vaginosis and candidiasis are generally advised to take measures to ↓ vulvar warmth and minimize moisture (e.g., losing weight; wearing cotton underpants and loose-fitting clothing).

### COMPLICATIONS

Bacterial vaginosis and trichomoniasis have been associated with an ↑ risk of preterm labor.

TABLE 16.14. Presentation and Treatment of Vulvovaginitides

| Cause | Symptoms | Exam | Bedside Tests | Treatment |
|---|---|---|---|---|
| Bacterial vaginosis (*Gardnerella* and other spp.) | Presents with a malodorous discharge. | Discharge is thin and yellowish-gray. A fishy odor may be noticeable without KOH. | pH > 4.5. Wet mount shows **clue cells** (see Figure 16.15). KOH whiff test is ⊕ for a fishy amine odor. | Metronidazole 500 mg PO BID × 7 days is most effective. Metronidazole gel 5 g PV QD × 5 days. Clindamycin 5 g PV QHS × 7 days. |
| Yeast infection (*Candida albicans*) | Presents with vaginal itching and burning accompanied by a cheesy white discharge. | Exam reveals a white discharge adherent to the introitus. The discharge is thick and cottage cheese–like. The perineum and vulva may be red and tender. | pH 3.5–4.5. KOH prep shows "budding" hyphae. | Intravaginal azole antifungals; oral fluconazole (avoid in pregnancy). Antifungal cream may be applied externally for symptom relief. |
| Trichomoniasis (*Trichomonas vaginalis*) | Presents with a copious green discharge. | Exam reveals a discharge that is frothy green. | See Table 16.13. | See Table 16.13. |
| Atrophic vaginitis | Vaginal irritation and pain with intercourse in postmenopausal women. | Exam reveals a clear, thin discharge and a pale vaginal epithelium with patches of erythema. | pH > 7. | Estrogen vaginal cream. If vaginal bleeding is present, rule out malignant causes. |

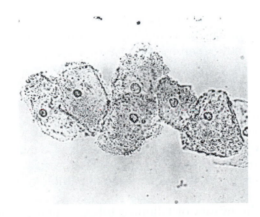

**FIGURE 16.15. Clue cells of bacterial vaginosis.**

Note the stippled appearance. (Reproduced, with permission, from DeCherney A, *Current Obstetrics and Gynecology Diagnosis and Treatment*, 8th ed. Stamford, CT: Appleton & Lange, 1994: 692.)

REPRODUCTIVE HEALTH

A 30-year-old woman complains of two years of intermittent bilateral pelvic pain. All lab tests are normal, and a pelvic ultrasound is normal as well. What is the next step in managing this patient? If the medical history is noncontributory and the patient is not depressed, consider a gynecology referral for possible laparoscopy.

Defined as episodic or continuous pain for six months or longer that is severe enough to affect daily functioning. Up to 20% of women of reproductive age are affected by pelvic pain. Although endometriosis is the most common associated condition, many women with pelvic pain have a history of abuse or depression. Etiologies are varied but include the following:

- **Gynecologic:**
    - **Uterine:** Adenomyosis, chronic endometritis, fibroids, IUD use, pelvic congestion, pelvic support defects, endometrial polyps.
    - **Extrauterine:** Adhesions, chronic ectopic pregnancy, chronic pelvic infection, endometriosis, ovarian neoplasm, imperforate hymen, cervical stenosis, chronic functional cyst.
- **Urologic:** Interstitial cystitis, urethral syndrome, chronic UTI, stones, ureteral diverticuli or polyps, bladder carcinoma, detrusor overactivity.
- **GI:** Chronic appendicitis, constipation, diverticular disease, IBS, IBD (Crohn's disease, ulcerative colitis), neoplasia.
- **Musculoskeletal:** Myofascial pain (trigger points, spasms), fibromyalgia, coccydynia, degenerative joint disease, low back pain, levator ani syndrome (spasm of the pelvic floor), nerve entrapment syndromes, osteoporosis (compression fractures), strains/sprains.
- **Other:** Abuse (physical or sexual, past or present), psychiatric disorders (depression, bipolar disorder), psychosocial stress (work stress, marital problems), herpes zoster, heavy metal poisoning (lead, mercury), lymphoma, sickle cell crisis, somatoform disorders, substance use (cocaine).

### SYMPTOMS

*Patients with chronic pelvic pain should be screened for depression.*

- In all patients, evaluate exacerbating or ameliorating factors; the relationship of the pain to the menstrual cycle; worsening or improvement of pain with work, exercise, stress, intercourse, or orgasm; and associated symptoms such as bleeding, discharge, constipation, or diarrhea.
- A thorough pregnancy, surgical, psychiatric, and substance abuse history is needed, including a depression screening test. Pain in other parts of the body should be explored as well, as some 90% of women with chronic pelvic pain have backaches, and up to 60% also have headaches.
- Specific symptoms to evaluate include the following:
    - Pain due to cervical, uterine, or vaginal pathology, often referred to the buttock or low back.
    - Pain from the ovaries or fallopian tubes, which is usually localized to one side and referred to the medial thigh.

### EXAM

Conduct a complete physical exam, focusing on abdominal, back, vulvar, perineal, vaginal, bimanual, and rectovaginal exams.

- **Labs:** CBC, ESR, UA and culture, stool guaiac, gonorrhea and chlamydia cultures, vaginal wet mount, pregnancy test.
- **Imaging:** Ultrasound, CT, MRI, hysterosonogram.
- **Surgical:** D&C, diagnostic laparoscopy, cystoscopy, colonoscopy.

## TREATMENT

- **Treat the underlying cause.**
- **Pharmacologic:** Pain medications and antidepressants.
- **Surgical:** Pelvic denervation procedures; hysterectomy with or without salpingo-oophorectomy; pelvic floor reconstruction.
- **Other:** Psychotherapy, marriage and sex counseling, biofeedback, physical therapy.

## CERVICAL CANCER SCREENING

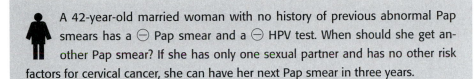

A 42-year-old married woman with no history of previous abnormal Pap smears has a ⊖ Pap smear and a ⊖ HPV test. When should she get another Pap smear? If she has only one sexual partner and has no other risk factors for cervical cancer, she can have her next Pap smear in three years.

## Screening Guidelines

- Current guidelines from the United States Preventive Services Task Force (USPSTF) recommend beginning Pap smears three years after a patient starts sexual intercourse but no later than age 21.
- Annual cytology testing is recommended until age 30.
- After age 30, options include continuing annual cytology screening, screening every 2–3 years after three ⊖ annual Pap smears, or cytology with the addition of an HPV DNA test with repeat testing every three years if both are ⊖.
- Annual screening after age 30 should continue for all women with a history of in utero DES exposure or HIV, as well as for all other immunocompromised patients.
- After a total hysterectomy (involving both the uterus and cervix), woman do not need to be screened unless the surgery was performed to treat cancer or a precancerous condition.
- After age 65–70, women with at least three normal and no abnormal Pap smears can consider stopping cervical cancer screening.

*Pap smear screening should begin three years after the first sexual intercourse or at age 21.*

## Management of Abnormal Cervical Cytology

- **Cytology ⊖, HPV ⊕:**
    - Associated with a 4% risk of developing cervical intraepithelial neoplasia (CIN) grade 2–3+ (includes CIN 2, CIN 3, adenocarcinoma in situ, and cancer).
    - Repeat cytologic and HPV testing in 6–12 months, as transient HPV infection may resolve; perform colposcopy if the repeat test is abnormal.
- **Atypical squamous cells of undetermined significance (ASCUS):**
    - Associated with a 6–12% risk of CIN 2–3+.

- Options include colposcopy, triage to colposcopy via HPV testing (if HPV ⊕, there is a 15–27% risk of CIN 2–3+; if HPV ⊖, there is less than a 2% risk), or repeat cytology at 6 and 12 months.
- Given their low risk of developing invasive cancer and the high probability of clearing HPV in their age group, adolescents with ASC and HPV ⊕ status can be monitored with repeat cytology at 6 and 12 months or with a single HPV test at 12 months, supplemented by colposcopy if either test is abnormal.

- **Low-grade squamous intraepithelial lesions (LSILs):**
  - Associated with a 15–30% risk of CIN 2–3+.
  - Perform colposcopy (adolescents can be monitored as outlined above for ASC and HPV ⊕).
- **ASC—cannot exclude high-grade intraepithelial lesion (ASC-H):**
  - Carries a 24–94% risk of CIN 2–3+.
  - Perform colposcopy.
  - If colposcopy is normal or shows CIN 1, repeat cytology at 6 and 12 months or HPV testing at 12 months; repeat colposcopy for ASC or higher or for those with HPV ⊕ status.
- **High-grade squamous intraepithelial lesions (HSILs):**
  - Associated with ≥ 70% risk of CIN 2–3+ and a 1–2% risk of invasive cancer.
  - Colposcopy with biopsy of visible lesions; endocervical biopsy (unless the patient is pregnant).
  - If colposcopy is ⊖, excision with LEEP or conization is recommended to ensure that no high-grade lesions are missed.
  - Adolescents with adequate colposcopy and ⊖ endocervical curettage can be followed with repeat cytology and colposcopy at 4–6 months.
- **Atypical glandular cells/adenocarcinoma in situ (AGC/AIS):**
  - Colposcopy with endocervical sampling for all patients; endometrial sampling is indicated if "atypical endometrial cells" are specified, for all women ≥ 35 years of age and those < 35 years of age with abnormal bleeding, obesity, or oligomenorrhea.
  - In patients with AGC and both a ⊖ initial evaluation and a ⊖ HPV status, repeat cytology and endocervical sampling in one year.
  - For AGC favoring neoplasia, AIS with a ⊖ initial evaluation, or a repeat AGC, excision with cold-knife conization is recommended.

## Management of Colposcopy Results

- **CIN grade 1:**
  - Most cases remit spontaneously over time.
  - Options include treatment (LEEP or cryotherapy) or observation, including two cytology screening tests six months apart or a single HPV test at 12 months, with colposcopy for ASC or higher or HPV ⊕ status.
- **CIN grade 2 or 3:** Although roughly 40% of CIN 2 cases regress over two years, regression of CIN 3 is rare.
  - Immediate treatment with excision or ablation is recommended in nonpregnant patients. For compliant adolescents with CIN 2, close follow-up may suffice; consider hysterectomy for persistent or recurrent CIN 2 or 3.

## Ovarian Cancer

The leading cause of gynecologic cancer death, with its high mortality rate attributable primarily to its often late-stage presentation. Risk factors include advancing age, family history, and nulliparity. Use of hormonal contraception provides significant and long-lasting protection. A history of tubal ligation and, to a lesser degree, hysterectomy appears to be protective.

### SYMPTOMS

- Initially asymptomatic, or may present with nonspecific symptoms such as pelvic fullness or dyspareunia.
- Rarely presents with acute abdominal pain from a torsed or ruptured mass.
- May → irregular menses or postmenopausal bleeding.
- Later, abdominal pain and swelling may result either from invasive tumor or from 2° ascites.

### EXAM

Symptoms should be evaluated with bimanual and rectovaginal exams, which may reveal a solid, irregular, fixed pelvic mass.

### DIFFERENTIAL

- Consider the broad differential diagnosis of abdominal pain and bloating.
- A palpable pelvic mass may be benign or may point to other malignancy.

### DIAGNOSIS

- Pelvic ultrasound reveals a solid or multilocular mass.
- CA-125 will be ↑ in the presence of malignancy and is useful for tracking the course of disease, but it is nonspecific and therefore not useful for screening asymptomatic women.

### TREATMENT

- Surgical excision and "debulking" of tumor burden.
- Chemotherapy if indicated.
- Women with a known hereditary syndrome may choose prophylactic oophorectomy.

*There is no effective way to screen for ovarian cancer, but suspicious symptoms should be evaluated by pelvic exam +/– transvaginal ultrasonography and CA-125.*

*The use of OCPs significantly reduces the risk of endometrial ovarian cancer.*

## Uterine Cancer

Endometrial cancer is the most common gynecologic malignancy in the United States. Since it often causes early symptoms, it tends to be diagnosed at a curable stage. Uterine sarcomas are rare but are more likely to be diagnosed late.

### SYMPTOMS

Presents with postmenopausal bleeding or, in premenopausal women, with heavy or irregular menses.

### EXAM

The uterus may be enlarged or normal. On general physical exam, look for signs associated with ↑ risk.

> **Risk factors for endometrial cancer—**
>
> **ENDOMET**
>
> **E**lderly
> **N**ulliparity
> **D**iabetes
> **O**besity
> **M**enstrual irregularity
> **E**strogen monotherapy
> Hyper**T**ension

### DIFFERENTIAL

- Benign causes of irregular or postmenopausal bleeding, such as atrophic vaginitis, endometrial hyperplasia, polyps, fibroids, trauma, infection, and hormonal medications.
- Other gynecologic cancers.

### DIAGNOSIS

- Suspicious symptoms should be evaluated with endometrial biopsy and/or transvaginal ultrasound.
- D&C with or without hysteroscopy may also assist in the workup.
- Pelvic masses suspicious on imaging but $\ominus$ on endometrial sampling should be excised to evaluate for sarcoma. Most are found incidentally at the time of surgery for fibroids or other benign indications.

### TREATMENT

- TAH-BSO is almost always indicated.
- Radiation, chemotherapy, and/or hormonal agents as indicated by the stage and type of cancer.

## Cervical Cancer

Since the introduction of the Pap smear, mortality from cervical cancer has greatly ↓ in the United States; see the discussion of cervical cancer screening for more information on the management of an abnormal Pap smear. It is now known that infection with a high-risk subtype of HPV is necessary for the development of cervical cancer. Risk factors include early sexual activity and multiple sexual partners. Smoking hastens the progression of cervical pathology.

### SYMPTOMS

- Preinvasive lesions (dysplasia and carcinoma in situ) are asymptomatic.
- Invasive carcinoma generally → abnormal vaginal bleeding +/− a foul-smelling discharge.
- Advanced disease may → pelvic pain, lower extremity edema, or urinary symptoms.

### EXAM

- Even invasive lesions may be invisible to the naked eye on speculum exam.
- If visible, tumors may appear ulcerated, necrotic, or exophytic.
- Bimanual +/− rectovaginal exam may reveal cervical distortion or a frank mass.
- Look for signs of disease extension such as inguinal lymphadenopathy, leg edema, ascites, or hepatomegaly.

### DIFFERENTIAL

- Benign causes of abnormal bleeding and discharge, such as atrophic vaginitis, endometrial hyperplasia, polyps, fibroids, trauma, infection, and hormonal medications.
- Other gynecologic cancers.

### DIAGNOSIS

Colposcopy with directed biopsy and endocervical curettage.

### TREATMENT

- Low-grade lesions can be followed without therapy, as > 90% will spontaneously regress.
- High-grade preinvasive lesions can be ablated or excised with cryotherapy, LEEP, or conization.
- Invasive disease requires radical hysterectomy and/or radiation therapy.

### COMPLICATIONS

- Most superficial therapies are safe and have little or no effect on future pregnancies.
- LEEP may modestly ↑ the risk of PROM and preterm delivery in future pregnancies.
- Conization ↑ the risk for cervical stenosis or incompetence.
- Pelvic radiation and radical surgery may have serious adverse effects.

All women who have had sex and who have a cervix should be routinely screened for cervical cancer. Cervical cytology (Pap smear) is the standard-of-care screening test.

A 60-year-old woman with a long-standing history of genital lichen sclerosus presents with ↑ vulvar itching, pain, and dysuria. What is the likely diagnosis, and how is it confirmed? Biopsy of the lesion confirms squamous cell carcinoma in situ arising in an area of lichen sclerosus (see Figure 16.16). Although itself a benign condition, lichen sclerosus → vulvar cancer in 4–6% of affected women.

## Vulvar and Vaginal Cancer

Vulvar and vaginal cancer is rare, but care should be taken not to miss the diagnosis, as the presenting symptoms can be nonspecific. In utero exposure to DES is an important risk factor for clear cell adenocarcinoma of the vagina. Other risk factors include HPV exposure, smoking, and advancing age.

### SYMPTOMS

- Many patients are asymptomatic.
- Vulvar itching is the most common presenting symptom.
- Less commonly, patients will see or feel a lesion.

### EXAM

- External genital and speculum exams may reveal a lesion that can vary in color, texture, and appearance.
- Paget's disease of the vulva, which is often associated with an underlying adenocarcinoma, appears as a well-demarcated, scaly lesion that may look like eczema.
- Skin cancers, including melanoma, may present on the vulva.

Malignant melanoma is the second most common vulvar cancer. In patients at ↑ risk of melanoma, the full-body skin check should truly include the entire body!

### DIFFERENTIAL

Genital warts; vaginitis; benign skin lesions, including lichen sclerosus and lichen planus.

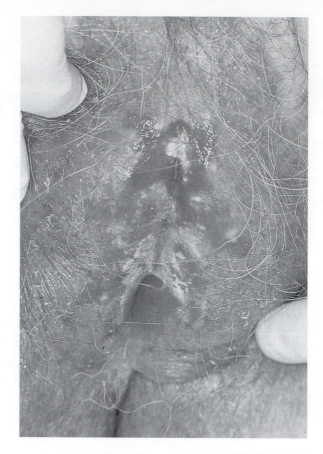

**FIGURE 16.16.** Squamous cell carcinoma of the vulva arising in an area of lichen sclerosus.

(Reproduced, with permission, from Wolff K et al. *Fitzpatrick's Color Atlas & Synopsis of Clinical Dermatology*, 5th ed. New York: McGraw Hill, 2005: 1047.) (Also see Color Insert.)

### DIAGNOSIS

- Vaginal malignancies may be detected on Pap smear.
- Biopsy, often guided by colposcopy, is required for definitive diagnosis.

### TREATMENT

Surgical excision +/− radiation.

## Gestational Trophoblastic Neoplasia

A malignancy arising from fetal tissue. This diagnosis includes a persistent or invasive mole and malignant choriocarcinoma. The majority of cases are curable, but metastases may be fatal. Although gestational trophoblastic neoplasia is most likely to occur after a molar pregnancy, 50% of cases occur after a normal pregnancy.

### SYMPTOMS

- Presents with persistent pregnancy symptoms and irregular vaginal bleeding for > 6 weeks following cessation of a term, preterm, ectopic, or molar pregnancy.
- Metastatic disease may present with pulmonary, GI, or neurologic symptoms.

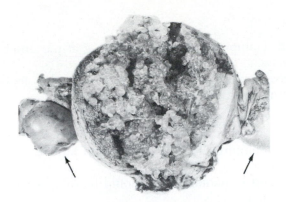

**FIGURE 16.17.   Complete hydatidiform mole with multiple edematous villi ("bunches of grapes" appearance) and no fetus.**

(Reproduced, with permission, from Cunningham FG et al. *Williams Obstetrics*, 22nd ed. New York: McGraw-Hill, 2005: 275.)

### EXAM

Exam reveals an enlarged uterus, adnexal fullness due to ovarian cysts, and RUQ pain from hepatic involvement.

### DIFFERENTIAL

Normal pregnancy; other pelvic masses.

### DIAGNOSIS

- Look for a rapidly rising β-hCG.
- Ultrasound reveals a "snowstorm" appearance.
- Pathologic diagnosis is made after surgical treatment. The characteristic "bunches of grapes" appearance is caused by hydropic villi (see Figure 16.17).

### TREATMENT

- D&C is curative in many cases. Rarely, hysterectomy is necessary.
- Chemotherapy in metastatic disease.
- Follow β-hCG levels to resolution.

### COMPLICATIONS

Molar pregnancy carries a 1% risk of recurrence with future pregnancies. Choriocarcinoma may metastasize to the lungs, vagina, brain, liver, kidney, or GI tract.

## MENSTRUAL DISORDERS

### Dysmenorrhea

Defined as pain during menses, likely caused by the release of prostaglandins. Dysmenorrhea is the leading cause of recurrent short-term absence from school in adolescent girls. 1° dysmenorrhea affects women with normal pelvic anatomy; risk factors include age < 20, nulliparity, heavy menses, depression, and smoking. 2° dysmenorrhea can be caused by endometriosis, adenomyosis, pelvic infection, IUD use, cervical stenosis, congenital vaginal or uterine abnormalities, or fibroids.

*SYMPTOMS/EXAM*

- Presents with crampy pelvic pain beginning at the onset of menses and lasting 1–3 days.
- A pelvic mass, abnormal vaginal discharge, or pelvic tenderness not limited to the time of menses suggest 2° dysmenorrhea.

*DIAGNOSIS*

- Can be treated empirically if the history and physical are consistent with 1° dysmenorrhea.
- A **speculum and bimanual exam** should be done on sexually active patients to evaluate for STIs.
- Ultrasound is useful in evaluating 2° dysmenorrhea; laparoscopy is best for the diagnosis of endometriosis.

*TREATMENT*

- NSAIDs are the best first-line treatment, as they have an analgesic effect while also decreasing the volume of menstrual flow.
- **Combined hormonal contraceptives** ↓ prostaglandin release during menses. Options include extended-cycle use (i.e., 12 continuous weeks of active hormones followed by one week off) to ↓ the number of menstrual periods.
- Depot medroxyprogesterone acetate → amenorrhea in most women.
- Levonorgestrel IUDs ↓ dysmenorrhea.
- Danazol or leuprolide acetate can be used to suppress the menstrual cycle, but both drugs are expensive and have side effects; thus, they are best reserved for refractory cases of 2° dysmenorrhea.
- Alternative therapies that may be effective include topical heat, vitamin E, thiamine, omega-3 fatty acids, and acupuncture.
- Hysterectomy is indicated only for severe, refractory cases.

*NSAIDs are first-line treatment for dysmenorrhea, as they ↓ both pain and volume of menstrual flow.*

## Abnormal Uterine Bleeding

Bleeding that deviates from the patient's normal pattern. Prior to the onset of menses, any vaginal bleeding should be considered abnormal with the exception of self-limited, physiologic withdrawal bleeding in some newborns. In women of childbearing age, abnormal uterine bleeding encompasses bleeding between cycles as well as any change that may occur in menstrual frequency, duration, or amount of flow. As a whole, bleeding may be classified as ovulatory or anovulatory based on the timing, duration, and amount of flow. Etiologies include the following:

- **Ovulatory bleeding:**
  - **Anatomic lesions:** Cervical disease (polyps, inflammation, cancer), PID, IUD use, uterine disease (fibroids, cancer).
  - **Concurrent disease:** Foreign body; coagulopathy; thyroid, hepatic, or renal disease.
  - **Medications:** Anticoagulants, antipsychotics, corticosteroids, herbal supplements (ginseng, gingko, soy), SSRIs, tamoxifen.
- **Anovulatory bleeding:**
  - **OCP use:** Inadequate estrogen dosage.
  - **Hypothalamic dysfunction:** PCOS; hypothyroidism; excess androgen, cortisol, or prolactin; situational stress; excess exercise or weight loss; puberty; perimenopause.

- **Dysfunctional uterine bleeding:** A diagnosis of exclusion that may be due to hormonal imbalances either at the pituitary level (anovulatory bleeding) or at the level of the endometrial lining (ovulatory bleeding). Pregnancy, iatrogenic causes, genital tract pathology, and systemic conditions must be ruled out before dysfunctional uterine bleeding is diagnosed.
- **Pregnancy:** Ectopic pregnancy, threatened abortion, incomplete abortion.
- **Postmenopausal bleeding:**
  - **Vaginal pathology:** Atrophic vaginitis.
  - **Cervical pathology:** Polyps, erosion, cancer.
  - **Uterine pathology:** Polyps, fibroids, cancer.

*Dysfunctional uterine bleeding is a diagnosis of exclusion and is due to hormonal imbalances.*

### SYMPTOMS

Clinical presentation varies according to the pattern of abnormal bleeding.

- **Ovulatory patterns:**
  - **Menorrhagia:** Excessive or prolonged bleeding during times of expected menstrual flow.
- **Anovulatory patterns:**
  - **Metrorrhagia:** Bleeding that occurs at abnormal times or more frequently than every 21 days.
  - **Menometrorrhagia:** Irregular, noncyclic bleeding characterized by heavy flow or duration.
  - **Oligomenorrhea:** Cycles lasting > 35 days.
  - **Amenorrhea:** Bleeding that is absent for at least six months.
- **Other:** Additional abnormalities of menstruation are defined as follows:
  - **Polymenorrhea:** Cycles < 21 days; usually due to luteal phase dysfunction.
  - **Midcycle spotting:** Physiologic spotting just before ovulation.
  - **Postmenopausal bleeding:** Bleeding that occurs in a menopausal woman more than one year after cessation of menses.

### EXAM

Exam may reveal postural signs, weight gain or loss, thyromegaly or thyroid tenderness, hirsutism, edema, petechiae, bruising, jaundice, enlargement of the liver or spleen, breast tenderness or discharge, an enlarged uterus, a firm or fixed uterus, cervical motion or uterine tenderness, or an adnexal mass (see Table 16.15).

### DIAGNOSIS

- **Always rule out pregnancy first.**
- **Labs:** hCG, CBC, LFTs, PT, TSH, prolactin, blood glucose, DHEA, free testosterone, Pap smear, gonorrhea and chlamydia cultures.
- **Imaging:** Transvaginal ultrasound, hysteroscopy for cases unresponsive to empiric treatment.
- Endometrial assessment (endometrial biopsy or D&C) is indicated for women < 35 years old with 2–3 years of untreated anovulatory bleeding, especially if they are obese; for any woman > 35 years of age with a change in bleeding pattern; and for all women with postmenopausal bleeding.

### TREATMENT

- **Acute anovulatory bleeding:** To stop bleeding, give high-dose oral or IV estrogen to build up the endometrial lining. Oral medroxyprogesterone or IM progesterone can also be used to convert proliferative endometrium to secretory endometrium. D&C or hysteroscopy is appropriate in refractory cases.

TABLE 16.15.    Exam Findings Associated with Abnormal Uterine Bleeding

| SYMPTOMS | CONDITION |
|---|---|
| Weight loss, stress | Hypothalamic suppression |
| Galactorrhea, headache, visual disturbance | Pituitary adenoma |
| Pelvic pain | Ectopic pregnancy, PID, trauma, miscarriage |
| Nausea, weight gain, fatigue, urinary frequency | Pregnancy |
| Weight gain, fatigue, constipation, cold intolerance | Hypothyroidism |
| Weight loss, palpitations, heat intolerance | Hyperthyroidism |
| Bleeding tendency, easy bruising | Coagulopathy |
| Jaundice, abdominal pain | Liver disease |
| Hirsutism, acne, acanthosis nigricans | PCOS |
| Postcoital bleeding | Cervical dysplasia, endocervical polyp |

- **Chronic anovulatory bleeding:** Treat the underlying cause, and add monthly progesterone therapy or combination hormonal contraceptives both to promote regular endometrial shedding and to prevent endometrial hyperplasia.
- **Ovulatory bleeding:** Treat the underlying cause and associated anemia. NSAIDs, combined hormonal contraceptives, or a levonorgestrel-releasing IUD can ↓ the duration and quantity of bleeding. Consider myomectomy in refractory cases associated with fibroids.
- In severe cases, surgical options such as endometrial ablation or hysterectomy may be indicated.

## Amenorrhea

Defined as the absence of menstrual periods. 1° amenorrhea is defined as failure of menses to appear by age 16 in a patient with normal 2° sexual characteristics or by age 14 in a patient with no 2° sexual characteristics. **2° amenorrhea** is defined as the absence of menses for three consecutive months in women with previous normal menstruation or for nine months in women with prior oligomenorrhea. Etiologies of **1° amenorrhea** include the following:

- **Hypothalamic/pituitary:**
  - **Hypothalamic dysfunction:** May be due to organic illness, vigorous exercise, stressful life events, or anorexia nervosa.
  - **Genetic gonadotropin deficiency:** Kallmann's syndrome.
  - **Hypothalamic lesions:** Craniopharyngioma.
  - **Pituitary tumors:** Prolactinoma.
  - **Endocrinopathies:** Cushing's syndrome, hypothyroidism.

- **Hyperandrogenism:** From adrenal, ovarian, or exogenous sources.
- **Ovarian:** Turner's syndrome, ovarian failure due to autoimmunity, ovarian steroidogenic enzyme deficiencies.
- **Uterine:** Congenital absence or malformation of the uterus; imperforate hymen.
- **Pseudohermaphroditism:** Absent uterus and intra-abdominal or cryptorchid testes due either to an enzymatic defect in testosterone synthesis or to complete androgen resistance (testicular feminization).

Etiologies of **2° amenorrhea** are as follows:

- Pregnancy.
- **Hypothalamic/pituitary:**
    - Emotional stress, illness, dieting, exercise, medications (phenothiazine, OCPs), anorexia nervosa, intensive exercise → extreme weight loss.
    - Cushing's syndrome; hypothyroidism.
    - Pituitary tumor (e.g., prolactinoma); pituitary infarction (e.g., Sheehan's syndrome).
    - Granulomatous disease (sarcoidosis).
- **Ovarian:**
    - PCOS.
    - Premature ovarian failure (autoimmune, radiation therapy, chemotherapy, endometriosis, oophoritis, idiopathic).
    - Hyperandrogenism (from adrenal, ovarian, or exogenous sources).
- **Uterine:** Asherman's syndrome (involves extensive intrauterine scarring and synechia formation); cervical scarring → closure of the os.

### SYMPTOMS

- Obtain a detailed menstrual history, including age at menarche, the character of normal cycles, and the timing of missed cycles, as well as a pregnancy history.
- Ask about the patient's psychosocial history, including situational stresses, emotional problems, dieting and nutritional issues, bulimia, weight loss, and exercise.
- Determine the patient's history of medication use, especially use of antipsychotics and OCPs.
- Ask about hormonal symptoms, including hot flashes, skin changes, hirsutism, headaches, breast changes, galactorrhea, and changes in libido.
- Inquire about previous CNS or pelvic chemoradiation.
- Determine if there is a family history of genetic defects or infertility; ask about the menstrual and pubertal history of the patient's mother and sisters.

### EXAM

Table 16.16 outlines physical exam findings that are commonly found in association with amenorrhea.

### DIAGNOSIS

- **1° amenorrhea:**
    - **Labs:** FSH, LH, prolactin, testosterone, TSH, free $T_4$, hCG. Virilized or hypertensive patients should have serum electrolytes and further hormonal evaluation.
    - **Imaging:** MRI of the hypothalamus and pituitary is indicated in girls with low to normal FSH and LH as well as high prolactin levels.

> **Causes of 2° amenorrhea—**
>
> **SOAP**
>
> **S**tress
> **O**CPs
> **A**norexia
> **P**regnancy

**TABLE 16.16.** **Exam Findings Associated with Amenorrhea**

| FINDING | RELATED DIAGNOSIS |
|---|---|
| Obesity, hirsutism, acne | PCOS |
| Webbed neck, widely spaced nipples, short stature | Turner's syndrome |
| Hypertension, buffalo hump, central obesity, easy bruising, striae | Cushing's syndrome |
| Pubic hair with absent uterus | Müllerian agenesis |
| Virilization, clitoral hypertrophy | Androgen-secreting tumor |
| Galactorrhea, visual field defects | Pituitary tumor |
| Enlarged thyroid | Hypothyroidism |
| Imperforate hymen, transverse vaginal septum | Outflow tract obstruction |
| Anosmia | Kallmann's syndrome |

- Karyotyping can diagnose X-chromosome mosaicism in patients with a normal uterus and high FSH without classic features of Turner's syndrome.

- **2° amenorrhea:**
  - Measure urine or serum hCG; if ↑, the most likely cause is pregnancy (although false ⊕ results are possible with ectopic hCG secretion, as occurs in choriocarcinoma or bronchogenic carcinoma).
  - Progestin challenge can be attempted; if withdrawal bleed occurs, the patient is likely anovulatory. If no withdrawal bleed occurs, an estrogen/progestin challenge can be used to distinguish a hypothalamic/pituitary disorder from outflow tract obstruction.
  - Labs that can be helpful include prolactin, FSH, LH, TSH, potassium, and renal and liver function tests.
  - MRI is indicated for ↑ prolactin or hypopituitarism.
  - In hirsute or virilized women, check serum testosterone.
  - In patients with signs of hypercortisolism, a 1-mg overnight dexamethasone suppression test is needed.

### TREATMENT

- **1° amenorrhea:** Treatment is based on the underlying cause.
- **2° amenorrhea:** Also directed at the cause. For reversible conditions, withholding therapy periodically is recommended to determine if periods return.
  - **Hypothalamic dysfunction:** Periods usually return when precipitants (exercise, dieting, situational stress) are withdrawn. Patients with anorexia nervosa often need to reach 90% of their normal weight prior to the return of menses. Chronic amenorrhea can be treated with medroxyprogesterone or combined hormones to bring on withdrawal bleeding every 1–3 months; efforts should also be made to protect the endometrial lining and promote healthy bones.

- **Pituitary disease:** Bromocriptine, a dopamine agonist, is used for hyperprolactinemia; larger pituitary tumors may require surgical intervention. Patients with destructive pituitary lesions may need replacement of estrogen, progesterone, thyroid hormone, or adrenal steroids.
- **Ovarian causes:** Estrogen/progesterone replacement is indicated for ovarian failure.
- **Uterine disease:** Asherman's syndrome can be treated with dilation and recurettage to sever bridging synechiae and with glucocorticoids to inhibit the formation of new scar tissue.

### COMPLICATIONS

Infertility, endometrial cancer, osteoporosis, heart disease.

## Polycystic Ovarian Syndrome (PCOS)

Characterized by androgen excess, insulin resistance, and gonadotropin abnormalities, PCOS is the most frequent cause of anovulatory infertility.

### SYMPTOMS/EXAM

May present with menstrual irregularities, infertility, hirsutism, acne, obesity, possible ovarian enlargement, and acanthosis nigricans.

### DIFFERENTIAL

- Pregnancy, premature ovarian failure, medications (progestational agents), pituitary adenoma, thyroid disorders, adrenal tumors, Cushing's syndrome, congenital adrenal hyperplasia.
- In patients with rapidly progressive hirsutism, ↑ DHEAS levels suggest a virilizing adrenal tumor.
- If congenital adrenal hyperplasia is suspected in patients with hypertension and potassium abnormalities, check serum 17-hydroxyprogesterone levels at 8 A.M.
- Patients with physical findings of cortisol excess (e.g., hypertension, easy bruising, central obesity, proximal muscle weakness) should have an overnight dexamethasone suppression test to rule out Cushing's syndrome.

### DIAGNOSIS

- Primarily a clinical diagnosis consisting of a combination of oligomenorrhea and hyperandrogenism.
- Laboratory findings can include ↑ testosterone, androstenedione, LH, estradiol, estrone, and fasting insulin; an ↑ ratio of LH to FSH (> 3:1); and ↓ sex hormone–binding globulin.
- Other important labs include hCG to rule out pregnancy, prolactin, fasting glucose, and a lipid panel.
- Diagnosis by ultrasound consists of more than eight follicles < 10 mm in diameter, but imaging is not necessary or sufficient for the diagnosis.

*PCOS is largely a clinical diagnosis, combining oligomenorrhea and clinical or laboratory hyperandrogenism.*

### TREATMENT

- **Oligomenorrhea:**
    - Combination OCPs (choose the least androgenic progestins; avoid norgestrel and levonorgestrel) prevent pregnancy and endometrial hyperplasia, normalize menstrual cycles, and treat hirsutism and acne.

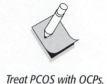

*Treat PCOS with OCPs.*

- Monthly DMPA is an option for contraception and endometrial protection but does not suppress ovarian androgen production.
- **Hirsutism:** Treat with antiandrogens such as spironolactone in combination with OCPs, or use OCPs with a progestin with antimineralocorticoid activity.
- **Anovulation/infertility:** Weight loss; clomiphene citrate +/– metformin. Surgical options (which are rarely used) include ovarian cautery or laser vaporization.
- **Weight loss:** ↓ serum androgen, insulin, and LH. Diet and exercise are recommended for all patients; metformin can help with weight loss.

### COMPLICATIONS

Chronic anovulation and amenorrhea, with associated long-term exposure to unopposed estrogen, can → endometrial hyperplasia and endometrial cancer. Lipid abnormalities and hyperinsulinemia can ↑ the risk for the development of cardiovascular disease.

## OTHER GYNECOLOGIC CONDITIONS

 A healthy 25-year-old woman asks you for a CA-125 test to screen for ovarian cancer. Should you order one? No, as the positive predictive value (PPV) in this patient is only 2.3%.

### Ovarian Mass

Most ovarian masses are found on physical exam in both symptomatic and asymptomatic women or are discovered incidentally on imaging. Types of benign ovarian masses include ovarian cysts, germ cell tumors (mature teratomas = dermoid cysts), stromal cell tumors (thecomas, fibromas), and epithelial cell tumors (serous or mucinous adenomas and Brenner tumors). The risk of malignancy ↑ significantly with age, from 13% in premenopausal women to 45% following the onset of menopause. Malignant adnexal lesions include 1° ovarian carcinoma and metastatic disease from the uterus, breast, or GI tract. Additional considerations are as follows:

- Newborns can have small functional cysts due to maternal hormones for a few months.
- In girls < 9 years of age, 80% of adnexal masses are malignant (usually germ cell tumors).
- In reproductive-age women, most adnexal masses are follicular and corpus luteum cysts of the ovary and benign tumors such as mature teratomas, endometriomas, and serous or mucinous cystadenomas.
- Nonmalignant masses in postmenopausal women include ovarian fibromas.

### SYMPTOMS

Many patients are asymptomatic, but symptoms may include urinary frequency, pelvic pressure or pain, dyspepsia, abdominal bloating, early satiety, constipation, and changes in stool caliber. Patients with ovarian cancer often complain of vague GI symptoms.

### EXAM

Evaluate for cervical, supraclavicular, and groin lymphadenopathy. Perform a breast exam, as the ovary is a common site of metastasis for breast carcinoma. Perform bimanual and rectovaginal exams as well.

### DIAGNOSIS

- **Imaging:** Ultrasound is the most important diagnostic study. Important characteristics include size, whether cystic or solid, and other signs suggestive of malignancy, such as internal septae/papillae or the presence of ascites.
- **Labs:** Lab tests include **β-hCG level** to rule out ectopic pregnancy. Serum tumor markers are useful in certain instances.
  - **α-fetoprotein:** For endodermal sinus tumors.
  - **LDH:** For dysgerminomas.
  - **β-hCG:** For nongestational choriocarcinomas.
  - **Serum CA-125:** ↑ in malignant conditions such as serous epithelial ovarian, breast, colon, lung, and pancreatic cancers. In the setting of a postmenopausal woman with an ultrasonographically suspicious pelvic mass, the PPV for malignancy is 97%. Because it can be ↑ in benign conditions, CA-125 is not recommended as a routine screening test (the PPV in healthy patients is only 2.3%).

*Ultrasound is the most important diagnostic test used in evaluating adnexal masses.*

### TREATMENT

- **Prepubertal patients:** All adnexal masses in prepubertal girls must be evaluated with ultrasound and referral.
- **Premenopausal patients:** Premenopausal women with cysts < 10 cm can be followed. Monophasic OCPs can suppress symptomatic functional cysts. All solid adnexal masses call for immediate surgical exploration, as does the presence of ascites.
- **Postmenopausal patients:**
  - Postmenopausal women with asymptomatic ovarian cysts < 3 cm in diameter and a normal serum CA-125 can be followed with serial ultrasounds, as such patients have a very low risk for malignancy. Larger cysts should be evaluated laparoscopically.
  - Symptomatic patients with an ultrasonographically suspicious mass and ↑ serum CA-125 should be referred for surgical evaluation.

> A 36-year-old woman with mild pelvic pain and moderately heavy periods but no anemia is found on pelvic ultrasound to have multiple small uterine fibroids. How would you manage this patient? As her symptoms are mild, the patient can be reassured and treated conservatively with pain medication and OCPs to ↓ menstrual flow. If she develops more severe symptoms, the ultrasound should be repeated and surgery considered.

## Fibroids

The most common benign neoplasm of the female genital tract. Also called uterine leiomyomas, fibroids are discrete, round, firm uterine tumors composed of smooth muscle and connective tissue. They are classified by anatomic location as intramural, submucous, subserous, intraligamentous, parasitic (deriving its blood supply from an organ to which it becomes attached), and cervical. Risk factors include nulliparity and obesity.

### SYMPTOMS

- Often asymptomatic, but may present with pelvic pain, dysmenorrhea, or menorrhagia (which may → anemia) as well as with urinary frequency, incontinence, or other complications stemming from the presence of an abdominal mass.
- Fibroids that distort the uterine cavity may → infertility or recurrent pregnancy loss.

### EXAM

Irregular enlargement of the uterus.

### DIFFERENTIAL

Pregnancy, adenomyosis, ovarian tumor, leiomyosarcoma.

### DIAGNOSIS

- **Labs:** Low hemoglobin results from blood loss, with rare cases of polycythemia from production of erythropoietin by the myomas.
- **Imaging:** Ultrasound can confirm the presence of fibroids and monitor their growth, and it can also be used to exclude ovarian masses. MRI is accurate in delineating intramural and submucous fibroids; hysteroscopy can confirm cervical or submucous fibroids.

### TREATMENT

- No treatment is necessary for small, asymptomatic fibroids. Most fibroids grow slowly until menopause, when they start to shrink.
- OCPs or progestins (including the levonorgestrel-releasing IUD) can be used to control menstrual bleeding, but they do not ↓ the size of fibroids.
- For severe anemia, ↓ bleeding with monthly depot medroxyprogesterone acetate or daily danazol.
- Surgery is indicated for rapid growth, severe bleeding → anemia, or pressure on the ureters, bladder, or bowel.
  - Surgical options include myomectomy (preferable during childbearing years), hysterectomy, uterine artery embolization, and MRI-guided focused ultrasound surgery.
  - Given that the risk of surgical complications ↑ with larger myomas, GnRH analogs (depot leuprolide, nafarelin) can be given preoperatively to ↓ the size of myomas.

## Endometriosis

The presence of endometrial tissue on the ovaries, fallopian tubes, or other abnormal sites → pain or infertility. Endometriosis is a progressive disease affecting 5–10% of women. Although its exact cause is not known, theories on its etiology include retrograde menstruation, transformation of peritoneal epithelium into endometrial tissue, and the differentiation of müllerian remnants into endometrial tissue.

### SYMPTOMS

Presents with dysmenorrhea, dyspareunia, and low back pain that worsens during menses. Rectal pain and painful defecation may also be seen. Infertility is often the presenting complaint. Many patients are asymptomatic.

### EXAM

- Exam is best performed during early menses, when implants are largest and most tender.
- Although most patients have normal pelvic exams, findings can include tenderness on bimanual exam, nodularity in the posterior cul-de-sac or along the uterosacral ligament, ↓ uterine mobility or retroversion, and adnexal masses.

### DIAGNOSIS

- No lab tests can help make the diagnosis, although CA-125 levels are sometimes ↑.
- If masses are present, CT, MRI, or ultrasound can be useful.
- Laparoscopy is required for definitive diagnosis, although lesions must be histologically confirmed, as they can be confused with a variety of lesions.
- Clinical manifestations and surgical findings often correlate poorly.

*Laparoscopy with histologic confirmation is needed for a definitive diagnosis of endometriosis*

### TREATMENT

- Medical treatment should be reserved for patients with symptoms other than infertility, as such treatment does not restore fertility.
- Combined hormonal contraceptives or progestin-only methods suppress LH and FSH and prevent ovulation, also → thinning of endometrial tissue and ↓ menstrual volume. May be used continuously.
- Danazol is an androgen derivative that inhibits LH and FSH and → endometrial atrophy. Androgenic side effects include acne, edema, hirsutism, and voice deepening; estrogen deficiency can → headache, flushing, sweating, and atrophic vaginitis.
- GnRH agonists (IM leuprolide, SQ goserelin, nasal nafarelin) inhibit gonadotropin secretion and produce pain relief in 90% of patients. Hypoestrogenic side effects, including bone loss, can be minimized by supplementing with low doses of estrogen.
- Surgical treatment is indicated for infertile patients with advanced endometriosis. Surgical ablation of lesions is often performed at the time of diagnostic laparoscopy. A combination of medical and surgical therapy may improve outcomes.
- Hysterectomy with oophorectomy can be performed in women with intractable pain who no longer want to become pregnant.

*Medical treatments for endometriosis include hormonal contraceptives, danazol, and GnRH agonists.*

### COMPLICATIONS

Without treatment, endometriosis progressively worsens in 65–80% of patients. Implants may grow and spread throughout the pelvis and to the urinary and intestinal tracts → pain, infertility, and obstruction.

REPRODUCTIVE HEALTH

## Vulvodynia

A syndrome of unexplained vulvar pain, often accompanied by physical disabilities, limitations in daily activities such as sitting or walking, sexual dysfunction, and psychological distress. Subtypes include the following:

- **Vulvar vestibulitis syndrome:** Usually premenopausal.
- **Cyclic vulvovaginitis:** Associated with pain that worsens during menses.
- **Dysesthetic or essential vulvodynia:** Usually peri- or postmenopausal.
- **Vulvar dermatoses.**
- **Papulosquamous vulvar dermatoses:** Itching is prominent.
- **Vesiculobullous vulvar dermatoses:** May present with itching or burning.
- **Vestibular papillomatosis:** A normal anatomic variant that is often asymptomatic.

### SYMPTOMS

- Usually acute in onset, becoming chronic and lasting months or years.
- Discomfort is often described as stinging or burning or, alternatively, a feeling of rawness or irritation. Itching may be prominent, and pain may be associated with menses, intercourse, or tampon use.
- Any history of vaginal infections, cryotherapy or laser therapy, and use of medications must be obtained.

### EXAM

- Some women have minimal findings.
- On pelvic exam, assess for **erythema, edema,** and **vaginal discharge,** and perform a swab test for vestibular point tenderness (vulvar vestibulitis).
- Also look for thickened or scaly lesions (papulosquamous vulvar dermatoses), blisters or ulcers (vesiculobullous vulvar dermatoses), or plaques (possible neoplasms), and assess for skin lesions elsewhere on the body.

### DIFFERENTIAL

Allergic vulvitis, chronic candidal vulvitis, lichen planus, lichen sclerosus, vulvar atrophy, vulvar intraepithelial neoplasia.

### DIAGNOSIS

- Fungal and bacterial cultures; KOH microscopic exam; biopsy of suspicious areas with acetowhitening and colposcopy to rule out dermatoses or neoplasm.
- The swab test involves palpation of the vestibulum with a moist, cotton-tipped swab to assess for point tenderness.

REPRODUCTIVE HEALTH

### TREATMENT

- **Oral medications:** Fluconazole for cyclic vulvovaginitis; TCAs, SSRIs, or gabapentin for essential vulvodynia; calcium citrate for cyclic vulvovaginitis or vulvar vestibulitis.
- **Topical medications:** Lidocaine or cromolyn cream; estradiol cream for vulvar vestibulitis; corticosteroids for papulosquamous dermatoses.
- Intralesional interferon injection for **vulvar vestibulitis.**
- Low-oxalate diet; physical therapy with biofeedback to ↓ vaginal spasms and strengthen weakened pelvic floor muscles; support groups.
- **Surgical treatment:** Vulvar vestibulectomy and excited dye laser surgery are reserved for severe cases in which all medical therapies have failed.

## Ovarian Torsion

Usually occurs in a pathologically enlarged ovary. Most common in the early reproductive years, with more than half of all cases affecting patients with ovarian masses (masses are usually benign, as malignant tumors often have adhesions that fix the ovary). Pregnant women with enlarged corpus luteum cysts, women undergoing ovulation induction, and patients with a history of pelvic surgery, especially tubal ligation, are at ↑ risk of ovarian torsion. Prepubertal patients with congenitally elongated fallopian tubes and normal ovaries are also at ↑ risk.

### SYMPTOMS

The classic presentation is sudden-onset, severe, unilateral pelvic pain that radiates to the back or thigh; however, pain can also be mild or bilateral. Most patients also complain of nausea and vomiting. Onset often occurs during exercise.

### EXAM

Most patients have a unilateral, tender adnexal mass, but up to 30% can have no tenderness on exam. In advanced cases, fever and peritoneal signs can be present.

### DIFFERENTIAL

Appendicitis, diverticulitis, endometriosis, mesenteric ischemia, bowel obstruction, ovarian cyst, PID, tubal ovarian abscess, ectopic pregnancy, renal calculi, UTI.

### DIAGNOSIS

- **Labs:** Rule out other diagnoses with a pregnancy test, UA, and gonorrhea and chlamydia cultures.
- **Imaging:** Ultrasound usually shows ovarian enlargement or an ovarian mass. Doppler flow imaging can be useful, but flow can be normal during transient periods of detorsing. CT can be used to rule out other causes of pain.

### TREATMENT

- Laparoscopy can be used to confirm the diagnosis as well as for treatment; conservative treatment consists of uncoiling the torsed ovary.
- Salpingo-oophorectomy is necessary in cases with severe vascular compromise, peritonitis, or tissue necrosis.

*While most patients with ovarian torsion have severe unilateral pain and tenderness, some patients present with mild or bilateral pain and no tenderness on exam.*

REPRODUCTIVE HEALTH

### COMPLICATIONS

Delayed diagnosis and treatment can → infarction and necrosis of the ovary.

## MENOPAUSE

Defined as permanent cessation of menses. The average age of menopause is 51. Most women experience vasomotor symptoms for about two years after their LMP, but 25% of women are asymptomatic.

### SYMPTOMS

- **Hot flashes:** Worsened by eating, exertion, emotional stress, and alcohol.
- **GU symptoms:** Vaginal atrophy → dryness, pruritus, and dyspareunia; urethral atrophy → stress incontinence, frequency, urgency, and dysuria.
- **Mood changes:** Irritability, anxiety, depression, sleep disturbance.
- **Perimenopause:** Precedes actual menopause; characterized by variable cycle length, often accompanied by the symptoms of menopause.

### EXAM

Exam reveals ↓ breast size, vaginal dryness, and urogenital atrophy.

### DIFFERENTIAL

Premature ovarian failure (cessation of menses in women < 40); infections such as TB; malignancy.

### DIAGNOSIS

↑ serum FSH can be indicative of menopause, although it is insensitive and is rarely needed for diagnosis.

### TREATMENT

- **Hormone replacement therapy (HRT):**
  - Associated with a significant ↓ in hot flash severity and frequency; also improves GU symptoms and can prevent osteoporosis.
  - HRT ↑ a woman's risk for coronary disease, stroke, DVT, and breast cancer, and therefore it is most appropriately used as a short-term treatment aimed at symptom relief. In order to prevent endometrial cancer, women with a uterus must be treated with a combination of estrogen and progestin.
  - HRT is contraindicated in patients with a history of breast cancer, premalignant breast lesions, endometrial cancer, unexplained vaginal bleeding, DVT or pulmonary embolism, liver disease, or CAD.
- Symptoms of **vaginal atrophy** can de controlled with topical estrogen cream, vaginal estradiol rings, and vaginal lubricants.
- Other oral medications that may ↓ hot flashes are SSRIs, including paroxetine, fluoxetine, and venlafaxine, as well as gabapentin and clonidine.
- Phytoestrogens, including soy and red clover, have not consistently been shown to help relieve menopausal symptoms, and studies of black cohosh have also yielded conflicting results.
- **Lifestyle interventions** to ↓ vasomotor symptoms include lowering room temperatures, consuming cold food and drinks, weight control, regular physical activity, tobacco avoidance, and relaxation techniques.

*HRT is best used as short-term treatment for menopausal symptom relief, as it ↑ the risk for coronary disease and breast cancer.*

*Alternatives to HRT in the treatment of hot flashes include lifestyle changes, SSRIs, gabapentin, and clonidine.*

### COMPLICATIONS

Long-term complications related to menopause and ↓ estrogen include cardiovascular disease and osteoporosis.

## FAMILY AND INTIMATE-PARTNER VIOLENCE

Affects individuals from all socioeconomic and cultural backgrounds and all family structures, including same-sex relationships, and is vastly underreported by victims and overlooked by physicians. Victims are more commonly women, and children of abused mothers are at ↑ risk for abuse or neglect. Additional risk factors include alcohol or drug abuse, social stressors (e.g., unemployment, poverty), and a family history of violence.

### SYMPTOMS

- Although there is insufficient evidence of the benefit of **universal screening,** experts recommend screening all women in the course of prenatal and routine well-woman care.
- In the outpatient setting, abuse may present as vague, recurrent somatic complaints, depressive symptoms, or ↑ use of medical services.
- Physical abuse is often preceded or accompanied by psychological abuse (insulting, controlling, denying of basic needs) and/or sexual abuse.

### EXAM

- Look for patterns of injuries, such as bruises in various stages of healing.
- If physical signs of abuse are present, document them in detail and take identifying photographs.

### DIFFERENTIAL

Bleeding disorder; affective, anxiety, and somatoform disorders.

### TREATMENT

- Validate the patient's right to be free from abuse (e.g., "You don't deserve to be hurt like this") and offer support.
- Recognize that abuse often occurs in repeated cycles: escalating tension → violence → remorse and reconciliation. Do not expect victims to leave right away, and avoid blaming or giving up on them if they return to the abuser.
- Help the patient establish a safety plan.
- If you suspect that children are being harmed or neglected, report to Child Protective Services.
- Know your state's laws with respect to reporting requirements for suspected abuse.

### COMPLICATIONS

Learned helplessness, low self-esteem, depression, anxiety, substance abuse, and PTSD; physical injury and disability; exacerbation of chronic medical conditions; death by suicide or homicide.

> **Questions for detecting domestic violence—**
>
> **SAFE**
>
> **S**tress/**S**afety?
> **A**fraid/**A**bused?
> **F**riends/**F**amily aware?
> **E**mergency plan?

*Pregnancy and attempted separation are especially high-risk times for abuse victims.*

REPRODUCTIVE HEALTH

Includes any actual or attempted sexual contact that is against the victim's will or that occurs when the victim is unable to consent because of age, disability, or impairment. At least one in three women and one in 33 men have been victims of rape or attempted rape. More than half of lifetime rapes occur before age 18.

### SYMPTOMS

- Patients who present acutely after sexual assault may have symptoms of trauma that are physical (**bruises, broken bones**), sexual (**genital lacerations, abrasions, bruises**), and/or psychological (**feeling fearful, withdrawn, angry**).
- Patients with a past or ongoing history of sexual violence may have symptoms of psychological sequelae such as **depression** or **PTSD**, or they may present with chronic somatic complaints such as **headache, nausea,** or **fatigue**.

### EXAM

- After an acute sexual assault, care should be taken to conduct the exam in a way that allows for adequate collection of forensic evidence and avoids retraumatizing the victim. If available, call on a certified sexual assault nurse examiner (SANE) or a rape victim's advocate.
- Document all signs of trauma and abuse.
- Patients with a past or ongoing history of sexual violence may experience added fear and anxiety with the routine physical (especially pelvic) exam. Limit invasive exams to those absolutely necessary, and offer to have a support person present.

### DIAGNOSIS

- Although there is insufficient evidence to recommend routine screening, all patients with suggestive signs or symptoms (physical or psychological) should be asked about their exposure to sexual violence.
- All victims of sexual assault should be offered testing for STIs (including oropharyngeal and anal sites if applicable) and pregnancy.

### TREATMENT

*Emergency contraception is the standard of care for women who are capable of becoming pregnant at the time they are raped. The sooner they get it, the more effective it will be at preventing pregnancy from the assault.*

- In the setting of acute assault, if clinically applicable, make sure to offer **emergency contraception** to prevent pregnancy, **postexposure HIV prophylaxis and HBV vaccination,** and **empiric STI treatment**.
- Compassion and advocacy throughout the clinical encounter tell victims that you are there to help. An independent victim's advocate, if available, should be provided.
- Work with law enforcement when applicable.
- Offer acute and ongoing psychological counseling.

### COMPLICATIONS

Undesired pregnancy; STIs; depression, anxiety, eating disorders, PTSD, and substance abuse; chronic headaches, sleep disturbance, and GI complaints; suicidal behavior.

## Female Sexual Dysfunction

Distress and impairment resulting from a disturbance in sexual desire and/or from emotional and physiologic changes in the sexual response cycle. Affects approximately 25–40% of women. Symptoms must → distress or significant interference in interpersonal relationships and social functioning. Factors that predict ⊕ sexual functioning include a general state of well-being and a quality relationship with a partner; dysfunction is generally **not** related to hormone levels. Subtypes include the following:

- **Hypoactive sexual desire disorder/low libido:** Absence of sexual fantasies and lack of desire to engage in sexual activity.
- **Sexual arousal disorder/excitement-phase dysfunction:** Inability to respond to sexual stimulation despite genital vasocongestion and lubrication.
- **Orgasmic dysfunction:** Inability to have an orgasm despite normal sexual desire and ability to enjoy intercourse.
- **Pain associated with sex:** Dyspareunia, vaginitis, incompletely ruptured hymen, Bartholin's gland cyst, postepisiotomy pain, vulvovaginal atrophy, vulvar vestibulitis, vaginismus (involuntary spasm of musculature of the outer third of the vagina, making penetration impossible), PID, ovarian cyst, endometriosis, fibroids, relaxation of pelvic support.

*Female sexual function is commonly related more to a state of well-being and relationship quality than to hormone levels.*

### SYMPTOMS

- Obtain a complete sexual history, including concerns, degree of satisfaction, sexual orientation, partner performance and satisfaction, contraception, and safe sex practices. Also elicit a psychiatric history (major depression, anxiety disorder, somatization disorder).
- Obtain a complete medical and surgical history to rule out 2° causes of sexual dysfunction (e.g., Cushing's disease, Addison's disease, DM, hyperprolactinemia, hypothyroidism, hypopituitarism, degenerative joint disease, MS, temporal lobe lesions, CAD).
- Explore the following:
  - **Interpersonal relationships:** Relationship quality and conflict.
  - **Psychology:** Depression, anxiety, past sexual or physical abuse, substance abuse.
  - **Sociocultural influences:** Stress, fatigue, lack of privacy, religion, lack of education.
  - **Physiology:** Medications, medical/neurologic problems, gynecologic/urologic problems, estrogen or androgen deficiency.

> **Sexual response cycle—**
>
> **EXPLORE**
>
> **EX**citement
> **PL**ateau
> **O**rgasm
> **RE**solution

### EXAM

Perform a pelvic exam to evaluate for vulvovaginitis, cervicitis, uterine masses or tenderness, cervical motion tenderness, and rectocele or cystocele.

### DIAGNOSIS

Diagnosis is primarily based on history, but some of the following may be indicated:

- **Labs:** CBC, ESR, FSH, estradiol, testosterone, TSH, prolactin, cervical cultures.
- **Imaging:** Pelvic ultrasound if exam is suspicious for a pelvic mass.

### TREATMENT

- Treat the underlying cause; counseling, sex therapy, and adjustment of life situation may be of benefit.
- **Estrogen/testosterone therapy:** Options include low-dose estrogen cream, an estradiol vaginal ring for postmenopausal vaginal dryness, combined estrogen/testosterone, DHEA, a transdermal testosterone patch, and testosterone vaginal cream.
- Risks of androgen therapy include hirsutism, acne, virilization, liver dysfunction, ↓ HDL, fluid retention, and psychological changes.

> A 68-year-old male smoker with hypertension and diabetes asks you to prescribe sildenafil for erectile dysfunction. The patient takes an ACEI, a diuretic, aspirin, a statin, metformin, and insulin. What do you tell him? Although sildenafil is absolutely contraindicated only in patients taking nitrates, you should make sure the patient understands the risks of sexual activity with his multiple cardiac risk factors before writing the prescription.

## Erectile Dysfunction (ED)

Repeated inability to achieve or sustain a penile erection sufficient for sexual intercourse. Affects up to 10% of men; more common in older men and smokers. Up to 50% of ED is due to organic causes (see Table 16.17).

**TABLE 16.17.    Etiologies of Erectile Dysfunction**

| DISORDER | EXAMPLES/COMMENTS |
|---|---|
| Psychogenic disorders | Performance anxiety, depression, mental stress. |
| Diabetes mellitus | ED is seen in up to 50% of DM cases. |
| Peripheral vascular disease | |
| Endocrine disorders | Hypogonadism, hyperprolactinemia, thyroid abnormalities, Addison's disease, Cushing's disease, acromegaly. |
| Pelvic surgery, spinal cord injury | |
| Drugs of abuse | Amphetamines, cocaine, marijuana, chronic alcoholism, tobacco, opiates, barbiturates. |
| Medications | Antihypertensives (thiazides, β-blockers, clonidine, methyldopa), antiandrogens (spironolactone, $H_2$ blockers, finasteride), antidepressants (TCAs, SSRIs), antipsychotics, benzodiazepines, opiates. |
| Prostate cancer | |
| Penile and urethral lesions | Pelvic fracture, hypospadias, priapism, Peyronie's disease, phimosis. |

- Obtain a thorough sexual history as well as a history of medications and substance abuse.
- Elicit a psychiatric, medical, and surgical history.
- Preservation of morning erections suggests psychogenic disease.
- Assess for atherosclerotic risk factors.

### EXAM

- **Vital signs:** Look for orthostatic changes in BP.
- **Skin:** Signs of endocrinopathies include palmar erythema, dryness, hyperpigmentation, and spider angiomata.
- **GU exam:** Inspect the penis for tumors, inflammation, discharge, phimosis, testicular masses, atrophy, or asymmetry; perform a prostate exam.
- **Vascular exam:** Assess peripheral pulses and evaluate for femoral and aortic bruits.
- **Neurologic exam:** Assess for pain sensation in the genital and perianal areas; test the bulbocavernosus reflex to evaluate the second, third, and fourth sacral segments of the spinal cord (the anal sphincter contracts around the examining finger as the glans is squeezed).
- **Other:** Thyroid exam; palpate the spine for tenderness and evidence of cord compression; examine for gynecomastia.

### DIAGNOSIS

- **Labs:** Depending on clinical presentation, consider glucose, lipids, TSH, testosterone, LH, and prolactin.
- Nocturnal penile tumescence testing; Doppler ultrasonography.

### TREATMENT

- Offer psychological support.
- Adjust medications that may be contributing to ED.
- Address the underlying cause, especially nicotine dependence.
- Medications include sildenafil, vardenafil, and tadalafil (has the longest duration of action). Side effects include flushing, headache, dyspepsia, and visual disturbance (sildenafil only); contraindicated if patients are on nitrates because of the risk of hypotension.
- Other treatments include intracavernosal injection with alprostadil and/or papaverine, transurethral alprostadil, penile prostheses, and vacuum constriction devices.

*Patients on nitrates should not take sildenafil, vardenafil, or tadalafil owing to the risk of hypotension.*

## INFERTILITY

A husband and wife present to your clinic appearing very anxious. They state that they have been married for almost two years and are eager to have a child but so far have not conceived. The woman, who is 33 years old, has been pregnant once and had an abortion. She reports regular menses every 30 days. The man, who is 38 years old, has two children from a previous marriage. Both travel frequently for work and report that they may go for 2–3 weeks at a time without having intercourse. What is the likely diagnosis, and how would you proceed? This couple is probably not experiencing true infertility, since they are not having regular intercourse reliably during fertile periods. They may have 2° or acquired infertility, but that diagnosis is not yet merited. Given that they have both been able to conceive in the past and that the woman has regular menstrual cycles, they have a high likelihood of being able to conceive together. Provide education about fertile times of the month, and encourage them to keep a journal of fertile periods and sexual activity to assist in the workup. At this visit, it would also be appropriate to provide the couple with pre-conception counseling regarding genetic risks, infection exposure, and nutrition.

Defined as the inability to conceive after one year of regular, unprotected vaginal intercourse. In 20% of cases, no cause is found. Among the rest, 40% are due to male factors, 40% to female factors, and 20% combined (see Table 16.18).

### SYMPTOMS

- Patients may present with a wide array of concerns that they associate with impaired fertility. Inquire about the frequency and timing of intercourse and how long the couple has been trying to conceive.

**TABLE 16.18. Causes of Infertility**

| | MALE FACTORS | FEMALE FACTORS |
|---|---|---|
| Anatomic (congenital or acquired) | Varicocele | Gonadal dysgenesis |
| | Cryptorchidism | Uterine anomalies |
| | History of orchitis | Endometriosis |
| | | Prior surgery affecting the reproductive organs |
| | | Prior tubal inflammation such as that associated with PID |
| | | Asherman's syndrome (uterine synechiae) |
| Endocrine/metabolic | Hypothalamic or pituitary dysfunction | Hypothalamic or pituitary dysfunction |
| | Hyperprolactinemia | Hyperprolactinemia |
| | Thyroid disease | Thyroid disease |
| | Adrenal disease | Premature ovarian failure |
| | | Androgen excess |
| | | Extremes of body weight |
| Functional | Erectile dysfunction | Sexual dysfunction |
| | Ejaculatory dysfunction | ↓ libido |
| | ↓ libido | |
| Exposures | Chemical, radiation, or heat effects on testes | DES in utero |
| | Exogenous androgens | Exogenous androgens |
| | | Chemical or radiation effects on ovaries |

- Take a complete menstrual and reproductive history. Irregular menses may indicate anovulatory cycles; prior conception rules out 1° infertility. A history of STIs or endometriosis predisposes women to 2° infertility.

### EXAM

- Perform a complete GU exam to look for anatomic abnormalities such as undescended testis or varicocele in men or large fibroids in women.
- Examine patients for 2° sexual characteristics as well as for signs of endocrine/metabolic disorders such as gynecomastia in men or hirsutism or extreme body weight in women.

### DIAGNOSIS

- Order a semen analysis to evaluate the male partner for ejaculatory function, sperm count, morphology, and motility.
- If hormonal/metabolic causes in the female partner are considered, check TSH, FSH, free testosterone, DHEAS, and an oral glucose tolerance test.
- If it is unclear whether the woman is ovulating, obtain a midcycle progesterone or home luteinizing hormone urine test kit. Daily basal body temperature readings can also be of benefit; a sustained rise of $\geq 0.4°F$ suggests that ovulation has occurred.
- If there is a concern for ↓ ovarian reserve, **obtain a day-3 FSH.**
- If anatomic causes in the female partner are considered, refer for appropriate imaging, which may include ultrasound, hysterosalpingography, hysteroscopy, and laparoscopy.

### TREATMENT

- Treatment should be targeted to the couple-specific cause of infertility.
- All couples should be advised to maximize fertility through lifestyle changes, including decreasing caffeine, alcohol, and tobacco and optimizing weight.
- Anovulation can be treated with clomiphene citrate.
- PCOS-related infertility should be addressed with weight loss. If this is unsuccessful, clomiphene citrate +/– metformin may be useful.
- Couples with irreversible or unidentified causes of infertility may still be able to conceive using intrauterine insemination, in vitro fertilization, or other assisted reproductive therapies.
- Couples may consider adoption as an alternative.
- Infertility and assisted reproductive therapy can be stressful and emotionally trying. For this reason, psychosocial support should be provided throughout the workup and treatment.

*Women with PCOS or metabolic syndrome ↑ their chance of conceiving by improving their insulin sensitivity.*

# MEN'S HEALTH

## EPIDIDYMITIS

The most common cause of scrotal inflammation in adults. Usually sexually transmitted in younger men; most often 2° to UTI or prostatitis in older men.

### SYMPTOMS

- Presents with a painful, swollen scrotum that is usually acute in onset. Pain may radiate to the groin, abdomen, or flank.

Differential
diagnosis of scrotal
swelling—

**THE THEATRES**

**T**orsion
**H**ernia
**E**pididymitis/orchitis
**T**rauma
**H**ydrocele, varicocele,
  hematoma
**E**dema
**A**ppendix testes
  (torsion, hemorrhage)
**T**umor
**R**ecurrent leukemia
**E**pididymal cyst
**S**yphilis, TB

- Dysuria and urinary frequency are common.
- Fever, chills, and malaise are seen.
- Urethral discharge is possible.

### EXAM

- Exam reveals a swollen, tender mass attached to the testicle. Inflammation may extend locally.
- Reactive hydrocele may be seen.
- Fever may be present, and patients may occasionally appear toxic.

### DIAGNOSIS

- UA and culture may reveal bacteriuria, pyuria, and hematuria.
- CBC and blood culture are indicated if the patient is febrile or toxic.
- Urine nucleic acid amplification tests or urethral culture for gonorrhea and chlamydia; offer testing for other STIs.

### TREATMENT

- Antibiotics to cover *N. gonorrhoeae* and *C. trachomatis* if sexual transmission is suspected; TMP-SMX or a fluoroquinolone if enteric gram-$\ominus$ organisms or staph are suspected.
- Hospitalization for IV therapy if the patient is febrile or toxic.
- NSAIDs, scrotal elevation, and cold packs are of benefit.

### COMPLICATIONS

Follow with periodic exams to exclude an underlying testicular mass.

## PROSTATITIS

A 65-year-old man comes to your office complaining of dysuria and deep rectal pain for the past two months. He is generally healthy and has no new sexual partners and no other urinary symptoms. On DRE, his prostate is found to be normal in size, shape, and consistency and is nontender. Urine culture is $\ominus$. Exam of expressed prostatic secretions reveals multiple WBCs, but culture is $\ominus$. What is the likely diagnosis, and how would you treat this patient? The patient has chronic nonbacterial prostatitis. Treatment is symptomatic, consisting of NSAIDs and sitz baths. $\alpha$-blockers or antispasmodics may provide additional relief.

An inflammatory disorder of the prostate that may be irritative or infectious. It may present as an acute febrile illness with risk of sepsis or may have a chronic, lingering course. Most chronic prostatitis is inflammatory with $\ominus$ cultures. Bacterial prostatitis stems from enteric gram-$\ominus$ organisms and/or from gonorrhea or chlamydia.

### SYMPTOMS

- Patients present with perineal, rectal, and/or low back pain.
- Urinary urgency, frequency, retention, nocturia, and dysuria are seen.

- Painful ejaculation is common.
- Fever, chills, malaise, and myalgias are seen in acute prostatitis.

### EXAM

- In acute prostatitis, the prostate feels boggy, swollen, warm, and tender, and the patient is febrile and appears toxic.
- Chronic prostatitis may present with a normal exam.

### DIFFERENTIAL

- Voiding symptoms may indicate UTI or BPH.
- Pain may be isolated prostatodynia with no exam or lab findings.
- Prostatic abscess, which is rare in nondiabetics, presents with high fever and nonresponse to treatment and requires surgical drainage.
- If the patient is not responding to antibacterial therapy, consider TB and *Cryptococcus*, especially in immunocompromised patients.

### DIAGNOSIS

- UA reveals bacteriuria, hematuria, and pyuria.
- Urine culture and sensitivity identifies the causal organism. If ⊖ in chronic prostatitis, prostatic secretions may be expressed by massage.
- In acute prostatitis, CBC reveals leukocytosis, and blood cultures may be ⊕.

### TREATMENT

- Acutely ill patients may require hospitalization and IV antibiotics. Ampicillin and an aminoglycoside are recommended until cultures can guide therapy.
- If IV therapy is not required, treat with a 21- to 30-day course of oral TMP-SMX, amoxicillin, or a fluoroquinolone.
- Adjuvant therapy includes analgesics (usually NSAIDs) and stool softeners for comfort.
- If chronic symptoms persist and cultures are ⊖, treatment is symptomatic with analgesics, anti-inflammatory agents, α-blockers, and sitz baths.

### COMPLICATIONS

- Acute prostatitis can seed the blood and → sepsis.
- Acute episodes may recur or become low-grade chronic prostatitis. A full month of therapy may ↓ the risk of recurrence. Occasionally patients may require chronic suppressive antibiotic therapy.
- Chronic prostatitis is the most common cause of recurrent UTI in men.

## BALANITIS

Inflammation of the glans penis, usually related to fungal organisms but sometimes due to bacteria from skin or sexually transmitted organisms. The condition is more common in uncircumcised men and diabetics.

### SYMPTOMS

- Presents with burning, irritation, and redness of the head of the penis.
- Dysuria may be present.
- A white, cheesy discharge may be seen if the cause is fungal.

*If you suspect acute prostatitis, avoid prostate massage and urethral catheterization if possible, as they may ↑ the risk of bacteremia.*

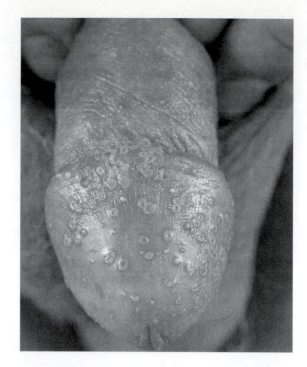

**FIGURE 16.18.** **Candidal balanitis.**

(Reproduced, with permission, from Wolff K et al. *Fitzpatrick's Color Atlas & Synopsis of Clinical Dermatology*, 5th ed. New York: McGraw-Hill, 2005: 727.) (Also see Color Insert.)

### EXAM

- Exam reveals a tender, erythematous, and swollen glans, prepuce, and urethral opening.
- Papules, pustules, or ulcerations may be seen (see Figure 16.18).
- If the patient is uncircumcised, retract the foreskin to reveal an adherent, cheesy discharge.

### DIFFERENTIAL

In prepubertal boys, rule out sexual abuse.

### DIAGNOSIS

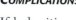

- The history and exam are usually diagnostic.
- Consider skin culture for fungus and bacteria; consider testing for STIs.

### TREATMENT

- Topical antifungals if a fungal source is suspected or proven.
- Recommend hygiene measures (keep the area clean and dry; avoid unnecessary foreskin manipulation) to prevent recurrence.
- Aggressive glycemic control in diabetics.
- Antibacterials against skin or STI organisms.
- If fungal infection recurs, consider treating the sexual partner to prevent reinfection.

*Diabetes is the most common condition underlying balanitis. Don't miss an opportunity to diagnose diabetes or motivate good glycemic control!*

### COMPLICATIONS

If balanitis recurs frequently in an uncircumcised patient, consider circumcision.

REPRODUCTIVE HEALTH

Infection of the testes, primarily caused by the mumps virus. Other causes include nonmumps viruses or, rarely, TB, fungi, or local bacterial spread from epididymitis.

### SYMPTOMS

- Presents with a painful, swollen testicle.
- If the infection is caused by mumps, associated symptoms include parotitis, fever, and malaise.

### EXAM

The testicle is tensely swollen and tender. Reactive hydrocele may be present.

### DIAGNOSIS

- The history and exam are usually diagnostic.
- Testicular masses of unknown etiology should be evaluated with ultrasound.
- In mumps, generalized symptoms and parotitis precede orchitis by 4–6 days.

### TREATMENT

- Supportive care with analgesics, scrotal support, and cold packs.
- If symptoms do not improve, consider abscess or other causes of testicular mass.

### COMPLICATIONS

Mumps → sterility in 10% of men affected.

*The key to preventing mumps is thorough vaccination. All children should receive two doses of MMR vaccine by kindergarten. Offer MMR to adults without proven immunity.*

## BENIGN SCROTAL MASSES

Hydrocele, varicocele, and spermatocele are relatively common scrotal swellings.

### SYMPTOMS

- Patients present with a scrotal swelling or lump.
- Also presents with scrotal discomfort or heaviness, occasionally with inguinal or low back pain.

### EXAM

- Hydrocele surrounds or sits below the testis and can be separated from it on exam.
- Spermatocele consists of one or several cysts of the epididymis and sits just above and attached to the testis.
- Varicocele consists of dilated veins of the spermatic cord, more commonly on the left side, and feels like a "bag of worms" on palpation. The mass enlarges when standing or with Valsalva and may disappear if the scrotum is elevated.
- Hydrocele and spermatocele transilluminate; varicocele does not.

REPRODUCTIVE HEALTH

### DIFFERENTIAL

Inguinal hernia must be considered as a source of a scrotal mass.

### DIAGNOSIS

If the exam is not definitive, imaging (usually ultrasound) is required to rule out testicular cancer.

### TREATMENT

- **Hydrocele and spermatocele** usually do not require treatment. If they become large or uncomfortable, surgical repair is offered.
- **Varicocele repair** is considered part of infertility treatment. If the mass was detected incidentally, repair may be advised to prevent infertility.

### COMPLICATIONS

By reducing spermatogenesis, varicocele may contribute to male fertility problems.

## TESTICULAR TORSION

A surgical emergency, as cessation of blood supply for 4–6 hours will → permanent loss of the testicle. Most common in infants, teens, and men < 30 years of age.

*Since testicular torsion can → complete loss of blood supply to the testicle if not surgically corrected, the "acute scrotum" should be treated as an emergency.*

### SYMPTOMS

Presents with abdominal pain, nausea, and vomiting. Scrotal pain is not always present.

### EXAM

The affected testicle is tender and elevated. The cremasteric reflex is absent.

### DIFFERENTIAL

Torsion of the appendix testis, appendicitis, epididymitis.

### DIAGNOSIS

- If torsion is considered, **do not delay consulting urology.**
- Ultrasound may help distinguish among the causes of scrotal pain but can be falsely ⊖ for torsion (approximately 10% of the time).
- UA is ⊖.

### TREATMENT

- Immediate surgical repair is the definitive treatment.
- Bilateral surgical fixation may be done to prevent recurrence.
- If surgical treatment is not available, manual detorsion may be attempted.
- Torsion of the appendix testis does not require treatment, but surgical exploration may be needed to rule out testicular torsion.

### COMPLICATIONS

- May → testicular infarction and impaired fertility if not corrected in time.
- If not surgically fixed, the testes have ↑ risk of recurrent torsion on the ipsilateral or contralateral side.

Enlargement of the prostate gland. BPH is common as men age and can cause partial urethral obstruction → urinary symptoms and occasionally impaired renal function. The severity of symptoms may not correlate with the size of the gland felt on exam.

### SYMPTOMS

- Presents with urinary frequency (every two hours or less) due to incomplete emptying; urinary hesitancy (difficulty initiating stream) or weak stream; and urinary dribbling or incontinence. Nocturia is common.
- Intermittence of voiding (starting and stopping urine flow during voiding) is also seen.

### EXAM

The gland feels smooth and symmetrically enlarged on DRE, and the bladder may be distended.

### DIFFERENTIAL

Prostate cancer, UTI.

### DIAGNOSIS

- The history and exam are usually diagnostic.
- Postvoid residual urine volume and urodynamic studies indicate the degree of obstruction.
- PSA may be ↑ but is nonspecific.
- Serum creatinine and other signs of renal impairment may be ↑ due to obstruction.
- Consider ultrasound +/– biopsy to evaluate for malignancy.

### TREATMENT

- Treatment is primarily symptomatic and is aimed at preventing or treating clinically significant urinary obstruction.
- α-blockers (doxazosin, terazosin, prazosin, tamsulosin) and 5α-reductase inhibitors (finasteride, dutasteride) can shrink the prostate medically. These two classes of medications can safely be used in combination.
- Transurethral resection of the prostate (TURP) and other minimally invasive surgical techniques have proven effective.
- Open prostatectomy is the treatment of last resort.

### COMPLICATIONS

Obstruction → hydronephrosis and chronic renal insufficiency; recurrent UTI may result from incomplete bladder emptying.

**Peyronie's disease** → "crooked" erections that may be painful due to thickening of the corpora tunica. **Priapism** is a prolonged, painful erection. It is most commonly related to medications such as chlorpromazine and sildenafil or to hematologic conditions such as sickle cell disease and leukemia. **Penile trauma** during erection can → rupture of the tunica albuginea, sometimes called penile fracture.

*The symptom severity of BPH may not correlate with gland size on exam. Once other causes of symptoms have been ruled out, treatment should be guided by the history.*

---

*Symptoms of BPH or "prostatism"—*

**HI FUN**

**H**esitancy
**I**ntermittence,
   **I**ncontinence
**F**requency, **F**ullness
**U**rgency
**N**octuria

---

REPRODUCTIVE HEALTH

### SYMPTOMS

- Peyronie's disease presents as a bent angle of the shaft that is often accompanied by pain during erection. The patient may also note subcutaneous nodules.
- The painful, prolonged erection of priapism may be accompanied by fever and by inability to urinate.
- Penile fracture is an acutely painful sensation that often occurs during sexual activity and may be accompanied by a popping sound.

### EXAM

- Peyronie's disease includes palpable, nontender plaques just beneath the skin of the penile shaft, usually on the dorsum.
- Priapism presents with an erect or semierect penis that may last for hours to days.
- Penile fracture is usually accompanied by a subcutaneous hematoma and by swollen "eggplant deformity" of the penis.

### DIAGNOSIS

- The history and exam are diagnostic.
- With penile injury, surgical exploration may be required to determine the extent of trauma.

### TREATMENT

- Peyronie's disease can be managed with verapamil injection, shock wave therapy, radiotherapy, or surgery. Many cases resolve without treatment.
- Priapism should be relieved as quickly as possibly to prevent cellular damage that can → functional impairment. Treatment is aspiration and irrigation.
- Penile trauma may require surgical repair. Rupture of the tunica albuginea is a surgical emergency.

### COMPLICATIONS

- Peyronie's disease may progress and → worsening pain and sexual dysfunction.
- Prolonged priapism can → erectile dysfunction.
- Untreated trauma to the corpora cavernosa or urethra can → permanent sexual and urinary dysfunction.

## PROSTATE CANCER

The most common malignancy among U.S. men, and the second most common cause of cancer death. Most cases remain latent, with only 10% progressing to clinically significant disease. Risk factors include advancing age, African-American ethnicity, and a ⊕ family history.

### SYMPTOMS

- Often asymptomatic, or may → urinary obstruction with symptoms of prostatism.
- Bony metastases can → vertebral or hip pain.

### EXAM

- DRE reveals areas of induration or nodules if the tumor is on the posterior aspect of the prostate.

- Anterior tumors will produce a normal exam.
- Palpate vertebrae for bony tenderness from metastases.

### DIFFERENTIAL

BPH.

### DIAGNOSIS

- There is insufficient evidence to support routine screening, but experts recommend discussing the risks and benefits of screening with all men starting at age 50, or at a younger age if risk factors are present.
- If PSA or DRE raises concern, ultrasound-guided biopsy is indicated.

### TREATMENT

- Treatment depends on the stage at diagnosis and on the patient's comorbidities and may include surgery, radiation, hormonal therapy, or watchful waiting.
- Close attention to pain control is essential, including management of bone pain from metastases with analgesics and bisphosphonates.

### COMPLICATIONS

Treatment (surgery or radiation) may → impaired sexual function and/or incontinence.

*Discuss the risks and benefits of prostate cancer screening with all men starting at age 50, or younger in African-American men or those with a family history.*

## TESTICULAR CANCER

Can occur at any age, but most commonly seen between the ages of 15 and 35. A history of undescended testis ↑ risk. All scrotal masses should be evaluated to rule out cancer.

### SYMPTOMS

- May be asymptomatic, or may present with a painless mass in the scrotum.
- Patients may have a dull ache in the lower abdomen or scrotum.

### EXAM

Exam reveals a nodular mass on the testis that does not transilluminate. May be accompanied by epididymitis.

### DIFFERENTIAL

Isolated epididymitis; benign scrotal mass.

### DIAGNOSIS

Any suspicious history or exam findings should be evaluated with ultrasound and possible referral to urology.

*There is no effective screening test for testicular cancer, but all suspicious masses should be considered cancerous until proven otherwise.*

### TREATMENT

- Depends on the tumor type. Orchiectomy +/− lymph node dissection in most cases. May include chemotherapy.
- Cure rates are high, with roughly 95% five-year survival.

### COMPLICATIONS

Impaired fertility after germ cell tumor; ↑ risk of cardiovascular disease and 2° malignancies.

## PENILE CANCER

A rare squamous cell cancer occurring largely in uncircumcised men. Appears to be associated with high-risk HPV infection.

*HPV-associated cancer is not for women only. Although rare, penile cancer is thought to be caused by HPV.*

### SYMPTOMS

Presents with an ulcer, erosion, or nodule on the glans or prepuce or, rarely, on the shaft. Often accompanied by phimosis, which masks the lesion.

### EXAM

Retract the foreskin to thoroughly examine the glans, prepuce, and shaft.

### DIFFERENTIAL

Genital warts, HSV, Peyronie's disease.

### DIAGNOSIS

Any suspicious lesion should be referred for biopsy.

### TREATMENT

- Depends on the stage at diagnosis.
- Local excision +/– lymph node dissection +/– radiation.
- Adjuvant chemotherapy may be advised.

### COMPLICATIONS

Urinary and sexual function after treatment depends on the extent of surgery and radiation required.

# CHAPTER 17

# Sports Medicine and Musculoskeletal Disorders

Tara Shaw, MD

## THE PREPARTICIPATION PHYSICAL EVALUATION (PPE)

The PPE is a screening tool used to evaluate athletes for injuries, illness, and other factors that might place them or others at risk during sports. Although there is no solid evidence that a screening PPE will reliably identify clinically silent conditions such as hypertrophic cardiomyopathy, a comprehensive PPE offers physicians the best opportunity to meet this objective.

*The most common presentation of a cardiac abnormality is sudden death.*

### Symptoms/Exam

- **History:** The history is the most important and highest-yield part of the PPE. Screen for the following conditions:
  - A history of sudden death in a family member < 50 years of age (hypertrophic cardiomyopathy is autosomal dominant).
  - A personal history of dizziness, palpitations, chest pain, or syncope with exertion.
  - A history of concussion, including confusion, memory loss, or headache with exertion (recent concussion ↑ the risk of recurrence).
  - A history of asthma or coughing/shortness of breath during or after exercise (may point to exercise-induced bronchospasm).
  - Rashes or skin problems, especially in close-contact sports such as wrestling.
  - Recent or current illnesses, infections, or fever.
- **Exam:**
  - Table 17.1 describes the standard components of a PPE.
  - Further testing is indicated for the following:
    - Systolic murmurs of grade 3/6 or more (atrial stenosis, mitral regurgitation).
    - Any diastolic murmur.
    - Any murmur that grows louder with ↓ venous return, as with Valsalva or with standing from a squat (hypertrophic cardiomyopathy).

*In light of the risk of splenic injury that occurs with mononucleosis (even in the absence of splenomegaly), sports should be avoided for 21–28 days from the start of infection.*

**TABLE 17.1. Components of the PPE**

| SYSTEM | COMPONENT |
|---|---|
| Vitals | Take routine vital signs (height, weight, pulse, BP, lungs) including BP in upper extremity. |
| Cardiovascular | Palpate pulses, auscultate for murmurs in both sitting and standing, and evaluate the effects of exercise on the individual. |
| Musculoskeletal | Determine strength, range of motion, flexibility, and previous injuries; assess range of motion (general, neck, shoulder/upper extremity, and back), gait/lower extremity, and asymmetry of muscle bulk/scarring/posture. |
| Skin | Check for contagious lesions and rashes. |
| Vision | General screening, look for evidence of retinal problems or eye injury. |
| Abdomen | Check for masses and evidence of hepatosplenomegaly. |
| Genitourinary—Males Only | Check for testicular abnormalities and hernias; note Tanner stage. |
| Neurologic | Rule out problems with coordination, gait, and mental processing. |

Based on data from Wilson PE, Matthews DJ. Rehabilitation and Sports Medicine. In Hay WW et al. *Current Pediatric Diagnosis and Treatment,* 18th ed. New York: McGraw-Hill, 2007.

*Myocarditis is an absolute contraindication for any sport in light of the risk of sudden death with exertion.*

### DIAGNOSIS

- No routine diagnostic testing is recommended.
- If the history and physical are suggestive of structural heart disease, the standard evaluation generally includes a 12-lead ECG, stress echocardiography, and graded exercise testing.

## CONCUSSION MANAGEMENT

You are serving as team physician for a high school football game. One of the players sustains a forceful tackle and falls to the ground unresponsive. You run onto the field and find him dazed but coherent. He reports a headache and dizziness. His teammates report that the player appeared to be unconscious for a few seconds before you reached him on the field. After clearing his C-spine, you help the player off the field and conduct a neurologic exam, which is normal. After 10 minutes, the player states that he feels fine and that his headache and dizziness are gone, and he asks to return to the game. What do you do? You inform the player and his coach that while the player may well feel better, he is at risk of sustaining a more severe head injury if he is hit again, so it is not safe for him to resume playing football today. You explain that you and the trainer will monitor him for symptoms over the next few days and will slowly ↑ his activity level if he remains symptom free. He will need to be able to exercise at game intensity without inducing any symptoms before he is safe to play again.

A concussion is defined as an alteration in cerebral function 2° to a direct or indirect (rotational) force on the brain. Concussions are classified as **simple,** in which symptoms progressively resolve without complication in 7–10 days, or **complex,** in which symptoms persist > 10 days and involve symptom recurrence with exertion, prolonged loss of consciousness (> 1 minute), and/or prolonged cognitive impairment after the injury. The 2004 Prague International Consensus statement on concussion eliminated the various concussion grading scales that had once been used to guide management. Therefore, return-to-play decisions can no longer follow specific guidelines based on concussion grade. Management is now more individualized, and amnesia is thought to be more indicative of concussion severity than loss of consciousness.

### SYMPTOMS/EXAM

- May present with headache, dizziness, nausea, confusion, irritability, double or blurry vision, sensitivity to light or noise, changes in sleep pattern (more or less), difficulty concentrating, memory problems, ↑ emotionality, and easy fatigability.
- Exam may reveal delayed verbal and motor responses, a vacant stare, disorientation, slurred or incoherent speech, incoordination, and memory deficits.

### DIFFERENTIAL

Structural injury or abnormalities such as cerebral hemorrhage or infection.

### DIAGNOSIS

- A clinical diagnosis.

- Any abnormalities found on neurologic exam are not normal for a concussion and should be emergently evaluated in the emergency department.

### TREATMENT

- Recommend complete mental and physical rest while the patient is symptomatic (including no homework or video games).
- Slow progression of activity from light aerobic exercise through the following stages: sport-specific exercise, noncontact drills, full-contact drills, and game play, with each stage lasting at least one day. Athletes must remain asymptomatic in order to progress to the next stage.

## SUPPLEMENTS AND STEROIDS

Table 17.2 outlines the uses and mechanisms of action of commonly used supplements.

**TABLE 17.2.** **Common Sports Supplements**

| | DESCRIPTION | SIDE EFFECTS |
|---|---|---|
| Glucosamine and chondroitin | Shown in some clinical trials to ↓ the symptoms of osteoarthritis. Glucosamine is an amino sugar that is thought to promote the formation and repair of cartilage. Chondroitin, a carbohydrate, is a component of cartilage that is thought to promote water retention and elasticity and to inhibit the enzymes that break down cartilage. | Considered safe, without significant side effects. |
| Creatine | A nutritional supplement used to promote protein synthesis and to provide a quick source of energy for muscle contraction (phosphocreatine supplies phosphate for the regeneration of ATP from ADP in muscle cells). Thought to enhance performance in short-duration, high-intensity exercise such as sprinting and weight lifting. | Associated with weight gain due to intracellular water retention. This can also → intravascular dehydration and → possible renal injury. |
| Androgens | "Nutritional supplements" (e.g., DHEA, a precursor to androgenic steroids) and synthetic agents used to stimulate muscle growth and strength. Banned by most competitive sports organizations. | Suppression of endogenous testicular function; diminishing spermatogenesis and fertility. Chronic use (over years) → loss of testicular size. Also associated with gynecomastia, erythrocytosis, hepatotoxicity, adverse effects on serum lipids, virilization of female athletes, premature epiphyseal fusion and stunting of growth, and psychological disorders (major mood disorders, aggressive behavior). |
| International Olympic Committee (IOC) doping classes | Stimulants, narcotics, anabolic agents, β2-agonists, β-blockers (used to stop trembling, calm, and ↓ BP and heart rate), diuretics (used to meet weight goals), peptide hormones and analogs (e.g., GH and erythropoietin), street drugs. | Banned by the IOC for use in athletic competition (except β2-agonists in the setting of documented asthma). |

Repetitive stress across a bone, tendon, or muscle without adequate healing time → tissue injury and degradation. The process can be largely inflammatory, as in carpal tunnel syndrome and de Quervain's tenosynovitis; largely degenerative, as in lateral epicondylitis; or due to incomplete remodeling, as seen in stress fractures.

## Stress Fractures

The majority of stress fractures (70–90%) occur in runners. Female runners are 12 times more likely to develop a stress fracture in their lifetimes than male runners. In athletes, the tibia is the most commonly involved bone, whereas in military recruits metatarsal and calcaneal stress fractures are more common 2° to the biomechanics of marching vs. running. Other affected areas include the fibula, femoral neck, and pelvis. Stress fracture development is usually related to an ↑ in the intensity, duration, or frequency of training. Other contributing factors include changes in technique, overly hard or irregular running surfaces, and footwear with poor shock absorption.

### SYMPTOMS

Presents with insidious onset of pain that occurs toward the end of a run, subsequently occurring earlier and earlier in the exercise period until pain occurs with activities of daily living.

### EXAM

Exam reveals focal tenderness over the area of the fracture as well as ↑ pain with vibratory testing and levered stress across the leg (for tibial stress fracture).

### DIFFERENTIAL

Shin splints; chronic exertional compartment syndrome (suggested by localized calf pain that progressively worsens with persistent running and is relieved with cessation of exercise); bony tumor (suggested by unusually severe bone pain and/or night pain).

### DIAGNOSIS

- X-rays may reveal periosteal reaction if the pain is of > 2–3 weeks' duration. If the suspected fracture is tibial, check for the **"dreaded black line"** of an anterior tibial cortex stress fracture, which can be prone to nonunion and progression to complete fracture.
- If x-rays are ⊖, bone scan or MRI is diagnostic.

### TREATMENT

- Cast or boot immobilization and crutches if pain relief is not obtained through resting.

*Multiple stress fractures, especially in female athletes, should prompt a workup for osteoporosis along with questioning regarding the female athlete triad (disordered eating, amenorrhea, osteoporosis).*

- Once the athlete is pain free with ambulation, cross-training such as swimming, biking, or weight lifting may be started.
- Reintroduction of running is done slowly and is advanced as the patient continues to remain pain free.

### Medial Tibial Stress Syndrome (Shin Splints)

- Diffuse stress reaction along the tibia; seen in runners and jumpers (basketball, dancing, racket sports).
- **Sx:** The onset of symptoms is insidious and is similar to that of tibial stress fractures, but pain often occurs at the beginning of a run, resolves as workout continues, and recurs after the workout. Alternatively, it may occur only at the end of the run.
- **Exam:** Reveals a more diffuse pattern of pain and tenderness along the medial border of the middle and distal thirds of the tibia (muscle attachment sites). Pain is noted with resisted plantar flexion and toe walking.
- **Dx:** Triple-phase bone scan or MRI can distinguish the injury from stress fracture if the exam is unclear.
- **Tx:** Treatment is similar to that of tibial stress fractures but is shorter and may begin with relative rest and cross-training (no immobilization).

### Tendinopathies

- Repetitive stress along a tendon (Achilles, patellar, medial and lateral elbow, rotator cuff) → collagen degeneration or tendinosis. Many studies have cast doubt on the role of inflammation (tendonitis). Overloading of the tendon due to poor biomechanics (e.g., muscle imbalances, foot overpronation) and repetitive stress → collagen breakdown and/or inflammation.
- **Tx:**
    - Treatment includes rest, cryotherapy/ice, unloading devices (e.g., counterforce straps for the elbow and patellar tendon; heel lifts for the Achilles tendon), and physical therapy.
    - The role of NSAIDs and corticosteroid injections is controversial, but treatment can often afford short-term relief.
    - Healing is slow and can take six months or longer.
    - Surgical debridement is a last resort but is usually effective.

*A fracture with any overlying laceration or abrasion should be considered an open fracture and requires further evaluation (the old term for this was a compound fracture).*

## PRINCIPLES OF IMAGING

### Standard Views

Radiographs must include a minimum of two views, AP and lateral, in order to fully evaluate patients for fractures. Table 17.3 describes additional views that may be useful.

**TABLE 17.3.  Radiologic Views and Key Points**

| REGION | VIEWS |
|---|---|
| Wrist | AP view of clenched fist with ulnar deviation to evaluate the scaphoid. |
| Elbow | Comparison views may be helpful. Look for an anterior **sail sign** (fat pad displaced by effusion), which is suggestive of fracture. |
| Cervical spine | The lateral view must include C1–C7 to fully clear C-spine. The swimmer's view (arm overhead) may help visualize C7. |
| Hip/pelvis | AP and frog-leg views. |
| Knee | Weight-bearing AP in full extension and 40° of flexion (notch view) if osteoarthritis is suspected; axial (Merchant) view to evaluate the patellofemoral joint. |
| Ankle | The mortise view allows for the evaluation of ankle joint integrity (symmetry of the mortise space). |

## Imaging of Fractures

### FRACTURE CATEGORIES

Fractures are categorized by location (e.g., distal radius, tibial plateau), type (see Table 17.4), and degree of displacement (see Table 17.5).

**TABLE 17.4.  Fracture Types**

| TYPE | DESCRIPTION |
|---|---|
| Transverse | Perpendicular to the shaft of the bone. |
| Oblique | Slanting or inclined fracture line. |
| Spiral | Multiplanar fracture line, caused by a torsional force. |
| Comminuted | Multiple fragments. |
| Segmental | Large, well-defined fragments (a type of comminuted fracture). |
| Intra-articular | Extends into the joint space. The general rule is that if the fracture includes more than one-third of the joint space, it requires surgical evaluation for possible fixation. |
| Avulsion | Bony fragment pulled away from its native bone. |
| Compression | Impaction of bone, such as in the vertebrae or proximal tibia. |
| Pathologic | Fracture through bone weakened by tumor or disease (e.g., osteoporosis). |

**TABLE 17.5.**  **Degrees of Fracture Displacement**

| TERM | DEFINITION |
|---|---|
| Displaced | When one fragment shifts in relation to the other through translation, angulation, shortening, or rotation. |
| Nondisplaced | A fracture in which the fragments are in anatomic alignment. |
| Translation | Movement in the AP (volar/dorsal in the forearm) or medial-lateral plane (ulnar/radial in the forearm.) |
| Angulated | Malalignment described using the direction the apex is pointing—e.g., apex dorsal angulation. |
| Bayonetted | The distal fragment longitudinally overlaps the proximal fragment. |
| Distracted | The distal fragment is separated from the proximal fragment by a gap. |

## IMAGING OF PEDIATRIC FRACTURES

Until late adolescence, tendons and ligaments are stronger than bones, so fractures are more common and true sprains are infrequent. Children's bones are also more malleable, creating a few fracture terms specific to pediatrics:

- **Torus or buckle fracture:** The periosteum bends but does not break.
- **Greenstick fracture:** The periosteum buckles on one side and breaks on the other, which can allow for angulation that may need to be reduced.
- **Salter-Harris classification:** Physeal injuries are unique to children, as their open growth plates allow for more fractures. Such fractures are classified using the Salter-Harris system (see Table 17.6 and Figure 17.1).

**TABLE 17.6.**  **Salter-Harris Classification of Fractures**

| TYPE | LOCATION | OUTCOME |
|---|---|---|
| I | Through the physis. | Associated with the best prognosis. |
| II | Through the physis and metaphysis. | Growth arrest may occur. |
| III | Through the physis and epiphysis. | Growth arrest is rare, but joint surface involvement requires close maintenance of anatomic reduction (referral). |
| IV | Through the metaphysis, across the physis, and through the epiphysis. | Associated with a risk for both growth arrest and articular cartilage damage (referral). |
| V | Crush injury to the physis. | Usually diagnosed retrospectively if growth arrest or angular deformity has occurred. |
| VI | Injury to the perichondrium. | May develop bony bridge across physis → angular deformity. |

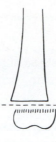
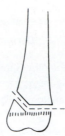
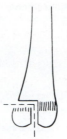
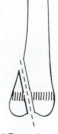
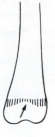

| I. Through growth plate | II. Through metaphysis and growth plate | III. Through growth plate and epiphysis into joint | IV. Through metaphysis, growth plate, and epiphysis into joint | V. Crush of growth plate. May not be seen on x-ray |

**FIGURE 17.1.** **Salter-Harris fractures, types I–V.**

(Reproduced, with permission, from Stone CK, Humphries RL. *Current Emergency Diagnosis & Treatment*, 5th ed. New York: McGraw-Hill, 2004: 513.)

## GENERAL APPROACH TO THE JOINT EXAM

- **Terms:** Anterior, posterior, medial, and lateral are equivalent in the forearm and hand to volar, dorsal, ulnar, and radial. Axial alignment is described in terms of the angle made by the proximal and distal segments.
    - **Valgus alignment:** Two limb segments create an angle that points toward midline.
    - **Varus alignment:** The angle formed by the two segments points away from midline.
- **Inspection:** Involves surface anatomy (muscle wasting, symmetry), alignment (e.g., genu valgum), gait, and active and passive ROM.
- **Palpation:** Performed to identify landmarks, localize tenderness, compare temperature to the contralateral side (to detect the warmth of infection or post-traumatic inflammation or to gauge the coolness of vasoconstriction or vascular compromise), and check pulses.
- **Manipulation:** Tests muscle strength, sensation, reflexes, stability, and special tests. Muscle strength is graded 0–5.

*In genu val**GUM**, the knees are stuck together with **GUM**.*

## SHOULDER INJURIES

Guidelines for the evaluation of shoulder injuries are as follows:

- **Inspection:** Note supraspinatus and infraspinatus atrophy seen on the posterior shoulder with **suprascapular nerve entrapment** or chronic rotator cuff tears.
- **Palpation:** Check for acromioclavicular (AC) joint tenderness (separation, arthritis).
- **ROM:** Watch for scapular dyskinesis or winging on abduction and forward flexion (rotator cuff disfunction).

Table 17.7 outlines special tests that can aid in the evaluation of injuries to the shoulder.

**TABLE 17.7.** Special Tests for the Diagnosis of Shoulder Injury

| EXAM | TECHNIQUE | INDICATIONS |
|------|-----------|-------------|
| Hawkins test | With the patient's elbow and shoulder flexed to 90° with the forearm parallel to the floor, the examiner passively internally rotates the shoulder. | Pain points to rotator cuff tendinosis/ impingement. |
| Neer impingement sign | The examiner passively flexes the patient's shoulder to the position of maximal forward flexion while stabilizing the patient's scapula with the other hand. | Pain points to rotator cuff tendinosis/ impingement. |
| Jobe test (empty can) | The arms are abducted 90° and brought forward 30°, thumbs down. The patient resists downward pressure. | Pain points to supraspinatus tendinosis; weakness suggests tear. |
| O'Brien test | Forward flex the shoulder to 90° with the elbow extended and the arm 15° toward the midline. The patient resists downward force with the thumb down and the thumb up. | Deep pain with the thumb down that improves with the thumb up suggests superior glenoid labrum (SLAP) lesions. |
| Apprehension test (crank test) | The shoulder is in 90° abduction and slight extension with the elbow flexed. The examiner externally rotates the arm. | Simulates the most common position of subluxation/dislocation. Pain or anxiety suggests anterior instability. |

## Rotator Cuff Tears and Impingement Syndrome

- The rotator cuff is made up of the supraspinatus (abduction), infraspinatus (external rotation), teres minor (external rotation), and subscapularis (internal rotation) muscles.
- **Sx/Exam:** Rotator cuff impingement and tearing usually begin in the supraspinatus tendon as it passes under the acromion. Patients are usually > 50 years of age and will often have significant pain with abduction above the head and internal rotation (reaching up the back). Hawkins and Neer tests are ⊕.
- **Dx/Tx:** Weakness on exam and lack of full improvement with rehabilitative exercises and subacromial corticosteroid injection suggest a tear rather than isolated impingement. Tears are diagnosed with MRI and often require surgical repair.

## Adhesive Capsulitis (Frozen Shoulder)

- Idiopathic loss of both active and passive motion of the shoulder that usually resolves over a period of **six months to two years.**
- Has a significant association with **diabetes, especially type 1;** 40–50% of diabetics will develop bilateral disease. Nondiabetics are also at ↑ risk for occurrence in the other shoulder.
- **Sx/Exam:** The initial "freezing" phase is progressive and painful, presenting with complaints similar to those of rotator cuff pathology (differentiated by loss of **passive** ROM). This is followed by a "thawing" phase with improvement in pain and ROM.

■ **Tx:** Treat with stretching exercises, glenohumeral corticosteroid injections, and, rarely, surgery.

### Acromioclavicular (AC) Joint Pathology

■ Degenerative **arthritis** of the AC joint is often a component of rotator cuff pathology and shoulder pain seen in patients > 50 years of age. For this reason, a distal clavicle resection often accompanies surgical repair of the rotator cuff.

■ AC injuries (**shoulder separations**) uaually occur with a fall onto the lateral aspect of the shoulder → stress and tearing of the AC ligaments and sometimes the coracoclavicular (CC) ligaments as well. Graded as types I–III.
  - ■ **Type I:** Partial or full disruption of the AC ligaments with CC ligaments intact → tenderness but no step-off on palpation.
  - ■ **Type II:** The AC ligaments are torn and the CC ligaments are partially disrupted, allowing for partial separation of the clavicle from the acromion on stress radiographs and palpation.
  - ■ **Type III:** Complete disruption of the AC and CC ligaments → complete separation of the clavicle from the acromion superiorly.

■ **Tx:** Types I and II are treated nonoperatively with a sling, analgesics, and ice followed by rehabilitative exercises. Type III injuries are sometimes treated conservatively and sometimes surgically.

### Glenohumeral Dislocations

*Glenohumeral dislocations are the most common type of major joint dislocation.*

■ The shoulder is at its most vulnerable when abducted and externally rotated. A fall or tackle with the arm in this position can → an anterior dislocation. Posterior dislocations are less common but can occur with a grand mal seizure or an electrical shock.

■ Recurrence rates after 1° traumatic dislocation are 65–95% in patients < 20 years of age; 60% in those 20–40 years of age; and 10% in patients > 40 years of age.

■ **Tx:**
  - ■ Treated initially with a sling and then physical therapy for strengthening.
  - ■ Surgical repair of the capsule integrity is required for recurrent dislocations.

### SLAP Lesions

■ Defined as an injury or tear of the superior labrum that extends anterior to posterior. The superior labrum is the upper portion of the cartilaginous ring that surrounds the glenoid fossa, increasing its depth and adding to shoulder stability.

■ **Sx/Exam:** SLAP lesions are most common in throwing athletes such as baseball pitchers. Patients experience a sense of catching or popping in the shoulder with loss of force and +/− pain.

■ **Dx/Tx:** Diagnosed with MRI or MR arthrography. Requires surgical repair.

### Fractures of the Shoulder

■ **Fractures of the clavicle:** Usually due to a fall onto the lateral aspect of the shoulder or a direct blow. Eighty percent affect the middle third of the clavicle. Most can be treated nonoperatively with either an arm sling or a figure-of-eight harness for 4–6 weeks (or 3–4 weeks for children < 12). Surgical referral is indicated for displacements greater than the width of the clavicle or for shortening > 20 mm.

- **Fractures of the scapula:** Usually due to high-energy trauma such as significant falls and motorcycle accidents. Ninety percent are associated with other injuries, such as rib fractures, pneumothorax, pulmonary contusion, and injuries of the head, spinal cord, and brachial plexus. Most are treated with a sling for comfort and early ROM.
- **Fractures of the proximal humerus:** Commonly occur in elderly patients with osteoporosis, especially women. Most are minimally displaced and can be treated with a sling and early motion.

## INJURIES OF THE ELBOW AND FOREARM

### Epicondylitis/Elbow Tendinosis

Due to repetitive stress across the common tendon of the wrist flexors (medial) or extensors (lateral) → collagen breakdown and a failure of tendon healing, resulting in a tendinosis. Not actually due to inflammation of the epicondyle as the classic name suggests. Medial epicondylitis is known as **golfer's elbow;** lateral epicondylitis is commonly called **tennis elbow.**

#### SYMPTOMS/EXAM

- Presents with activity-related pain progressing to pain at rest and functional strength loss.
- Exam reveals tenderness over the medial or lateral tendon origins and pain with resisted wrist flexion/pronation (medial) or resisted wrist and middle finger extension/supination (lateral).

#### DIAGNOSIS

- Clinical diagnosis is based on the history and exam.
- Histopathology of resected tissue does not reveal inflammatory cells, instead showing disruption of the normal collagen matrix with invasion by fibroblasts and vascular granulation. The bone (epicondyle) is not involved.

#### TREATMENT

- Promotion of tendon healing with rest from inciting trauma and rehabilitative exercises.
- Anti-inflammatory medications can control pain and allow for rehabilitative exercises.
- Therapeutic modalities such as high-voltage electrical stimulation, ultrasound, heat/cold, and steroid iontophoresis aid in pain relief.
- Control of force loads across the tendon with use of counterforce strap bracing and improvements in technique.
- Corticosteroid injections under the flexor pronator mass (medial) or the extensor carpi radialis brevis origin (lateral) are effective in pain control and may stimulate healing via ↑ blood flow to the area.
- Surgical debridement of the tendon is appropriate if conservative measures fail.

### Ulnar Nerve Compression

Chronic or post-traumatic compression of the ulnar nerve near or at the elbow → an ulnar neuritis. May occur in multiple sites, the most common of which is the "cubital tunnel," where the nerve passes through the groove on the posterior aspect of the medial epicondyle.

### SYMPTOMS/EXAM

- Presents with aching pain in the medial aspect of the elbow along with numbness and tingling into the fourth and fifth fingers.
- A later finding is weakness of the intrinsic muscles, which can interfere with activities such as opening jars or turning a key.
- Exam reveals pain and paresthesias in an ulnar distribution with tapping on the nerve in the cubital tunnel (⊕ **Tinel's test**).

### DIAGNOSIS

Nerve conduction velocity studies can confirm the clinical diagnosis and may provide an objective measure of nerve impairment. A reduction in velocity of ≥ 30% suggests significant compression.

### TREATMENT

- Activity modification to limit elbow flexion and direct pressure on the ulnar nerve.
- A nighttime splint is used to prevent full flexion (nerve stretch).
- Surgical decompression or transposition of the nerve for failure of conservative measures after 3–4 months.

### COMPLICATIONS

Loss of grip and pinch strength with numbness in the ring and little fingers can become permanent in long-standing cases.

## Pediatric Injuries of the Elbow and Forearm

### FRACTURES

- Supracondylar fractures of the distal humerus are the most common elbow fractures in children, typically affecting those 2–12 years of age.
- Associated with a high incidence of neurovascular injuries and therefore always requires referral.
- Medial and lateral epicondyle fractures are unique to pediatrics due to growth plate weakness.

### LITTLE LEAGUE ELBOW

- Medial epicondyle apophysitis seen in young throwers due to repetitive valgus stress across the elbow.
- **Dx:** Clinical; rule out ulnar nerve involvement and ligamentous instability.
- **Tx:** Responds well to rest and conservative measures. Indications for surgical intervention include ulnar neuropathy with displaced fracture and valgus instability.

### NURSEMAID'S ELBOW/SUBLUXATION OF THE RADIAL HEAD

- The most common elbow injury in children < 5 years of age. Associated with ↑ ligamentous laxity.

- **Sx/Exam:** Occurs with a pull on the forearm in an extended, pronated position, allowing the annular ligament to slip proximally and to become stuck between the radius and ulna. The child holds the forearm slightly flexed and pronated and refuses to use it.
- **Tx:** Reduction is achieved with supination and flexion of the forearm.

## INJURIES OF THE HAND AND WRIST

Table 17.8 outlines special tests that may facilitate the diagnosis of wrist and hand injuries. The presentation and treatment of specific wrist and hand injuries are described in the sections that follow.

### Carpal Tunnel Syndrome

Compression of the median nerve in the carpal tunnel at the wrist due to direct trauma, repetitive use, or anatomic anomalies. Most commonly affects middle-aged or pregnant women.

#### SYMPTOMS/EXAM

- Presents with a vague ache into the thenar eminence and sometimes the forearm.
- Numbness, tingling, and pain occur in a median nerve distribution (the thumb, index, long, and radial half of the ring fingers).
- Nighttime pain and paresthesias occur 2° to sleeping with the wrists flexed.
- Late symptoms include weakness, dropping objects, persistent numbness, and thenar atrophy.
- Reproduction of these symptoms with Tinel's and/or Phalen's test is suggestive.
- ↓ two-point discrimination can be seen on sensation testing.

#### DIFFERENTIAL

- **DM** with neuropathy.
- **Flexor carpi radialis tenosynovitis:** Presents with tenderness near the base of the thumb.

**TABLE 17.8.** Special Tests for the Diagnosis of Wrist and Hand Injuries

| EXAM | TECHNIQUE | INDICATIONS |
|------|-----------|-------------|
| Finkelstein test | With the hand in a neutral position, the patient flexes the thumb across the palm and then ulnar-deviates the wrist. | Pain along the first dorsal compartment indicates de Quervain's tenosynovitis. |
| Tinel's test | The examiner taps over the median nerve in the wrist. | Pain and tingling into the hand is suggestive of carpal tunnel syndrome. |
| Phalen's test | The patient compresses the backs of both hands against each other so that the wrists are flexed 90° for one minute. | Reproduction of the patient's symptoms and aching or tingling in a median nerve distribution are suggestive of carpal tunnel syndrome. |

- **Cervical radiculopathy affecting the C6 nerve:** Presents with neck pain and numbness in the thumb and index finger only.
- **Hypothyroidism:** Detected by laboratory testing.
- **Arthritis of the wrist or carpometacarpal joint of the thumb:** Presents with painful, limited motion; evident on radiographs.

### DIAGNOSIS

- EMG (median nerve conduction velocity study) confirms the diagnosis and indicates severity (important if surgery is being considered).
- Some 5–10% of patients with carpal tunnel syndrome have normal EMG results.

### TREATMENT

- Wrist splints for night and provocative activities with a short course of NSAIDs and ergonomic modifications if indicated.
- Corticosteroid injection into the carpal canal (avoid the median nerve).
- Surgical decompression is appropriate for those who fail conservative treatment or who have weakness or atrophy.

## de Quervain's Tenosynovitis

Swelling and stenosis of the sheath that surrounds the abductor pollicis longus and extensor pollicis brevis tendons (the first extensor compartment). More common in middle-aged women. Often precipitated by repetitive use of the thumb and activities requiring a forceful grip (cleaning tasks, racket sports).

### SYMPTOMS/EXAM/DIAGNOSIS

- Presents with pain and tenderness over the radial styloid, especially with use of the thumb and ulnar deviation of the wrist (pulls tendons through the inflamed sheath). There may also be some swelling and triggering symptoms.
- A ⊕ Finklestein test is pathognomonic.

### TREATMENT

- Treated with a thumb spica splint to immobilize both the wrist and the thumb along with a two-week course of NSAIDs.
- Corticosteroid injection into the tendon sheath.
- Surgical decompression is appropriate if no improvement is seen with conservative measures.

## Thumb and Finger Injuries

### ULNAR COLLATERAL LIGAMENT (UCL) TEAR

- A fall onto an abducted thumb → an acute rupture of the UCL of the thumb metacarpophalangeal (MCP) joint. Also known as **skier's** or **gamekeeper's thumb.**
- **Sx/Exam:** Patients present with pain and swelling over the ligament along with laxity with abduction across the MCP joint. Up to 70% of full ruptures are associated with a **Stener lesion,** in which the torn end of the UCL is displaced superficially to the aponeurosis, preventing healing and

requiring surgical repair. This is suggested by a palpable lump or gross instability.

- **Tx:** In the absence of a Stener lesion, many injuries heal well in a thumb spica cast for four weeks followed by protective splinting during competitive activities for 2–4 months.

### MALLET FINGER

- Forced flexion of an actively extended distal interphalangeal (DIP) joint (e.g., "jammed finger") → disruption of the extensor mechanism at its insertion into the distal phalanx.
- **Sx/Exam:** The patient will have full passive ROM but an inability to actively extend at the DIP joint.
- **Dx:** Based on physical exam, but x-rays should be obtained to evaluate for bony avulsion vs. tendon rupture as the cause.
- **Tx:** Treatment involves continuous extension splinting for at least six weeks followed by four weeks of nighttime splinting. Surgical referral for large bony avulsion or failure to heal with splinting.

### JERSEY FINGER

- Forced extension of an actively flexed DIP joint (e.g., grabbing someone's jersey) → an avulsion of the flexor digitorum profundus tendon from its insertion on the distal phalanx. Some 75% of cases involve the ring finger.
- **Tx:** All cases require surgical repair, but the urgency depends on the degree of tendon retraction (the more retracted, the more urgent).

### BOUTONNIÈRE DEFORMITY

- Rupture of the central slip of the extensor tendon at its insertion into the middle phalanx. If not properly treated, the head of the middle phalanx may buttonhole through the defect between the lateral bands of the extensor tendon mechanism → fixed flexion at the proximal interphalangeal (PIP) joint (see Figure 17.2).
- **Dx:** Radiographs are required to rule out fracture.

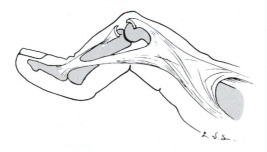

**FIGURE 17.2.** **Boutonnière deformity.**

Avulsion or laceration of the central extensor mechanism results in a flexion deformity at the PIP joint and hyperextension of the DIP joint—the boutonnière, or buttonhole, deformity. (Reproduced, with permission, from Doherty GM, Way LW. *Current Surgical Diagnosis & Treatment,* 12th ed. New York: McGraw-Hill, 2006: 1256.)

- **Tx:** The finger is treated with extension splinting of the PIP while allowing DIP motion for six weeks. Surgical repair is required for large bony fragments or with lack of improvement with splinting.

### TRIGGER FINGER

- Inflammation of the flexor tendon and thickening and stenosis of the first annular (A1) pulley → pain and catching with flexion/extension of the finger. Most cases are degenerative, although there is an association with rheumatoid arthritis.
- **Dx:** Observation of catching as the patient extends a fully flexed finger. A nodule (the thickened A1 pulley) is often palpable at the level of the distal palmar crease.
- **Tx:** Treatment is with corticosteroid injection into the tendon sheath at the level of the A1 pulley. Surgical release is appropriate for stubborn lesions.

## Fractures of the Hand and Wrist

In a fall onto an outstretched hand, approximately 80% of the weight-bearing load across the wrist is through the radial side. Subtypes of wrist fractures include the following:

- **Distal radius fractures:** The most frequently occurring fracture in adults.
    - **Colles fracture:** The distal fragment is tilted dorsally, e.g., from a fall on an outstretched hand. The most common type; may be associated with an ulnar styloid fracture.
    - **Smith fracture:** The distal fragment is tilted volarly. Less angulation is tolerable in this direction.
- **Scaphoid fractures:**
    - The most common carpal bone to be fractured. Young adult males are most likely to sustain this injury. Not as common in children and older adults because the distal radius is the weak point in these two populations.
    - Has a high incidence of nonunion and osteonecrosis due to poor blood supply, which enters the bone only in the distal third.
    - Any pain in the anatomic snuff box, when seen in the setting of trauma, should be assumed to be due to a scaphoid injury and the wrist immobilized until repeat x-rays are performed after two weeks.
    - If pain persists and x-rays are nondiagnostic, an MRI or CT is indicated.
    - Many patients will require surgical fixation.
- **Metacarpal fractures:**
    - More common in adults (vs. phalangeal fractures, which are more common in children).
    - **Boxer's fracture** is a fracture of the neck of the fifth metacarpal. It is the most common fracture in the hand and results from a closed fist striking an object. Up to 40° of angulation can be tolerated if there is no extensor lag (the patient can fully extend the finger). Treated with an ulnar gutter cast for 2–3 weeks.
    - Less angulation is tolerated in fractures of the other metacarpals 2° to less mobility of the bones in the hand structure

Low back pain affects 60–80% of adults at some point in their lives, and most episodes of back and neck pain resolve within a few weeks. Nonetheless, it is important to fully evaluate each case.

### EXAM

- Exam includes inspection (e.g., loss of normal lordosis), palpation (e.g., midline tenderness vs. paraspinal tenderness), ROM, muscle testing, reflexes, and sensation (see Table 17.9).
- **Red flags** in conjunction with neck or back pain include night pain and weight loss (think tumor); fevers, chills, and sweats (think bone or disk infection); acute bony tenderness (think fracture); morning stiffness lasting > 30 minutes in young adults (think seronegative spondyloarthropathy); and any neurologic deficit or bowel/bladder involvement (think nerve root compromise).
- **Spurling test:** The patient extends the neck and tilts the head to the side while the examiner presses down on the head. This narrows the patient's neural foramen and will worsen or reproduce radicular pain due to disk herniation or cervical spondylosis.
- **Straight-leg raise:** With the patient supine, the straight leg is raised (many variations), placing the L5 and S1 nerve roots and the sciatic nerve under tension. ⊕ with reproduction or worsening of radicular symptoms. Dorsiflexion of the foot should worsen symptoms.

## Herniated Disk

Bulging or herniation of the **nucleus pulposus** (a gel-like substance that cushions axial compression) through the surrounding **annulus fibrosus** (the outer,

**TABLE 17.9.   Nerve Root Testing**

| NERVE ROOT | MOTOR TESTING | REFLEX | SENSATION |
|---|---|---|---|
| C5 | Deltoid, biceps | Biceps | Lateral shoulder |
| C6 | Biceps, wrist extensors (extensor carpi radialis longus and brevis) | Brachioradialis | Radial side of the forearm, thumb, and index finger |
| C7 | Triceps, wrist flexors, finger extensors | Triceps | Middle finger |
| C8 | Finger abduction and adduction (interosseous muscles), finger flexors | – | Ulnar side of the forearm and ring and pinky fingers |
| L4 | Foot dorsiflexion (tibialis anterior) | Patellar | Medial side of the big toe and lower leg |
| L5 | Big toe dorsiflexion (extensor hallucis longus) | – | Dorsum of the foot from the lateral side of the big toe to the medial side of the little toe |
| S1 | Foot eversion (peroneus longus and brevis), plantar flexion (gastrocsoleus) | Achilles tendon | Lateral side of the little toe and lower leg |

ligamentous portion of the intervertebral disk) into the spinal canal → nerve root irritation and compression. Also known as herniated nucleus pulposus. Lumbar disk herniations affect 2% of the population, but only 10–25% of these patients have symptoms that persist > 6 weeks.

### SYMPTOMS/EXAM

- Often presents with abrupt onset of unilateral radicular leg pain with low back pain that is worsened by sitting, walking, standing, coughing, or sneezing.
- Most commonly occurs at the L4–L5 or L5–S1 level.

### DIFFERENTIAL

- **Lateral femoral cutaneous nerve entrapment:** Involves the lateral thigh; sensory only.
- **Spinal stenosis:** Affects the older population; associated with relief with flexion.
- **Cauda equina syndrome:** Bilateral involvement; presents with perianal numbness with possible ↓ sphincter tone along with urinary overflow incontinence or retention.
- **Demyelinating conditions:** Can present with clonus.

### DIAGNOSIS

- Obtain plain radiographs to evaluate vertebral alignment and disk space. Imaging is likely to show degenerative changes in older patients.
- MRI is necessary only for progressive neurologic changes or preoperative planning.

### TREATMENT

- Acute use of NSAIDs, muscle relaxants, and/or narcotics with 1–3 days of bed rest if needed followed by slow progression of activity.
- A short course of oral steroids or an epidural steroid injection may be necessary.
- Surgical evaluation is appropriate for patients who show no improvement or have progressive neurologic symptoms.

## Degenerative Disk Disease

- Refers to age-related degenerative changes of the intervertebral disks with loss of disk height and hydrophilic properties of the nucleus pulposus. The amount of degeneration may be modified by factors such as injury, repetitive trauma, infection, heredity, and smoking.
- **Sx/Exam:** Presents with recurrent, episodic low back pain that radiates to one or both buttocks with or without intermittent sciatica.
- **Dx:** AP and lateral radiographs may reveal anterior osteophytes, loss of disk height, and a "vacuum sign" showing apparent air (nitrogen) in the disk space.
- **Tx:** Treat with intermittent NSAIDs, weight reduction, and core strengthening.

## Lumbar Spinal Stenosis (Neurogenic Claudication)

Narrowing of one or more levels of the spinal canal with resultant compression of the nerve roots. Up to 30% of adults > 60 years of age have lumbar stenosis anatomically, but many are asymptomatic because the stenosis is usually anatomically severe before symptoms develop.

### SYMPTOMS/EXAM

- Presents with radicular symptoms with or without back pain that starts gradually or following a minor trauma and usually progresses from proximal to distal.
- Pain is aggravated by extension, and patients have poor walking tolerance.
- Walking and prolonged standing → fatigue and leg weakness.
- Leg pain due to vascular claudication resolves when the patient stops walking; neurogenic claudication does not immediately subside.

### DIFFERENTIAL

Vascular claudication, DM, folic acid or vitamin $B_{12}$ deficiency, infection, tumor, degenerative disk disease.

### DIAGNOSIS

- Obtain AP and lateral x-rays to look for contributing degenerative factors such as spondylolisthesis, narrowing of the intervertebral disk spaces, osteoporosis, osteophytic changes, or an old burst fracture of a vertebral body.
- Usually diagnosed on MRI.

### TREATMENT

- Physical therapy focusing on flexion exercises and core/abdominal strengthening.
- Surgical decompression.

## Pediatric Injuries of the Back and Spine

Back pain is uncommon in children and always warrants evaluation when it does not rapidly resolve.

### SPONDYLOLISTHESIS

- Slippage of one vertebral body forward in relation to the vertebral body below it. In children, this is most often a movement of L5 forward on S1 due to a congenital defect or stress fracture through the pars interarticularis (**spondylolysis**) (see Figure 17.3).
- **Sx:** Presents with localized back pain at the site of spondylolysis. May have radicular symptoms if slippage is present. Pars injuries are more common in youth sports involving significant hyperextension, such as gymnastics and football.
- **Exam:** The "stork test" can localize a pars defect. Extension of the back while standing on one foot → localized pain in the back on the side of the spondylolysis. ↑ lordosis, ↓ ROM, and tight hamstrings may also be seen.
- **Dx:** Oblique radiographs can show a break in the neck of the "**Scottie dog**," which represents the pars defect (spondylolysis). If radiographs are ⊖, bone scan and MRI are more sensitive. If spondylolisthesis (slippage) is present, it will be evident on lateral radiographs.
- **Tx:** Usually treated conservatively (with rest, core strengthening, and monitoring) unless patients have documented progression of a slip > 50%, in which case bracing or spinal fusion may be considered.

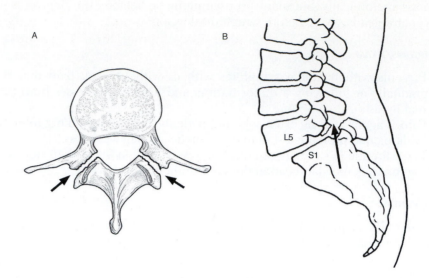

**FIGURE 17.3.** **A. Spondylolysis (defect or fracture through the pars, can be unilateral). B. Spondylolisthesis (slippage that can occur as a result of bilateral spondylolysis).**

(Reproduced, with permission, from Imboden J et al. *Current Rheumatology Diagnosis & Treatment,* 1st ed. New York: McGraw-Hill, 2004: 89.)

## SCOLIOSIS

- Lateral curvature of the thoracic or lumbar spine > 10°. Usually idiopathic, but can be 2° to neuromuscular disease (cerebral palsy, spinal muscular atrophy, myelomeningocele) or vertebral disease (tumor, infection). Can also be disease associated (e.g., neurofibromatosis or Marfan's syndrome).
- **Sx:** Usually develops in early adolescence. Mild cases (curves < 20°) have an equal male-to-female ratio, but girls are seven times more likely to have progressive disease requiring treatment. Usually asymptomatic unless there is underlying disease.
- **Exam:** Use a forward bending test to assess for vertebral and rib rotation. Evaluate for associated conditions such as skin lesions, cavus feet, limb-length discrepancy, abnormal joint laxity, and neuromuscular abnormalities.
- **Dx:** Order PA and lateral full-length spinal radiographs to measure the **Cobb angle.** Unusual findings such as pain, convex left thoracic curves, foot deformities, or neurologic abnormalities require evaluation for underlying etiologies.
- **Tx:** Monitor for progression of curvature (progression frequency depends on the degree of curvature and the amount of growth remaining). Bracing is appropriate for progressive curves in the range of 20–45°; spinal fusion is indicated for curves > 50°. If the curve is < 50° at skeletal maturity, progression usually ceases.
- **Cx:** An idiopathic thoracic curve > 60° often progresses in adulthood and can compromise respiratory function.

## INJURIES OF THE HIP AND THIGH

Pain from actual hip pathology such as osteoarthritis localizes to the anterior groin or thigh and is exacerbated with internal rotation of the hip. Lateral hip pain is much more likely to be 2° to soft tissue pathology such as trochanteric bursitis/iliotibial band (ITB) tightness. ROM and resisted muscle testing will often identify the source of pain in soft tissue injuries. Special tests are listed in Table 17.10.

## Iliotibial Band (ITB)–Related Pathology

The ITB is a large, flat, fascial band that runs from the iliac crest down the lateral thigh and inserts onto the lateral condyle of the tibia at the knee (Gerdy's tubercle). Tightness of this band can → pain and bursitis as it rubs over bony prominences both proximally (at the greater trochanter) and distally at the lateral knee.

### SNAPPING HIP

- A snapping or popping sensation that occurs as a tendon "snaps" across a bony prominence. Most commonly due to the ITB snapping over the greater trochanter, but can also be due to the iliopsoas tendon sliding over the pectineal eminence of the pelvis or from labral tears of the acetabulum.
- **Sx/Exam:**
  - Presents with a snapping sensation at the lateral hip that can often be reproduced in the office with rotation of the hip. If the trochanteric bursa has become inflamed, there will be tenderness with palpation.
  - Snapping of the iliopsoas tendon is felt in the groin as the hip extends from a flexed position (e.g., with rising from a chair).
- **Dx:** If not evident on exam, obtain AP pelvis and lateral hip radiographs to exclude bony pathology. If the diagnosis remains unclear, MR arthrography may be needed to rule out a labral tear or an intra-articular loose body.
- **Tx:** Physical therapy for stretching of the ITB, hip abductors, adductors, and flexors. If the injury is painful, corticosteroid injection into the trochanteric bursa or psoas sheath may be needed.

**TABLE 17.10. Special Tests for the Diagnosis of Hip and Thigh Injuries**

| EXAM | TECHNIQUE | INDICATIONS |
|---|---|---|
| Ober's test | The patient lies on his or her side with the affected side up. The knee is flexed 90° and hip is abducted, extended, and then allowed to drop down toward the table. | ⊕ if the knee does not drop past the midline, suggesting a tight ITB. |
| Trendelenburg test | The patient is observed from behind while standing on one foot and then the other. Pelvic stability is noted. | ⊕ if an unsupported hemipelvis droops, suggesting hip abductor weakness on the other side. |
| FABER (Flexion, **AB**duction, External **Rotation**) test | The patient is supine and places the leg of the affected side into the figure-four position with the ankle resting above the contralateral knee. The examiner presses down on the ipsilateral knee, stressing the sacroiliac joint and stretching the psoas. | Posterior hip pain suggests sacroiliac pathology; anterior pull suggests psoas involvement. |

## TROCHANTERIC BURSITIS

- Inflammation, swelling, and hypertrophy of the greater trochanteric bursa can develop with direct injury, with ITB tightness/overuse, or in association with pathology that changes the mechanics of the hip, such as lumbar spine disease, intra-articular hip pathology, or significant limb-length inequalities.
- **Sx/Exam:** Presents with pain and tenderness at the lateral hip directly over the greater trochanter that can make rising from a chair or sleeping on the affected side intensely painful. Point tenderness is diagnostic, but radiographs may be used to rule out bony and articular pathology.
- **DDx:** Osteoarthritis of the hip, trochanteric fracture, sciatica, tumor.
- **Tx:** Treated with stretching of the ITB, NSAIDs, rest, activity modification, and corticosteroid injection.

## Fractures of the Hip and Thigh

*A femoral neck fracture in a patient < 60 years of age is a surgical emergency because nondisplaced hip fractures have the potential to displace, which can → avascular necrosis of the femoral head.*

- Hip fractures are a common problem in the elderly, occurring with equal frequency in the femoral neck with twisting injuries and in the intertrochanteric region with a fall onto the greater trochanter.
- Age is the most important risk factor, with the frequency of hip fractures doubling with each decade beyond 50 years. Other risk factors include being white, female, sedentary, a smoker, or an alcoholic.
- **Sx/Exam:** Patients with a displaced fracture will present with the limb externally rotated, abducted, and shortened. Femoral neck stress fractures will have gradual onset of groin pain, antalgic gait, and pain on internal rotation.
- **Dx:** AP pelvis and cross-table lateral radiographs are usually diagnostic for complete fractures. Stress fractures may require MRI for diagnosis.
- **Tx:**
  - Most hip fractures require operative management.
  - Compression-side stress fractures (those on the inferior surface) can be managed with non-weight-bearing status until there is radiographic evidence of healing.
  - The more uncommon tension-side femoral neck stress fractures (those on the superior surface) often require internal fixation, as they are more likely to progress to full fractures.

## Pediatric Injuries of the Hip and Thigh

> 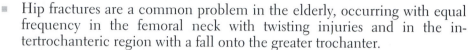 A 13-year-old overweight boy is brought to your office for evaluation of anterior thigh and knee pain. He does not remember sustaining any injury, but his mother has noticed that he has been limping intermittently over the past few weeks. His knee exam is normal, but when you flex his hip and knee to 90° and attempt to internally rotate the hip, he has pain and loss of internal rotation compared to the other side. What is the likely diagnosis? Slipped capital femoral epiphysis. Once the diagnosis is confirmed with radiographs, you make him non–weight bearing and arrange for urgent surgical evaluation. You tell the patient and his mother that the same problem may develop on the other side at some point in the future.

## SLIPPED CAPITAL FEMORAL EPIPHYSIS (SCFE)

Displacement of the femoral head due to microfracture through the physis that usually occurs during the adolescent growth spurt. Predisposing factors include obesity, male gender, and involvement in sports activities. The typical age range is 10–14 years for girls and 11–16 years for boys. Onset outside the normal age range suggests an underlying endocrine disorder. Bilateral involvement over time is seen in 40–50% of patients.

### SYMPTOMS/EXAM

- Presents with pain exacerbated by activity that localizes to the anterior proximal thigh or knee.
- Loss of hip internal rotation, especially with the hip flexed, is both sensitive and specific.
- Patients typically walk with the involved extremity externally rotated.

### DIAGNOSIS

- AP and frog-leg radiographs show "ice cream falling off the cone" (see Figure 17.4).
- Early diagnosis is critical, as the degree of displacement correlates with the duration of symptoms.

### TREATMENT

- All cases warrant urgent orthopedic evaluation for stabilization surgery.
- Inability to walk or severe pain after a fall suggests an unstable SCFE and requires emergent reduction and stabilization.

### COMPLICATIONS

Surgically stabilized mild or moderate SCFEs usually have good long-term function. More severe disease can progress to arthritis, chondrolysis, and osteonecrosis.

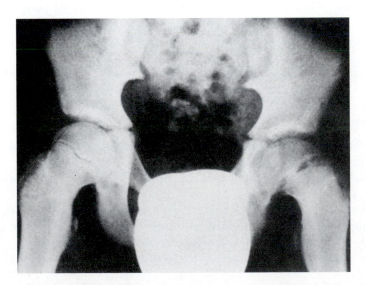

**FIGURE 17.4.  SCFE of the left hip.**

(Reproduced, with permission, from Tintinalli JE et al. *Emergency Medicine: A Comprehensive Study Guide*, 6th ed. New York: McGraw-Hill, 2004: 883.)

### LEGG-CALVÉ-PERTHES DISEASE

- Idiopathic osteonecrosis of the femoral head typically occurring in children 4–8 years of age but ranging from 2 to 12 years of age. Ninety percent of cases are unilateral. The disorder is four times more common in boys and is uncommon in blacks.
- **Sx/Exam:** Presents with a limp that worsens with activity, possibly accompanied by an ache in the groin or proximal thigh. Restricted hip abduction is also seen (vs. the ↓ internal rotation seen in SCFE). Bilateral involvement should prompt screening for thyroid disease and epiphyseal dysplasia (AP radiographs of the hand and knee).
- **Dx:** AP and frog-leg radiographs of the pelvis show ↑ density of the femoral head early on and the **crescent sign** once a shear fracture has occurred in the subchondral bone. Obtain an MRI if radiographs are ⊖.
- **Tx:** The younger the patient, the better the healing process, but no single treatment modality consistently prevents deformity of the femoral head. Children < 6 years of age are usually monitored, while older children may need bed rest, abduction bracing, or osteotomy to alter the area of the weight-bearing surface of the femoral head.
- **Cx:** Residual deformity can progress to osteoarthritis of the hip.

## KNEE INJURIES

### Meniscal Tears

The medial and lateral menisci are fibrocartilaginous disks that provide shock absorption and stability between the femur and tibia. The blood supply to the menisci is very poor, especially to the inner portion, so tears do not usually heal and can predispose the knee to degenerative arthritis.

#### SYMPTOMS/EXAM

- Traumatic tears usually occur with a sudden twisting injury and have slow development of swelling and stiffness over a few days. Symptoms can then wax and wane.
- Pain is localized to the medial (more common) or lateral joint line and often recurs with twisting or squatting motions such as getting out of a car.
- Mechanical symptoms such as locking, catching, and popping can also develop.
- Moderate effusion, joint line tenderness, pain with forced flexion, and meniscal rotation signs on exam (McMurray's sign) are suggestive.

#### DIFFERENTIAL

- **Anterior cruciate ligament (ACL) tear:** Sudden; characterized by larger swelling and instability.
- **Medial collateral ligament (MCL) injury:** Presents with pain with valgus stress.
- **Osteoarthritis:** Loss of joint space is seen on weight-bearing radiographs.
- **Pes anserine bursitis:** Medial tenderness distal to the joint line at the attachment of the sartorius, gracilis, and semitendinosus tendon.
- **Bony pathology:** Tibial plateau fracture; osteonecrosis of the femoral condyle.
- **Patellar subluxation or dislocation:** Presents with tender patellar facets and apprehension sign.
- **Saphenous neuritis:** Tenderness along the course of the saphenous nerve.

### DIAGNOSIS

- Radiographs to rule out bony conditions.
- MRI is used for diagnosis, as it is highly sensitive and specific for meniscal pathology.

### TREATMENT

- Arthroscopic partial meniscectomy (debridement) or repair is the treatment of choice for traumatic tears in the younger, active population.
- For degenerative tears (more likely in the older population) or in the absence of mechanical symptoms, conservative measures (e.g., rest, ice, NSAIDs, corticosteroid injection) can initially be tried.

## Ligamentous Injuries

### ANTERIOR CRUCIATE LIGAMENT (ACL) TEAR

The ACL is the 1° stabilizer of the knee. It resists anterior translation of the tibia on the femur and is the most frequently injured major ligament of the knee. The most common mechanism of injury is a rotational/pivot injury on a planted/stationary foot (common in skiing, football, and soccer) followed by hyperextension with internal rotation (e.g., landing from a rebound in basketball). Seventy percent of ACL injuries occur during sporting activities.

### SYMPTOMS/EXAM

- Forty percent of patients report feeling or hearing a pop (the most reliable factor).
- There is usually rapid development of hemarthrosis → significant swelling.
- The Lachman test is the most sensitive test (87–98%), showing ↑ anterior tibial displacement and a soft end point.

### DIAGNOSIS

- Radiographs should be closely evaluated for an avulsion of the tibial spine, a **Segond fracture** (an unusual lateral capsule avulsion associated with ACL injury), or a tibial plateau fracture.
- The history and exam remain key diagnostic tools, but MRI is increasingly used for confirmation as well as for the evaluation of associated injuries, such as injury of the menisci, posterior cruciate ligament (PCL), and collateral ligaments.

*The most common cause of an acute hemarthrosis after a sports-related knee injury is an ACL tear.*

### TREATMENT

- Treatment decisions depend on patient preference, age, activity level, knee instability, and associated injuries.
- Some older, less active patients can have satisfactory outcomes with rehabilitation alone (the ACL does not heal, but patients can develop muscular stability). Younger, more active patients are more likely to undergo reconstruction in order to continue to remain active.

### COLLATERAL LIGAMENT (MCL AND LCL) INJURIES

- Most often caused by a direct blow to the lateral aspect of the knee → valgus stress and medial collateral ligament (MCL) injury. Isolated lateral collateral ligament (LCL) injuries are rare.

649

- Sx/Exam:
  - Presents with pain +/− laxity on valgus (MCL) or varus (LCL) stress testing at 30° of flexion (relaxes the cruciate ligaments).
  - LCL injuries should be thoroughly evaluated for accompanying injuries (ACL, PCL, posterolateral corner injuries).
- **Tx:** Nonoperative management with a hinged knee brace and ROM exercises usually suffices for isolated MCL or LCL injuries. Rehabilitation can take 6–8 weeks.

## Patellofemoral Pain Syndrome

Patella-related pain is the single most common cause of knee pain. Patellofemoral pain syndrome is a multifactorial syndrome characterized by aching anterior knee pain that worsens with activities that stress the patellofemoral joint (e.g., climbing stairs, kneeling).

### SYMPTOMS/EXAM

- Presents with diffuse, aching anterior knee pain that is exacerbated by loaded flexion activities such as stair climbing, jumping, or prolonged sitting (theater sign).
- Note any patellar crepitation or tenderness of the patellar retinaculum or facets.
- Evaluate for contributing factors, including ↑ Q angle at the knee (more common in women owing to their wider pelvises), patellar tilt or malalignment, excessive lateral patellar mobility, tight hamstrings, weak quadriceps, and excessive femoral anteversion.

### DIFFERENTIAL

- **Patellar tendonitis (jumper's knee):** Point tenderness over the inferior pole of the patella.
- **Patellofemoral osteoarthritis:** Diagnosed by radiographic changes on sunrise view; affects older patients.
- **Synovial plica:** A redundant fold of synovial lining that can become painfully inflamed and fibrotic, most commonly occurring along the medial border of the patella.
- **Chondromalacia patellae:** Disruption in the articular cartilage of the patella (painful or nonpainful), with possible etiologies including trauma, malalignment, and biomechanical or metabolic factors.
- **Patellar instability:** Transient displacement (usually laterally) of the patella either partially (subluxation) or completely (dislocation) → acute and/or chronic patellar pain. Associated with a ⊕ apprehension sign when displacing the patella laterally.

### DIAGNOSIS

A clinical diagnosis. AP, lateral, and sunrise radiographs can evaluate for articular cartilage loss, tilt, and subluxation.

### TREATMENT

- Treated with activity modification and an exercise program consisting of quadriceps strengthening (especially the medial quadriceps) and hamstring flexibility with avoidance of open-chain knee extension exercises.
- Use of a knee sleeve with patellar cutout or a patellar stabilizing brace.

## Iliotibial Band Syndrome

- An overuse tendinopathy of the ITB as it passes over the lateral femoral condyle.
- **Sx/Exam:** Presents with lateral knee pain and crepitus at the lateral femoral condyle or insertion on Gerdy's tubercle. A tight ITB is seen on Ober's test. Check for contributing mechanics such as genu varus, excessive foot pronation or supination, and weak hip abductors/pelvic stabilizers.
- **Tx:** ITB stretching, foam roller exercises for soft tissue work to relax the ITB, rest, ice, NSAIDs, iontophoresis.

*ITB syndrome is the leading cause of lateral knee pain in runners.*

## Quadriceps and Patellar Tendon Ruptures

Typically occur with a fall onto a knee that is partially flexed while the quadriceps muscle is forcibly contracting to break the fall. Patellar tendon ruptures typically occur in younger patients (< 40 years of age) and are frequently associated with sporting activities. Quadriceps tendon ruptures usually occur in patients > 40 years of age and are three times more common than patellar tendon ruptures.

### Symptoms/Exam

Patients often feel a pop at the time of injury and have a palpable defect in one tendon with an inability to extend the knee against gravity or perform a straight-leg raise.

### Diagnosis

- Radiographs of the knee can rule out patellar fracture and will show patella alta (patellar tendon rupture) or patella baja (quadriceps rupture).
- MRI to confirm the diagnosis and for surgical planning.

### Treatment

- Immediate surgical repair is indicated for complete ruptures of either tendon.
- Partial tears with little loss of strength and maintenance of the ability to extend the knee can be treated conservatively with a cylinder cast in full extension for 4–6 weeks (uncommon).

## Pediatric Knee Injuries

### Osgood-Schlatter Disease

- Traction apophysitis of the tibial tubercle that occurs in rapidly growing adolescents. A repetitive stress injury to the 2° ossification center of the tibial tubercle where the patellar tendon inserts. It is five times more common among those active in sports and 2–3 times more common in boys, typically occurring in those 10–15 years of age.
- **Sx/Exam:** Presents with pain and tenderness at the tibial tubercle that is exacerbated by running, jumping, and kneeling. May be bilateral, but one side is usually worse.
- **Dx:** Radiographs can be normal or may show small spicules of heterotopic ossification anterior to the tibial tuberosity.

- **Tx:** Relative rest/activity modification; quadriceps stretching and strengthening; icing after activity; analgesics. Apophysitis will resolve once growth is complete.

### OSTEOCHONDRITIS DISSECANS

- Osteonecrosis of subchondral bone (most commonly on the medial femoral condyle) that → separation from underlying well-vascularized bone and eventual fragmentation if progression occurs. Thought to be due to repetitive small stresses to the subchondral bone.
- Onset in most cases is during childhood, although patients may not become symptomatic until late adolescence or early adulthood. Early diagnosis is critical, as the injury has a better potential to heal while the bones are still growing.
- **Sx/Exam:** Presents with gradual onset of vague knee pain and intermittent swelling after running and sports activities.
- **Dx:** Usually visible on plain radiographs (especially the tunnel view). MRI is used to assess the stability of the fragment as well as the viability of subchondral bone.
- **Tx:**
  - Younger patients with smaller, stable lesions are most likely to heal well with conservative measures. Activity modification (no running or jumping; possible crutch use) minimizes shear forces and allows for new bone formation.
  - If the overlying articular cartilage is disrupted, a loose body is present, or the patient is skeletally mature, evaluation for operative management is appropriate.

## INJURIES OF THE FOOT AND ANKLE

### Ankle Sprains

*The ATFL is the most commonly sprained ligament in the ankle or foot.*

Partial or complete tearing of one or more of the ligaments that support the ankle joint. Most often due to an inversion mechanism → injury to the lateral ligaments (see Figure 17.5). The anterior talofibular ligament (ATFL) is the first ligament to be injured, followed by the calcaneofibular ligament (CFL) and, finally, in the most severe lateral sprains, the posterior talofibular ligament (PTFL). A syndesmotic ankle sprain involving the anterior tibiofibular ligament that forms the distal portion of the syndesmosis between the tibia and fibula (**a high ankle sprain**) is less common and more severe. Isolated deltoid ligament sprains (medial ankle) are uncommon and are usually accompanied by a lateral malleolar fracture and/or by syndesmotic injury.

#### SYMPTOMS/EXAM

- Lateral ankle swelling and ecchymosis are proportional to the degree of ligament damage, as is the number of ligaments involved.
- Tenderness of the anterior tibiofibular ligament and pain with the **squeeze test** (compressing the tibia and fibula at midcalf stresses the distal syndesmosis) suggest a high ankle sprain.

#### DIFFERENTIAL

- Fracture of the lateral malleolus, calcaneus, talus, or base of the fifth metatarsal.
- Peroneal tendon tear or subluxation (retrofibular tenderness and swelling).

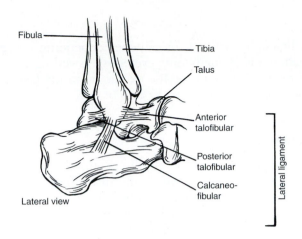

**FIGURE 17.5.** **Lateral ligament of the ankle joint.**

(Reproduced, with permission, from Tintinalli JE et al. *Emergency Medicine: A Comprehensive Study Guide*, 6th ed. New York: McGraw-Hill, 2004: 1737.)

## DIAGNOSIS

The need for radiographs to rule out fracture is based on the **Ottawa ankle rules** (see Figure 17.6). Indicated if the patient is unable to bear weight for four steps immediately after injury or in the office, or if there is lateral or medial malleolar bone tenderness; does not apply for patients < 18 years of age.

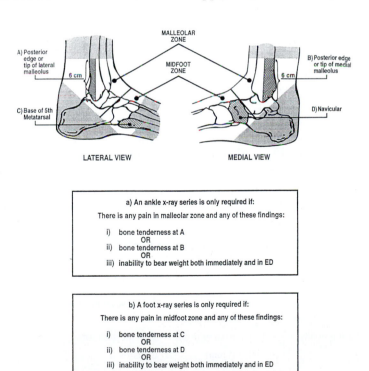

**FIGURE 17.6.** **Ottawa ankle rules for ankle and midfoot injuries.**

(Reproduced, with permission, from Tintinalli JE et al. *Emergency Medicine: A Comprehensive Study Guide*, 6th ed. New York: McGraw-Hill, 2004: 1738.)

### TREATMENT

- Treat with a brace, an air cast, or crutches depending on severity, with early mobilization and strengthening exercises as swelling ↓.
- The speed of recovery depends on the degree on injury (see Table 17.11).
- Residual symptoms can occur in up to 40% of patients.

## Achilles Tendon Rupture

- Disruption of the Achilles tendon usually occurs 5–7 cm proximal to its insertion onto the calcaneus. Most commonly affects middle-aged men who play quick stop-and-go sports such as tennis, squash, and basketball.
- **Sx/Exam:** Presents with sudden, severe calf pain with swelling and a palpable defect in the tendon. Exam shows lack of plantar flexion with manual squeezing of the calf (⊕ **Thompson test).**
- **DDx:** Achilles tendinosis (gradual onset), medial gastrocnemius tear (more proximal tenderness), DVT (no history of injury; ⊖ Thompson test).
- **Tx:** Nonoperative or surgical repair. Both require a program of graduated casting or bracing to allow for healing.

## Plantar Fasciitis

*Plantar fasciitis is the most common cause of heel pain in adults.*

- An overload injury (inflammation, degeneration, and tearing) of the plantar fascia, most commonly occurring at its calcaneal insertion. Contributing factors include a tight gastrocnemius-soleus complex, tight plantar fascia, a rigid rear foot, and overpronation or supination.
- **Sx/Exam:** Presents with pain and tenderness at the plantar medial heel that worsens with the first few steps in the morning, after rest, and with extended walking.
- **Dx:** A clinical diagnosis, but radiographs show a plantar heel spur in 50% of patients with plantar fasciitis and in 15% of asymptomatic patients. A bone scan can differentiate plantar fasciitis from calcaneal stress fracture.
- **Tx:**
  - Achilles stretching, activity modification, cushioned heel cups, ice massage, NSAIDs, and night splints can help maintain Achilles and plantar stretch. Repetitive corticosteroid injections can → fat pad insufficiency.

**TABLE 17.11. West Point Ankle Sprain Grading System**

|  | GRADE 1 | GRADE 2 | GRADE 3 |
|---|---|---|---|
| Edema/ecchymosis | Localized/slight | Localized/moderate | Diffuse/significant |
| Weight-bearing ability | Full or partial without significant pain | Difficult without crutches | Impossible |
| Ligament pathology | Ligament stretch | Partial tear | Complete tear |
| Instability testing | None | None or slight | Definite |
| Time to return to sports | 11 days | 2–6 weeks | 4–26 weeks |

- Ninety-five percent of patients will have resolution of symptoms within 12–18 months. For those with persistent symptoms, surgical release of plantar fascia is usually effective.

## Morton's Neuroma

- A perineural fibrosis of the common digital nerve as it passes between the metatarsal heads. Most commonly occurs between the third and fourth toes; five times more common in women (thought to be due to compression resulting from tight shoe wear).
- **Sx/Exam:** Presents with forefoot plantar pain +/– dysesthesias that can be reproduced with pressure to the plantar aspect of the third web space while squeezing the metatarsals together.
- **DDx:**
    - **Metatarsalgia:** Presents with tenderness over the metatarsal heads.
    - **Hammer toe:** Flexion deformity of the proximal interphalangeal joint.
    - **Metatarsophalangeal (MTP) synovitis:** Characterized by tenderness and swelling over the MTP joint.
    - **Stress fracture:** Dorsal metatarsal tenderness.
- **Tx:** Use of shoes with low heels and a wide toe box; metatarsal pads to spread the metatarsal heads; lidocaine/corticosteroid injection.

## Fractures of the Foot and Ankle

### MALLEOLAR FRACTURES

- The ankle joint is considered stable with an isolated malleolar fracture (usually lateral). When combined with an injury to the other side of the ankle (e.g., lateral malleolus fracture and deltoid ligament disruption), the ankle joint becomes unstable.
- **Sx/Exam:** Patients present with a history of trauma with swelling, tenderness, and possible deformity at the site of the fracture.
- **Dx:** AP, lateral, and mortise views can evaluate for fracture and widening of the mortise, which suggest an unstable ankle joint.
- **Tx:**
    - **Stable fractures of the distal fibula:** Use of a weight-bearing cast or a brace for 4–6 weeks.
    - **Unstable, nondisplaced fractures:** Use of a non-weight-bearing short- or long-leg cast for a longer period with close orthopedic follow-up.
    - Unstable, displaced fractures usually require open reduction.

### MAISONNEUVE FRACTURE

- A fracture of the proximal fibula that is associated with disruption of the tibia-fibula syndesmosis and fracture of the medial malleolus or rupture of the deltoid ligament.
- Occurs with significant torsional force to the ankle, which is transmitted up the syndesmosis to the proximal fibula.
- **Dx:** It is important to palpate the proximal fibula if there is tenderness over the medial ankle.

## FRACTURE OF THE BASE OF THE FIFTH METATARSAL

There are three types of proximal fifth metatarsal fractures:

- **Avulsion fracture of the tuberosity:** The most common type; generally extra-articular and rarely displaced. Generally treated with weight bearing in a walking cast or hard-soled shoes until pain subsides.
- **Jones fracture:** Fracture just distal to the tuberosity at the neck. Associated with a higher rates of nonunion; treated with intramedullary fixation or a non-weight-bearing short-leg cast for 6–8 weeks.
- **Diaphyseal stress fracture:** Treated with a non-weight-bearing short-leg cast for 6–8 weeks.

## RHEUMATOLOGY

## Systemic Lupus Erythematosus (SLE)

A chronic inflammatory disease that can affect multiple organ systems, including the skin, joints, kidneys, lungs, nervous system, and serous membranes. The disease course can include episodes of remission as well as chronic or acute flare-ups. The female-to-male ratio is 9:1, with onset often occurring in the 20s and 30s. Three times more common among African-Americans.

### SYMPTOMS/EXAM

See Table 17.12. Nearly 90% of patients have joint symptoms.

### DIAGNOSIS

- See Table 17.12.
- ANA testing is close to 100% sensitive but is not specific, whereas antibodies to dsDNA and Smith are specific but not sensitive (can be confirmatory if ⊕). Titers of dsDNA antibodies generally correlate with disease activity.

### TREATMENT

- Sun and stress avoidance; skin protection.
- Pharmacologic treatment depends on the severity of the disease and the degree of organ involvement; can include NSAIDs, topical and systemic steroids, antimalarials, methotrexate, and IVIG.

### COMPLICATIONS

Organ-specific damage plus accelerated atherosclerosis and opportunistic infections.

## DRUG-INDUCED LUPUS

- Presentation is similar to that of SLE, but has equal prevalence among men and women, and symptoms resolve with withdrawal of the offending medication.
- The most commonly associated drugs are hydralazine, procainamide, INH, quinidine, methyldopa, and chlorpromazine.

**TABLE 17.12. Diagnostic Criteria for SLE (4 of 11 Needed for Diagnosis)**

| VARIABLE | SYMPTOMS |
|---|---|
| **S**kin/**S**unlight | 1. Malar rash<br>2. Discoid rash<br>3. Photosensitivity |
| **S**erosa/mucous membranes | 4. Oral ulcers<br>5. Serositis (pleuritis/pericarditis) |
| **S**ynovitis | 6. Arthritis |
| **S**eizures, "**S**"ychosis | 7. Neurologic disease (seizures, psychosis) |
| "**S**"ellular casts, proteinuria | 8. Renal disease (any one of the following):<br>a. > 0.5 g/day proteinuria<br>b. ≥ 3+ dipstick protein<br>c. Cellular casts |
| "**S**"ytopenias | 9. Hematologic disorders (any one of the following):<br>a. Hemolytic anemia<br>b. Leukopenia (< 4000/mL)<br>c. Lymphopenia (< 1500/mL)<br>d. Thrombocytopenia (< 100,000/mL) |
| **S**erologies | 10. ⊕ ANA<br>11. Immunologic abnormalities (any one of the following):<br>a. Antibodies to native DNA<br>b. Anti-Smith antibodies<br>c. Antiphospholipid antibodies:<br>  i. False-⊕ serologic test for syphilis<br>  ii. Evidence of anticardiolipin antibodies<br>  iii. Evidence of lupus anticoagulant |

Adapted, with permission, from Le T et al. *First Aid for the Internal Medicine Boards,* 1st ed. New York: McGraw-Hill, 2006: 588.

## Rheumatoid Arthritis

A chronic systemic inflammatory disease that primarily affects the joints. Affects 1–2% of the U.S. population, with a female-male ratio of 3:1 and a typical age of onset of 20–40 years.

### SYMPTOMS/EXAM

- Presents with symmetric, inflammatory joint pain, most commonly of the PIP and MTP joints, wrists, ankles and knees. Inflammatory characteristics include morning stiffness and pain; improvement of symptoms with use of the joint; and possible erythema, warmth, and/or swelling of the joint.
- Patients with long-standing, erosive, RF-⊕ disease can also develop extra-articular disease, including vasculitis, interstitial lung disease, serositis, ocular disease, Sjögren's syndrome, and amyloidosis.

### DIFFERENTIAL

Osteoarthritis (affects the DIP joints; lacks inflammatory characteristics).

### DIAGNOSIS

- Diagnostic criteria are as follows (four of seven criteria lasting > 6 weeks must be met for diagnosis):
  - Morning stiffness
  - Arthritis involving three or more joint areas
  - Arthritis involving the hands
  - Symmetric arthritis
  - Serum RF
  - Radiographic changes consistent with disease
  - Rheumatoid nodules (subcutaneous nodules over the extensor surfaces or bony prominences)
- Classic radiographic findings include periarticular osteopenia, joint space narrowing, and juxta-articular erosions.
- RF is ⊕ in 70–80% of patients but is not specific.

### TREATMENT

The American College of Rheumatology recommends starting disease-modifying antirheumatic drugs (DMARDs) within three months of diagnosis. NSAIDs are appropriate for symptom flares.

## Seronegative Spondyloarthropathies

A group of disorders characterized by ⊖ serologies for ANA and RF, a strong association with the HLA-B27 antigen, and spinal arthritis. Consist of ankylosing spondylitis, psoriatic arthritis, reactive arthritis (Reiter's syndrome), and IBD-associated arthritis.

### ANKYLOSING SPONDYLITIS

- Particularly involves the sacroiliac joints and the spine.
- Affects 1 in 2000 people, with men having more severe disease than women.
- **Sx:** Presents with progressive pain and stiffening of the spine with low back pain that worsens in the morning and with inactivity but improves with exercise.
- **Exam:** Exam reveals tenderness of the sacroiliac joints with ↓ lumbar lordosis and cervical motion.
- **Dx:** Diagnosed by the classic "bamboo-like" appearance of the spine on radiographs and/or sacroiliitis on radiographs or MRI. ⊖ RF with ↑ ESR.
- **Tx:** NSAIDs, physical therapy, methotrexate, spinal fusion.

### PSORIATIC ARTHRITIS

- Affects 10–20% of patients with psoriasis; usually preceded by skin disease.
- Has significant association with nail disorders (pitting, ridging, onycholysis).
- **Sx/Exam:** Has multiple patterns of presentation, including mono- and polyarticular types.

- **Dx:** Characteristic radiographic changes are seen, such as marginal erosions and "pencil-in-cup" deformities of the distal digits.
- **Tx:** NSAIDs, DMARDs.

### REACTIVE ARTHRITIS (REITER'S SYNDROME)

- Develops within days to weeks of antecedent infection with *Salmonella, Shigella, Campylobacter, Yersinia, Chlamydia,* or unknown pathogens.
- **Sx/Exam:** Presents with the classic triad of **conjunctivitis, urethritis, and arthritis** (more commonly of the larger peripheral joints than of the spine). Patients may also have systemic symptoms such as fever and weight loss.
- **Dx:** Arthrocentesis with an inflammatory pattern and a ⊖ culture.
- **Tx:** NSAIDs; antibiotics as indicated; DMARDs if arthritis does not improve.
- **Cx:** Rare aortitis and aortic regurgitation.

### IBD-ASSOCIATED ARTHRITIS

- Twenty percent of patients with IBD (Crohn's > ulcerative colitis) will develop associated arthritis.
- **Sx/Exam:** Peripheral arthritic flares are associated with GI disease. Presents with asymmetric, oligoarticular, large joint involvement peripherally. Spinal involvement mimics ankylosing spondylitis and is independent of intestinal disease.
- **Tx:** NSAIDs. Treatment of GI disease can control peripheral arthritis.

## Crystalline-Induced Arthropathies

Deposition of crystals in the synovium and other tissues → an inflammatory response. Characterized by episodes of abrupt-onset, severe, and usually monoarticular joint pain.

### HYPERURICEMIA

- Due to overproduction of uric acid (glycogen storage diseases, psoriasis, myeloproliferative disorders, large tumor burden) or underexcretion of uric acid (renal disease, thiazide or loop diuretics, lactic acidosis, alcoholism, ketoacidosis).
- ↑ the risk of gout, but the majority of patients do not actually develop gout.

### GOUT

- Deposition of uric acid crystals in the synovium, bursae, tendon sheaths, skin, heart valves, and kidneys → arthritis, tophi, renal stones, and gouty nephropathy.
- Onset is usually after age 30, with a male-to-female ratio of 9:1. Women affected are almost always postmenopausal.
- **Sx/Exam:** Presents with sudden-onset, self-limited, recurrent, acute mono- or oligoarticular arthritis events → a "red-hot" joint. The first MTP joint is most commonly affected, but the knees, ankles, feet, elbows, and hands may also be involved. Nodular deposits of uric acid crystals, or **tophi,** may be seen in subcutaneous tissues, tendons, cartilage, and bone.

- **Dx:** Negatively birefringent, needle-like crystals are seen in synovial fluid aspiration. Cultures are sterile. "Rat-bite" erosions may be seen on joint radiographs. Serum uric acid is ↑ in 95% of cases, but this is not diagnostic and is not required for the diagnosis.
- **Tx:**
    - Acute attacks are usually treated with colchicine, an NSAID such as indomethacin, or an intra-articular corticosteroid.
    - Diet modification to ↓ purine intake, including alcohol avoidance, is also recommended.
    - Patients with recurrent attacks can be treated with daily colchicine, allopurinol for overproducers, or probenecid for underexcretors.

### CALCIUM PYROPHOSPHATE DEPOSITION DISEASE (CPPD)

*Rapid or unusual distribution of degenerative joint disease should raise suspicion for CPPD.*

- Crystalline arthropathy → a spectrum of disease ranging from asymptomatic chondrocalcinosis (calcification of the articular cartilage surface) to **pseudogout.**
- **Sx/Exam:** Presents with a monoarticular inflammatory arthropathy similar to gout.
- **Dx:** Weakly ⊕ birefringent rhomboid-shaped crystals are seen on synovial fluid aspiration. Radiographs can show the white lines of chondrocalcinosis in joint spaces.
- **Tx:** NSAIDs; corticosteroid injections; colchicine for chronic cases.

## Infectious Arthritis

### GONOCOCCAL ARTHRITIS (DISSEMINATED INFECTION)

- Arthritis and arthralgias are the principal manifestations of disseminated gonococcal infection, which occurs in 1–3% of patients infected with *Neisseria gonorrhoeae.* Most common in patients < 40 years of age.
- **Sx/Exam:** Presents with migratory polyarthralgias and tenosynovitis with fever and a papulopustular rash that can involve the palms and soles.
- **Dx:** Blood, rectal, throat, and urethral cultures are 70–80% sensitive, whereas synovial fluid culture is < 50% sensitive.
- **Tx:** Treat with IV antibiotics (third-generation cephalosporin) until clinical improvement is seen, followed by oral antibiotics for a 7- to 10-day total course. Empiric treatment for chlamydia.

### NONGONOCOCCAL ARTHRITIS (SEPTIC JOINT)

*Prosthetic infections–think S. epidermidis.*

- Inoculation of bacteria into a joint from hematogenous spread, direct penetration of the joint, or spread from an adjacent focus of infection. The most common organisms are gram-⊕ species (*S. aureus, Streptococcus*). Gram-⊖ organisms such as *E. coli* or *Pseudomonas* are less common. There is an ↑ risk with previous joint damage, IV drug use, endocarditis, and prosthetic joints.
- **Sx/Exam:** Presents with acute-onset, monoarticular joint pain with swelling, warmth, and erythema as well as fevers and chills.
- **Dx:** Fifty percent of patients have ⊕ blood cultures, and 75% have ⊕ synovial fluid cultures and a ⊕ Gram stain. Radiographs can show joint erosions, osteomyelitis, demineralization, or periostitis.
- **Tx:** IV antibiotics (often needed for up to six weeks).
- **Cx:** Articular destruction; septicemia.

## Inflammatory Myopathies

### POLYMYOSITIS

- A systemic inflammatory disease characterized by proximal muscle weakness. Women are affected twice as often as men; average age of onset is 40–60 years.
- **Sx/Exam:** Presents with progressive muscle weakness of the neck and proximal musculature of the limbs along with difficulty swallowing. Pain is not pronounced.
- **DDx:** Inclusion body myositis (distal muscles are more affected), polymyalgia rheumatica (pain is more common), myopathy or myositis 2° to malignancy, medications, toxins, endocrine/metabolic disorders.
- **Dx:** ↑ muscle enzyme markers (CK and/or aldolase); muscle biopsy. EMG shows nonspecific changes.
- **Tx:** Corticosteroids, DMARDs.

### DERMATOMYOSITIS

- A systemic inflammatory disease with proximal muscle weakness and characteristic skin rashes. Often associated with occult malignancy.
- **Sx/Exam:** Similar to polymyositis plus rashes.
  - **Gottron's papules:** A scaly rash over the extensor surfaces.
  - **Shawl sign:** Erythema in a sun-exposed V-neck or shoulder distribution.
  - **Heliotrope rash:** A violaceous rash over the eyelids +/− periorbital edema.
  - **Facial erythema:** A diffuse, dusky facial rash.
- **Dx:** Similar to polymyositis with a different lymphocytic inflammatory infiltrate pattern on muscle biopsy.
- **Tx:** Corticosteroids, DMARDs, IVIG for refractory cases.

*A diagnosis of dermatomyositis warrants an investigation for occult malignancy.*

## Systemic Sclerosis (Scleroderma)

- An autoimmune disorder characterized by **CREST** syndrome (**C**alcinosis, **R**aynaud's phenomenon, **E**sophageal dysmotility, **S**clerodactyly, and **T**elangiectasias). The majority of cases (80%) are limited scleroderma, which has a better prognosis; progressive systemic sclerosis can have kidney, heart, lung, and GI tract involvement in addition to CREST syndrome.
- Both types are ANA ⊕, with anticentromere antibodies in limited scleroderma and anti-SCL-70 antibodies in the progressive type.
- **Tx:** Treatment of CREST is symptomatic; progressive disease also requires corticosteroids and immunosuppressants.

## Vasculitis

- Infiltration of leukocytes into vessel walls with resultant reactive damage to mural structures. Can be 1° or 2°.
- **Sx/Exam:**
  - Presentation depends on the structures involved.
  - 1° vasculitis can be categorized according to the size of the involved vessels (see Figure 17.7). 2° vasculitis can be due to infection (especially indolent infections such as subacute bacterial endocarditis and

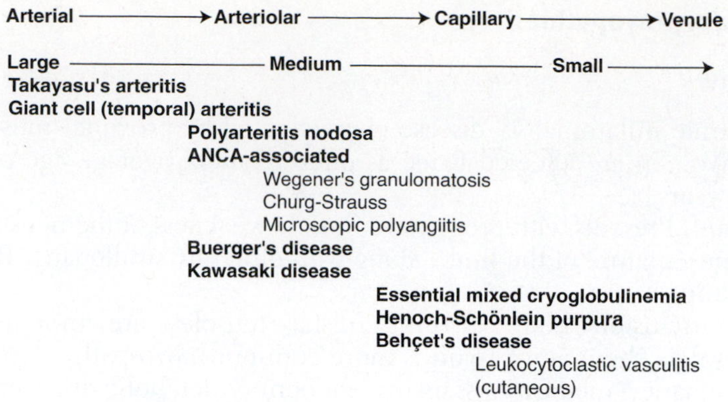

Arterial ⟶ Arteriolar ⟶ Capillary ⟶ Venule

Large ⟶ Medium ⟶ Small ⟶
**Takayasu's arteritis**
**Giant cell (temporal) arteritis**
> **Polyarteritis nodosa**
> **ANCA-associated**
>> Wegener's granulomatosis
>> Churg-Strauss
>> Microscopic polyangiitis
**Buerger's disease**
**Kawasaki disease**
> **Essential mixed cryoglobulinemia**
> **Henoch-Schönlein purpura**
> **Behçet's disease**
>> Leukocytoclastic vasculitis
>> (cutaneous)

**FIGURE 17.7. Classification of 1° vasculitis according to size of vessel involved.**

(Reproduced, with permission, from Le T et al. *First Aid for the Internal Medicine Boards*, 1st ed. New York: McGraw-Hill, 2006: 602.)

HCV), medications (→ hypersensitivity vasculitis, ANCA-associated vasculitis), collagen vascular disease, or malignancy.

- **Tx:** Treatment usually includes corticosteroids and/or immunosuppressants.

# Emergency/Urgent Care

Grace Chen Yu, MD

> A 78-year-old woman with a history of dementia and DM is sent to the ER from her nursing home because of fever, lethargy, and hypotension. Her caregiver gives a recent history of foul-smelling urine, ↓ mentation, and urinary incontinence. In the ER, the patient is found to have a temperature of 39.2°C and a BP of 72/35. What is her most likely diagnosis? Distributive shock due to urosepsis. If diagnosed early, fluid resuscitation, prompt initiation of IV antibiotics, and pressor support may → resolution of her symptoms.

A physiologic state in which alterations in tissue perfusion → ↓ tissue $O_2$ delivery. Although initially reversible, untreated or refractory shock → permanent organ damage, failure of multiple organ systems, and eventually death. Shock can be broadly classified into three categories on the basis of etiology: hypovolemic, cardiogenic, or distributive (vasodilatory) (see Table 18.1).

**Types of shock –**

- *Hypovolemic: Blood* **Volume** *problem*
- *Cardiogenic: Blood* **Pump** *problem*
- *Distributive: Blood* **Vessel** *problem*

### SYMPTOMS

Presents with hypotension (SBP < 90 mmHg or a ↓ in SBP > 40 mmHg), oliguria, and changes in mental status.

### EXAM

- Findings depend on the etiology, but almost all patients have tachycardia, tachypnea, altered mental status, and cool, clammy skin (except in distributive shock).
- The history may reveal food and medicine allergies, recent changes in medications, drug intoxication, preexisting illnesses, immunosuppressed states, or hypercoagulable conditions.

### DIFFERENTIAL

See Table 18.1 for the different etiologies of shock.

### DIAGNOSIS

- Generally diagnosed through the history and physical exam.
- CBC with differential, complete metabolic panel, amylase/lipase, cardiac enzymes, toxicology screen, UA, CXR, and ABG can help determine the etiology.
- Mixed venous oxygen saturation ($SvO_2$) and pulmonary artery catheterization (PCWP, CO/CI, SVR) can also help distinguish hypovolemic from cardiogenic and distributive shock (see Table 18.2).

### TREATMENT

- Regardless of the cause of shock, the ABCs must initially be evaluated and stabilized.
- If the patient is in respiratory distress, consider intubation and mechanical ventilation, which can facilitate elimination of $CO_2$ and compensate for any coexisting metabolic acidosis.
- Circulatory improvement can be achieved through aggressive volume resuscitation with isotonic fluids and blood products if indicated, as well as

**TABLE 18.1.**   **Etiologies and Mechanisms of Shock**

| Type | Mechanism of Action | Common Etiologies |
|---|---|---|
| Hypovolemic | Absolute deficiency in intravascular blood volume caused by hemorrhage or fluid loss. | Trauma, GI bleed, ruptured aneurysm, fractures, diarrhea, vomiting, heat stroke, inadequate replacement of insensible losses, burns, "third spacing" (seen in intestinal obstruction, pancreatitis, and cirrhosis). |
| Cardiogenic | Impaired cardiac contractility and pump failure. | Cardiomyopathies; arrhythmias; ischemic heart disease; mechanical (valvular) abnormalities; extracardiac (obstructive) disorders such as massive pulmonary embolus, tension pneumothorax, or pericardial tamponade. |
| Distributive | Inappropriate relaxation of peripheral vascular tone often associated initially with ↑ cardiac output. | Sepsis, anaphylaxis, neurologic injury, drug-related causes. |

through pharmacologic therapy with vasopressors and cardiac inotropic agents once coexisting hypovolemia has been addressed.

- If sepsis is a concern, early coverage with empiric broad-spectrum antibiotics is essential.
- Sodium bicarbonate may be indicated in patients with marked hypoperfusion → lactic acidosis and a reduction in pH below 7.1.
- Pharmacotherapy depends on the etiology. Table 18.3 lists the common pharmacologic agents used in shock along with their indications and predominant effects.

## TOXICOLOGY

### Common Ingestions

Ingestions may be asymptomatic on initial presentation depending on the time and the amount of ingestion. Timely consultation with a regional poison control center (1-800-222-1222), gut decontamination, and administration of an antidote (if available) can ↓ morbidity and mortality. Table 18.4 lists common ingestions and their treatment. Gut decontamination measures include the following:

**TABLE 18.2.**   **Hemodynamic Features of Shock[a]**

| Type of Shock | Preload (PCWP) | Pump Function (CO) | Afterload (SVR) | Tissue Perfusion (SvO$_2$) |
|---|---|---|---|---|
| Hypovolemic | ↓ | ↓ | ↑ | ↓ |
| Cardiogenic | ↑ | ↓ | ↑ | ↓ |
| Distributive | ↓ or ↔ | ↑ | ↓ | ↑ (peripheral) and ↓ (central) |

[a] PCWP = pulmonary capillary wedge pressure; SVR = systemic vascular resistance; CO = cardiac output; SvO$_2$ = mixed venous O$_2$ saturation.

TABLE 18.3. Pharmacologic Agents Used in Shock

| PHARMACOLOGIC AGENT | RECEPTOR ACTIVITY | | | | PREDOMINANT EFFECTS | INDICATIONS |
|---|---|---|---|---|---|---|
| | $\alpha_1$ | $\beta_1$ | $\beta_2$ | DA | | |
| Phenylephrine | +++ | 0 | 0 | 0 | SVR ↑↑, CO ↔/↑ | Sepsis, neurogenic shock |
| Norepinephrine | +++ | ++ | 0 | 0 | SVR ↑↑, CO ↔↓↑ | Sepsis |
| Epinephrine | +++ | +++ | ++ | 0 | CO ↑↑, SVR ↓ (low); SVR ↔/↑ (high) | Anaphylaxis, ACLS, sepsis |
| **Dopamine** | | | | | | |
| Low-dose (0.5–2) | 0 | + | 0 | ++ | CO ↑, SVR ↑↓ | Sepsis, cardiogenic shock |
| Mid-dose (5–10) | + | ++ | 0 | ++ | CO ↑ | |
| High-dose (10–20) | ++ | ++ | 0 | ++ | SVR ↑↑ | |
| Dobutamine | 0/+ | +++ | ++ | 0 | CO ↑, SVR ↓ | Cardiogenic shock |
| Isoproterenol | 0 | +++ | +++ | 0 | CO ↑, SVR ↓ | Cardiogenic shock with bradycardia |

■ **Ipecac:** Not useful for gut decontamination, and no longer recommended for ingestions.

■ **Gastric lavage:** Not effective beyond 1.0–1.5 hours after ingestion, but may be useful in severely ill patients. Should be combined with activated charcoal and used only in patients who are intubated or able to protect their airway.

■ **Activated charcoal:** The treatment of choice for most ingestions (except metals). Best if used within the first hour of overdose, but may be administered in all ingestions unless the agent is nontoxic or not bound by activated charcoal. The usual doses are 50–100 g in adults and 10–25 g in pediatric patients.

■ **Whole bowel irrigation:** May be useful after the ingestion of enteric-coated and timed-release medications and in body packers. The usual dose is 3–8 L of GoLytely.

## Food Poisoning

An acute illness caused by ingestion of food contaminated by bacteria, bacterial toxins, viruses, parasites, natural poisons, or harmful chemical substances. Characterized by a short incubation period of hours up to one week, most cases of food poisoning are mild and improve with supportive care, antiperistaltic or antisecretory agents, absorbents, and volume repletion. Some patients, however, may have severe disease requiring hospitalization, aggressive rehydration therapy, antibiotic treatment, and avoidance of antiperistaltic agents. Table 18.5 lists the common etiologies of food poisoning.

## Substance Abuse

A maladaptive pattern of substance use → significant impairment or distress. DSM-IV criteria include one of the following within a 12-month period:

EMERGENCY/URGENT CARE

667

**TABLE 18.4.** **Common Ingestions and Toxidromes**

| INGESTION | SYMPTOMS/EXAM | DIAGNOSIS | TREATMENT | COMPLICATIONS |
|---|---|---|---|---|
| Acetaminophen | Nausea, vomiting, jaundice. | History of acute overdose (> 140 mg/kg) or chronic overuse (> 4 g/day). ↑ liver enzymes; toxic serum level on nomogram (see Figure 18.1). | Activated charcoal if within 1–2 hours of ingestion. N-acetylcysteine (PO or IV) for 72 hours if serum level is toxic. | Metabolic acidosis, hepatic encephalopathy, fulminant hepatic failure, renal failure, death. |
| Acids or alkalies (commonly found in household cleaners) | Throat pain, abdominal pain, bloody emesis or stools, nausea, vomiting, difficulty swallowing or breathing, discoloration of skin and oral mucosa. | History of ingestion; prompt EGD to determine the extent of injury; CXR and abdominal x-ray (AXR) to evaluate for esophageal or gastric perforation. | Do **not** induce emesis. Dilute with milk or water to drink. Gastric lavage for liquid acid ingestion. | Respiratory failure, ARDS, local tissue necrosis, burns, death. |
| Anticholinergics (atropine, scopolamine, belladonna alkaloids, antihistamines, antipsychotics) | Mydriasis, dry mucous membranes, urinary retention, flushing, altered mental status ("dry as a bone, red as a beet, mad as a hatter"). | History of ingestion. | Activated charcoal, gastric lavage. Benzodiazepines for agitation; physostigmine in severe cases (may induce seizures or arrhythmias). | Status epilepticus, hyperthermia, hypertension, coma, respiratory failure, death. |
| Carbon monoxide | Confusion, coma, seizures, headache, fatigue, nausea. | History of exposure to furnace or car exhaust. ↑ carboxyhemoglobin level; normal $O_2$ saturation. | Give 100% $O_2$ or hyperbaric $O_2$ in patients with evidence of CNS impairment, myocardial ischemia, or carboxyhemoglobin level > 30%. | Arrhythmias, myocardial ischemia, rhabdomyolysis, death. |
| Cholinergics (organophosphates, pilocarpine, carbamates) | Diaphoresis, salivation, lacrimation, defecation, urination, miosis, nausea, altered mental status, weakness ("blind as a mole, moist as a slug, weak as a kitten"). | History of ingestion; farming or industrial work exposure; ↑ serum cholinesterase levels. | Skin decontamination with alkaline soap, then ethanol. Activated charcoal, gastric lavage. Atropine to dry secretions (may → ileus); pralidoxime in symptomatic patients. | Seizures; respiratory failure; cranial nerve palsies; impaired hearing, visual memory, reaction time, dexterity, and problem solving; delayed peripheral neuropathy; death. |

TABLE 18.4. **Common Ingestions and Toxidromes (continued)**

| INGESTION | SYMPTOMS/EXAM | DIAGNOSIS | TREATMENT | COMPLICATIONS |
|---|---|---|---|---|
| Iron | Nausea, vomiting, diarrhea, hypotension, acidosis. | History of ingestion. Serum levels > 350–500 µg/dL. | IV fluids, whole bowel irrigation. Deferoxamine to chelate the iron. | GI bleeding, metabolic acidosis, peritonitis, sepsis, fulminant hepatic failure, death. |
| Lead | Colicky abdominal pain, constipation, headache, irritability, seizures, motor neuropathy, learning disorders, microcytic anemia with basophilic stippling. | History of chronic repeated exposure (rare in acute ingestions). **Mild:** 10–50 µg/dL. **Moderate:** 50–70 µg/dL. **Severe:** 70–100 µg/dL. | Edetate calcium disodium (EDTA) +/– dimercaprol (BAL) for severe toxicity. Dimercaptosuccinic acid (DMSA) or EDTA for chelation in mild to moderate toxicity. | Learning disorders, motor neuropathy, anemia. |
| Salicylates | Nausea, vomiting, hyperpnea, tachycardia, tinnitus, coma, seizures, anion-gap metabolic acidosis, hyperthermia. | History of acute overdose (> 200 mg/kg) or chronic overmedication. Serum level > 100 mg/dL in acute, 60–70 mg/dL in chronic. | Activated charcoal, gastric lavage, hemodialysis. Sodium bicarbonate to treat metabolic acidosis and to alkalinize the urine. | Coma, cardiovascular collapse, pulmonary edema, death. |
| Theophylline | Nausea, vomiting, tachycardia, tremulousness, hypotension, seizures, hypokalemia, hyperglycemia, metabolic acidosis. | History of acute overdose or chronic overmedication. Serum level > 100 mg/L in acute, 40–60 mg/L in chronic. | Activated charcoal, whole bowel irrigation, hemodialysis. Benzodiazepines or barbiturates for seizure treatment. | Ventricular arrhythmias, status epilepticus, death. |
| TCAs | Mydriasis, tachycardia, dry mouth, flushing, muscle twitching, ↓ peristalsis, QRS widening and QT prolongation, seizures, diaphoresis, hypotension. | History of ingestion. | Do **not** induce emesis. Activated charcoal, gastric lavage. Sodium bicarbonate boluses to reverse cardiotoxicity. | Ventricular arrhythmias, hyperthermia, status epilepticus, death. |

EMERGENCY/URGENT CARE

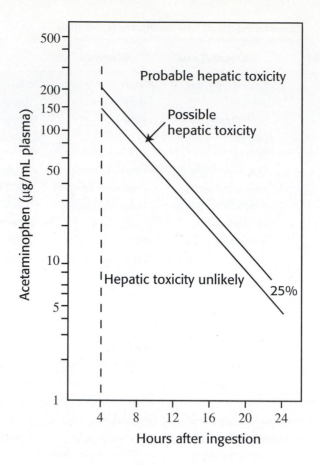

**FIGURE 18.1.** **Nomogram for predicting acetaminophen toxicity.**

(Reproduced, with permission, from Smilkstein MJ, Bronstein AC, Linden C, et al. "Acetaminophen Overdose: A 48-Hour Intravenous N-Acetylcysteine Treatment Protocol," *Ann Emerg Med* 1991;20(10): 1058, with permission from the American College of Physicians. As adapted from Rumack BH, Matthew H. Acetaminophen poisoning and toxicity. *Pediatrics* 1975;55: 871–876.)

recurrent substance use → failure to fulfill major obligations at work, school, or home; recurrent use in situations where use is hazardous; recurrent substance abuse–related legal problems; or continued use despite knowledge of having a persistent social or interpersonal problem caused by substance use. See the section on intoxication and withdrawal for the symptoms and treatment of illicit substance use.

### Bioterrorism

Includes a spectrum of natural organisms or toxins that can be used to incapacitate, kill, or otherwise harm individuals. Characterized by low visibility, high potency, substantial accessibility, and easy delivery, biological weapons can cause widespread destruction. Typical biological weapons and the syndromes they cause are listed in Table 18.6.

TABLE 18.5. **Common Causes of Food Poisoning**

| SUBSTANCE | FOODS | SX/EXAM | ONSET | TREATMENT |
|---|---|---|---|---|
| *Bacillus cereus* | Fried rice. | Vomiting, diarrhea. | 1–6 hours | Supportive care. |
| Ciguatera | Red snapper, grouper, warm-water fish. | GI symptoms followed by perioral numbness, hot-cold reversal on the face, cranial nerve palsies, hallucinations, and hypotension. | Minutes to hours | Supportive care, gut decontamination, calcium gluconate or atropine as needed. |
| *Campylobacter jejuni* | Untreated water; undercooked meat, milk, or shellfish. | Foul-smelling watery diarrhea followed by bloody diarrhea, cramps, fever, and headache. | 2–10 days | Supportive care; erythromycin for invasive disease. |
| *Clostridium perfringens* | Undercooked meat or poultry. | Watery diarrhea, nausea, cramps. | 6–12 hours | Supportive care. |
| *Clostridium botulinum* | Improperly canned foods, honey. | Diplopia, ptosis, descending weakness and paralysis, respiratory difficulties. | 4–72 hours | Supportive care, airway management, antitoxin. |
| Enterotoxic *E. coli* | Contaminated water and food. | Watery diarrhea, vomiting, cramps. | 8–12 hours | Supportive care. |
| *E. coli* O157:H7 | Untreated water, raw beef, unpasteurized milk. | Cramps, bloody diarrhea, nausea, vomiting, fever. | 3–4 days | Supportive care; treatment of hemolytic-uremic syndrome if present. |
| *Salmonella* | Eggs, poultry. | Bloody diarrhea, cramps, low-grade fever, vomiting. | 8–48 hours | Supportive care; antibiotics for systemic infection. |
| *Shigella* | Undercooked food, egg salad. | Nausea, vomiting, fever, bloody diarrhea, neurologic symptoms, tenesmus. | 36–72 hours | Supportive care; antibiotics for severe infection. |
| *Staphylococcus* spp. | Improperly stored meats, dairy, or bakery products. | Vomiting, cramps, mild diarrhea. | 1–2 hours | Supportive care. |
| *Vibrio cholerae* | Contaminated water and food. | Profuse rice-water stools, cramps. | 8–24 hours | Supportive care, tetracycline. |
| *Giardia lamblia* | Contaminated ground water. | Watery +/− bloody diarrhea, cramps, fatigue, bloating, weight loss. | 2–3 days | Supportive care, metronidazole. |
| Hepatitis A virus | Contaminated food. | Fatigue, fever, nausea, vomiting, cramps, anorexia, jaundice, darkened urine. | 14–50 days | Supportive care; prophylaxis with immunization; liver transplant for liver failure. |

EMERGENCY/URGENT CARE

**TABLE 18.6.** **Effects of Exposure to Biological Agents**

| AGENT | DESCRIPTION | SYMPTOMS/EXAM | DIAGNOSIS | TREATMENT |
|---|---|---|---|---|
| Anthrax (*Bacillus anthracis*) | A large, aerobic, gram-⊕, spore-forming nonmotile bacillus causing a zoonotic disease in domesticated and wild animals. | **Cutaneous (> 95% of cases):** Fever, malaise, and headache; a painless papule or vesicle that later turns into a necrotic ulcer with a characteristic 1- to 5-cm black eschar; extensive surrounding edema; local lymphadenitis. **Inhalation:** Headache, fever, myalgias, fatigue, nonproductive cough, chest discomfort, increasing respiratory distress. **Oropharyngeal/GI:** Oral ulcer from ingestion of infected and undercooked meat; fever, neck swelling, dysphagia, nausea, vomiting, respiratory distress, hematemesis, massive ascites, diarrhea. | ⊕ Gram stain or culture of cutaneous lesion or peripheral blood; mediastinal widening and pleural effusion on CXR. | Penicillin and doxycycline are FDA approved (but may have resistance in terrorist attacks); fluoroquinolones in suspected inhalation anthrax infections. |
| Brucellosis (*Brucella* spp.) | A small, aerobic, nonmotile, gram-⊖ coccobacillus causing a zoonotic disease in wild and domesticated animals; transmitted via skin abrasions, the conjunctivae, and the GI or respiratory tracts. | May present as an acute, systemic febrile illness, an insidious chronic illness, or a localized inflammatory process. Fever, diaphoresis, fatigue, anorexia, arthralgias, depression, headache, irritability, cough; focal pain in the bones, joints, or GU tract with localized infection. | ⊕ tube agglutination test; ⊕ cultures of blood, bone marrow, or body fluid samples. | Relapse is common, so combined regimens are recommended: doxycycline + streptomycin or rifampin. |
| Plague (*Yersinia pestis*) | A gram-⊖ nonmotile coccobacillus causing a zoonotic disease spread by the flea bites of an infected animal (usually a rat) or inhalation of an infectious aerosol. | **Bubonic (85–90%):** High fevers, chills, headache, nausea, vomiting, painful lymphadenopathy, severe malaise, altered mental status, cough, presence of buboes. **Septicemic (10–15%):** Fevers, chills, nausea, vomiting, diarrhea, DIC, acrocyanosis, purpura. **Pneumonic (1%):** Cough with blood-tinged sputum; bilateral alveolar infiltrates on CXR. | Presence of the organism in bubo aspiration; ⊕ cultures of blood, bubo aspirate, sputum, and CXR; fourfold rise in antibody titers. | Isolation; streptomycin +/− chloramphenicol (in patients with meningitis or hemodynamic instability). |

TABLE 18.6. **Effects of Exposure to Biological Agents (continued)**

| AGENT | DESCRIPTION | SYMPTOMS/EXAM | DIAGNOSIS | TREATMENT |
|---|---|---|---|---|
| Tularemia (*Francisella tularensis*) | A gram-$\ominus$, nonmotile, intracellular coccobacillus causing a zoonotic disease spread by the tick bites of an infected animal (usually a rabbit). | **Ulceroglandular (75%):** Fever, localized skin or mucous membrane ulceration, regional lymphadenopathy > 1 cm, cough, malaise. **Typhoidal (25%):** Fever, cough, shortness of breath, malaise, hemoptysis. | $\oplus$ cultures of blood, sputum, ulcers, pharyngeal and conjunctival exudates, and gastric washings; $\oplus$ ELISA or bacterial agglutination. | Streptomycin (drug of choice), gentamicin, tetracycline, chloramphenicol. |
| Q fever (*Coxiella burnetii*) | A rickettsia-like organism with high infectivity causing illnesses in livestock and the humans who are exposed to them. | May present acutely or insidiously. Fever, chills, headache, diaphoresis, malaise, fatigue, anorexia, pneumonia, acute hepatitis, heart failure, clubbing, and splenomegaly in acute endocarditis. | $\oplus$ serologic studies (ELISA is the most sensitive method). | Tetracycline (drug of choice), erythromycin, azithromycin. |
| Botulism (*Clostridium botulinum*) | An anaerobic, gram-$\oplus$, spore-forming bacillus that produces toxins causing neuromuscular blockade. | Diplopia, mydriasis, ptosis, dysphagia, dysphonia, muscle weakness, symmetric descending flaccid paralysis, cranial nerve palsies, respiratory failure. | $\oplus$ ELISA analysis of nasal swabs. | Trivalent antitoxin, supportive care, botulinum immunization. |
| Smallpox (variola) | A highly infectious member of the poxvirus family that is spread to humans by aerosol. | High fever, headache, rigors, vomiting, malaise, abdominal pain, altered mental status, synchronous exanthem with a centrifugal distribution. | Demonstration of virions on electron microscopy of vesicular scrapings; $\oplus$ silver stain or gel diffusion test. | Respiratory isolation, supportive treatment, prophylaxis with smallpox vaccine. |
| Ricin | Plant protein toxin derived from beans of the castor plant. | **Inhalation:** Sudden onset of nasopharyngeal congestion, nausea, vomiting, urticaria, chest tightness, and respiratory distress. **Ingestion:** Less toxic due to poor absorption; nausea, vomiting, diarrhea, fever, cramps, hematochezia, shock. | $\oplus$ ELISA analysis of nasal swab sample; bilateral infiltrates on CXR. | Supportive treatment; activated charcoal and gastric lavage. |

EMERGENCY/URGENT CARE

Failure to respond to the external environment in an appropriate manner despite verbal or physical stimulation. Altered mental status, which may range from delirium to coma, consists of an impairment of arousal or consciousness and is estimated to prompt 25% of all acute visits among the elderly population. Because the differential diagnosis is far-reaching, it is helpful to consider altered mental status in the context of multiple different systems, as listed in Table 18.7.

### SYMPTOMS/EXAM

Presentation depends on the underlying disorder, but almost all patients exhibit disorientation, confusion, irritability, fluctuating levels of consciousness, mental slowing, agitation, and inattention.

### DIAGNOSIS

- Generally diagnosed through comprehensive history and physical exam, including the Mini-Mental Status Exam to assess cognitive function and to rule out dementia.
- **Routine laboratory testing:** Comprehensive chemistry panel, LFTs, TFTs, ABGs, CBC, blood cultures, UA, LP, and toxicology screen.
- **Imaging studies:** EEG, CT, MRI, CXR, ECG.
- Figure 18.2 shows an algorithm for assessing altered mental status.

### TREATMENT

- The first priorities include stabilization and reversal of acutely life-threatening conditions, followed by correction of the underlying problem.
- General principles include discontinuation of medications that may exacerbate the problem; establishment of a comfortable, nonthreatening environment with adequate nursing; fluid resuscitation; and behavioral control with medications (haloperidol, risperidone) or physical restraints (should not substitute for a diagnostic workup).

TABLE 18.7. **Causes of Altered Mental Status**

| | ETIOLOGIES | SYMPTOMS/TREATMENT |
|---|---|---|
| Drugs | 1. Intoxication or withdrawal from alcohol, sedative-hypnotics, analgesics, psychedelic drugs, stimulants, household solvents, or corticosteroids.<br>2. Anticholinergic drugs, antidepressants, $H_2$ blockers, digoxin, salicylates (chronic use), antiemetics, antiparkinsonian agents, muscle relaxants, polypharmacy. | See the sections on toxicology and intoxication/withdrawal for further details. |
| Metabolic | 1. Electrolyte imbalance (hypo-/hypernatremia, hypercalcemia, hypo-/hypermagnesemia)<br>2. Thyroid dysfunction<br>3. Hypo-/hyperglycemia<br>4. Renal failure (uremia)<br>5. Hepatic encephalopathy<br>6. Wernicke's encephalopathy<br>7. Nutritional deficiencies: vitamin $B_1$ (beriberi), vitamin $B_{12}$ (pernicious anemia), folic acid, nicotinic acid (pellagra)<br>8. Seizures or postictal states<br>9. Hypercapnea<br>10. Hypoxia | 1–3. Correction of underlying abnormality<br>4. Hemodialysis<br>5. Lactulose<br>6. Thiamine<br>7. Nutritional supplementation<br>8. Anticonvulsant therapy<br>9. Assisted ventilation<br>10. $O_2$ supplementation |
| Vascular | 1. Hypertensive encephalopathy<br>2. Arrhythmias (may → diminished $O_2$ delivery to the brain)<br>3. Stroke/TIA<br>4. Thrombotic thrombocytopenic purpura<br>5. CNS vasculitis<br>6. Subarachnoid hemorrhage | 1. BP control to DBP < 100<br>2. Antiarrhythmic agents or cardioversion<br>3. Evaluation for embolic source +/− anticoagulation<br>4. Plasma exchange transfusion +/− prednisone, immunosuppressants, aspirin<br>5. Steroids, immunosuppressants<br>6. Surgical drainage +/− clipping |
| Infectious | 1. Meningitis, encephalitis<br>2. Bacteremia, UTI, pneumonia<br>3. AIDS, neurosyphilis | 1–3. Treatment of underlying infection |
| Structural | 1. Space-occupying lesion (tumor, may be 1° malignancy or metastatic)<br>2. Hydrocephalus<br>3. Subdural hematoma | 1. Surgical decompression, radiation therapy, chemotherapy<br>2. Ventriculoperitoneal shunt<br>3. Craniotomy and evacuation |
| Neuropsychiatric | 1. Sundowning<br>2. Schizophrenia, depression<br>3. Alzheimer's disease, parkinsonism, Huntington's chorea, Pick's disease | 1. Antipsychotics (e.g., haloperidol)<br>2. Psychiatric medications<br>3. Neurologic medications as indicated |
| Environmental | 1. Hypo-/hyperthermia<br>2. ICU psychosis | 1. Maintenance of euthermia<br>2. Normal sleep-wake cycle, calm environment +/− sedatives |

EMERGENCY/URGENT CARE

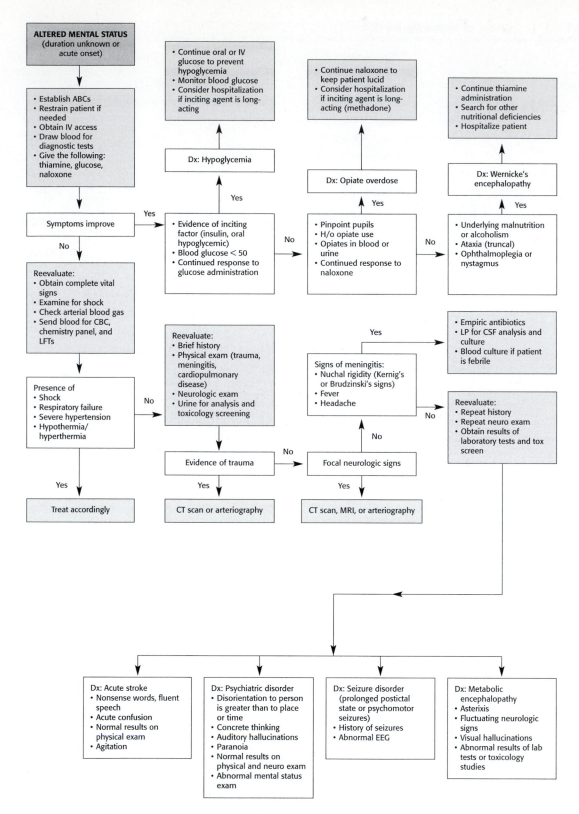

**FIGURE 18.2.** **Algorithm for the assessment of altered mental status.**

(Adapted, with permission, from Stone CK, Humphries RL. *Current Emergency Diagnosis & Treatment*, 6th ed. New York: Mc-Graw-Hill, 2006: Figure 20-1.)

A common chief complaint seen in the ER or urgent care setting; can be due to a multitude of benign or malignant etiologies. Structural headaches caused by head trauma that → space-occupying hematomas and elevation of ICP are considered neurosurgical emergencies and warrant immediate diagnosis and intervention.

## Epidural Hematoma

An accumulation of blood in the potential space between the dura and bone due to disruption of interposed vessels. Intracranial epidural hematomas are considered the most serious complication of head injury and are most commonly due to tearing of the middle meningeal artery. They are associated with skull fractures in 85–95% of adult cases.

### SYMPTOMS

Headache, nausea, vomiting, seizures, focal neurologic deficits occurring within hours of the injury.

### EXAM

- Directed toward the evaluation of traumatic sequelae and associated neurologic deficits.
- Findings include bradycardia and/or hypertension due to ↑ ICP, anisocoria, skull fractures or lacerations, CSF rhinorrhea or otorrhea, hemotympanum, altered mental status, facial nerve injury, and vertebral column instability.

### DIAGNOSIS

- Noncontrast head CT shows a hyperdense, lens-shaped mass between the brain and skull (see Figure 18.3).
- Conventional angiography, MRA, or CT angiography may be used to confirm the presence of an underlying vascular malformation.

### TREATMENT

- As with all traumatic injuries, establishment of the ABCs with immobilization of the spine is the first priority.
- Additional measures include correction of any coexisting coagulopathy; osmotic diuretics; hyperventilation to achieve a $Pco_2$ of 28–32 mmHg; and elevation of the head of the bed to 30 degrees for patients with ↑ ICP.
- Systemic arterial blood pressure control; isotonic fluids; seizure treatment or prophylaxis.
- Although conservative management may be a reasonable option in mild cases, craniotomy followed by evacuation of the hematoma is the definitive treatment.

### COMPLICATIONS

Post-traumatic seizures, postconcussion syndrome, neurologic deficits, death.

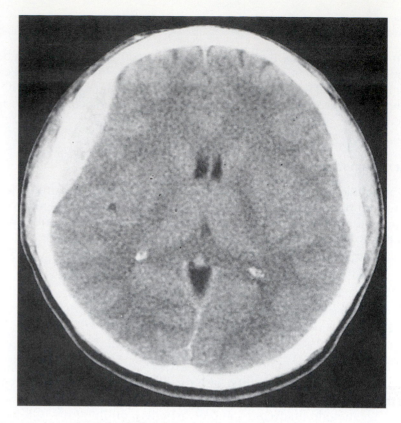

**FIGURE 18.3.** **Classic lenticular-shaped epidural hematoma.**

(Reproduced, with permission, from Kasper DL et al. *Harrison's Principles of Internal Medicine,* 16th ed. New York: McGraw-Hill, 2005: 2450.)

## Subdural Hematoma

A collection of venous blood below the inner layer of the dura but external to the brain and arachnoid membrane. Usually caused by blunt head trauma that → disruption of bridging veins; more frequently found in patients > 60 years of age. If left untreated, acute subdural hematomas can progress to subacute (3–7 days after injury) and chronic (2–3 weeks after injury) stages. Alcoholics, hemophiliacs, and patients on chronic anticoagulation therapy are considered at risk in light of their ↑ risk of bleeding.

### SYMPTOMS/EXAM

- Presents with headache, loss of consciousness, mental status changes, and a history of blunt head trauma.
- Exam reveals impaired mental status, focal neurologic deficits, and a Glasgow Coma Scale (GCS) score of < 15.

### DIFFERENTIAL

Child or elder abuse, epidural hematoma, meningitis, stroke, SAH, dementia.

### DIAGNOSIS

- Noncontrast head CT shows a hyperdense crescentic mass along the inner table of the skull, most commonly in the parietal region (see Figure 18.4).
- Contrast-enhanced CT or MRI is recommended for imaging 48–72 hours after head injury.

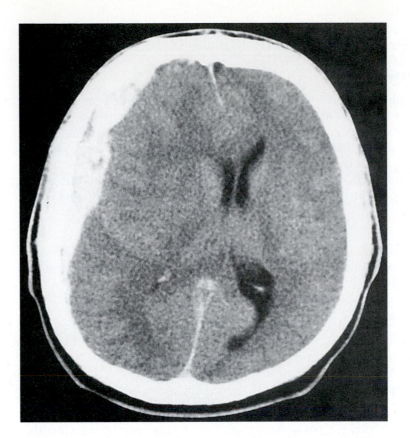

**FIGURE 18.4.** **Hyperdense, crescent-shaped subdural hematoma with midline shift.**

(Reproduced, with permission, from Kasper DL et al. *Harrison's Principles of Internal Medicine*, 16th ed. New York: McGraw-Hill, 2005: 2450.)

### TREATMENT

- Consider endotracheal intubation in patients with a GCS score of < 10 to guarantee airway protection.
- Additional measures include correction of any coexisting coagulopathy; elevation of the head of the bed to 30 degrees for patients with ↑ ICP; and, if the patient is intubated, mild hyperventilation to achieve a $P_{CO_2}$ of approximately 30 mmHg.
- Systemic arterial blood pressure control; isotonic fluids; seizure treatment or prophylaxis.
- Conservative management may be sufficient for small, asymptomatic subdural hematomas, but patients with focal findings or midline shift require craniotomy and evacuation.
- Burr holes are a temporizing option before definitive surgery if herniation syndrome is evident.

### COMPLICATIONS

↑ ICP, brain edema, recurrent hematoma, infection, seizures.

## Subarachnoid Hemorrhage (SAH)

The presence of blood within the subarachnoid space resulting from a pathologic process, usually rupture of a berry aneurysm or an AVM. SAH carries a significant risk of morbidity and mortality and is commonly associated with uncontrolled hypertension, smoking, alcohol use, and cerebral AVMs.

### SYMPTOMS

- Sudden onset of a severe headache (described as a "thunderclap" headache or "the worst headache of my life") that may be accompanied by loss of consciousness, nausea and vomiting, focal neurologic deficits, signs of meningeal irritation such as neck stiffness or low back pain, photophobia, and seizure activity.
- Prodromal symptoms from minor blood leakage ("sentinel" headache) are reported in 30–50% of aneurysmal SAHs and are not due to ↑ ICP.

### EXAM

Exam reveals global or focal neurologic abnormalities, syndromes of cranial nerve compression, seizures, papilledema, retinal hemorrhages, ↑ BP, and tachycardia.

### DIFFERENTIAL

Encephalitis, hypertensive emergency, meningitis, stroke, TIA, temporal arteritis, tension/migraine/cluster headache.

### DIAGNOSIS

- Noncontrast head CT is most sensitive within 24 hours after the event and shows SAH with or without evidence of associated hydrocephalus.
- If CT is ⊖, LP should be performed to look for the presence of RBCs and xanthochromia in the CSF.
- Cerebral angiography, CT angiography, or MRA may be used to evaluate the vascular anatomy and localize the site of the bleed.

### TREATMENT

- Stabilize the patient and establish the ABCs, avoiding sedation if possible.
- Additional measures include osmotic diuretics; elevation of the head of the bed to 30 degrees to ↓ ICP in patients with signs of herniation; and, if the patient is intubated, mild hyperventilation to achieve a $P_{CO_2}$ of approximately 30 mmHg.
- Systemic arterial blood pressure control to keep mean arterial pressure < 130; seizure prophylaxis; calcium channel blockers (nimodipine) to ↓ cerebral vasospasm; isotonic fluids.
- Ventriculostomy placement to address coexisting hydrocephalus.
- Definitive treatment involves surgical clipping or endovascular treatment (coiling) of the ruptured berry aneurysm.

### COMPLICATIONS

Hydrocephalus, rebleeding, intraventricular or intracerebral hemorrhage, cerebral ischemia, hyponatremia from cerebral salt wasting, hypothalamic dysfunction, seizures, ↑ ICP, neurologic deficits, death.

## Increased Intracranial Pressure

- A pathologic state that indicates an ↑ in the normal brain pressure (8–18 mmHg in adults); often caused by intracranial hematomas or cerebral edema. Can → midline shift of brain structures and herniation syndrome, all → an ischemic cascade that may eventually end in death.

- Common etiologies include severe head injury, epidural hematoma, subdural hematoma, hydrocephalus, brain tumor, hypertensive hemorrhage, intraventricular hemorrhage, meningitis, encephalitis, SAH, status epilepticus, and stroke.
- **Sx:** Nausea, vomiting, headache, mental status changes.
- **Exam/Dx:** Papilledema on funduscopic exam, papillary dilation, global neurologic abnormalities, ↑ opening pressure on LP, Cushing's response (hypertension and bradycardia), respiratory changes.
- **Tx:** Removal of the underlying cause. Temporizing measures include osmotic diuretics (mannitol); adequate analgesia; elevation of the head of the bed to 30 degrees; and, if the patient is intubated, mild hyperventilation to achieve a $P_{CO_2}$ of roughly 30 mmHg.
- **Cx:** Permanent neurologic deficits, death.

## CHEST PAIN

A common chief complaint seen in the ER or urgent care setting; can be due to many benign or serious etiologies that are differentiated mostly through a history and physical along with careful assessment of risk factors. Additional studies may be performed to supplement and/or confirm the diagnosis.

### Aortic Dissection

Most common in men > 60 years of age. Uncontrolled hypertension is the most important risk factor; less common associations include Marfan's syndrome, congenital bicuspid aortic valves, aortic coarctation, pregnancy, and cocaine use.

#### SYMPTOMS

- Presents with sudden, tearing pain felt in the anterior chest (ascending dissection) or posterior chest (descending dissection), neck, throat, or jaw.
- May be associated with syncope, CVA symptoms, CHF, MI, or abdominal pain.

#### EXAM

Exam reveals hypertension or hypotension, asymmetrical pulses, asymmetrical BP, syncope, altered mental status, dyspnea, dysphagia, a new diastolic murmur, and findings suggestive of cardiac tamponade.

#### DIFFERENTIAL

Myocardial ischemia, pericarditis, pulmonary embolus, aortic regurgitation, aortic aneurysm, musculoskeletal pain, mediastinal tumors, pleuritis, cholecystitis, PUD, acute pancreatitis, acute coronary syndrome.

#### DIAGNOSIS

- Diagnosed by clinical symptoms suggestive of aortic dissection, mediastinal widening on CXR, variation in pulse (absence of a proximal extremity pulse), and a BP difference of > 20 mmHg between the right and left arm.
- Thoracic MRI or CT, transesophageal echocardiography (TEE), aortography.

### TREATMENT

- Admit to the ICU and administer medications to ↓ cardiac contractility and control systemic arterial pressure (nitroprusside, β-blockers, calcium channel blockers).
- Ascending aortic dissections are treated with immediate surgical correction, whereas surgery for descending aortic dissections is indicated only in patients with persistent pain, aneurysmal dilation > 5 cm, end-organ ischemia, or evidence of retrograde dissection to the ascending aorta.

### COMPLICATIONS

MI, stroke, pericardial tamponade, claudication, compressive symptoms, acute aortic regurgitation, aortic rupture, aneurysmal dilation, mesenteric or renal ischemia, death.

## Myocardial Infarction (MI)

Rapid development of myocardial necrosis caused by an imbalance between myocardial $O_2$ supply and demand. Usually results from plaque rupture with thrombus formation in a coronary vessel. Considered part of the acute coronary syndrome spectrum that includes ST-segment-elevation MI (STEMI), non-ST-segment-elevation MI (NSTEMI), and unstable angina.

### SYMPTOMS

Presents with prolonged substernal pressure radiating to the left arm or neck associated with nausea, vomiting, diaphoresis, or dyspnea. However, some patients, especially women or diabetics, may present atypically with only nausea, dyspnea, or neck pain.

### EXAM

Exam reveals hypotension or hypertension, cool and clammy skin, systolic murmur (if valvular defects develop), S4, and signs of CHF.

### DIFFERENTIAL

Cardiac ischemia without infarction, aortic dissection, aortic stenosis, cholecystitis, esophageal spasm, esophagitis, gastritis, GERD, pneumothorax, pulmonary embolism, acute pericarditis, anxiety disorder, pneumonia, pancreatitis.

### DIAGNOSIS

- ↑ cardiac enzymes measured serially over a 24-hour period (CK-MB and troponin are most specific).
- ECG; echocardiogram showing wall motion abnormalities; myocardial perfusion imaging or cardiac angiography showing ↓ blood flow to portions of the myocardium.

### TREATMENT

- Antiplatelet therapy with aspirin and/or clopidogrel; β-blockers; nitrates (contraindicated in RV infarction, hypotension, and phosphodiesterase inhibitor use within the last 24 hours).
- Morphine for pain control; supplemental $O_2$; ACEIs within the first 24 hours of STEMI in the absence of hypotension and as long-term therapy if

LV dysfunction is present; angiotensin receptor blockers if left if LV dysfunction is present and the patient and patient is intolerant of ACEIs.

- Glycoprotein IIb/IIIa receptor antagonists and heparin are appropriate in patients with continuing ischemia and in whom percutaneous intervention (PCI) is planned.
- Thrombolytic therapy is appropriate in patients with ST-segment elevation, new left bundle branch block, or anterior ST-segment depression consistent with posterior infarction if presenting within 12 hours of onset of symptoms and if PCI is not readily available within 90 minutes.
- PCI is considered the treatment of choice assuming a door-to-needle time of < 90 minutes.
- Coronary artery bypass graft (CABG) surgery is appropriate for patients who fail PCI or who develop mechanical complications.

### COMPLICATIONS

Arrhythmias, recurrent ischemia, CHF, cardiogenic shock, acute valvular abnormalities, pericarditis, ventricular aneurysms, mural thrombi, hypertension.

## ABDOMINAL PAIN

### Appendicitis

Acute inflammation of the vermiform appendix.

### SYMPTOMS

Presents with abdominal pain, initially periumbilical and then migrating to the RLQ, along with anorexia, nausea, and vomiting.

### EXAM

Exam reveals low-grade fever, maximal tenderness at McBurney's point, Rovsing's sign, psoas sign, and obturator sign. Peritoneal signs (guarding and rebound tenderness) are seen in appendiceal perforation; inability to jump up and down is a fairly sensitive test for peritonitis.

### DIFFERENTIAL

Cholecystitis, biliary colic, constipation, diverticular disease, gastroenteritis, mesenteric ischemia, IBD, endometriosis, ovarian cysts or torsion, intussusception, PID.

### DIAGNOSIS

- Generally diagnosed clinically, as lab studies are not specific for appendicitis.
- Look for leukocytosis, mild pyuria, and ↑ inflammatory markers.
- Abdominal ultrasound; CT scan with IV, oral, or rectal contrast.

### TREATMENT

Appendectomy with antibiotic treatment until the patient is afebrile and the WBC count normalizes.

### COMPLICATIONS

Although the prognosis is usually excellent, wound infections, abscess formation, persistent ileus, or cecal fistulas can occur.

## Ischemic Bowel

Also called mesenteric ischemia; caused by a ↓ in intestinal blood flow, usually arising from occlusion, vasospasm, or hypoperfusion of the mesenteric vasculature. It can be categorized as acute or chronic based on the rapidity and degree to which blood flow is impaired. Clinical consequences of acute mesenteric ischemia can be catastrophic, making rapid diagnosis and treatment imperative. Risk factors include advanced age, atherosclerosis, low cardiac output states, cardiac arrhythmias, recent MI, severe cardiac valvular disease, and intra-abdominal malignancy.

### SYMPTOMS

- Rapid onset of severe periumbilical pain out of proportion to findings on the physical exam.
- Nausea, vomiting, anorexia, and diarrhea progressing to obstipation.
- Presentation may be more insidious in patients with chronic mesenteric ischemia or in those with thrombotic causes, vasculitis, or nonocclusive ischemia.
- Colonic (vs. small bowel) ischemia is usually associated with hematochezia and less pain.

### EXAM

- Exam may initially be normal or may reveal only mild abdominal distention or occult blood in the stool.
- As ischemia progresses and infarction occurs, peritoneal signs develop and a feculent odor to the breath may be noted.

### DIFFERENTIAL

Abdominal abscess, abdominal aneurysm, aortic dissection, appendicitis, biliary disease, diverticular disease, ectopic pregnancy, MI, pancreatitis, renal calculi, acute intermittent porphyria, bowel obstruction.

### DIAGNOSIS

- Accurate diagnosis depends on a high index of suspicion in patients with known risk factors, since early signs are nonspecific and definitive diagnosis often requires invasive testing.
- Often associated with leukocytosis and metabolic acidosis.
- Angiography, although invasive, remains the gold standard.
- MRA, CT angiography, or duplex sonography may also be considered.

### TREATMENT

- The goal of treatment is to restore intestinal blood flow as rapidly as possible. Measures include the following:
  - Aggressive hemodynamic monitoring and support, correction of metabolic acidosis, initiation of broad-spectrum antibiotics, and placement of an NG tube for gastric decompression.
  - Systemic anticoagulation to prevent thrombus formation or propagation unless contraindicated.
- Medical treatment with close observation may be considered for patients who lack peritoneal signs and who have good mesenteric blood flow as demonstrated by angiography.
- Intra-arterial vasodilators or thrombolytic agents, angioplasty, stent placement, embolectomy, or exploratory laparotomy with resection of necrotic bowel may be necessary if indicated.

### COMPLICATIONS

Bowel necrosis, septic shock, death.

## Ruptured Abdominal Aortic Aneurysm (AAA)

A degenerative process of the abdominal aorta often attributed to atherosclerosis → focal dilation with at least a 50% ↑ over normal arterial diameter. An estimated 65% of patients with ruptured AAAs die from sudden cardiovascular collapse before arriving at a hospital.

### SYMPTOMS

- Presents with sudden onset of abdominal, back, or flank pain associated with hypotension, tachycardia, or temporary loss of consciousness.
- Symptoms may be milder if the rupture is contained.

### EXAM

Exam reveals hypotension, tachycardia, the presence of an abdominal bruit, or a pulsatile abdominal mass.

### DIFFERENTIAL

Appendicitis, biliary disease, diverticular disease, gastritis, PUD, MI, bowel obstruction or infarction, pancreatitis, URI, nephrolithiasis.

### DIAGNOSIS

Abdominal CT or MRI is considered most sensitive. Angiography is no longer routinely recommended.

### TREATMENT

Initial management includes hemodynamic support, blood transfusions, and immediate consultation for surgical repair.

### COMPLICATIONS

Hemorrhage; death from exsanguination.

## ANAPHYLAXIS

A severe allergic reaction involving more than one organ system; caused by the release of mediators from mast cells and basophils. An anaphylactic reaction occurs through an immunologic mechanism involving prior sensitization to an allergen with later re-exposure, with symptoms ranging from urticaria to angioedema with hypotension and bronchospasm (see Table 18.8).

### SYMPTOMS

- Urticaria (hives), flushing, conjunctival and/or cutaneous pruritus, angioedema, warmth, nasal congestion, rhinorrhea, dyspnea, throat tightness, wheezing, weakness, dizziness, chest pain, palpitations, nausea and vomiting (particularly in cases of food allergy).
- Symptoms usually begin within 5–30 minutes of allergen exposure, although in rare cases symptom onset can be delayed for several hours.

### EXAM

Although exam findings depend on the affected organ systems and on the severity of the attack, common findings include nonpitting angioedema, hoarseness, wheezing, stridor, hypoxia, tachycardia, hypotension, flushing, urticaria, frank cardiovascular collapse, and respiratory arrest.

### DIFFERENTIAL

Angioedema, anxiety, asthma, conversion disorder, carcinoid syndrome, epiglottitis, tracheal foreign bodies, MI, pulmonary embolism, idiopathic urticaria.

### DIAGNOSIS

- Diagnosed on the basis of the clinical history and exam; does not rely on laboratory testing.
- Skin testing and/or in vitro IgE testing may aid in the confirmation of clinical reactivity.

### TREATMENT

- As with all medical emergencies, initial stabilization and establishment of the ABCs are crucial.
- Removal of the antigen source or tourniquet placement on the extremity with the antigen source (do not leave in place > 30 minutes) followed by immediate administration of IM epinephrine into a different extremity.
- Adjuvant medications include antihistamines (both $H_1$ and $H_2$ blockers), inhaled β-agonists, corticosteroids (to prevent late-phase reactions), and IV fluids for BP support.
- In cases of respiratory failure, endotracheal intubation, cricothyrotomy, or tracheotomy may be required.

TABLE 18.8. **Common Classes of Allergens Causing Anaphylaxis**

| ALLERGEN | COMMON OFFENDERS | SYMPTOMS/DIAGNOSIS |
| --- | --- | --- |
| Medications | Penicillin and cephalosporin antibiotics (most common). IV radiocontrast media; aspirin and NSAIDs. | May occur without a prior history of drug exposure. Desensitization or prophylactic pretreatment protocols may be instituted if there is no alternative to the particular allergenic medication. |
| Foods | Tree nuts, legumes, fish and shellfish, milk, soy, eggs. | Quite common and usually limited to mild GI symptoms, although full-blown anaphylaxis can occur. |
| Bites/stings | Insect stings (*Hymenoptera* venom). | Local reactions and urticaria are much more common than full-blown anaphylactic reactions. Consider referral to an allergist for desensitization or a treatment kit with epinephrine and oral antihistamines for patients with a history of anaphylaxis or generalized urticaria following insect stings. |
| Latex | Surgical gloves, Foley catheters. | Reactions are usually cutaneous or involve the mucous membranes, although anaphylactic reactions can occur. |

An algorithm used to treat adult cardiopulmonary arrest. ACLS requires knowledge of basic life support and the use of advanced equipment and techniques for establishing effective ventilation and circulation, including airway management, establishment of IV access, arrhythmia recognition, and use of medications for cardiac and respiratory arrest. Four rhythms produce cardiac arrest: ventricular fibrillation (VF), unstable ventricular tachycardia (VT), pulseless electrical activity (PEA), and asystole. Figures 18.5 and 18.6 show the guidelines for basic life support and the management of cardiac arrest in adults.

## Airway Management

Adequate ventilation and oxygenation are crucial for the survival of cardiopulmonary arrest victims, beginning with proper airway-opening techniques such as head tilt and chin lift, or jaw thrust if trauma is suspected. Bag-mask ventilation should be started immediately, with the use of oropharyngeal or nasopharyngeal airway adjuncts as necessary.

An advanced airway (endotracheal tube, Combitube, or laryngeal mask airway) may be considered in patients in whom bag-mask ventilation is inadequate or in prolonged resuscitative efforts. In such cases, it is crucial to confirm tube placement with both clinical assessment and the use of confirmatory devices such as exhaled $CO_2$ detectors or esophageal detector devices.

Rapid-sequence intubation (see Table 18.9) should be attempted only in patients in whom control of the airway is certain, since the patient will be paralyzed and unable to breathe. Indications include respiratory failure, acute intracranial lesions, some drug overdoses, status epilepticus, and combative trauma patients.

TABLE 18.9. Rapid-Sequence Intubation

| PREPARATION | INDUCTION | PARALYSIS | INTUBATION |
|---|---|---|---|
| ■ Preoxygenation, IV lines, monitor, oximetry, equipment. <br> ■ Lidocaine 1–2 mg/kg (100 mg usual adult dose)—may be omitted in non-head-injury cases. <br> ■ Atropine 0.01 mg/kg (0.5 mg usual adult dose)—may be omitted if bradycardia is absent or if the patient is > 8 years of age. <br> ■ Sellick maneuver (cricothyroid pressure to prevent vomiting and aspiration). | ■ Etomidate 0.3 mg/kg (20 mg usual adult dose), **or** <br> ■ Midazolam 0.1 mg/kg (7 mg usual adult dose). | ■ Succinylcholine 1.5 mg (100 mg usual adult dose), **or** <br> ■ Rocuronium 0.6–1.2 mg/kg (70 mg usual adult dose), **or** <br> ■ Vecuronium 0.1 mg/kg (10 mg usual adult dose). | ■ Endotracheal tube, laryngeal mask airway, or Combitube. <br> ■ Approximate endotracheal tube size for children = (age/4) + 4. <br> ■ Confirm tube placement after intubation. |

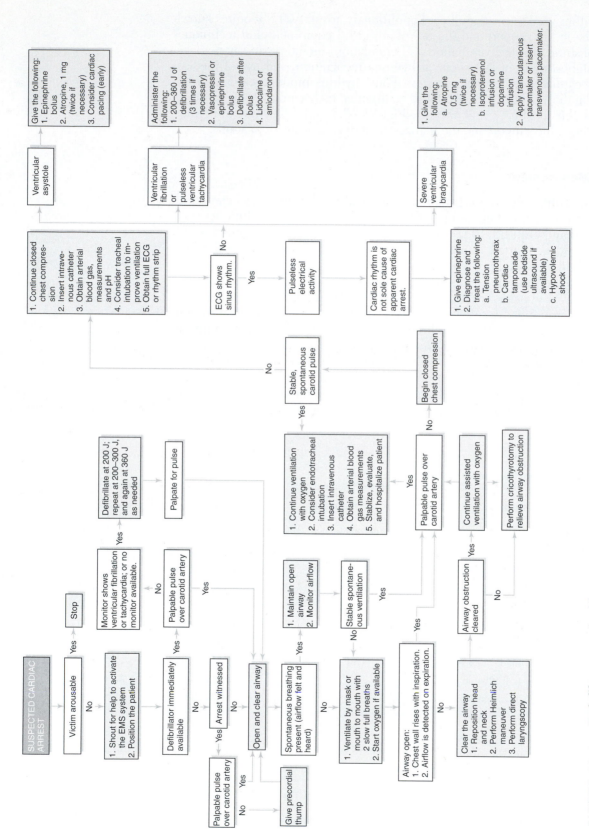

**FIGURE 18.5. Basic life support algorithm.**

(Reproduced, with permission, from Stone CK et al. *Current Emergency Diagnosis & Treatment*, 5th ed. New York: McGraw-Hill, 2004: 148.)

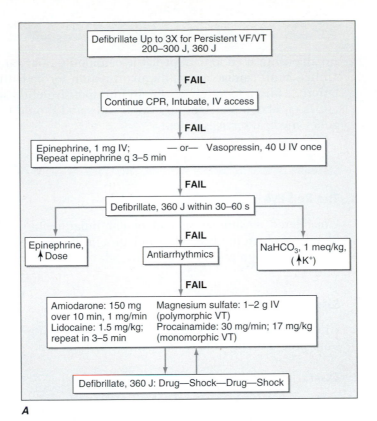

**FIGURE 18.6.** Ventricular fibrillation and pulseless ventricular tachycardia algorithm.

(Reproduced, with permission, from Kasper DL et al. *Harrison's Principles of Internal Medicine,* 16th ed. New York: McGraw-Hill, 2005: 1623.)

## PEDIATRIC ADVANCED LIFE SUPPORT (PALS)

An algorithm used to treat pediatric cardiopulmonary arrest (see Figure 18.7). Unlike adult cardiac arrest, the main reason for pediatric arrest is respiratory failure. Thus, a lone rescuer for an unresponsive child should begin with five cycles of 30 compressions and two breaths and should then activate the emergency medical services system.

## OCULAR DISORDERS

### The Red Eye

Considered a cardinal sign of ocular inflammation; caused by dilation of blood vessels in the eye. The etiologies of the red eye are multiple, but most cases are benign and may be managed effectively by the primary care physician.

*The following symptoms occur in ocular emergencies and warrant immediate ophthalmologic consultation:*

- *Severe pain or photophobia*
- *Systemic symptoms (fever, nausea/vomiting)*
- *Acute changes in vision*

#### SYMPTOMS

Clinical manifestations depend on the underlying etiology but may range from mild discomfort to severe pain with vision loss.

#### EXAM

- Eyelid inspection; visual acuity testing; examination for extraocular movements, pupil shape and reactivity, photophobia, presence of pain, and discharge; eversion of the upper lid to look for foreign body; fluorescein exam. A thorough exam is best done after application of topical anesthetic drops.
- If available, slit-lamp examination of the cornea, anterior chamber evaluation, ophthalmoscopy, and intraocular pressure measurements can facilitate diagnosis.

#### DIFFERENTIAL

Blepharitis, chemical burns, orbital or preseptal cellulitis, chalazion or hordeolum, conjunctivitis (allergic, bacterial, viral, and giant papillary types), corneal abrasion, corneal erosion, foreign body, dacryocystitis, dry eye syndrome, ectropion, entropion, endophthalmitis, episcleritis, iritis, acute angle-closure glaucoma, HSV, herpes zoster, pterygium, subconjunctival hemorrhage.

#### DIAGNOSIS

Usually diagnosed by clinical history and exam.

#### TREATMENT

Depends on the underlying disease process.

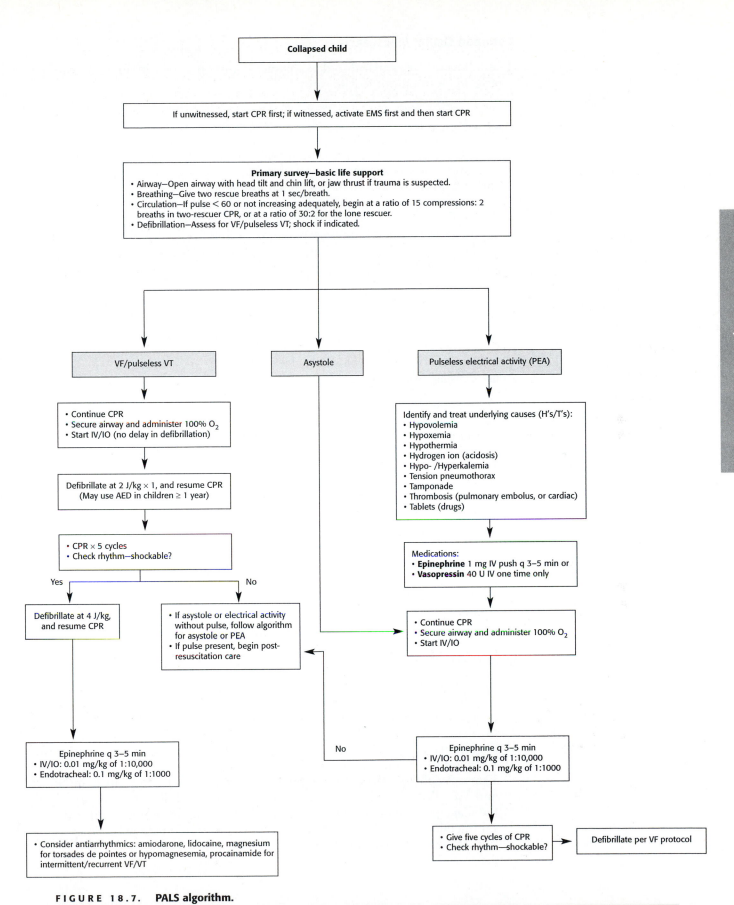

**Collapsed child**

If unwitnessed, start CPR first; if witnessed, activate EMS first and then start CPR

**Primary survey—basic life support**
- Airway—Open airway with head tilt and chin lift, or jaw thrust if trauma is suspected.
- Breathing—Give two rescue breaths at 1 sec/breath.
- Circulation—If pulse < 60 or not increasing adequately, begin at a ratio of 15 compressions: 2 breaths in two-rescuer CPR, or at a ratio of 30:2 for the lone rescuer.
- Defibrillation—Assess for VF/pulseless VT; shock if indicated.

**VF/pulseless VT**

**Asystole**

**Pulseless electrical activity (PEA)**

- Continue CPR
- Secure airway and administer 100% $O_2$
- Start IV/IO (no delay in defibrillation)

Defibrillate at 2 J/kg × 1, and resume CPR (May use AED in children ≥ 1 year)

- CPR × 5 cycles
- Check rhythm—shockable?

Yes                No

Defibrillate at 4 J/kg, and resume CPR

- If asystole or electrical activity without pulse, follow algorithm for asystole or PEA
- If pulse present, begin post-resuscitation care

Identify and treat underlying causes (H's/T's):
- Hypovolemia
- Hypoxemia
- Hypothermia
- Hydrogen ion (acidosis)
- Hypo- /Hyperkalemia
- Tension pneumothorax
- Tamponade
- Thrombosis (pulmonary embolus, or cardiac)
- Tablets (drugs)

Medications:
- **Epinephrine** 1 mg IV push q 3–5 min or
- **Vasopressin** 40 U IV one time only

- Continue CPR
- Secure airway and administer 100% $O_2$
- Start IV/IO

No

Epinephrine q 3–5 min
- IV/IO: 0.01 mg/kg of 1:10,000
- Endotracheal: 0.1 mg/kg of 1:1000

Epinephrine q 3–5 min
- IV/IO: 0.01 mg/kg of 1:10,000
- Endotracheal: 0.1 mg/kg of 1:1000

- Consider antiarrhythmics: amiodarone, lidocaine, magnesium for torsades de pointes or hypomagnesemia, procainamide for intermittent/recurrent VF/VT

- Give five cycles of CPR
- Check rhythm—shockable?

Defibrillate per VF protocol

**FIGURE 18.7.** **PALS algorithm.**

## Common Ocular Emergencies

The following are ocular disorders that are commonly seen in an acute care setting and warrant immediate care.

### ORBITAL CELLULITIS

- A potentially devastating infection that can rapidly progress to blindness, meningitis, or death. Most cases develop from the direct spread of untreated sinusitis. Considered an **ocular emergency.**
- **Sx:** Erythema, eye pain, fever, photophobia, chemosis, lid edema, visual loss.
- **Exam:** Directed toward localizing the source of infection.
- **DDx:** Distinguished from preseptal or periorbital cellulitis by involvement of the orbit, which → chemosis, proptosis, or visual loss.
- **Dx:** Leukocytosis; ⊕ blood cultures; CT scan of the orbit, sinus, and head.
- **Tx:** IV antibiotics or antifungals; nasal decongestants; ophthalmologic or ENT consultation for possible surgical drainage.
- **Cx:** Visual loss, cavernous sinus thrombosis, brain abscess or meningitis, death.

### ANGLE-CLOSURE GLAUCOMA

- A rare condition in which the iris blocks the aqueous humor outflow tract when the pupil becomes mid-dilated, causing an abrupt ↑ in intraocular pressure. Susceptible eyes have a shallow anterior chamber (more common in patients of East Asian origin). Also known as acute narrow-angle glaucoma.
- Considered an **ocular emergency;** prompt treatment is essential to prevent permanent optic nerve damage and vision loss.
- **Sx:** Sudden onset of severe eye pain, blurred vision, nausea/vomiting, and headache.
- **Exam:** Shallow, occluded anterior chamber on gonioscopy; ↑ intraocular pressure; diffuse lacrimation; swollen optic disk; mid-dilated pupil (see Figure 18.8). May be precipitated by pupillary dilation.
- **Tx:** Topical agents to constrict the pupil and ↓ intraocular pressure until the patient can get laser iridotomy or surgical iridectomy.
- **Cx:** Visual loss.

### CORNEAL ABRASION

- Disruption in the integrity of the corneal epithelium, often as a result of external physical forces. Frequently caused by dry eye, foreign body injuries, and wearing of contact lenses. One of the most common, yet often overlooked, eye injuries.
- **Sx:** Eye pain, foreign body sensation, photophobia, tearing, history of traumatic injury or contact lens use.
- **Exam:** A defect in the corneal epithelium is seen with fluorescein staining and Wood's lamp. Slit-lamp examination is helpful but not necessary in the diagnosis of corneal abrasions. Also characterized by bulbar conjunctival injection, normal visual acuity, and possible foreign body seen on eversion of the eyelids (see Figure 18.9).

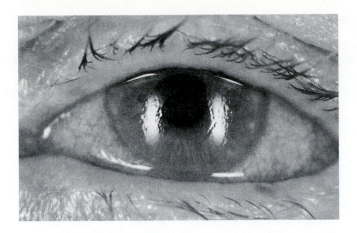

**FIGURE 18.8.** Angle-closure glaucoma.

(Reproduced, with permission, from Knoop KJ et al. *Atlas of Emergency Medicine,* 2nd ed. New York: McGraw-Hill, 2002: 49.) (Also see Color Insert.)

- **Tx:**
    - Local anesthetic +/− cycloplegic agents, tetanus immunization, topical antibiotics.
    - Ophthalmologic referral if a retained foreign body or corneal ulcer is suspected; follow up every two days until resolved.
    - Eye patching is no longer routinely recommended in view of the ↑ risk of infection, especially among contact lens wearers.
    - Systemic analgesics are preferred over local anesthetic drops for patient use in light of the potential for causing inadvertent damage to an insensate cornea.
- **Cx:** Usually minimal, although recurrent epithelial erosions or corneal ulcers may occur → permanent loss of visual acuity.

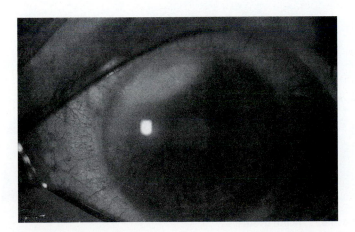

**FIGURE 18.9.** Corneal abrasion.

(Reproduced, with permission, from Knoop KJ et al. *Atlas of Emergency Medicine,* 2nd ed. New York: McGraw-Hill, 2002: 98.) (Also see Color Insert.)

### ACUTE UVEITIS

■ Inflammation of one or all parts of the uveal tract, including the iris and the anterior chamber (iritis), ciliary body (iridocyclitis), and posterior chamber (choroiditis or chorioretinitis) (see Figure 18.10).
■ **Sx:** Unilateral, painful red eye; blurred vision; tearing; photophobia.
■ **Exam:**
  ■ Perilimbal injection increasing toward the limbus (vs. conjunctivitis); normal or slightly ↓ visual acuity; direct and consensual photophobia; constricted pupils; normal or slightly ↓ intraocular pressure; keratitic precipitates, cells, or flare on slit-lamp exam.
  ■ The presence of associated conjunctivitis, urethritis, and polyarthritis suggests Reiter's syndrome.
■ **Dx:** No further workup is indicated for the first episode of simple acute uveitis, although bilateral, granulomatous, or recurrent uveitis merits a workup to exclude uncommon etiologies (CBC, ESR, ANA, RPR, PPD, CXR, Lyme titer).
■ **Tx:** Cycloplegics to ↓ pain and inflammation; ophthalmologic referral within 24 hours. Topical steroids should be initiated only by the consulting ophthalmologist.
■ **Cx:** An acute ↑ in intraocular pressure → optic nerve atrophy and permanent vision loss.

### ORBITAL FRACTURE

■ Fracture of any of the six facial bones comprising the orbit: the frontal bone, zygoma, maxilla, maxillary sinus, lacrimal bone, ethmoid bone, and sphenoid bone. Due to traumatic injuries, blowout fractures occur when a blow to the eye ↑ pressure in the orbit → a fracture of the weakest portion of the orbit, the thin orbital floor (maxilla) and lamina papyracea (ethmoid bone).

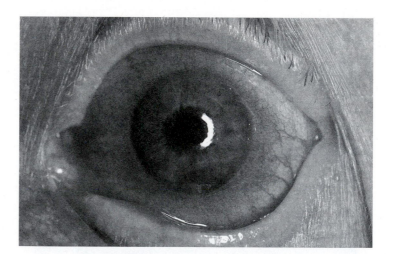

**FIGURE 18.10.   Acute uveitis.**

(Reproduced, with permission, from Knoop KJ et al. *Atlas of Emergency Medicine*, 2nd ed. New York: McGraw-Hill, 2002: 52.) (Also see Color Insert.)

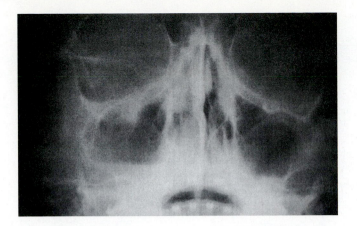

FIGURE 18.11. **Orbital fracture.**

(Reproduced, with permission, from Knoop KJ et al. *Atlas of Emergency Medicine*, 2nd ed. New York: McGraw-Hill, 2002: 15.)

- **Sx:** ↓ visual acuity; enophthalmos; paresthesia of the cheek on the affected side; periorbital ecchymosis and edema; diplopia; symptoms of associated eye injuries.
- **Exam:** Full ophthalmologic exam plus evaluation for facial asymmetry, tenderness, or step-offs over the orbital bones, as well as for CSF leak and septal hematoma.
- **Dx:** CT of the face and sinus is considered the test of choice. Plain films (Waters, Caldwell, and lateral views) may suffice in the absence of associated ocular injury (see Figure 18.11). Opacification of the maxillary sinus (teardrop sign) is a sign of blowout fracture.
- **Tx:** ABCs and trauma survey. Nasotracheal intubation may be contraindicated in severe facial injuries. Appropriate surgical referrals if indicated.
- **Cx:** Corneal abrasion, lens dislocation, tears of the uveal tract, retinal detachment, hyphema, ocular muscle entrapment, globe rupture.

## EAR, NOSE, AND THROAT DISORDERS

### Septal Hematoma

- A blood-filled cavity between the cartilage and supporting perichondrium resulting from nasal trauma. Left untreated, septal hematomas can easily become infected, causing necrosis of the underlying cartilage and permanent saddle-nose deformity.
- **Sx/Exam:** Presents with a history of nasal trauma, pain, progressive nasal obstruction, and reddish-purple areas of fluctuance lying on one or both sides of the nasal septum obstructing the nostril (see Figure 18.12).
- **DDx:** Nasal polyps, deviated septum, enlarged nasal turbinates.
- **Dx:** Usually made clinically; requires a high index of suspicion.
- **Tx:** Aspiration with or without placement of a sterile drain; splints applied to both sides of the septum to provide pressure and support.
- **Cx:** Avascular necrosis of the cartilage; infection or abscess formation; saddle-nose deformity.

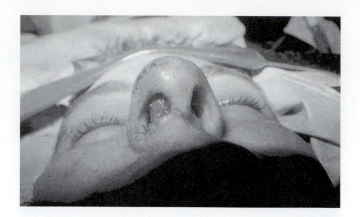

**FIGURE 18.12.    Septal hematoma.**

(Reproduced, with permission, from Knoop KJ et al. *Atlas of Emergency Medicine*, 2nd ed. New York: McGraw-Hill, 2002: 9.)

## Blowout Fractures

See the discussion of orbital fractures for further details.

## Epistaxis

An acute hemorrhage from the nostril, nasopharynx, or nasal cavity. Frequently encountered in the ER or urgent care setting, epistaxis may be due to anterior hemorrhage from Kiesselbach's plexus or from the anterior end of the inferior turbinate, or it may result from posterior hemorrhage from branches of the sphenopalatine artery in the posterior nasal cavity or nasopharynx.

### SYMPTOMS/EXAM

- Presents with a history of frequent epistaxis, anticoagulation use or coagulopathy, vascular abnormalities, or trauma.
- Bleeding from one or both nares is seen.
- Visualize anterior epistaxis using a nasal speculum or blood draining in the posterior pharynx indicative of posterior epistaxis.

### DIFFERENTIAL

Barotrauma, foreign bodies, hemophilia (or other coagulopathy), sinusitis, cocaine use, anticoagulation, hemoptysis, hematemesis.

### DIAGNOSIS

- Usually made clinically, but a CT scan or nasopharyngoscopy may be indicated if a neoplasm is suspected.
- CBC, type and cross, bleeding time, and coagulation studies are warranted if the following are suspected: massive or recurrent epistaxis, anticoagulation use, liver failure, coagulopathy, neoplasm, or a platelet disorder.

- Establish ABCs.
- Maintain continuous pressure over the entire nose for 10 minutes, and insert pledgets soaked with anesthetic-vasoconstrictor solution into the nasal cavity. Gently cauterize using silver nitrate if the bleeding site is easily identified, and if pressure or cautery fails, apply nasal packing using a compressed sponge, Vaseline gauze, or epistaxis balloons. Give empiric antibiotics with staphylococcal and streptococcal coverage if nasal packing is placed.
- ENT consultation and hospital admission are indicated in cases of posterior epistaxis that require packing.

### COMPLICATIONS

Sinusitis, septal hematoma or perforation, aspiration, mucosal pressure necrosis, external nasal deformity.

## CARDIAC DISORDERS

### Myocardial Infarction (MI)

See the discussion of chest pain for further details.

### Arrhythmias

Abnormalities of cardiac rhythm and conduction that can be lethal and may be symptomatic or asymptomatic. Arrhythmias typically arise in patients with ↑ susceptibility due to structural heart disease, electrolyte imbalances, hormonal imbalances, hypoxia, drug effects, or myocardial ischemia. They may be classified as either tachyarrhythmias (see Figure 18.13) or bradyarrhythmias. Tachyarrhythmias may be further divided into supraventricular (narrow-QRS) or ventricular (wide-QRS) tachycardias. Although the symptoms and treatment differ depending on the underlying arrhythmia, some general rules apply:

- Assess whether the patient has a stable or an unstable arrhythmia.
- Obtain a complete history, including onset of symptoms, duration and frequency of episodes, pattern of symptoms over time, effect of any treatment, aggravating or alleviating factors, and family history of a similar problem.
- Complete a thorough physical examination, making special note of orthostatic hypotension, syncope, carotid bruits, ↓ pulses, peripheral vascular disease, signs of pulmonary disease, heart murmurs, the patient's gender and age, and comorbidities.
- Document the cardiac rhythm with an ECG and a rhythm strip.

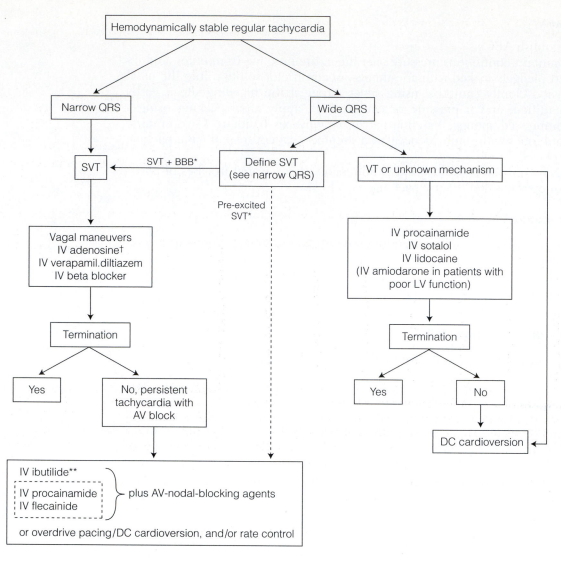

**FIGURE 18.13.** **Stable tachycardia algorithm.**

(Reprinted, with permission, from ACC/AHA/ESC Guidelines for the Management of Patients with Supraventricular Arrhythmias. A Report of the American College of Cardiology/American Heart Association Task Force and the European Society of Cardiology Committee for Practice Guidelines [Writing Committee to Develop Guidelines for the Management of Patients with Supraventricular Arrhythmias]. Copyright © 2003 by the American College of Cardiology Foundation, the American Heart Association, Inc., and the European Society of Cardiology.)

## FLUIDS, ELECTROLYTES, AND NUTRITION

## Dehydration

A loss of free water disproportionate to the loss of sodium. Dehydration may exist with or without volume depletion, a contraction of the total intravascular plasma pool. Although dehydration can present in any age group, the highest morbidity and mortality occur in the pediatric population, usually as a result of gastroenteritis and other diarrheal illnesses.

### SYMPTOMS/EXAM

Table 18.10 lists the presenting symptoms and corresponding exam based on the degree of dehydration.

TABLE 18.10.    Symptoms and Exam Findings of Dehydration

| DEGREE OF DEHYDRATION | SYMPTOMS/EXAM |
|---|---|
| 5–6% | Slightly dry mucous membranes, thirst, concentrated urine, normal tear production, tachycardia 10–15% above baseline. |
| 7–8% | Irritability, lethargy, dry skin, dizziness, flushing, headaches, very dry mucous membranes, ↓ tear production, resting tachycardia, weak peripheral pulses, ↓ skin turgor, oliguria, sunken eyeballs, sunken anterior fontanelle (in infants), tachypnea. |
| >9% | Resting tachycardia or bradycardia, weak central pulses, cold and mottled skin, hypotension, delayed capillary refill, spastic muscles, lethargy, coma. |

## DIAGNOSIS

BUN/creatinine ratio of > 20, ↑ urine specific gravity, ↑ serum osmolarity, ↓ arterial pH.

## TREATMENT

- Oral rehydration therapy in cases of mild to moderate dehydration, given at doses of 50–100 cc/kg over four hours.
- IV rehydration (with calculation of electrolyte and free-water deficits, maintenance requirements, and replacement of ongoing losses) in cases of severe dehydration. Begin with isotonic fluids in 20 cc/kg boluses.
- Follow the "4-2-1 rule" for estimating maintenance fluid requirements: 4 cc/kg/hr for the first ten kilograms of weight; 2 cc/kg/hr for the second ten kilograms of weight; and 1 cc/kg/hr for each additional kilogram thereafter— e.g., the maintenance rate for a child weighing 24 kg is $(4 \times 10) + (2 \times 10) + (1 \times 4) = 64$ cc/hr.

## COMPLICATIONS

Iatrogenic electrolyte imbalances, CNS sequelae from overly aggressive replacement of volume deficits, coma, death.

## DERMATOLOGIC DISORDERS

Erythema multiforme (EM), Stevens-Johnson syndrome (SJS), and toxic epidermal necrolysis (TEN) are thought to be variants of the same disease spectrum, whose features include widespread distribution of skin and mucosal lesions. Commonly affected sites include the torso, face, palms, soles, and extensor surfaces. SJS and TEN are the more serious variants and carry mortality rates of 5% and 40%, respectively (see Table 18.11). The conditions are distinguished as follows:

- **Erythema multiforme:** A generally benign process characterized by target lesions in a symmetric acral distribution (see Figure 18.14), often involving the oral mucosa. Usually 2° to prior infection with a herpesvirus, EM has very low morbidity and is often recurrent.
- **Stevens-Johnson syndrome:** An immune complex–mediated hypersensitivity reaction involving the skin and mucous membranes (see Figure 18.15).

**TABLE 18.11.** Stevens-Johnson Syndrome vs. Toxic Epidermal Necrolysis

| | STEVENS-JOHNSON SYNDROME | TOXIC EPIDERMAL NECROLYSIS |
|---|---|---|
| Symptoms | **Chief complaint:** Pain associated with a rash.<br>Has a 1- to 14-day prodrome consisting of fever, sore throat, cough, malaise, arthralgias, chills, headache, vomiting, and diarrhea.<br>Nonpruritic mucocutaneous lesions last 2–4 weeks. | **Chief complaint:** Pain associated with a rash.<br>Has a two- to three-day prodrome consisting of fever, sore throat, cough, malaise, arthralgias, and anorexia.<br>Has an 8- to 12-day acute phase consisting of persistent fevers, generalized epidermal sloughing, and mucosal involvement. |
| Exam | A nonpruritic macular rash develops into papules, vesicles, bullae, and confluent erythema with a characteristic target appearance.<br>Less than 10% of body surface area (BSA) is affected.<br>Associated findings include fever, tachycardia, orthostasis, hypotension, altered mental status, epistaxis, conjunctivitis, erosive vulvovaginitis or balanitis, seizures, and coma. | An erythematous maculopapular rash with bullae, erosions, and targetlike lesions rapidly → confluent blisters that easily slough off.<br>More than 30% of BSA is affected.<br>⊕ Nikolsky's sign—epidermis separation when pressure is applied laterally to the epidermal surface.<br>Associated findings are the same as those for SJS. |
| History | Drug exposure (sulfa, phenytoin, allopurinol, and penicillin are most commonly implicated), malignancies, vaccinations, and infections. | Same as that of SJS, but drugs are almost always the cause of TEN. |
| Differential | Chemical or thermal burns, exfoliative dermatitis, EM, pemphigus, cutaneous T-cell lymphoma, staphylococcal scalded skin syndrome, toxic shock syndrome. | Same as that for SJS. |
| Diagnosis | Skin biopsy shows subepidermal bullae +/– epidermal cell necrosis and lymphocytic infiltration of perivascular areas. | Skin biopsy shows full-thickness epidermal necrosis with little dermal and epidermal inflammation. |
| Treatment | Supportive treatment with airway management, fluid replacement, electrolyte correction, wound care, and pain control. | Same as that for SJS, but referral to a burn center and treatment with plasmapheresis or IVIG may also be indicated in TEN. |
| Complications | Depends on the organ system involved, but may include 2° infection, corneal ulceration, anterior uveitis, blindness, renal tubular necrosis, renal failure, vaginal or penile scarring, esophageal strictures, GI hemorrhage, respiratory failure, and cosmetic deformity. | Same as those for SJS. |

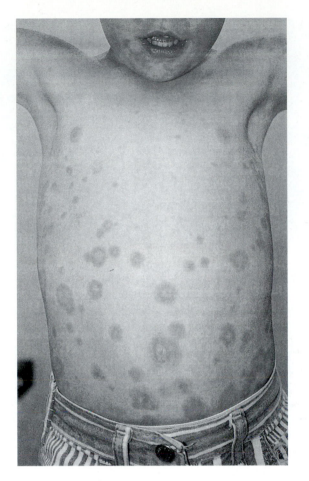

**FIGURE 18.14.    Erythema multiforme.**

(Reproduced, with permission, from Knoop KJ et al. *Atlas of Emergency Medicine,* 2nd ed. New York: McGraw-Hill, 2002: 378.) (Also see Color Insert.)

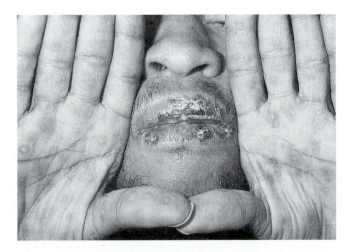

**FIGURE 18.15.    Stevens-Johnson syndrome.**

(Reproduced, with permission, from Knoop KJ et al. *Atlas of Emergency Medicine,* 2nd ed. New York: McGraw-Hill, 2002: 379.) (Also see Color Insert.)

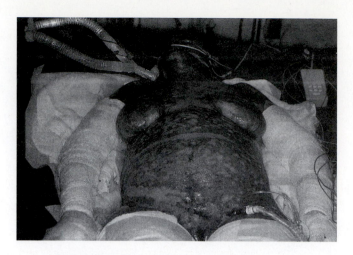

**FIGURE 18.16.** **Toxic epidermal necrolysis.**

(Reproduced, with permission, from Knoop KJ et al. *Atlas of Emergency Medicine*, 2nd ed. New York: McGraw-Hill, 2002: 380.) (Also see Color Insert.)

Also known as erythema multiforme major, SJS is a serious systemic illness that → significant morbidity and mortality.

- **Toxic epidermal necrolysis:** A rapidly evolving mucocutaneous reaction characterized by widespread erythema, necrosis, and bullous detachment of the epidermis (see Figure 18.16). More often seen in adults, TEN is potentially life-threatening and is a true dermatologic emergency requiring prompt diagnosis and treatment.

## ENVIRONMENTAL STRESSORS

### Hypothermia

A decline in core temperature below 35°C (95°F) due to either accidental exposure to cold (1°) or a failure of thermoregulatory function (2°). Most cases in the United States occur in an urban setting and are related to homelessness, coexisting psychiatric illness, trauma, substance abuse, or the elderly.

### SYMPTOMS/EXAM

Table 18.12 lists the symptoms and exam findings for the different degrees of hypothermia. To ensure appropriate diagnosis, a true core temperature should be measured using a low-reading temperature probe in the bladder, esophagus, or rectum.

### DIFFERENTIAL

Stroke, drug toxicity, hypothyroidism, hypopituitarism, frostbite, alcoholism, septic or hemorrhagic shock, delirium, anorexia nervosa, spinal cord injury, MI, CNS trauma.

### DIAGNOSIS

↑ hematocrit (↑ 2% for each 1°C drop in core temperature) due to volume contraction; electrolyte abnormalities; hypoglycemia or hyperglycemia; ↑ pH and ↓ $PaO_2$ and $PaCO_2$ on ABG; prolonged bleeding time; PR, QRS, and QTc prolongation and Osborn (J) waves on ECG.

**TABLE 18.12.** Symptoms and Exam Findings of Hypothermia

| DEGREE OF HYPOTHERMIA | SYMPTOMS | EXAM |
|---|---|---|
| Mild (32°–35°C) | Lethargy, confusion, shivering, loss of fine motor coordination. | Shivering, altered mental status, tachypnea, tachycardia, vasoconstriction, dysarthria, ataxia, lethargy. |
| Moderate (28°–32°C) | Delirium, slowed reflexes. | Bradycardia, cessation of shivering, stupor, dilated pupils, arrhythmias. |
| Severe (< 28°C) | Unresponsiveness, coma, respiratory difficulties. | Rigidity, apnea, hypotension, very cold skin, areflexia, fixed pupils, unresponsiveness, VF. |

### TREATMENT

▪ **Rewarming measures:** Removal of wet clothing; heat packs or warmed blankets applied to the axillae, groin, and abdomen; provision of warmed, humidified $O_2$ and heated IV saline; warmed gastric, thoracic, and/or peritoneal lavage; warm-water immersion; initiation of CPR as needed; hemodialysis; cardiopulmonary bypass.
▪ Patients with hypothermia may appear dead; therefore, patients are not considered dead until they are warm and dead.

### COMPLICATIONS

Cardiac arrhythmias, hypotension due to marked vasodilation during rewarming, aspiration pneumonia, pulmonary edema, peritonitis, acute tubular necrosis, metabolic acidosis, rhabdomyolysis, gangrene, compartment syndrome, death.

*Patients with hypothermia are not considered dead until they are warm and dead.*

## Hyperthermia

Represents a continuum of illness ranging from heat exhaustion to heatstroke. Heat exhaustion, the most common heat-related illness, involves a mild to moderate dysfunction of temperature control caused by ↑ ambient temperatures and/or strenuous exercise → dehydration and salt depletion. Heatstroke, which is associated with a systemic inflammatory response, is extreme hyperthermia (> 41.1°C, or > 106°F) that → end-organ damage and significant morbidity and mortality.

### SYMPTOMS

Depends on the degree of heat illness, but may include fatigue, weakness, nausea and vomiting, headache, muscle cramps, irritability, altered mental status, coma, sweating, and, later, anhidrosis.

### EXAM

↑ temperature (usually > 41°C), tachycardia, orthostatic pulse and BP changes, piloerection, tachypnea, hyperventilation, CNS dysfunction, muscle tenderness, signs of DIC, and GU symptoms (hematuria, oliguria, or anuria) that may occur due to concurrent acute renal failure (ARF).

### DIFFERENTIAL

Delirium, DKA, DTs, hepatic or uremic encephalopathy, hyperthyroidism, encephalitis, meningitis, neuroleptic malignant syndrome, tetanus, status epilepticus, septic shock, cerebral malaria, drug toxicity (especially cocaine, amphetamine, phencyclidine, salicylates, anticholinergics, and MAOIs).

### DIAGNOSIS

- **Labs:** Laboratory studies are used primarily to detect end-organ damage and include CBC, a coagulation panel (abnormal in concurrent DIC), a metabolic panel, UA, hepatic enzymes (almost universally ↑ in heatstroke), CK (↑), serum glucose (reveals hypoglycemia), and ABG (reveals respiratory alkalosis and/or metabolic acidosis).
- **Imaging:** CXR, head CT to rule out other causes of altered mental status.

### TREATMENT

- Heatstroke is a medical emergency requiring rapid reduction of core body temperature, as the duration of hyperthermia is the main determinant of outcome.
- The ideal goal rate for decreasing core temperature is 0.2°C/min; the target goal is 39°C.
- Rapid cooling measures include removal of clothing, covering the patient with ice water–soaked sheets or ice packs, ice water immersion, and evaporative techniques.
- Supportive measures include infusing $D_{50}W$ in IV lines to prevent hypoglycemia, placing an NG tube to monitor for GI bleeding and fluid losses, constant core temperature monitoring, inserting a Foley catheter to monitor urine output, placing a Swan-Ganz catheter to guide fluid management, and mechanical ventilation if indicated.
- Useful adjunctive medications include benzodiazepines to stop agitation, shivering, and seizures, as well as barbiturates for refractory seizures.
- Avoid anticholinergics, α-adrenergic agonists, and antipyretics.

### COMPLICATIONS

Seizures, neurologic deficits, rhabdomyolysis, ARF, hepatic failure, DIC, ARDS, pulmonary edema, respiratory alkalosis, electrolyte imbalances, death.

A 21-year-old medical student from New Orleans, Louisiana (below sea level), traveled to Cusco, Peru (approximately 11,000 feet), to hike the Inca trail to Machu Picchu. After spending a restless night at altitude, she awoke the next morning with a severe headache. Throughout the day, she felt lethargic and nauseated and vomited twice. By the next morning, her symptoms

## Altitude Sickness

One of a group of syndromes resulting from altitude-induced hypoxia. Acute mountain sickness (AMS) is caused by a fundamental lack of $O_2$ related to both the ascent rate and the maximum altitude achieved and represents the mildest and most common form of altitude illness. Other diseases in the spectrum include high-altitude pulmonary edema (HAPE) and high-altitude cerebral edema (HACE), which generally occur at elevations of 3500–5500 m (11,000–18,000 feet).

### SYMPTOMS

Headache, anorexia, nausea, vomiting, weakness, lightheadedness, fluid retention with ↓ urination.

### EXAM

There are no characteristic physical findings in AMS, but patients appear ill. Ataxia and altered mental status are suggestive of HACE; cough, rales or wheezing, dyspnea, tachypnea, tachycardia, and low-grade fevers are suggestive of HAPE.

### DIFFERENTIAL

Anxiety, asthma, COPD, dehydration, MI, pneumonia, pulmonary embolism.

### DIAGNOSIS

Usually made by clinical history and exam, but ↓ arterial $O_2$ saturation and a CXR showing unilateral or bilateral fluffy infiltrates are characteristic of HAPE.

### TREATMENT

- For HAPE and HACE, definitive treatment is descent, but supplemental $O_2$, nifedipine, and portable hyperbaric chambers may be useful adjunctive treatments.
- For AMS, slow, gradual ascent with time for acclimatization, supplemental $O_2$, acetazolamide, and dexamethasone help both to prevent and to treat symptoms.

## Frostbite

A cold-related injury due to formation of ice crystals within tissues and cellular death. Common sites of injury include the hands, the feet, and exposed tissue such as the ears, nose, and lips.

### SYMPTOMS

Coldness, stinging, numbness, burning, clumsiness, throbbing or burning pain on rewarming.

### EXAM

- As in thermal burns, findings depend on the degree of injury, but all injuries may cause joint pain, hyperhidrosis, bluish discoloration, hyperemia, skin necrosis, or gangrene.
- Distinguished as follows:
  - **First degree:** Erythema, edema, nonsensate white plaque with surrounding hyperemia.
  - **Second degree:** Clear blisters with surrounding erythema within 24 hours of injury.
  - **Third degree:** Hemorrhagic blisters followed by eschar formation over several weeks.
  - **Fourth degree:** Focal necrosis with tissue loss.

### DIAGNOSIS

No routine laboratory tests of radiographs are indicated, but technetium scintigraphy or MRI may aid in visualization of nonviable tissue earlier than clinical examination.

### TREATMENT

- Rapid rewarming of affected parts (as long as it can be maintained) in circulating warm water at 40°–42°C (104°–108°F) for 15–30 minutes until thawing is complete.
- Topical application of aloe vera to debrided clear blisters and intact hemorrhagic blisters; elevation of affected parts; tetanus prophylaxis; analgesia as needed; daily hydrotherapy.
- Optional antibiotic coverage to prevent infection.
- Surgical debridement should be delayed for 3–4 weeks to prevent removal of viable tissue.

### COMPLICATIONS

Sensory deficits, hyperhidrosis or anhidrosis, abnormal color changes, phantom pain of amputated extremities, cold sensitivity, joint pains, wound infection, tetanus, gangrene, death.

## Burns

May be classified by etiology into thermal, chemical, or radiation burns. Thermal burns are most common and occur when soft tissue is exposed to temperatures > 45.5°C (> 114°F). Regardless of the mechanism of thermal burn (scald, contact, steam, flame, gas, flash, or electrical), the injury involves ↑ capillary permeability, fluid loss, and ↑ plasma viscosity → microthrombus formation.

### SYMPTOMS/EXAM

- **First degree:** Red, warm, painful tissue involving the epidermis that blanches with pressure.
- **Second degree:** Red, wet, painful tissue with or without blisters involving the epidermis and portions of the dermis.
- **Third degree:** Dry, insensate, waxy, leathery tissue with or without overlying blisters involving the epidermis, the dermis, and possibly underlying subcutaneous fat tissue, muscle, and bone.

## DIAGNOSIS

- Evaluation of the extent (in BSA) and depth of burn are crucial for appropriate management.
- The extent of injury in adults may be estimated using the "rule of nines" (see Figure 18.17).
- Severe burns necessitate a CBC, chemistry panel, ABG with carboxyhemoglobin, coagulation panel, UA, type and screen, CPK and urine myoglobin (in electrical burns), and CXR for suspected inhalational injuries.

## TREATMENT

- Superficial burns may be managed in an outpatient setting with wound cleansing, pain control, topical dressing, and appropriate follow-up care.
- Deeper or more extensive burns should be managed in an inpatient setting (preferably a burn center) with establishment of the ABCs, fluid resuscitation using isotonic crystalloid solution for the first 24 hours (may use modified Brooke or Parkland formulas to calculate fluid deficit), wound excision and grafting if necessary, and rehabilitation.
- Topical medications include silver sulfadiazine, aqueous 0.5% silver nitrate, petrolatum, debriding enzymes, and topical antibiotic ointments.

## COMPLICATIONS

Scarring, cosmetic deformity, burn infections, ARDS, sepsis, death.

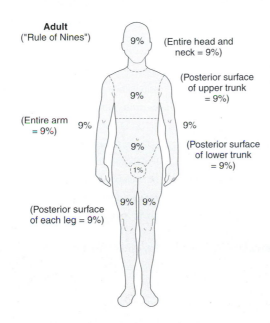

**FIGURE 18.17.** Adult "rule of nines" for burn evaluation.

Common presentations of substance use disorders in the acute setting. Drug dependency ranges from habituation to addiction and can encompass a spectrum of symptoms depending on the amount of drug used, the duration of usage, and the presence of polysubstance abuse. Tables 18.13 and 18.14 list the intoxication and withdrawal syndromes of the most commonly abused substances.

**TABLE 18.13.** Common Intoxication Syndromes[a]

|  | OPIOID | SEDATIVE | STIMULANT | HALLUCINOGEN |
|---|---|---|---|---|
| Symptoms | Altered mental status, euphoria, drowsiness, pruritus, nausea, abdominal pain, constipation, vomiting, urinary retention. | Altered mental status, slurred speech, ataxia, ↓ fine motor function, disinhibition, anxiety, drowsiness, hallucinations, coma. | Altered mental status, paranoia, seizures, hypervigilance, euphoria, chest pain, agitation, flushing, stroke symptoms, epistaxis, cough with black sputum. | Altered mental status, visual hallucinations, disorientation, sweating, mood lability, acute panic symptoms. |
| Exam | Respiratory depression, miosis, hypoxia, pulmonary rales. | Nystagmus, hypotonia, respiratory depression. | Seizures, diaphoresis, hyperthermia, dyspnea, tachycardia, mydriasis, hypertension. | Diaphoresis, tachycardia, mydriasis, tachypnea. |
| Treatment | Airway management and supportive care; naloxone for reversal; activated charcoal if recent oral overdose. | Airway management and supportive care; activated charcoal for acute benzodiazepine ingestion; flumazenil for benzodiazepine reversal; seizure and hypoglycemia treatment. | Airway management and supportive care; benzodiazepines for seizures and sedation; cooling measures; sedation; avoidance of nonselective β-blockers; activated charcoal for acute ingestion. | Supportive care in a nonstimulating environment; benzodiazepines if needed for sedation; cooling measures. |
| Complications | Pulmonary edema, hypotension, respiratory failure, death. | **Benzodiazepines:** Aspiration pneumonia, respiratory failure, death. **Alcohol:** Holiday heart, DTs, hypoglycemia, cardiomyopathy, liver failure, behavioral toxicity. | MI, cardiomyopathy, hypertensive crisis, pulmonary edema, behavioral toxicity, death. | Respiratory arrest, coma, hyperthermia, behavioral toxicity. |

[a] Examples of opioids include morphine and heroin; sedatives, benzodiazepine and alcohol; stimulants, cocaine and amphetamine; and hallucinogens, LSD.

EMERGENCY/URGENT CARE

TABLE 18.14.    Common Withdrawal Syndromes[a]

| | OPIOID | SEDATIVE | STIMULANT | HALLUCINOGEN |
|---|---|---|---|---|
| Symptoms | Sneezing, yawning, lacrimation, leg and abdominal cramps, nausea, vomiting, diarrhea. | Tremor, anxiety, nausea, disorientation, agitation, insomnia, hallucinations, sensory hyperacuity, seizures. | Dysphoria, craving, sleep disturbances, hunger, depression. | No true withdrawal state, but dysphoria may occur after discontinuation of chronic use. |
| Exam | Rhinorrhea, mydriasis, tachycardia, tachypnea, hypertension, piloerection, hyperthermia. | Tachypnea, tachycardia, diaphoresis, hyperthermia, hyperreflexia. | Psychomotor retardation. | |
| Treatment | Long-acting opioid agonist (methadone) or buprenorphine taper; clonidine, naltrexone for maintenance. | Benzodiazepines or barbiturates for withdrawal symptoms and seizures; dextrose, thiamine, clonidine, β-blockers. | Bromocriptine for withdrawal symptoms; desipramine for maintenance. | |

[a] Examples of opioids include morphine and heroin; sedatives, benzodiazepine and alcohol; stimulants, cocaine and amphetamine; and hallucinogens, LSD.

## PSYCHIATRIC DISORDERS

### Psychosis

Defined as an impaired sense of reality → an inability to communicate, emotional turmoil, and impaired cognitive abilities. Not a diagnosis in itself, psychosis is often linked to schizophrenia, severe clinical depression, bipolar disorder, drug intoxication and withdrawal (in particular, cocaine, amphetamines, PCP, and hallucinogens), SLE, dementia, traumatic brain injury, and electrolyte imbalances in the elderly.

#### SYMPTOMS/EXAM

Hallucinations, delusions, personality changes, disorganized thinking, lack of insight.

#### DIAGNOSIS

Usually made clinically, but laboratory testing and head imaging may be indicated to rule out organic causes of acute psychosis (e.g., CBC, UA, LFTs, chemistry panel, TFTs, VDRL, HIV, and toxicology screen; heavy metal screen and ceruloplasmin level are rarely indicated).

#### TREATMENT

- Antipsychotics are given initially to control behavior, followed by hospitalization and long-term treatment directed toward the underlying etiology.
- Rapid tranquilization is necessary for violent, extremely agitated patients:
  - **Typical antipsychotics** (e.g., droperidol, haloperidol, chlorpromazine): Given with diphenhydramine or benztropine to prevent extrapyramidal reactions.

EMERGENCY/URGENT CARE

- **Atypical antipsychotics** (e.g., olanzapine, risperidone).
- **Benzodiazepines:** May be used as adjuncts to antipsychotics for sedative effects; the drugs of choice for alcohol and benzodiazepine withdrawal.

## Suicidal Ideation

Risk factors associated with completed suicide include male gender, white ethnicity, advancing age, widowed or divorced status, living alone, access to firearms, coexisting psychiatric disorders or substance abuse, major life stressors, and a prior history or family history of suicide attempt.

### SYMPTOMS/EXAM

Anhedonia, hopelessness, insomnia, anxiety, impaired concentration, psychomotor agitation.

### DIAGNOSIS

Made clinically through a thorough psychiatric history, including discussion of the following:

- **Extent of suicidal ideation:** When suicidal thoughts began, precipitating factors, frequency of thoughts, aggravating/alleviating factors, formulation of suicidal plan, ability to control suicidal thoughts, deterrents to carrying out plan.
- **Lethality of suicidal plan:** Access to firearms and harmful medications, recent changes in will or life insurance policy, prior attempts.

### TREATMENT

- Immediate hospitalization is indicated for all patients with a plan, access to lethal means, recent social stressors, and symptoms indicative of a psychiatric disorder.
- Involuntary commitment may be made if a person poses an imminent danger to self or others or displays an inability to care for himself or herself.
- Outpatient treatment may be an option if the patient is able to make a contract for safety, displays good judgment, and has adequate social support.
- Antidepressant therapy (in particular, SSRIs) and close monitoring are essential, as patients may be at ↑ risk for suicide as their energy level improves while the depressed mood persists. MAOIs are contraindicated in suicidal ideation owing to their lethal potential in the event of an overdose.

## Homicidal Ideation

### SYMPTOMS/EXAM

Prior history of violence, coexisting psychiatric disorder, substance abuse, access to weapons.

### DIAGNOSIS

As with suicide, no clinician is able to predict what will happen. Thus, the goal is accurate risk assessment in order to develop a reasonable treatment plan and to prevent injury.

*When someone's life is in imminent danger, the physician is allowed (and is in fact obligated) to breach the patient's confidentiality if it is necessary to intervene.*

## TREATMENT

- Immediate hospitalization in all patients with a plan, access to lethal means, and symptoms indicative of a psychiatric disorder.
- Involuntary commitment may be made if a person poses an imminent danger to self or others or displays an inability to care for him/herself.
- Initiation of appropriate psychiatric intervention, depending on the underlying diagnosis.

## TRAUMA

The fourth leading killer among Americans and the main cause of death in those < 45 years of age. Trauma care should be predicated on the concepts of rapid triage, diagnosis, resuscitation, and therapeutic intervention. Trauma evaluation can be broken down into two main surveys: the 1° survey and the 2° survey.

- **1° survey (ABCDE):**
  - **A**irway: Establish an airway using a jaw thrust maneuver.
  - **B**reathing: Ventilate with 100% $O_2$ and check for breathing compromise.
  - **C**irculation: Apply pressure to sites of external bleeding, place two large-bore IV lines, assess blood volume status, and begin fluid resuscitation if hypovolemia is present.
  - **D**isability: Document functional status and perform a brief neurologic examination.
  - **E**xposure: Completely disrobe the patient and logroll to inspect the back.
- **2° survey:**
  - Perform a head-to-toe examination to search for other injuries and to set further priorities.
  - May include trauma series imaging, Foley catheter placement, gastric tube placement, splinting of unstable fractures/dislocations, tetanus prophylaxis, surgical consultation, and medications.

## Head Trauma

The cause of death in one-third of all traumatic deaths in persons < 45 years of age. Traumatic brain injury can result from direct injury caused by the force of an object striking the head, or it may represent indirect injury from acceleration/deceleration forces. The GCS should be used to assess all patients with head trauma (see Table 18.15).

### SYMPTOMS/EXAM

- **Low-risk injuries:** Characterized by minor trauma, scalp wounds, a GCS score of 15, a normal neurologic exam, and the absence of signs of intracranial injury.
- **Moderate- to high-risk injuries:** Characterized by loss of consciousness, persistent nausea and vomiting, seizures, severe headaches, focal neurologic signs, presence of penetrating skull injuries, evidence of basilar skull fracture (e.g., CSF rhinorrhea, Battle's sign, raccoon eyes, hemotympanum), a GCS score < 14, and altered mental status.

**TABLE 18.15.** Glasgow Coma Scale for All Age Groups

| | FOUR YEARS TO ADULT | CHILDREN < 4 YEARS | INFANTS |
|---|---|---|---|
| **Eye opening** | | | |
| 4 | Spontaneous | Spontaneous | Spontaneous |
| 3 | To speech | To speech | To speech |
| 2 | To pain | To pain | To pain |
| 1 | No response | No response | No response |
| **Verbal response** | | | |
| 5 | Alert and oriented | Oriented, social, interacts | Coos, babbles |
| 4 | Disoriented conversation | Confused speech, disoriented, consolable, aware | Irritable cry |
| 3 | Speaking but nonsensical | Inappropriate words, inconsolable, unaware | Cries to pain |
| 2 | Moans or unintelligible sound | Incomprehensible, agitated, restless, unaware | Moans to pain |
| 1 | No response | No response | No response |
| **Motor response** | | | |
| 6 | Follows commands | Normal, spontaneous movements | Normal, spontaneous movements |
| 5 | Localizes pain | Localizes pain | Withdraws to touch |
| 4 | Withdraws to pain | Withdraws to pain | Withdraws to pain |
| 3 | Decorticate flexion | Decorticate flexion | Decorticate flexion |
| 2 | Decerebrate extension | Decerebrate extension | Decerebrate extension |
| 1 | No response | No response | No response |

### DIAGNOSIS

Head CT and skull radiographs are generally not indicated in adults unless depressed fracture is suspected and palpation of the skull is not possible.

### TREATMENT

- Establish ABCs, including cervical spine immobilization and intubation if the patient is unable to protect the airway.
- Prompt neurosurgical consultation if a high-risk injury is suspected.
- Hyperventilation to maintain a $P_{CO_2}$ of 25–30, maintenance of normal cardiac output, mannitol, and elevation of the head of the bed to 30 degrees to ↓ ICP.

### COMPLICATIONS

Postconcussion syndrome, seizures, neurologic deficits, death.

## Neck Trauma

May be classified as penetrating or blunt trauma, half of which is due to motor vehicle accidents. Optimal management of patients with neck trauma is challenging, since seemingly minor injuries can rapidly become life-threatening.

### Symptoms/Exam

- Depends on the type of injury but may include active bleeding, large or expanding hematomas, diminished pulses or bruits, lateralizing signs, tracheal deviation, subcutaneous emphysema, cranial nerve palsies, stridor, hoarseness, vocal cord paralysis, hemoptysis, or hematemesis.
- To clear cervical spine fractures clinically, patients must meet all of the following criteria: no neck pain or tenderness on palpation, no history of loss of consciousness, no altered mental status, no symptoms referable to a neck injury (e.g., paralysis, sensory changes), and no other distracting painful injuries.

### Diagnosis

- Three-view radiographs showing all seven cervical vertebrae, the C7–T1 interspace, and a lateral view.
- A full spine series is indicated in patients with one spinal fracture.
- Consider CT angiography in the presence of a penetrating neck trauma close to the arterial blood supply.

### Treatment

Establish airway (orotracheal intubation, cricothyroidotomy, or tracheostomy); stop bleeding; stabilize the cervical spine until clearance can be definitively made.

## Spinal Cord Trauma

One of the most devastating trauma-related injuries. The majority of spinal cord trauma cases are caused by blunt trauma from motor vehicle accidents and occur most frequently on weekends and holidays and during summer months.

### Symptoms/Exam

Depends on the degree of injury but may include flaccid paralysis and loss of sensation below the level of the lesion, urinary and fecal retention, loss of reflex activity, spastic paraplegia or quadriplegia, hyperreflexia and extensor plantar responses, priapism, paralytic ileus, vasomotor instability due to spinal neurogenic shock, loss of temperature and pain appreciation, or hypoventilation and hypoxia if above C5.

### Diagnosis

Complete spinal series, portable CXR and pelvic radiograph, CT, MRI.

### Treatment

Prompt neurosurgical consultation, methylprednisolone 30 mg/kg within eight hours of injury, anatomic realignment of the spinal cord, immobilization.

### Complications

Decubitus ulcers, URI, depression, paralysis, sensory deficits, incontinence, death.

### Ophthalmologic Trauma

Commonly manifests as orbital floor ("blowout") fractures resulting from blunt anteroposterior force directed against the eyeball. An ↑ in intraocular pressure exerted in all directions leads the orbital floor to give way, as it is the weakest component of the orbital skeleton. See the discussion of ocular complaints for more details.

Other common consequences of ocular trauma necessitating immediate consultation include hyphema (post-injury accumulation of blood in the anterior chamber) and ruptured globe (disruption of the integrity of its outer membranes by blunt or penetrating trauma).

### Maxillofacial Trauma

Includes injuries to any bony or fleshy structure of the face caused by physical force, foreign objects, or burns. Maxillofacial trauma is most often due to athletic injuries, assaults, or motor vehicle accidents and should raise the question of domestic violence.

#### SYMPTOMS/EXAM

- Pain, swelling, bleeding, ecchymosis, bony deformity, paresthesias, epistaxis, CSF rhinorrhea, difficulty breathing.
- A patient's description of malaligned teeth is a very sensitive indicator that a mandibular or maxillary fracture is present.

#### DIAGNOSIS

Can be made clinically, but plain film radiographs and CT scans may aid in the diagnosis of fractures.

#### TREATMENT

Depends on the type of injury, but may include establishment of an airway; realignment and immobilization of fractures; pain control; and prompt referral to an otolaryngologist, a plastic surgeon, or an oral and maxillofacial surgeon if indicated.

#### COMPLICATIONS

Permanent facial deformity, chronic sinusitis, nonunion of fractures, hemorrhage, scars, nerve damage, infection, airway compromise, chronic pain.

### Abdominal Trauma

A leading cause of morbidity and mortality among all age groups. Abdominal trauma may be due to blunt injuries, the majority of which are from motor vehicle accidents, or penetrating injuries, which are predominantly due to gunshot or stab wounds. Initial evaluation should be directed toward diagnosing hemorrhage, solid organ injury, or bowel rupture.

#### SYMPTOMS/EXAM

Lap-belt ecchymosis, abdominal pain, tenderness over the ribs, referred pain to the left (splenic injury) or right (biliary injury) shoulder, hypotension, gross hematuria, flank discoloration, acute abdomen.

## DIAGNOSIS

CXR, AXR, abdominal CT with triple contrast, ultrasound, IVP, diagnostic peritoneal lavage (to detect the presence of intraperitoneal blood), exploratory laparotomy.

## TREATMENT

Blood transfusions, pain control, fluid resuscitation, prompt surgical referrals if indicated.

## COMPLICATIONS

Intra-abdominal sepsis, hemorrhage or abscess formation, delayed rupture of solid organs, infection, death.

## Chest Trauma

Present in half of all patients with trauma-related injuries. Around 25% of all trauma deaths are directly attributable to chest trauma. Table 18.16 lists immediately and potentially life-threatening thoracic injuries.

**TABLE 18.16.   Traumatic Chest Injuries**

| TYPE OF INJURY | PRESENTATION | TREATMENT |
|---|---|---|
| Flail chest | Paradoxical chest wall motion due to multiple fractured ribs, chest pain, tachypnea, shallow respirations, crepitus. | Intubation if ventilation is compromised, supplemental $O_2$, pain control. |
| Tension pneumothorax | ↓ breath sounds, dyspnea, tracheal deviation, distended neck veins, chest pain, hypotension. | Needle thoracostomy in the second intercostal space and midclavicular line followed by chest tube placement. |
| Open pneumothorax | ↓ breath sounds, open thoracic wound, dyspnea, chest pain. | Occlusive dressing taped on three sides, followed by chest tube placement and wound closure. |
| Massive hemothorax | ↓ breath sounds, dyspnea, chest pain, **no** midline shift, dullness to percussion on affected side. | Chest tube placement, surgical repair, blood transfusion. |
| Cardiac tamponade | JVD, muffled heart sounds, pulsus paradoxus, hypotension, tachycardia. | Pericardiocentesis, fluid infusion. |
| Myocardial contusion | Blunt trauma to the heart causing episodes of chest pain, paroxysmal supraventricular tachycardia, or self-limited ventricular tachycardia; abnormal ECG. | Supportive care. |
| Aortic disruption | Chest and back pain, dyspnea, hypotension, enlarged aortic knob, widened mediastinum, and rightward esophageal deviation on CXR. | BP control, surgical repair. |

## Chest Wall Trauma

A significant source of morbidity and mortality in the United States, blunt injury to the chest includes chest wall fractures, dislocations, barotraumas, or injuries to the pleurae, lungs, digestive tract, heart, great vessels, or lymphatics. The most common cause of blunt chest trauma is motor vehicle accidents.

### SYMPTOMS

- Symptoms may range from minor pain to florid shock, depending on the mechanism of injury and the organ systems involved.
- Rib fractures (ribs 4–10) are the most common blunt thoracic injuries.

### EXAM

Clinical findings depend on the organ systems affected.

### DIAGNOSIS

ECG, CXR, chest CT, TEE or transthoracic echocardiography (TTE), esophagoscopy (if esophageal injury is suspected), bronchoscopy (if tracheobronchial injury is suspected), aortography (if aortic injury is suspected).

### TREATMENT

- Most patients do not require surgical treatment and can be treated with supportive measures and simple interventions such as tube thoracostomy.
- Regardless of the type of injury, all patients require initial establishment of their ABCs and a trauma survey.
- Immediate surgery is indicated for patients with loss of chest wall integrity; blunt diaphragmatic injuries; massive air leak following chest tube insertion; massive hemothorax; cardiac tamponade; pulmonary or cardiac emboli; or confirmed tracheal, major bronchial, esophageal, or great vessel injury.

### COMPLICATIONS

Wound infection, MI, arrhythmias, septal defects, valvular insufficiency, aneurysm formation, respiratory infections, hemothorax, fistula formation, stroke, DVT.

## Hand Injuries

Common injuries presenting to the ER or urgent care setting but seldom life-threatening, hand injuries may → significant disability and include soft tissue injuries, nerve damage, sprains, dislocations, and fractures. Hand injuries may be isolated or part of multisystem trauma.

### SYMPTOMS/EXAM

- A full examination of the upper extremity is warranted, with special attention paid to asymmetry, anatomical deformities, color changes, ↓ range of motion against resistance, ↓ muscle strength, muscle wasting, and sensory deficits.
- Patients with injuries to the dorsum of the hand should be questioned about the possibility of a closed-fist injury with a human bite. Exam reveals a small laceration over the dorsal MCP joint +/– fracture of the fifth metacarpal bone.

*It is important to test resistance when assessing tendon function because up to 90% of a tendon can be lacerated with preservation of function.*

*The combination of a fifth metacarpal fracture and lacerations over the dorsal MCP joints is a closed-fist injury until proven otherwise and should be treated as a human bite wound.*

Plain film radiographs are indicated if fracture or occult foreign body is suspected; MRI may be helpful in detecting tendon rupture, but not on an emergent basis.

***TREATMENT***

Depends on the type of injury, but may include laceration repair if the wound is < 12 hours old, antibiotic prophylaxis in closed-fist injuries and cat and human bites, irrigation and debridement of open wounds, analgesics and anti-inflammatory agents, reduction of dislocations, splinting, and prompt referral to a hand surgeon if indicated.

***COMPLICATIONS***

Pain, joint stiffness, nonunion of fractures, infection, scar formation, loss of extremity use.

## Wound Care

Chronic wounds can arise from a number of causes, including pressure (decubitus) ulcers, diabetic foot ulcers, venous stasis ulcers, arterial insufficiency ulcers, neoplasms, atheroembolic disease, pyoderma gangrenosum, anticoagulant-induced skin necrosis, radiation damage, and various infections. Table 18.17 lists treatment strategies for common chronic wounds. Basic principles governing wound care are as follows:

- Accurately assess the entire patient.
- Ensure adequate oxygenation and nutrition.
- Treat underlying infections.
- Irrigate and remove foreign bodies.
- Provide a moist wound bed.
- Consider compression therapy.
- Provide proper pain control.

**TABLE 18.17.** **Management of Common Wounds**

| WOUND | HISTORY/PRESENTATION | TREATMENT |
|---|---|---|
| Animal bite | Type of animal and status, foreign body in wound, tendon or tendon sheath involvement, bone injury, joint space violation, neurovascular status. | Irrigation, debridement, 1° closure if clean or facial wound (otherwise delayed 1° closure), tetanus +/− rabies prophylaxis, antibiotics (amoxicillin-clavulanate) for cat bites. |
| Human bite | Tendon or tendon sheath involvement, crepitus, tissue loss, foreign body in wound. | Irrigation, tetanus prophylaxis, fracture treatment if necessary, delayed closure, IV antibiotics (amoxicillin-clavulanate). |
| Pressure ulcer, stage 1 | Nonblanchable erythema of intact skin. | Transparent dressings. |
| Pressure ulcer, stage 2 | Partial-thickness skin loss of epidermis, dermis, or both with superficial ulcer formation. | Hydrocolloid or transparent dressings. |
| Pressure ulcer, stage 3 | Full-thickness skin loss involving damage to subcutaneous tissue and extending into, but not through, underlying fascia. | Debridement, irrigation, hydrocolloid or transparent dressings. |
| Pressure ulcer, stage 4 | Full-thickness skin loss with extensive involvement of underlying tissues, including muscle, bone, or supportive structures. | Surgical debridement, irrigation, advanced topical dressings +/− antibiotics, flap closure to cover defect. |
| Diabetic foot ulcer | Diabetes control, neurovascular status, presence of Charcot foot deformity. | Appropriate footwear and prevention, maintenance of moist wound environment, debridement, antibiotic therapy, blood glucose control. |
| Venous stasis ulcer | Due to ambulatory venous hypertension, brawny induration in extremities, shallow ulcer with weeping discharge. | Compression, debridement, maintenance of moist wound environment +/− skin grafting. |
| Arterial insufficiency ulcer | Pulselessness, cool skin, delayed capillary refill, atrophic skin, loss of hair, well-circumscribed punctate ulcers. | Debridement, maintenance of moist wound environment, surgical or medical treatment to ↑ arterial circulation. |

# Index

Peripartum complications (*continued*)
  meconium-stained amniotic fluid, 563
  operative vaginal delivery, 562
  placental pathology, 563–564
  shoulder dystocia, 560–561
  vaginal birth after C-section (VBAC), 562
Peripheral vascular disease, 72–73
Peritoneal carcinomatosis, 128
Peritonitis
  chlamydial, 128
  as complication of appendicitis, 391
  spontaneous bacterial (SBP), 129
Personality disorders, 496–497
Pertussis, 421
Peyronie's disease, 619–620
Phalen's sign, 352
Pharyngitis, 156–157
Phentermine, 15
Pheochromocytoma, 100
Phobias, 491–492
*Phthirus pubis*, 583
Pica, 199
Pilonidal disease, 398–399
Pituitary apoplexy, 84
Pituitary disorders, 81–86
  diabetes insipidus (DI), 82–83
  growth hormone (GH) excess, 85
  hyperprolactinemia, 85–86
  hypopituitarism, 83–85
  tumors, 81–82
Pituitary hormones, 81
Pityriasis rosea, 302–303
*Pityrosporum orbiculare*, 311
Placenta previa, 540
Placental abruption, 540
Placental pathology, 563–564
Plantar fasciitis, 654–655
*Plasmodium falciparum*, 21
Platelet disorders, 206–209
  hemolytic-uremic syndrome (HUS), 206–207
  heparin-induced thrombocytopenia (HIT), 208–209
  idiopathic thrombocytopenic purpura (ITP), 208
  thrombotic thrombocytopenic purpura (TTP), 206–207
*Plesiomonas shigelloides*, 179
Pleural effusion, 172, 258–259
Plummer-Vinson syndrome, 199
*Pneumococcus*, 129, 191, 421, 439, 465
*Pneumocystis jiroveci* cystic pneumonia (PCP), 191
Pneumonia
  in children, 439
  community-acquired (CAP), 168–172
    causative organisms and historical features of, 169
    criteria for discharge in, 171
    recommendations for site of care for, 171
    recurrent, 172

    scoring system for risk class assignment of, 170
  health care–associated (HAP), 172–173
  ventilator-associated, 173
Pneumothorax, 259–260, 715
Poisoning, 445
Polio vaccine, 421
Polycystic ovarian syndrome (PCOS), 599–600
Polycythemia vera, 50, 216–217
Polyhydramnios, 543–544
Polymyositis, 359, 661
Polyneuropathies, peripheral, 350–351
  chronic inflammatory demyelinating polyneuropathy, 351
  Guillain-Barré syndrome (acute idiopathic polyneuropathy), 168, 180, 289, 350–351
Polypharmacy, 521
Polyps
  adenomatous, 138
  nasal, 251
Pompholyx (dyshidrotic eczema), 300
Portal hypertension, 128, 129, 130
Postherpetic neuralgia (PHN), 520–521
Postoperative care, 381
  convalescent period, 383–384
  immediate postoperative period, 381
  intermediate postoperative period, 381–383
    antibiotics, 383
    fluid and electrolyte management, 382
    fluid requirements, estimating, 382
    gastrointestinal care, 382–383
    pain management, 383
    pulmonary care, 382
Postpartum care, routine, 564–565
  counseling, 565
  labs, 565
  physical exam, 564–565
Postpartum complications, 565–567
  breast-feeding issues, 567
  endometritis, 565
  hemorrhage, 566
  retained placenta, 567
Postpartum major depression (PMD), 487–488, 570–571
Poststreptococcal glomerulonephritis (PSGN), 279
Post-traumatic stress disorder (PTSD), 490–491
Potassium disorders, 286–287
  hyperkalemia, 286
  hypokalemia, 286–287
Pott's disease, 185
Powassan virus, 152
Pravastatin, 53
Precholecystectomy syndrome, 132
Prednisone, 106
Preconception issues, 530–531
  interventions, 531

  lab workup, 530–531
  risk assessment, 520
Preeclampsia, 548
Pregnancy and breast-feeding, psychotropic medications during, 500–501
Premature rupture of membranes (PROM), 545–546
Premenstrual dysphoric disorder (PMDD), 486–487
Preoperative evaluation, 377–379
  anticoagulation, management of, 378
  cardiac risk evaluation, 377
  perioperative β-blockers, 377–378
  pulmonary risk evaluation, 378–379
Pressure ulcers, 519–520, 717, 718
Preterm labor, 544–545
  algorithm for treatment of contractions, 545
  risk factors for, 545
Preventive medicine, 9
  cancer screening, 9–11
    breast cancer, 10
    cervical cancer, 9
    colon cancer, 11
    ovarian cancer, 10
    prostate cancer, 10
  dental care, 11–13
    dental caries in preschoolers, prevention of, 11
    endocarditis prophylaxis, 12–13
  health maintenance, adult, 11
    clinical preventive services for, recommended, 12, 13
  immunizations, adult, 9
  indications for, 10
Priapism, 619–620
Proguanil, 21
Prolactinomas, 81, 85–86, 596
Prostate cancer, 620–621
Prostatitis, 614–615
Protease inhibitors (PIs), 190
*Proteus mirabilis*, 181
*Proteus vulgaris*, 177
Pruritic urticarial papules and plaques of pregancy (PUPPP), 549–550
Pseudohypoparathyroidism, 95
*Pseudomonas*, 388, 410, 433
*Pseudomonas aeruginosa*, 155, 172, 173, 185, 307
Psoriasis, 301–302
Psychiatry, therapeutic drugs in, 499–501
  adverse effects of, 499
  drug-drug interactions, 501
  pregnancy and breast-feeding, psychotropic medications during, 500–501
Psychosis, 485, 709–710
Psychotic disorders, 492–494
  delusional disorder, 492
  schizophrenia, 493–494
Pubic lice (crabs), 583

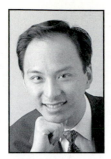
Tao Le, MD, MHS

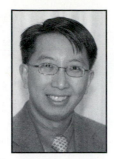
Michael Mendoza, MD, MPH

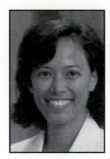
Cynthia Ohata, MD

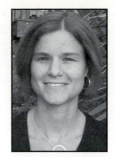
Christine Dehlendorf, MD

**Tao Le, MD, MHS**

Dr. Le has been a well-recognized figure in medical education for the past 14 years. As senior editor, he has led the expansion of *First Aid* into a global educational series. In addition, he is the founder of the *USMLERx* online test bank series as well as a cofounder of the *Underground Clinical Vignettes* series. As a medical student, he was editor-in-chief of the University of California, San Francisco *Synapse,* a university newspaper with a weekly circulation of 9000. Dr. Le earned his medical degree from the University of California, San Francisco, in 1996 and completed his residency training in internal medicine at Yale University and fellowship training at Johns Hopkins University. At Yale, he was a regular guest lecturer on the USMLE review courses and an adviser to the Yale University School of Medicine curriculum committee. Dr. Le subsequently went on to cofound Medsn and served as its chief medical officer. He is currently conducting research in asthma education at the University of Louisville.

**Michael Mendoza, MD, MPH**

Dr. Mendoza is a clinical assistant professor in the Department of Family Medicine at the Pritzker School of Medicine at the University of Chicago. Dr. Mendoza is actively involved in medical student education and research. His research focuses on community-based curricular reform and practice innovations to eliminate health disparities, particularly with respect to the prevention and management of chronic illness. He earned his medical degree from the University of Chicago and his master's degree in public health from the University of Illinois at Chicago. He completed his residency training and served an additional year as chief resident in family and community medicine at the University of California, San Francisco, and San Francisco General Hospital. Dr. Mendoza has served as a national officer in the American Medical Student Association and the Committee of Interns and Residents and, more recently, as a founding member of the National Physicians Alliance. A devoted father and husband, Dr. Mendoza is an award-winning amateur photographer and spends his free time racing sailboats on Lake Michigan.

**Cynthia Y. Ohata, MD**

After attending the University of Washington School of Medicine in Seattle, Washington, Dr. Ohata entered the University of Washington Family Medicine Residency. As a resident and as a fourth-year chief resident, she has lectured on primary care topics such as clinical management of diabetes mellitus, prenatal care, and abnormal uterine bleeding. She is currently in clinical practice in a University of Washington neighborhood clinic in Seattle. She has done research on long-term care in geriatrics and in house officer morale.

**Christine Dehlendorf, MD**

Christine Dehlendorf attended the University of Washington School of Medicine and completed a residency in family and community medicine at the University of California, San Francisco/Community Health Network. Following a year as a fourth-year chief resident, she entered a family planning fellowship at UCSF. Her research interests include disparities in access to and use of contraception and integrating abortion care into primary care practices.

# ABOUT THE AUTHORS